For Reference

Not to be taken from this room

Atlas of
Surgical
Techniques

ATLAS OF
SURGICAL
TECHNIQUES

Steven G. Economou, MD
Professor of Surgery,
Rush Medical College of Rush University
Chairman Emeritus and Senior Attending Surgeon,
Department of General Surgery
Rush–Presbyterian–St. Luke's Medical Center
Chicago, Illinois

Tasia S. Economou, MD
Department of Otolaryngology—Head and Neck Surgery
Kaiser Foundation Hospital—West Los Angeles
Los Angeles, California

W.B. SAUNDERS COMPANY
A *Harcourt Health Sciences Company*
Philadelphia London New York St. Louis Sydney Toronto

W.B. SAUNDERS COMPANY
A *Harcourt Health Sciences Company*

The Curtis Center
Independence Square West
Philadelphia, Pennsylvania 19106

Library of Congress Cataloging-in-Publication Data

Economou, Steven G.
    Atlas of surgical techniques / Steven G. Economou, Tasia S.
Economou.

        p.   cm.

    ISBN 0–7216–1611–9

    1. Surgery, Operative—Atlases.   I. Economou, Tasia S.
II. Title
    [DNLM: 1.   Surgery, Operative—atlases.   WO 517 E19a 1996]

RD41.E26   1996
617.91—dc20

DNLM/DLC   95–30944

ATLAS OF SURGICAL TECHNIQUES   ISBN 0–7216–1611–9

Printed in the United States of America.

Last digit is the print number: 9   8   7   6   5   4   3   2

This book is dedicated to
Kathryn Dotska Economou,
whose endless, silent sacrifices as wife and mother
have made it possible for others
in the family to pursue their own ambitions.

PREFACE

A surgical atlas should differ from a surgical textbook in several significant ways, and we made a concerted attempt to address these differences in this work.

An atlas should not be simply a series of illustrations, however attractive they may be. It was our paradoxical good fortune to work with talented artists. Many of the illustrations are remarkable in themselves, and it would have been easy to expect the reader to admire them for their dazzling appearance alone. It was important, however, for every illustration to serve a practical purpose.

There should not be so few illustrations that one can see the beginning and the end of an operation but too little of what happened in the process. A dispassionate examination of many atlases revealed just this shortcoming in some. An author must recognize that an operation is being illustrated primarily for those who are unlikely to be familiar with all the steps in its performance. If the author assumes otherwise, a neophyte could read a chapter to learn about an operation and be satisfied initially but realize when attempting to actually perform the operation that something was lacking in the exposition of the practical steps of it.

Even if the above pitfalls are avoided, the author must recognize the impracticality of illustrating every minute detail of an operation, so the question of which parts to omit, which to include, and which to emphasize specifically is important. The reader thus realizes that not all steps in an operation are of equal importance. Likewise, the author should attempt to make the reader aware of steps that may be done in several different but equally effective ways. Certainly, a demonstration of steps because they work for the author, even though they are unsound, should be avoided.

The spatial layout of an atlas can influence the ease with which it is used. All of the copy can be on one page and the illustrations on the facing page. This plan has the advantage of grouping more illustrations on each page, but the eye must always shift back and forth between pages in order to follow each step. We chose to place illustrations and the text that describes them on the same page. After all, the atlas attempts to teach the step-by-step approach to an operation rather than to present a sweep of illustrations whose explanation is a number of eye spans away.

There is also the question of which surgical procedures to include, especially when the atlas encompasses general surgery, whose boundaries are poorest defined of all. With the current swift advances in surgical knowledge and technology, this decision is more difficult than ever. A traditional list of procedures is included in practically all atlases of general surgery. In reality, however, most atlases include some procedures whose main justification for being selected speaks mainly to the author's interest in some narrower aspects of general surgery, or they feature one or more operations that the author has always performed well but that are now done largely by specialists. This atlas is no exception.

In the end, an atlas is valuable to the extent that it fulfills the desires of the reader. We earnestly hope this particular atlas meets those expectations.

STEVEN G. ECONOMOU
TASIA S. ECONOMOU

ACKNOWLEDGMENTS

This book is infused throughout with the incomparable artistry of Mr. Alfred Teoli, whose renditions rival those of the masters of medical illustration. Following innumerable working sessions and countless revisions, he always came back with a fresh eagerness and invariably brought forth truly marvelous and imaginative work, much of it unique and all of it having a quality that rivets the attention of the reader. We extend to Al our deep and warmest gratitude.

As is often necessary with a work of this size, other artists participated in a more minor yet significant way. We are particularly thankful that Mr. Michael Dulude applied himself with such energy and talent. Also, we are fortunate that he and the other artists, Mr. Richard Gersony, Mrs. Kim Combs Gersony, and Mrs. Corrine Sandone, had artistic styles that blended so well with the whole. A number of sweeping insightful illustrations by Mrs. Joanne Goldin from two decades ago still provided a backdrop for some of these pages.

STEVEN G. ECONOMOU
TASIA S. ECONOMOU

Consultants

It would not have been possible to create this work without the help of talented colleagues. Superior technical surgeons and dedicated teachers of interns and residents, they brought these qualities to bear in ways that immeasurably elevated the art and science of surgery. We are sincerely indebted to all of them for their insight, clarity, and unselfish devotion.

Daniel J. Deziel, M.D.
Associate Professor of Surgery, Rush
 Medical College of Rush University;
 Associate Attending Surgeon,
 Department of General Surgery,
 Rush–Presbyterian–St. Luke's Medical
 Center, Chicago, Illinois

Alexander Doolas, M.D.
Professor of Surgery, Rush Medical
 College of Rush University; Associate
 Dean for Surgical Sciences and
 Services, Associate Vice President of
 Medical Affairs, Senior Attending
 Surgeon, and Associate Chairman,
 Department of General Surgery,
 Rush–Presbyterian–St. Luke's
 Medical Center, Chicago, Illinois

James S. Economou, M.D., Ph.D.
Louis P. Beaumont Professor of Surgery,
 Division of Surgical Oncology,
 Department of Surgery, University of
 California, Los Angeles, UCLA School of
 Medicine, Los Angeles, California

S. Renée Edwards, M.D.
Assistant Professor, Department of
 Obstetrics and Gynecology, Section of
 Urogynecology and Reconstructive Pelvic
 Surgery, Rush–Presbyterian–St. Luke's
 Medical Center, Chicago, Illinois

Preston F. Foster, M.D.
Assistant Professor of Surgery, Rush
 Medical College of Rush University;
 Assistant Attending Surgeon, Department
 of General Surgery, Section of
 Transplantation, Rush–Presbyterian–
 St. Luke's Medical Center, Chicago,
 Illinois

Jerome Hoeksema, M.D.
Assistant Professor of Urology, Rush
 Medical College of Rush University;
 Director, Urologic Education,
 Department of Urology, and Associate

Attending Surgeon, Rush–Presbyterian–
 St. Luke's Medical Center, Chicago,
 Illinois

James A. Hunter, M.D.
Professor of Cardiovascular Surgery,
 Rush Medical College of Rush
 University, Chicago, Illinois

Robert A. March, M.D.
Assistant Professor of Cardiovascular
 Surgery, Rush Medical College of
 Rush University; Assistant Attending
 Surgeon, Department of Cardiovascular
 and Thoracic Surgery, Rush–
 Presbyterian–St. Luke's Medical Center,
 Chicago, Illinois

Lawrence P. McChesney, M.D.
Assistant Professor of Surgery, Rush
 Medical College of Rush University;
 Assistant Attending Surgeon, Department
 of General Surgery, Section of
 Transplantation, Rush–Presbyterian–
 St. Luke's Medical Center, Chicago,
 Illinois

Keith W. Millikan, M.D.
Assistant Professor of Surgery and Director
 of Undergraduate Surgical Education,
 Rush Medical College of Rush
 University; Assistant Attending Surgeon,
 Department of General Surgery,
 Rush–Presbyterian–St. Luke's Medical
 Center, Chicago, Illinois

Richard A. Prinz, M.D.
Helen Shedd Keith Professor and Chairman,
 Department of General Surgery, Rush
 Medical College of Rush University;
 Senior Attending Surgeon, Rush–
 Presbyterian–St. Luke's Medical Center,
 Chicago, Illinois

Theodore J. Saclarides, M.D.
Associate Professor of Surgery, Rush
 Medical College of Rush University;

Head, Section of Colon and Rectal Surgery and Associate Attending Surgeon, Department of General Surgery, Rush–Presbyterian–St. Luke's Medical Center, Chicago, Illinois

Howard N. Sankary, M.D.
Associate Professor of Surgery, Rush Medical College of Rush University; Associate Attending Surgeon, Department of General Surgery, Section of Transplantation, Rush–Presbyterian–St. Luke's Medical Center, Chicago, Illinois

Edgar D. Staren, M.D., Ph. D.
Associate Professor of Surgery, Rush Medical College of Rush University; Assistant Dean, Clinical Curriculum, and Associate Attending Surgeon, Rush–Presbyterian–St. Luke's Medical Center, Chicago, Illinois

Wayne M. Swenson, M.D.
Professor and Regional Assistant to the Chairman, Department of Surgery, University of North Dakota School of Medicine, Bismarck, North Dakota

Van L. Vallina, M.D.
Assistant Professor of Surgery, Rush Medical College of Rush University;

Assistant Attending Surgeon, Department of General Surgery, Rush–Presbyterian–St. Luke's Medical Center, Chicago; Associate Director of Critical Intensive Care Unit, Rush North Shore Medical Center, Skokie, Illinois

José M. Velasco, M.D.
Professor of Surgery, Rush Medical College of Rush University; Senior Attending Surgeon, Department of General Surgery, Rush–Presbyterian–St. Luke's Medical Center, Chicago; Chairman, Department of Surgery, Rush North Shore Medical Center, Skokie, Illinois

Thomas R. Witt, M.D.
Associate Professor of Surgery, Rush Medical College of Rush University; Associate Attending Surgeon, Department of General Surgery, Rush–Presbyterian–St. Luke's Medical Center, Chicago, Illinois

Norman L. Wool, M.D.
Assistant Professor of Surgery and Director, Residency Clinical Activities, Department of General Surgery, Rush Medical College of Rush University; Associate Attending Surgeon, Rush–Presbyterian–St. Luke's Medical Center, Chicago, Illinois

Contents

ATLAS OF
SURGICAL
TECHNIQUES

SALIVARY GLANDS

A SUPERFICIAL PAROTID LOBECTOMY

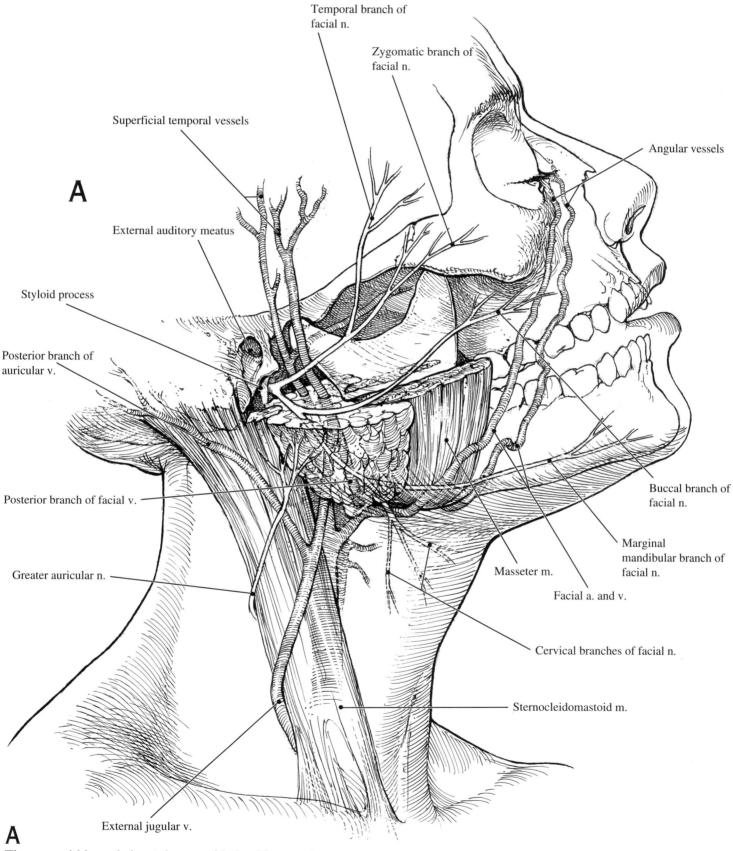

A

Temporal branch of facial n.

Zygomatic branch of facial n.

Superficial temporal vessels

Angular vessels

External auditory meatus

Styloid process

Posterior branch of auricular v.

Posterior branch of facial v.

Buccal branch of facial n.

Greater auricular n.

Marginal mandibular branch of facial n.

Masseter m.

Facial a. and v.

Cervical branches of facial n.

Sternocleidomastoid m.

External jugular v.

A

The area within and about the parotid gland is one of moderate anatomic complexity. This illustration, with some areas cut transversely, helps to demonstrate some of the anatomic relationships more clearly.

B

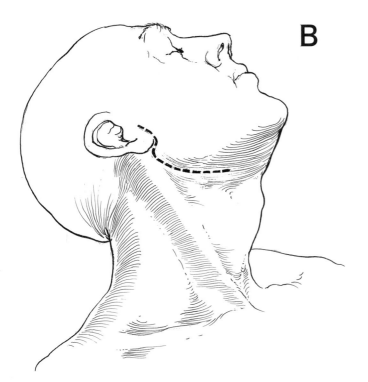

General anesthesia administered endotracheally is used routinely. With the exception of a dose during intubation, no muscle relaxants should be used. A small sandbag is placed under the patient's shoulders, and the head is rotated away from the side being operated on. A pledget of sterile cotton is placed in the external auditory canal to prevent blood from entering, with subsequent encrusting; the area is then painted and draped to leave the side of the face and the entire ear exposed. A number of skin incisions are suitable. We prefer one that is begun in front of the tragus, goes under and very close to the crease under the base of the earlobe, and then extends downward and forward, preferably in a natural skin crease, skirting the angle and horizontal ramus of the mandible by several centimeters. It is terminated in accordance with the extent of intended exposure. An injection of approximately 5 ml of 1 : 50 epinephrine in the preauricular crease near the stylomastoid foramen is very helpful in controlling bleeding.

C

The skin flaps are developed by applying upward traction to the skin edges with small rakes and performing the separation with either a small Metzenbaum scissors or round-tipped manicure scissors, or even a scalpel with a no. 10 blade. The plane of the dissection proceeds between the subcutaneous fat and the superficial parotid fascia. To skirt a more superficial tumor adequately, it is safe to leave some fat on the fascia during the dissection; the skin flap will not be compromised. Small but distinct fibrous septa from the surface of the parotid are encountered and divided while the flap is developed. Hemostasis can easily be achieved utilizing bipolar cautery. The anterior margins of the mobilization extend to just short of the gland periphery. The earlobe is mobilized to the external auditory canal, folded upward, and held in this position with a single stitch. The edges of the skin flaps can be held in position in a similar manner or with the help of rakes, as the surgeon prefers.

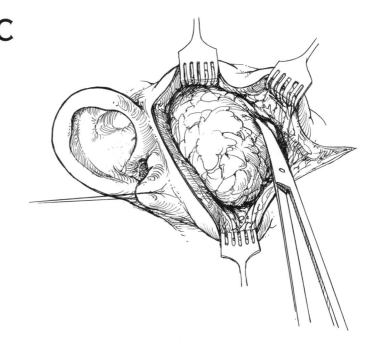

D

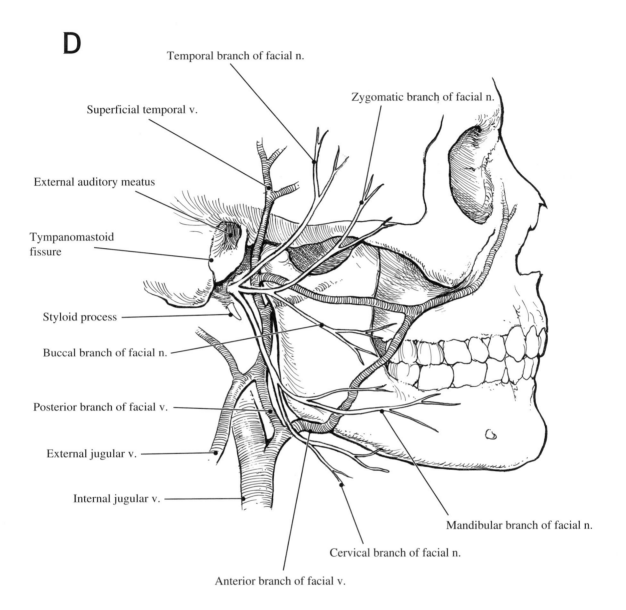

Temporal branch of facial n.

Zygomatic branch of facial n.

Superficial temporal v.

External auditory meatus

Tympanomastoid fissure

Styloid process

Buccal branch of facial n.

Posterior branch of facial v.

External jugular v.

Internal jugular v.

Mandibular branch of facial n.

Cervical branch of facial n.

Anterior branch of facial v.

D

Two important objectives in performing a superficial parotid lobectomy are the adequate removal of the lobe and the incorporated tumor and the proper safeguarding of the facial nerve. The nerve can be identified either peripherally or centrally, certain factors favoring each approach. Given a choice, the surgeon should identify the main nerve trunk and dissection should proceed peripherally. The following important bony landmarks are the most reliable for localizing and identifying the main trunk of the facial nerve. The facial nerve can be found approximately 1 cm medial and inferior to the often prominent tympanomastoid suture, or "pointer." Deeper still is the styloid process, which can be quite prominent but sometimes is almost absent. The nerve always exits the stylomastoid foramen but assumes a more superficial position within a centimeter.

E

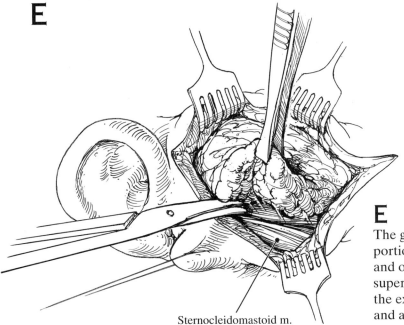

Sternocleidomastoid m.

E

The greater auricular nerve emerges from the posterior portion of the sternocleidomastoid muscle at its midpoint and on its upward course swings around to lie on the superficial surface of the muscle parallel and posterior to the external jugular vein. It trifurcates into mastoid, facial, and auricular branches. Most of the time it is not necessary to divide the main trunk; severing just the facial branch permits the other branches to be retracted posteriorly. The hypesthesia this often produces is incomplete or temporary, or both, and therefore more desirable than permanent anesthesia over a wider area. The external jugular vein is divided. Bleeding vessels on the gland can be tied with 4-0 chromic catgut, coagulated with bipolar cautery, or often controlled by applying pressure with gauze while other areas of the operative field are attended to. The dissection proceeds as the posterior belly of the digastric muscle is sought.

F

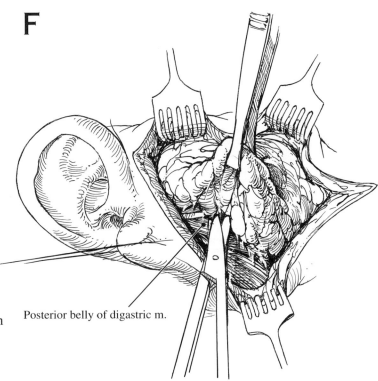

Posterior belly of digastric m.

F

The capsule at the inferoposterior margin of the parotid gland is grasped with an Allis forceps and retracted anteriorly and superiorly while it is separated from the sternocleidomastoid muscle and the origin of the posterior belly of the digastric muscle deep along the anterior margin of the mastoid process. Using the landmarks already mentioned, the facial nerve can be found approximately 1 cm deep to this point.

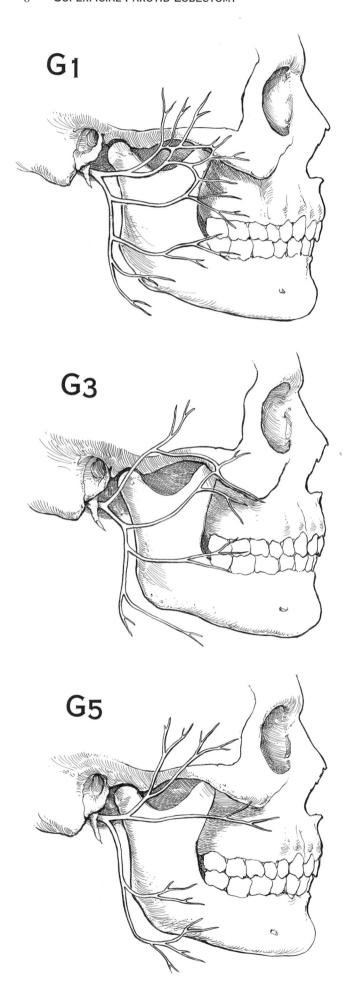

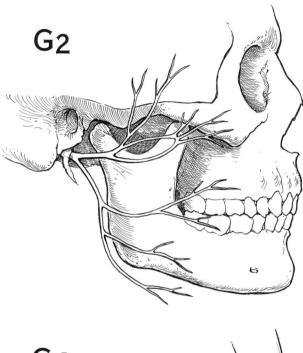

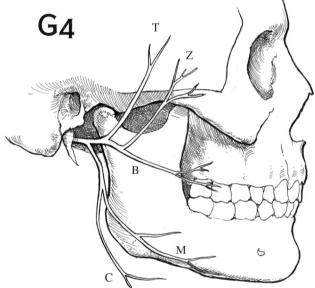

G₁, G₂, G₃, G₄, G₅

The facial nerve is constant in emerging as a single trunk from the stylomastoid foramen and then dividing into temporofacial and cervicofacial branches, which divide further into (T) temporal, (Z) zygomatic, (B) buccal, (M) mandibular, and (C) cervical branches. Beyond this, there is considerable variation in the method and course of its subsequent ramifications. (This knowledge is of value to the surgeon choosing to begin by isolating a peripheral branch; care must be taken to locate the branches terminally, where they measure about 1 mm in diameter.)

These drawings also show the variation in anastomoses among the branches. Of note, the mandibular branch anastomoses with other branches least commonly, so that injury to it is more certain to result in permanent paresis of the affected muscles. Thus, extreme care is warranted in first isolating a peripheral branch and then following its course through to the terminal, thread-like branches.

H

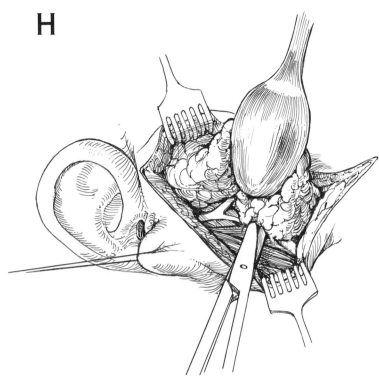

H, I

As dissection continues, the gland is retracted anteriorly and superiorly and the nerve uncovered from greater to lesser tributaries. A spoon is shown being used because it can be an ideal retractor and is often held by the surgeon's free hand. A definite plane of dissection exists where the nerve traverses the gland. The surgeon should strive to remain in this plane, as it offers an easier dissection and keeps the nerve in constant view. Alternatively, a clamp may be spread over the nerve and a no. 12 scalpel blade used—cutting edge facing up—to divide tissue with the nerve in full view.

Venous bleeding from the deep lobe is stopped by compression as other areas are attended to or is done directly with bipolar cautery. If bleeding vessels must be individually secured, fine ligature should be used, and no tissue whose identity is not certain is to be included. Suture ligatures ("stick-ties") are to be avoided, as the deep sweep of the needle may snare a nerve filament.

I

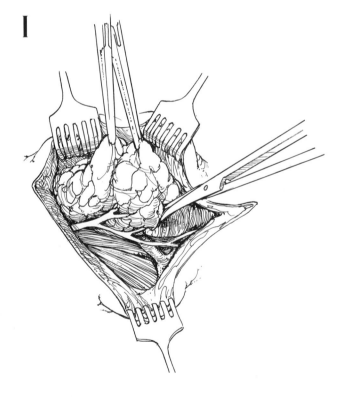

J

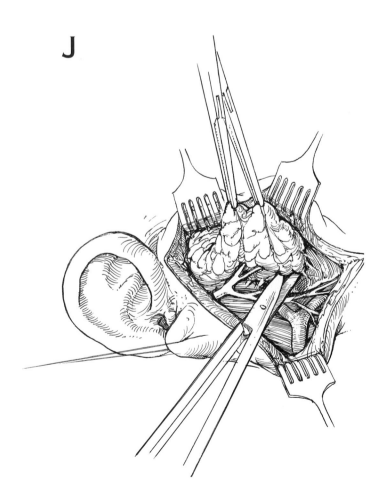

J

At about this point, the salivary duct is encountered as it traverses the buccal tissue in its course toward the oral cavity. It is ligated with catgut and divided.

K

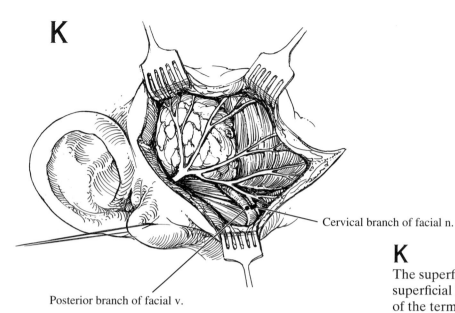

Cervical branch of facial n.

Posterior branch of facial v.

K

The superficial lobe has now been removed. Usually, the superficial lobe need not be removed to the very extremes of the terminal filaments as shown here.

L

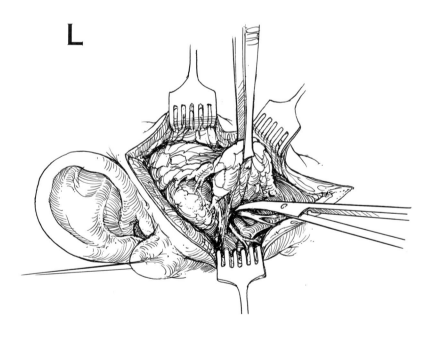

L

Sometimes the tumor is situated in the posterior portion of the superficial lobe and thus is so "socked in" that it effectively thwarts the use of this route for a safe exposure and dissection of the main trunk of the nerve. In such instances, a retrograde dissection from a peripheral branch is necessary. We prefer to use the cervical branch of the facial nerve for this purpose. It lies in proximity to, and runs in the same direction as, the posterior facial vein, which is relatively easy to find. Also, should the nerve be damaged in the course of initial dissection, the paralysis of the platysma muscle is of no significant consequence.

M

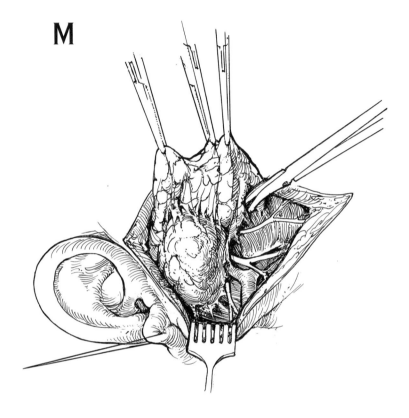

M

The posterior facial vein is identified and, along with it, the cervical branch of the facial nerve. The nerve is exposed retrograde to a bifurcation, at which point this newly found branch is followed distally. In the process, the superficial lobe of the parotid and the contained tumor are reflected superiorly. The process of progressive retrograde-antegrade dissection is continued until the main trunk of the nerve is identified. The superior half of the dissection is now begun, proceeding in a peripheral direction until the superficial lobe is removed. Once hemostasis is assured, a small caliber suction drain is exteriorized through an inferiorly placed counterincision. Alternatively, a small Penrose drain is exteriorized through the incision, and a pressure dressing is applied. The subcutaneous tissue is approximated with 4-0 absorbable suture and the skin with interrupted vertical mattress stitches of 5-0 nylon, or subcuticularly with 5-0 Prolene. The patient is observed immediately on awakening to determine that all branches of the nerve are functioning, because some hours later, weakness or paresis of one or several branches may be present. Thus, if adequate function is observed immediately postoperatively, the patient and the surgeon can feel more assured that the paresis is probably temporary.

B SUBMANDIBULAR SALIVARY GLAND—RESECTION

A

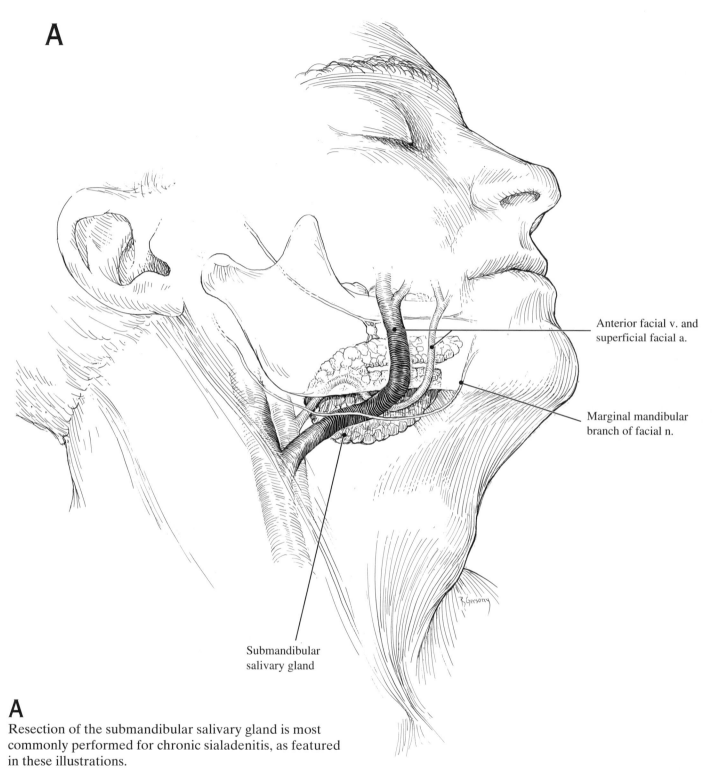

Anterior facial v. and
superficial facial a.

Marginal mandibular
branch of facial n.

Submandibular
salivary gland

A

Resection of the submandibular salivary gland is most
commonly performed for chronic sialadenitis, as featured
in these illustrations.

It is important to remember that the marginal mandibular
branch of the facial nerve has a loose course caudal to the
horizontal ramus of the mandible; its caudal position is
accentuated when the neck is hyperextended and the head
turned away from the operative site. The nerve is motor to
the platysma, which, along with the depressor labii
inferioris and the depressor anguli oris into which it inserts,
aids in depressing the lower lip. Injury to the nerve
produces a most unwelcome deformity.

B

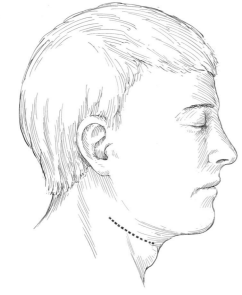

B

The procedure is performed using general anesthesia with the patient in the supine position, the neck hyperextended, and the head turned away from the operative site. The incision should be in a natural crease, if possible, and about 2 to 4 cm caudal to the horizontal ramus of the mandible.

C

The incision is carried through the skin, platysma muscle, and superficial layer of the cervical fascia. Even the generous 4 cm distance of the incision from the horizontal ramus of the mandible is no assurance that the nerve will not lie just deep to the platysma at this point. The surgeon must not incise boldly until the nerve is actually visualized.

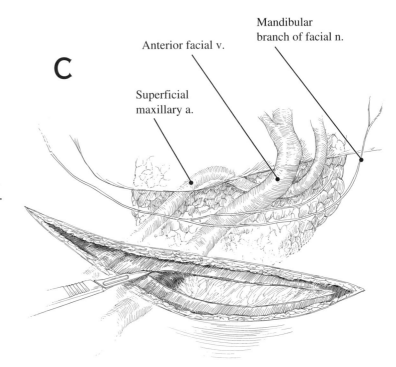

Anterior facial v.

Mandibular branch of facial n.

Superficial maxillary a.

C

D

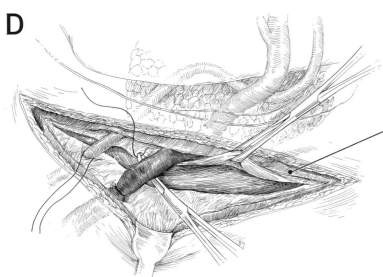

Platysma m.

D

The facial artery and the anterior facial vein are ligated with 3-0 chromic catgut and divided; the mandibular branch of the facial nerve runs deep to the platysma. An Allis forceps is applied to the superficial cervical fascia on the cephalic flap, which is then retracted.

E

Gentle cephalad traction on the Allis forceps effectively takes the tissue and nerve with them. The artery is deep to the gland, often passing through part of it; the vein usually is superficial to and free of the gland.

E

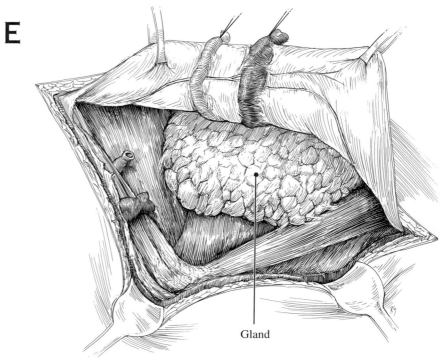

Gland

F

The anterior gland lies on the underside of the mylohyoid muscle. A Babcock forceps is applied to the gland and used to retract it as the dissection is begun along its inferior border.

F

Mylohyoid m.

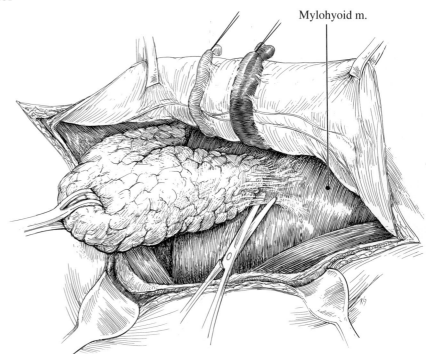

G

This semidiagrammatic rendition is a view from the inside of the oral cavity and shows how the submandibular gland extends to lie on top of the mylohyoid muscle.

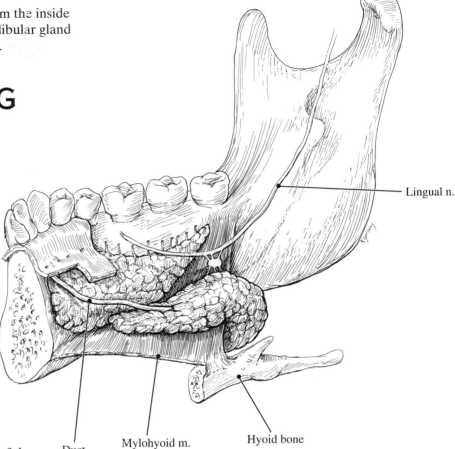

G

Lingual n.

Duct

Mylohyoid m.

Hyoid bone

H

The gland is fully freed to the posterior edge of the mylohyoid muscle. As traction is applied to the gland to facilitate deep dissection, the attached lingual nerve may be pulled down with it; inadvertent division of the lingual nerve is a serious complication. As Wharton's duct comes into view, it is tied with 3-0 chromic catgut and divided. The mylohyoid muscle may need to be retracted anteriorly to obtain a clear view of the operative field. The dissection is completed by separating the gland from the dorsal surface of the mylohyoid muscle. The hypoglossal nerve can be seen coursing between the muscle and the gland inferiorly and deep to the digastric muscle. This should be identified and protected before the final removal of the gland.

The platysma is reapproximated with interrupted simple stitches of 4-0 chromic catgut. The skin is closed with a subcuticular stitch using fine suture material.

H

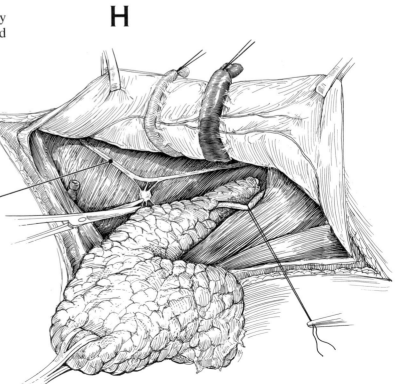

Lingual n.

Chapter

2

NECK

A RADICAL NECK DISSECTION

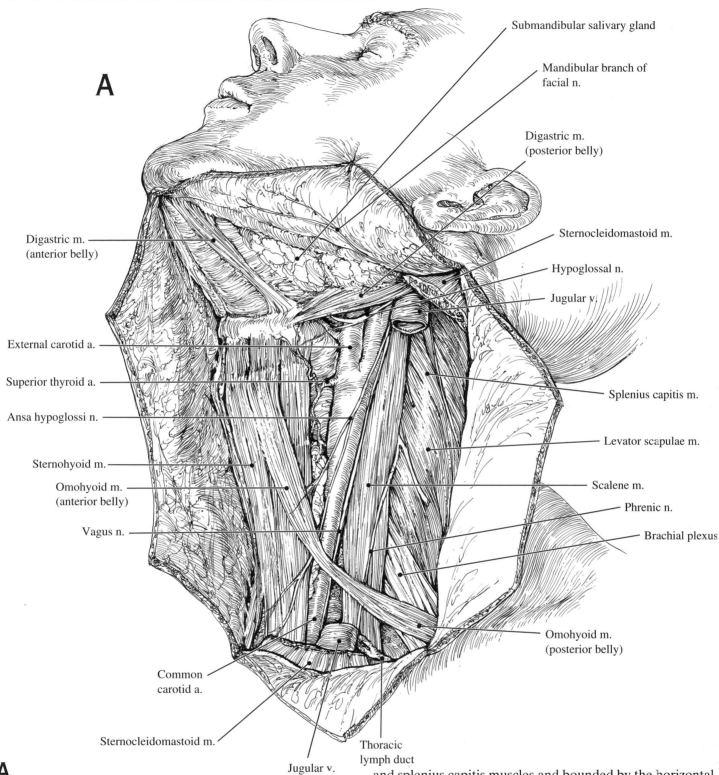

A

Submandibular salivary gland

Mandibular branch of
facial n.

Digastric m.
(posterior belly)

Sternocleidomastoid m.

Hypoglossal n.

Jugular v.

Splenius capitis m.

Levator scapulae m.

Scalene m.

Phrenic n.

Brachial plexus

Omohyoid m.
(posterior belly)

Digastric m.
(anterior belly)

External carotid a.

Superior thyroid a.

Ansa hypoglossi n.

Sternohyoid m.

Omohyoid m.
(anterior belly)

Vagus n.

Common
carotid a.

Sternocleidomastoid m.

Jugular v.

Thoracic
lymph duct

A

The neck is almost unmatched in the number of anatomic structures within or passing through it. These structures affect the transport of food, blood, air, and nerve impulses. The neck is also the seat of important endocrine organs.

Radical neck dissection means different things to different surgeons, as is true of many operations that deal with the wide excision of certain areas of the body rather than with a single organ. Here, the term is used to designate the unilateral removal of all lymph node–bearing tissue in the cervical area superficial to the scalenus, levator scapulae,

and splenius capitis muscles and bounded by the horizontal ramus of the mandible superiorly, the anterior border of the trapezius posteriorly, the clavicle inferiorly, and the midline anteriorly. Included in the removed tissue are the sternocleidomastoid and omohyoid muscles, the internal jugular vein, and the contents of the submandibular triangle.

In the accompanying illustration, the major portions of the sternocleidomastoid muscle and the underlying internal jugular vein have been removed to show more clearly the other anatomic structures.

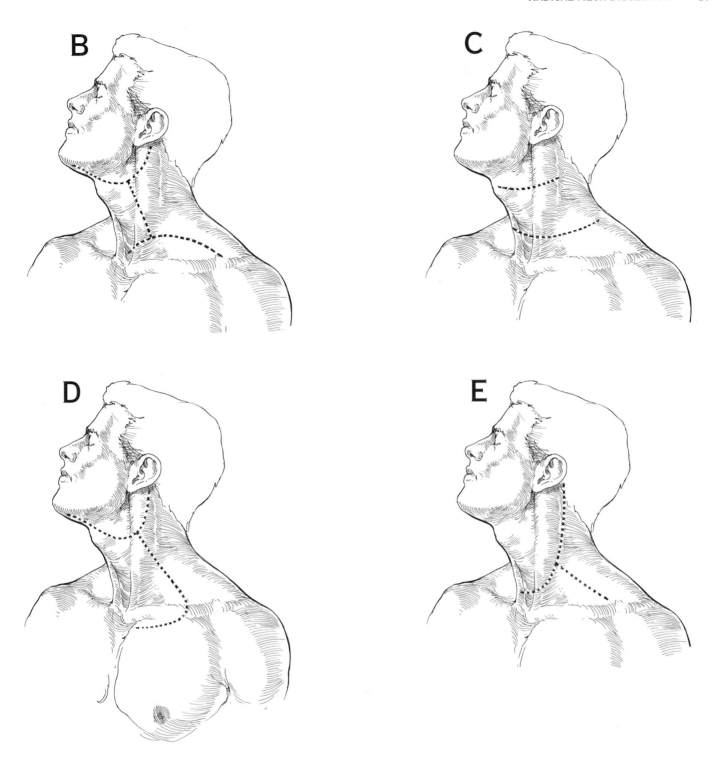

B, C, D, E

We favor the Hayes Martin incision as modified by Slaughter (*B*). Although it does not offer ideal protection of the underlying artery, it eliminates the sharp acute angles at both bifurcations of the Martin incision and the risk of their becoming avascular and necrotic. The extremes of the arms of the upper Y are the mastoid process posteriorly and the symphysis menti anteriorly. Those of the inferior Y are the junction of the trapezius and clavicle posteriorly and the midline anteriorly. If only the upper neck is involved, the lower arm of the Y incision need not be made. As with several other incisions, the modified Hayes Martin can be adapted to concomitant work on intraoral tissue. The MacFee incision (*C*), may seem an awkward choice for access to adequate exposure and meaningful dissection, especially without its upper arm. Yet it can be surprisingly

suitable if the incision is placed slightly more cephalad and the length of the lower arm is extended significantly. It can be ideal for thyroid surgery, especially as the submandibular triangle need not be addressed. The flaps of the Loré incision (*D*) have a good blood supply and offer satisfactory protection of the carotid artery. It is versatile and can be used with virtually any head and neck operation. The Lahey incision (*E*) is best suited to radical thyroid or laryngeal surgery and to bilateral neck dissection. Although it offers good protection of the carotid artery, it is not well suited to concomitant intraoral surgery.

Regardless of the type of incision, flaps should be elevated in the subplatysmal plane to maintain viability unless the extent of the tumor dictates otherwise.

F

F

The posterior flap is developed to the anterior border of
the trapezius muscle. At its cephalic aspect, fibers of the
sternocleidomastoid are in intimate association with the
dermis. Toward the lower half of the anterior border of the
trapezius muscle, the spinal accessory nerve is encountered
and should be isolated and preserved if possible. The
medial flap is developed to the midline; this area is devoid
of significant structures. The inferior flap is developed to
the clavicle and the superior one to the horizontal ramus of
the mandible.

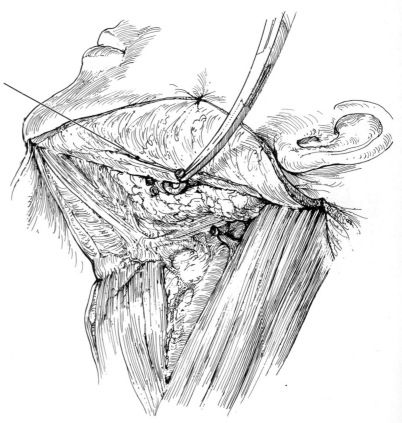

Marginal mandibular
branch of facial n.

G

G

As the superior flap is developed, extra care should be
taken to identify and preserve the marginal mandibular
branch of the seventh nerve. By placing gentle traction
superiorly on the flap and applying countertraction on the
neck tissue, an attentive, restrained dissection of the flap
with the scalpel in this relatively bloodless field reveals the
nerve. Once the mandibular branch of the facial nerve has
been found, the facial artery and vein are identified, ligated
inferior to the nerve, and retracted superiorly, restricting
further manipulation of this delicate structure.

H

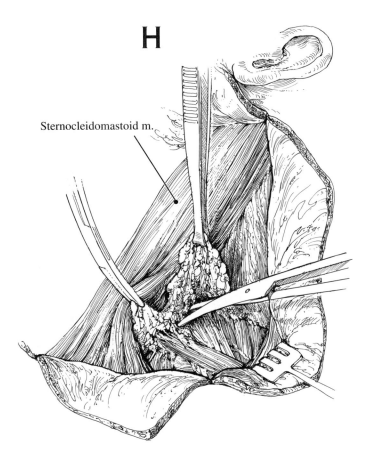

Sternocleidomastoid m.

The beginning of the formal dissection is often dictated by clinical considerations; electively, we begin at the inferolateral aspect. As the dissection is carried toward the posteroinferior edge of the sternocleidomastoid muscle, the inferior belly of the omohyoid muscle is encountered. The phrenic nerve to be spared is visible overlying the anterior scalene muscle in the window between this and the lateral edge of the sternocleidomastoid muscle.

I

The inferior belly of the omohyoid muscle is ligated and divided at a point just above the clavicle. As this muscle and the fatty areolar tissue with the associated lymph nodes are retracted medially, a portion of the brachial plexus is exposed. If the brachial plexus is not readily visible or is situated more medially, it can be located by running a finger transversely over its expected course and feeling the usually taut nerve trunks. This concern for locating the plexus is not an idle one, as the nerve trunks in some older individuals can be tented by the retraction and brought into the path of the dissecting scissors. The apical pleura is deep and inferior to this point but may extend superficially to near—or even above—the clavicle and thus could be inadvertently cut.

The dissection continues along the anterior border of the trapezius muscle up to the mastoid process with constant retraction medially of the tissues to be removed. Venules in this area can be expected to ooze throughout the operation if they are not diligently electrocoagulated.

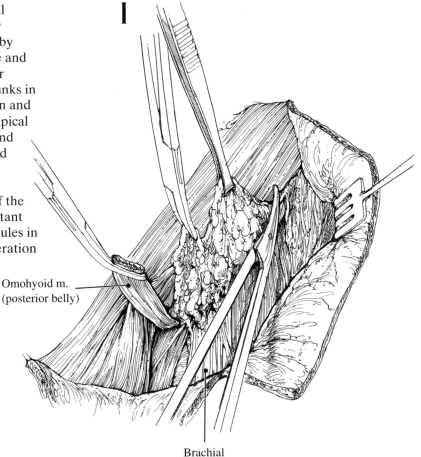

Omohyoid m.
(posterior belly)

Brachial
plexus

J

Sternocleidomastoid m.
(being divided)

J

Attention is now shifted to the sternocleidomastoid muscle, which inserts by a sternal and a clavicular head. It is separated from the underlying jugular vein by blunt finger dissection and then slowly cauterized or cut above its insertion. Bleeding is minimal, and hemostasis should be selective rather than a ligation of the entire muscle mass. The sternocleidomastoid muscle can then be retracted superiorly with a 6-inch hemostat to provide countertraction.

K

K

The previous step exposes the jugular vein, which is a cardinal point in beginning the inferior aspect of the dissection. This and the previous steps will also expose the subclavian vessels if they curve above the clavicle; awareness of this possibility can prevent their inadvertent injury. If injury occurs, blind clamping and use of regular hemostats only invite bigger tears. Instead, vascular clamps should be used and the repair done with fine vascular suture material.

The internal jugular vein should be carefully freed from the fatty areolar tissue overlying the carotid sheath. A curved forceps and then a right-angled clamp are used to isolate the vein fully to allow passage of a 0 silk tie for ligation. Before ligation, care should be exercised first to avoid injury to the vagus nerve, which lies medially and slightly deep to the internal jugular vein and lateral to the carotid artery.

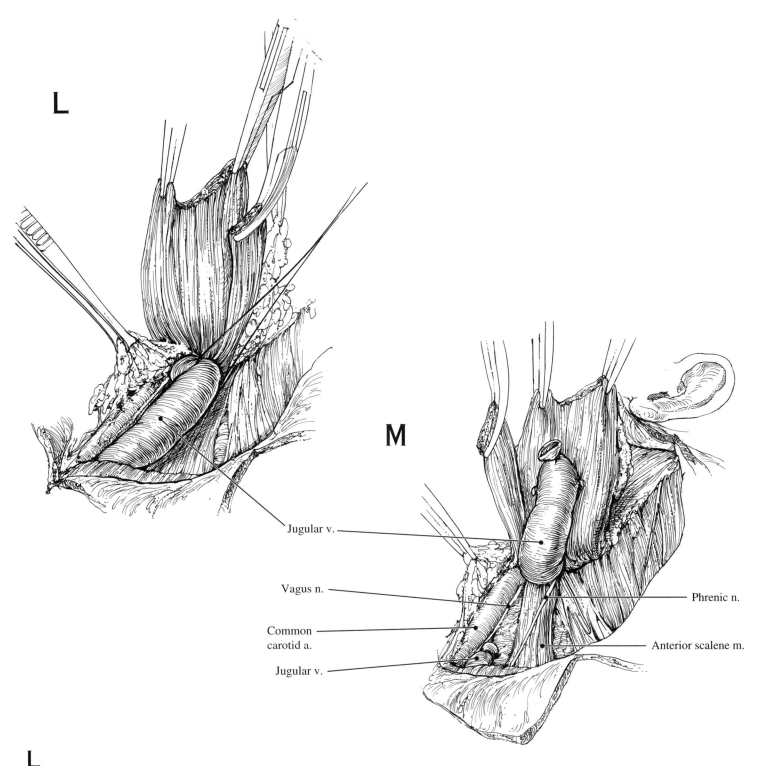

L

M

Jugular v.

Vagus n.

Common
carotid a.

Jugular v.

Phrenic n.

Anterior scalene m.

L

The jugular vein is doubly ligated with 0 silk just above the
clavicle. A stick tie of 2-0 silk is used to further secure the
transected vein on the thoracic side.

M

The dissection continues along the carotid artery with
awareness that the vagus nerve usually lies superficial and
anterior to it and the cervical sympathetic chain lateral and
deep to it. The thoracic duct can usually be seen if it is
sought just above the clavicle, where it enters the internal
jugular vein. This translucent, tortuous duct is 2 to 4 mm in
diameter and is occasionally recognized only after it is
inadvertently torn. The presence in the wound of milky
chyle signals this mishap. The duct should then be
thoroughly oversewn with fine vascular suture.

N

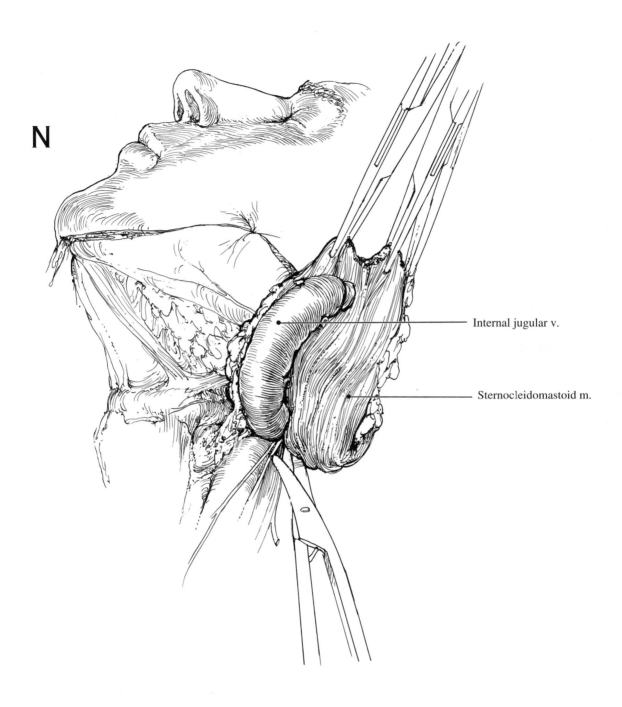

Internal jugular v.

Sternocleidomastoid m.

N

During the lateral aspect of the dissection, branches from the transverse cervical and scapular vessels are encountered and ligated individually or caught along with fatty areolar tissue and secured. Once again, the spinal accessory nerve is located at the anterior border of the trapezius muscle and halfway between the clavicle and mastoid process. Often, contraction of the trapezius muscle in the nonparalyzed patient may be the first sign that the spinal accessory nerve has been encountered. If permitted by the clinical circumstances, it is possible, using meticulous technique, to dissect the nerve free as it courses superiorly through the sternocleidomastoid muscle to the jugular foramen.

O

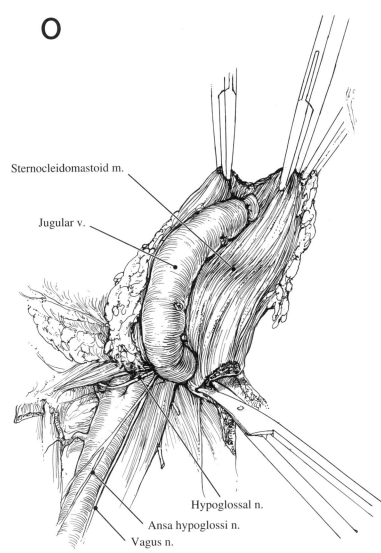

Sternocleidomastoid m.

Jugular v.

Hypoglossal n.

Ansa hypoglossi n.

Vagus n.

O

The dissection proceeds cephalad along the carotid artery. Within the carotid sheath, a tunnel may be created with blunt dissection by using the index finger to push tissues superiorly in the carotid sheath, separating tissues from the carotid artery up to the base of the skull. This facilitates faster subsequent dissection. As the branches of the cervical plexus are sectioned, the mobilization of the specimen improves perceptibly. The ansa hypoglossi nerve is expendable if necessary. As the omohyoid muscle is detached from the hyoid bone, the structures in the area of the carotid bifurcation are readily exposed. The other strap muscles are not disturbed. We do not practice routine anesthetization of the carotid bulb. The hypoglossal nerve is found approximately 2 cm cephalad to the carotid bifurcation; it loops in a direction transverse to the internal and external carotid arteries. Pharyngeal branches from the jugular vein are encountered medially and superficial to the nerve. They are quite short and often sizable; if torn, they are difficult to secure without risk to the adjacent hypoglossal nerve. It is prudent to tie them in continuity before dividing them. The superior laryngeal nerve is more medially situated but is usually not encountered in a standard dissection.

P

A 6-inch curved hemostat can now be advanced just superficial to the posterior belly of the digastric muscle to the mastoid tip. Electrocoagulation of the issue superficial to the clamp will quickly free the superior portion of the sternocleidomastoid muscle, a relatively bloodless dissection except for the posterior facial vein. The greater auricular nerve can be seen coursing over the sternocleidomastoid muscle at this point and is taken with the specimen.

The jugular vein is isolated by carefully passing a Mixter forceps around it just cephalad and deep to the lower border of the posterior belly of the digastric muscle. Care must be taken to again identify the vagus, spinal accessory, and hypoglossal nerves as they all course toward the base of the skull to enter the jugular foramen and hypoglossal canal, respectively. The digastric muscle is retracted to permit higher ligation of the vein and may be sacrificed if necessary for exposure or tumor resection. The jugular vein has a low pressure here and can be secured with a single tie of 0 silk.

P

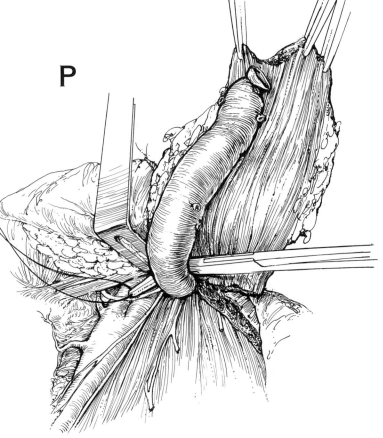

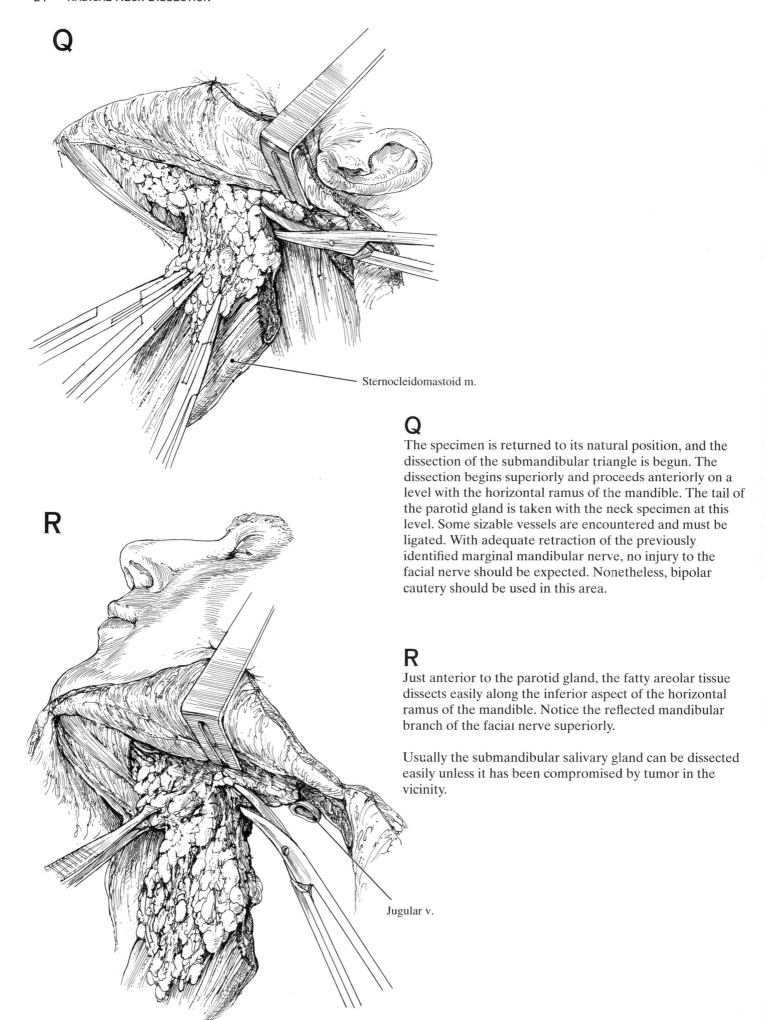

Q

Sternocleidomastoid m.

Q

The specimen is returned to its natural position, and the dissection of the submandibular triangle is begun. The dissection begins superiorly and proceeds anteriorly on a level with the horizontal ramus of the mandible. The tail of the parotid gland is taken with the neck specimen at this level. Some sizable vessels are encountered and must be ligated. With adequate retraction of the previously identified marginal mandibular nerve, no injury to the facial nerve should be expected. Nonetheless, bipolar cautery should be used in this area.

R

R

Just anterior to the parotid gland, the fatty areolar tissue dissects easily along the inferior aspect of the horizontal ramus of the mandible. Notice the reflected mandibular branch of the facial nerve superiorly.

Usually the submandibular salivary gland can be dissected easily unless it has been compromised by tumor in the vicinity.

Jugular v.

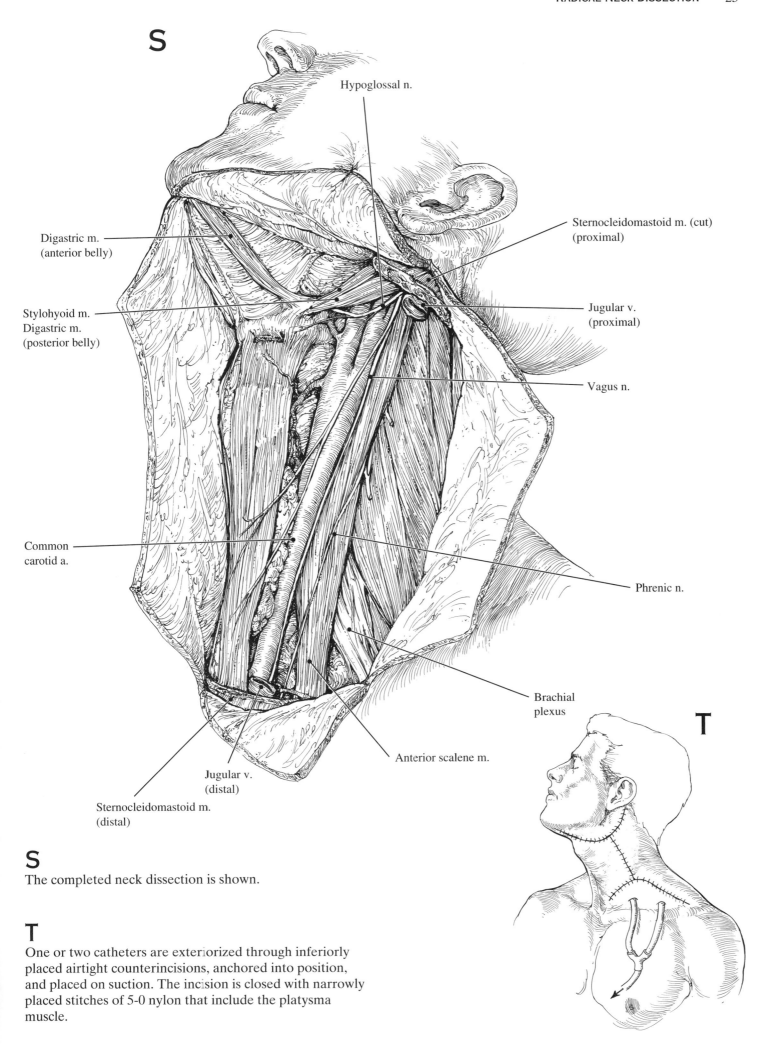

S

Hypoglossal n.

Digastric m.
(anterior belly)

Stylohyoid m.
Digastric m.
(posterior belly)

Common
carotid a.

Sternocleidomastoid m. (cut)
(proximal)

Jugular v.
(proximal)

Vagus n.

Phrenic n.

Brachial
plexus

Anterior scalene m.

Jugular v.
(distal)

Sternocleidomastoid m.
(distal)

T

S

The completed neck dissection is shown.

T

One or two catheters are exteriorized through inferiorly
placed airtight counterincisions, anchored into position,
and placed on suction. The incision is closed with narrowly
placed stitches of 5-0 nylon that include the platysma
muscle.

DELTOPECTORAL FLAP

A deltopectoral flap has limited but important applications. In this instance, the clinical scenario is such that irradiated affected skin and underlying soft tissue have been excised in the course of the neck dissection, creating a wound that exposes the carotid artery and cannot be closed primarily. The intent here is to cover the defect (and the exposed vessels) with a healthy, full-thickness skin pedicle graft. A deltopectoral flap is a full-thickness flap of the anterior chest wall that includes the pectoralis fascia and is medially based with its blood supply from the first to fourth internal mammary arteries and their branches. Except for very long flaps or other special circumstances, mobilization and placement of the flap do not need to be delayed.

A

Creation of the flap is not begun until after all of the destructive aspects of the operation are completed. There is not much concern about the ratio of the width of the base to the length of the flap. The skin incision is carried down to the muscle, and the flap is mobilized along with the surface fascia. The perforating vessels should be meticulously coagulated with fine-tipped cautery. Twisting, excessive tension, acute angulation, and gross ligation of tissue along with the vessels are to be avoided, as they encourage necrosis of the flap.

A

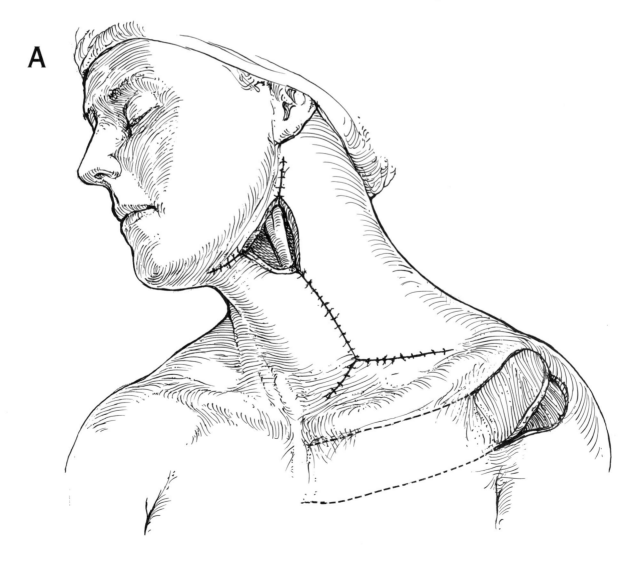

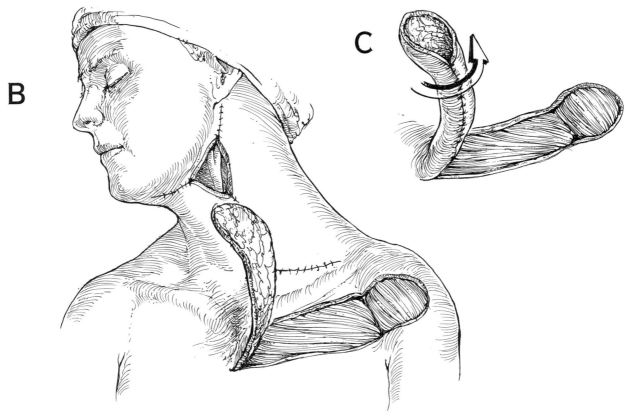

B

C

B, C

The flap is elevated off its bed, and the portion of it that will not lie on the raw recipient site is fashioned into a tube by coapting the skin with a continuous simple stitch of 5-0 nylon.

D

The spatulated pedicle that has been created is now turned 180 degrees on itself, and the spatulated portion is sutured to the neck defect with interrupted 5-0 nylon. The donor site is covered with a thin split-thickness skin graft.

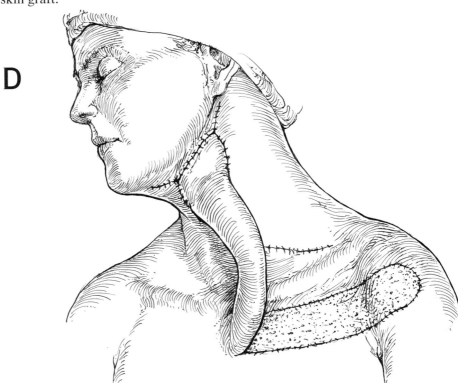

D

E

When the "paddle" part of the tube flap is deemed secure and flourishing—usually 6 weeks or longer—it is detached from the tubular portion. The tube flap is then reopened into its original flat configuration and replaced on the donor site, from which an appropriate amount of the temporary skin graft has been removed. Usually the skin graft over the shoulder remains. Attention is returned to the spatulated portion in the neck; it will need to be trimmed and its incised border secured to the adjacent native skin.

E

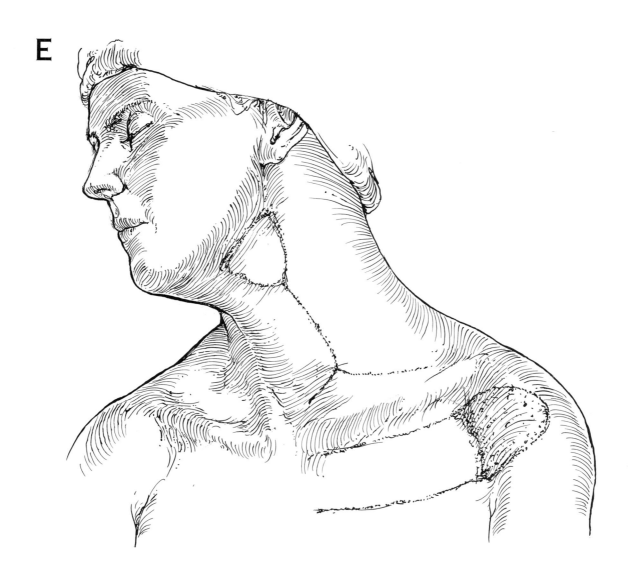

B THYROGLOSSAL DUCT CYST—EXCISION

A

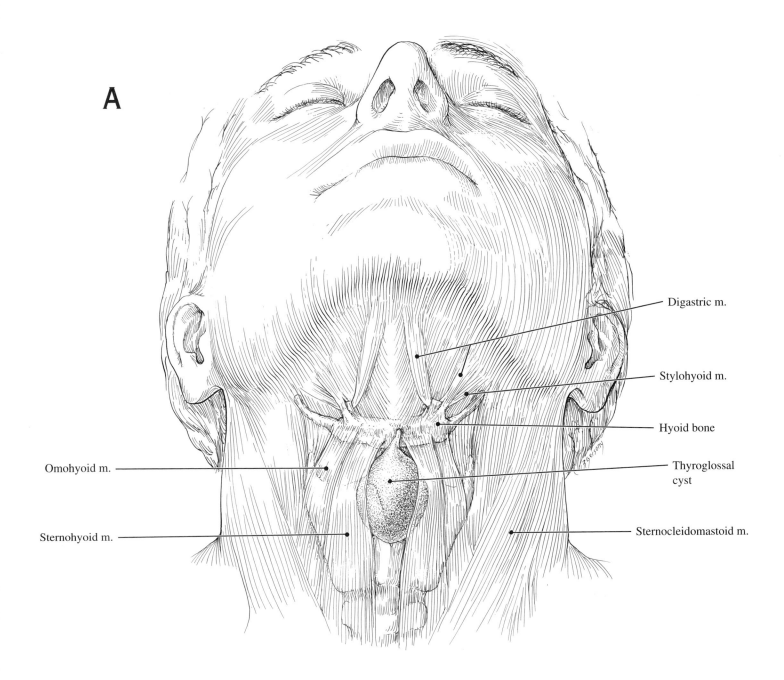

Digastric m.

Stylohyoid m.

Hyoid bone

Thyroglossal cyst

Omohyoid m.

Sternohyoid m.

Sternocleidomastoid m.

A

The thyroglossal duct cyst can be nonpalpable and nonvisible and located just caudal to the hyoid bone, or it can be present as a swollen, infected, painful mass in the anterior neck. Excising the cyst can be as simple as removing a mass superficial to the hyoid bone or as complex as identifying and excising a thyroglossal tract extending to the foramen cecum, making it necessary to excise a button of the base of the tongue.

The hyoid bone does not have direct attachment to any other bone; it is held in position by a number of muscles with opposing forces, as shown in this illustration.

B

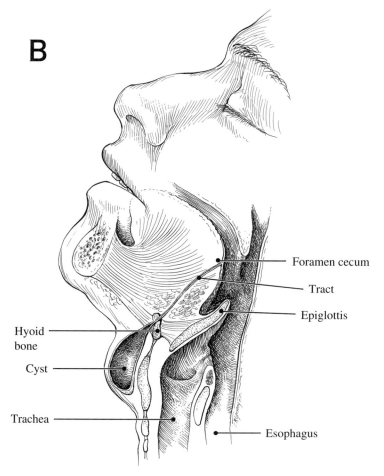

Foramen cecum

Tract

Epiglottis

Hyoid bone

Cyst

Trachea

Esophagus

B

The sagittal view shows one possible course of this epithelially lined cyst. Clearly, if the duct is not completely excised and the foramen cecum retains its patency, an anterior neck abscess can form.

The skin incision should be transverse and a centimeter or so cephalad to the mass; this location will position the surgeon advantageously with the dissection should the tract extend beyond the hyoid bone.

C

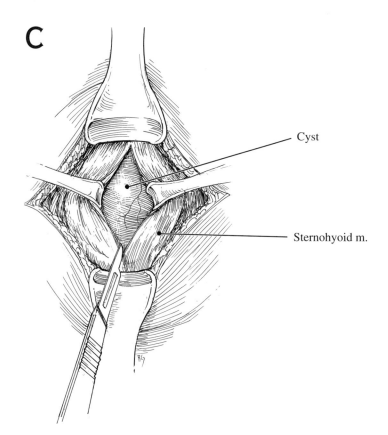

Cyst

Sternohyoid m.

C

The dissection is carried directly down to the mass and is maintained on the (pseudo) capsule from this point on. The sternohyoid and omohyoid muscles will have been retracted laterally, thus requiring minimal additional dissection to free them from the sides of the cyst.

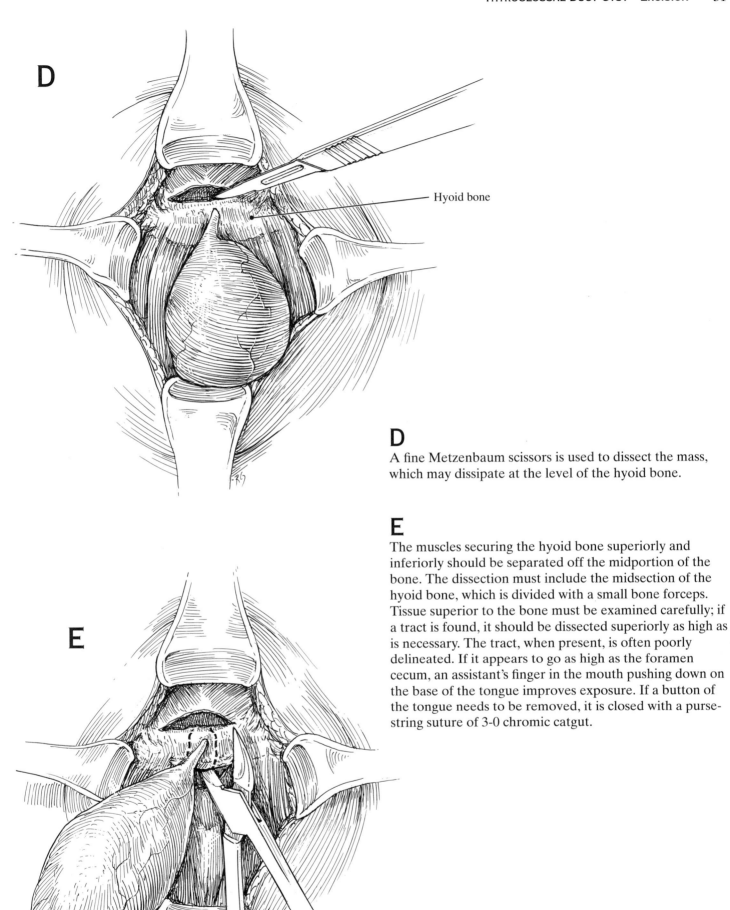

Hyoid bone

D

A fine Metzenbaum scissors is used to dissect the mass, which may dissipate at the level of the hyoid bone.

E

The muscles securing the hyoid bone superiorly and inferiorly should be separated off the midportion of the bone. The dissection must include the midsection of the hyoid bone, which is divided with a small bone forceps. Tissue superior to the bone must be examined carefully; if a tract is found, it should be dissected superiorly as high as is necessary. The tract, when present, is often poorly delineated. If it appears to go as high as the foramen cecum, an assistant's finger in the mouth pushing down on the base of the tongue improves exposure. If a button of the tongue needs to be removed, it is closed with a purse-string suture of 3-0 chromic catgut.

F

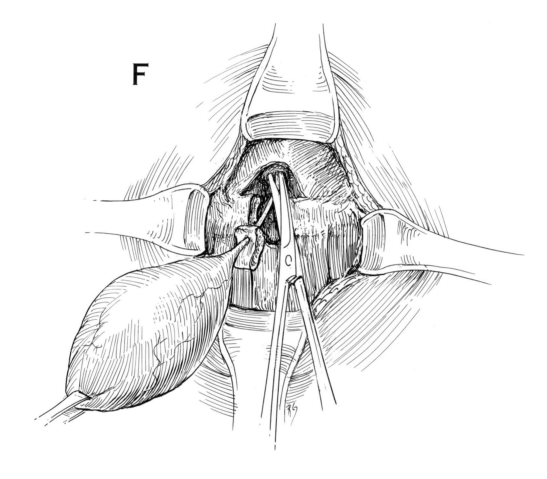

F
The tissue is reapproximated with interrupted stitches of
4-0 chromic catgut and the skin with a continuous
subcuticular stitch of fine monofilament suture.

C BRANCHIAL CLEFT CYST—EXCISION

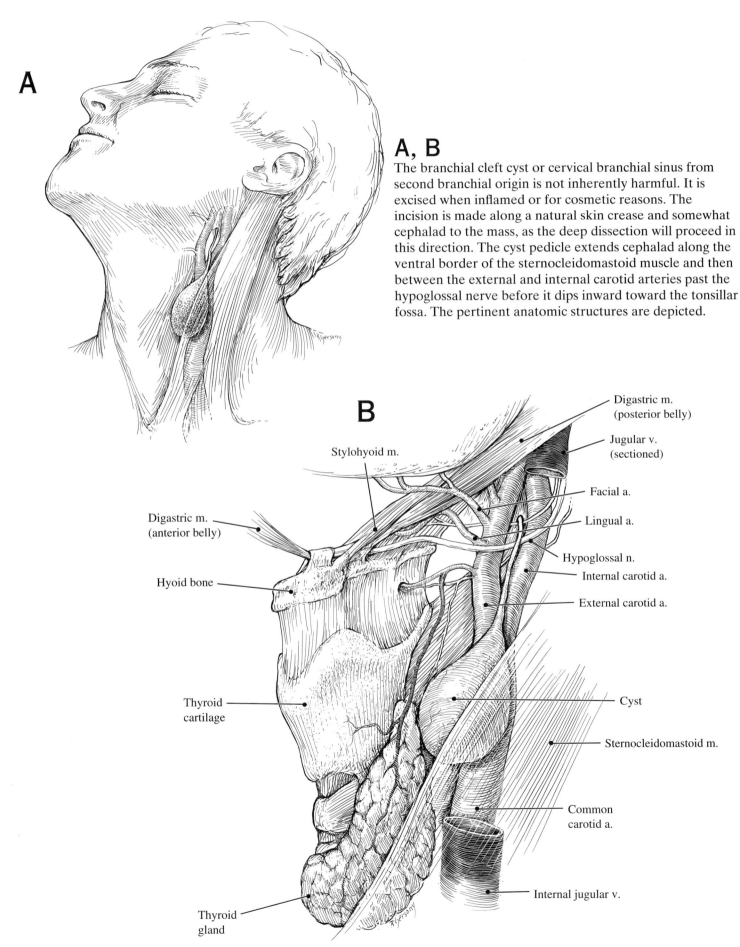

A

A, B

The branchial cleft cyst or cervical branchial sinus from second branchial origin is not inherently harmful. It is excised when inflamed or for cosmetic reasons. The incision is made along a natural skin crease and somewhat cephalad to the mass, as the deep dissection will proceed in this direction. The cyst pedicle extends cephalad along the ventral border of the sternocleidomastoid muscle and then between the external and internal carotid arteries past the hypoglossal nerve before it dips inward toward the tonsillar fossa. The pertinent anatomic structures are depicted.

B

Stylohyoid m.

Digastric m. (anterior belly)

Hyoid bone

Thyroid cartilage

Thyroid gland

Digastric m. (posterior belly)

Jugular v. (sectioned)

Facial a.

Lingual a.

Hypoglossal n.

Internal carotid a.

External carotid a.

Cyst

Sternocleidomastoid m.

Common carotid a.

Internal jugular v.

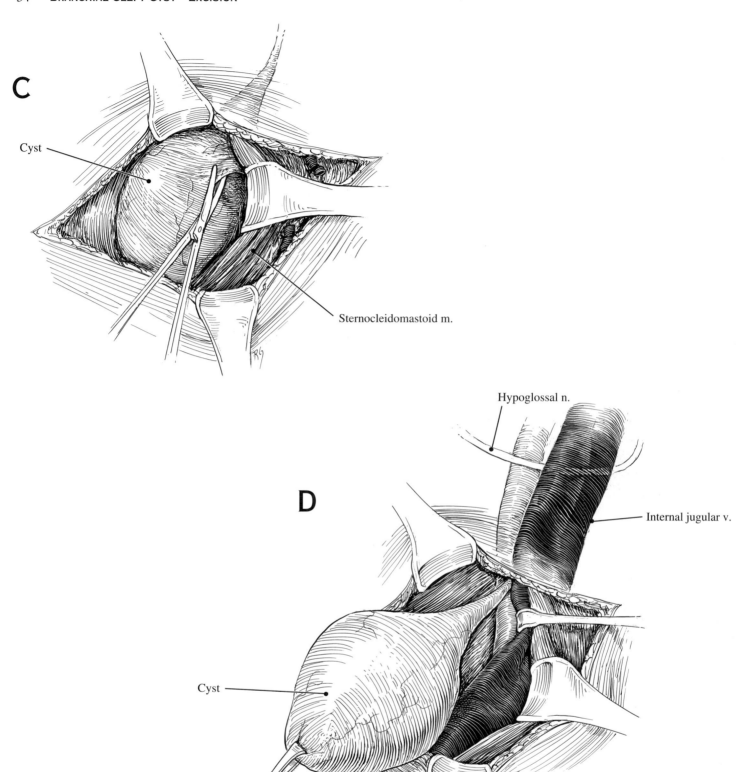

C

The incision is carried through the skin and platysma down to the deep cervical fascia. The sternocleidomastoid muscle is suffficiently mobilized along its anterior border that it can be retracted dorsally. The exposed cyst is dissected with a fine Metzenbaum scissors.

D

The body of the cyst is dissected free to position it out of the depth of the field. Keep in mind that the cyst lies on the jugular vein, which must not be entered.

E

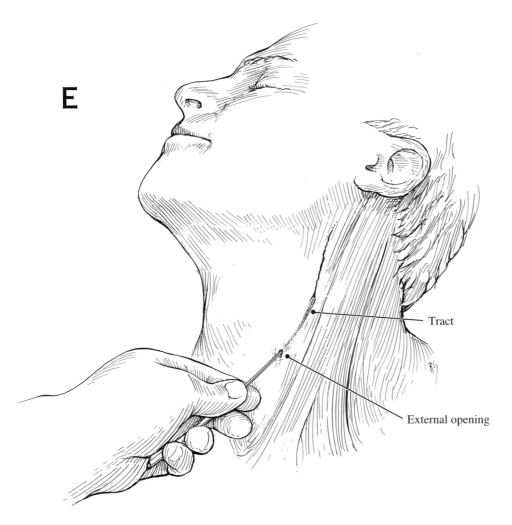

Tract

External opening

E

The dissection proceeds cephalad with the scissors in intimate contact with the pedicle, which early becomes a narrow strand of tissue. It is ligated with 4-0 chromic catgut and the specimen removed. The platysma is reapproximated with interrupted 4-0 chromic catgut, and a fine monofilament stitch is used for the subcuticular closure of the skin.

F

In planning excision of a cervical branchial sinus, the path of the sinus (expected to be along the ventral border of the sternocleidomastoid muscle) is confirmed by inserting a malleable, smooth-tipped probe through the external opening. A narrow ellipse of skin, oriented in the direction of a natural skin crease, is carried through the skin and platysma to the deep cervical fascia. If the fistulous opening is rather high and the anticipated length of the tract not too long, the entire procedure can be performed through an extension of the incision encompassing the external opening. If the tract is long, then the external opening is encircled through a limited incision and the dissection continued through a second incision at a point about halfway between the external opening and the tonsillar fossa. The dissection continues as before, closely hugging the tract as it courses toward the tonsillar fossa. At its farthest extreme, the tract is ligated with 4-0 chromic catgut and divided. No drain is used, and a plastic closure terminates the operation.

F

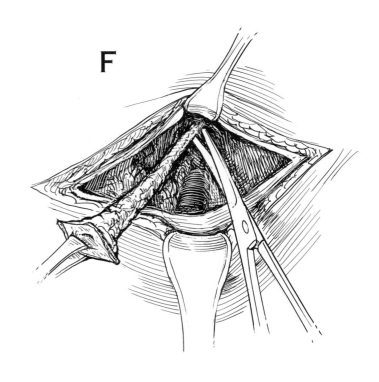

D TRACHEOSTOMY

Tracheostomy is performed for acute or chronic airway obstruction from a variety of causes, under elective or emergency conditions. Thorough familiarity with the anatomy of this area is the best insurance for performing this operation with confidence.

A

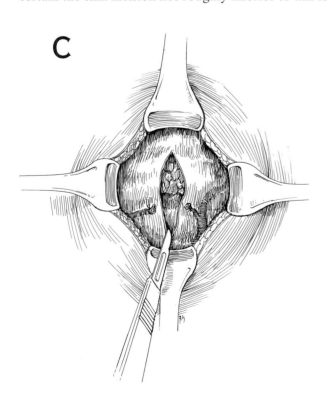

The pertinent anatomic landmarks of this area are highlighted. The surgeon should be aware that the trachea may be pushed to one side or compressed by the same process that prompted the tracheostomy, making it difficult to locate under certain emergency conditions. Sometimes an obstructing mass may lie anterior to the trachea and will need to be cut through to reach the airway.

Thyroid cartilage
"Strap" muscles

Crycoid cartilage
Thyroid isthmus
Thyroid gland (left lobe)

Trachea

B

The patient is positioned with the neck extended to bring the trachea closer to the surface, making it tauter and less likely to move from side to side. The incision should be transverse and about 2 to 3 cm above the sternal notch. It is helpful to palpate and mark the level of the cricoid to make certain the skin incision lies roughly inferior to this level.

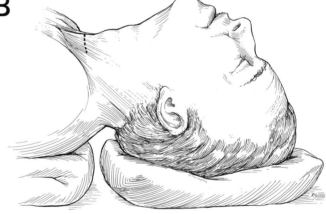

C

The skin incision is carried deep to the platysma with sufficient mobilization of the flaps to expose only that portion of the trachea above and below the second tracheal ring. Often a tributary of the inferior thyroid vein crosses at this level. If it cannot be retracted, the vein should be secured with a stick tie and divided.

The strap muscles are bluntly separated at the median raphe and retracted laterally to expose the trachea for introduction of the tube. The thyroid isthmus often crosses the trachea at this level and must be freed from surrounding tissue and retracted superiorly with a vein retractor. If especially large, it may need to be divided and secured with a stick tie to expose the trachea. The trachea is then cleared of loose adventitial tissue with a "peanut."

D

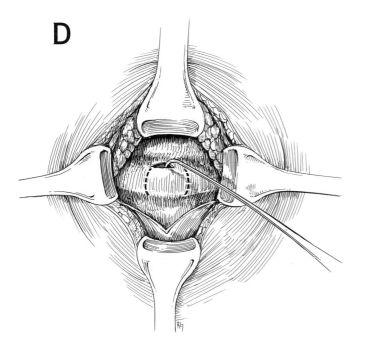

D

If the tracheostomy is being done in the unintubated patient, 1 ml of lidocaine without epinephrine may be instilled directly into the trachea with a syringe to anesthetize the trachea and decrease discomfort during this difficult time. The second tracheal ring is secured with a tracheal hook, and the tissue just above this hook is cut transversely. The cartilaginous ring on either side of the hooked portion is cut vertically, creating a flap that can be either used to steady the trachea as the tube is introduced or amputated immediately before introduction of the tube. Alternatively, the inferiorly based flap can be sewn to the skin with absorbable suture. This not only steadies the trachea for tube insertion but ensures that if the tube is accidentally dislodged in the first few days, a ready passage is available for reinsertion.

E

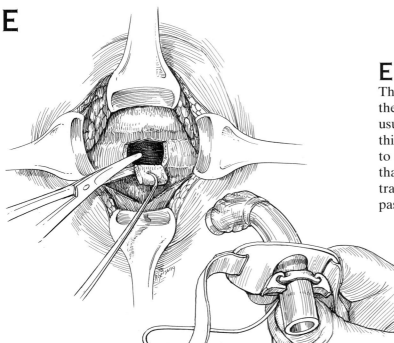

E

The tube is introduced facing directly dorsally. As it enters the trachea, the tip is directed downward. Copious mucus is usually present and is both coughed up and aspirated at this time. A small suction catheter should be advanced fully to aspirate the trachea distal to the tube and to guarantee that the tracheostomy tube is incontrovertibly in the trachea; occasionally a distorted anatomy exists, and false passage must be avoided.

F

A stitch of 4-0 nylon placed on each side of the skin opening encourages the development of a more pleasing scar postoperatively. The tracheostomy tube should be tied in place securely while the patient's neck is in the flexed position if possible. Alternatively, the tracheal tube can be sutured to the skin. A square piece of slit gauze is placed under the tube at the tracheostomy site and is changed as needed.

F

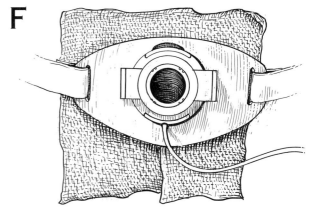

3

NECK AND MANDIBLE

A EN BLOC RESECTION

A

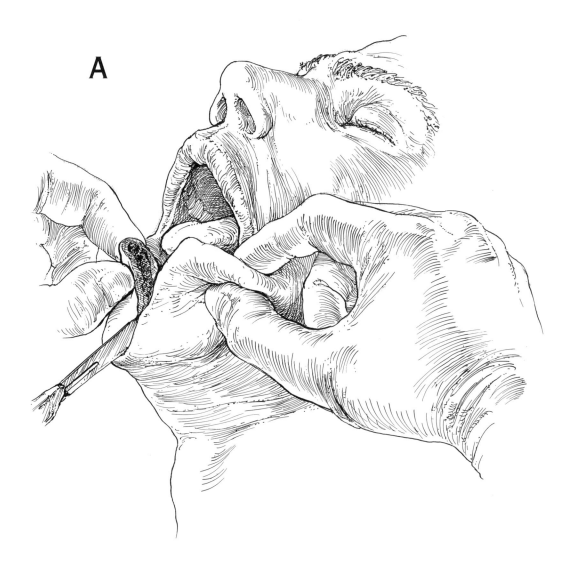

A

The standard radical neck dissection will have been performed in the manner already described in Chapter 2. Anesthesia is administered nasotracheally because a tube inserted orotracheally would interfere with the oral aspects of the operation. Alternatively, a tracheostomy can be performed early in the operation, depending on the site of the tumor. The lip is divided to enhance exposure of the intraoral area. Holding the lip firmly with the fingers as shown helps stabilize the tissue and provides hemostasis until the labial artery coursing through the lip is secured with a suture ligature or electrocoagulation. The anterior limb of the upper horizontal neck incision is carried to the lower point of the symphysis menti, and when the buccogingival sulcus is reached and divided (shown in *B*) the entire cheek flap can be retracted cephalad.

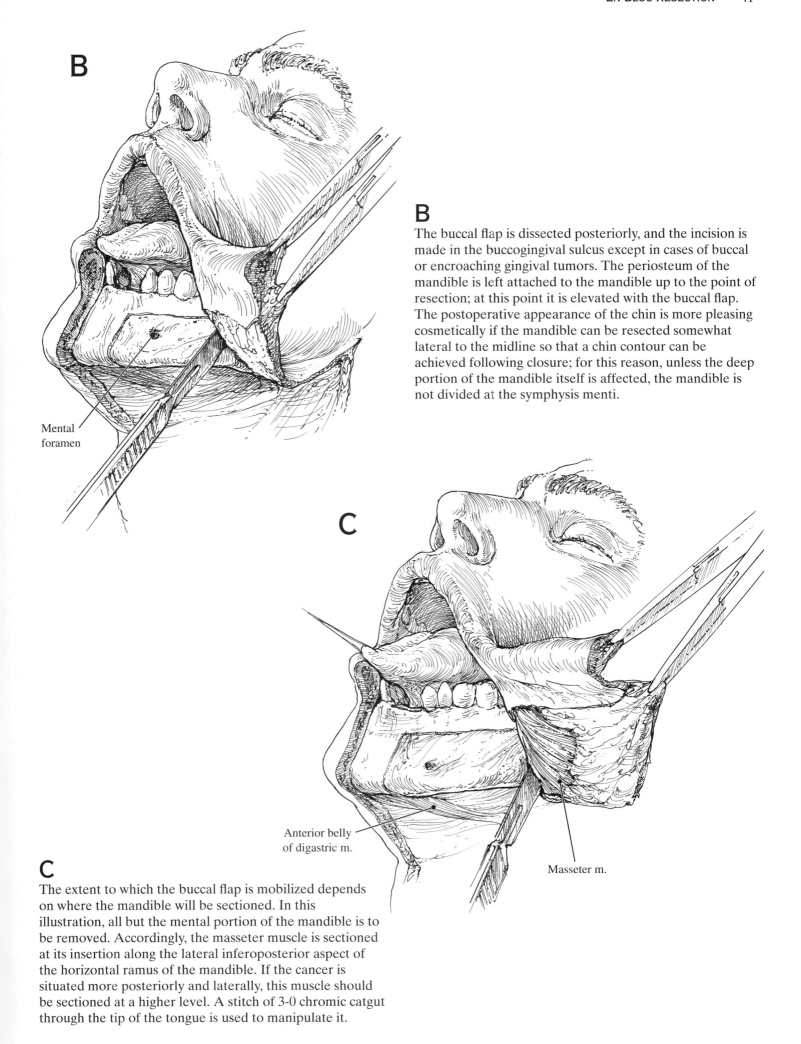

B

Mental
foramen

C

Anterior belly
of digastric m.

Masseter m.

B

The buccal flap is dissected posteriorly, and the incision is made in the buccogingival sulcus except in cases of buccal or encroaching gingival tumors. The periosteum of the mandible is left attached to the mandible up to the point of resection; at this point it is elevated with the buccal flap. The postoperative appearance of the chin is more pleasing cosmetically if the mandible can be resected somewhat lateral to the midline so that a chin contour can be achieved following closure; for this reason, unless the deep portion of the mandible itself is affected, the mandible is not divided at the symphysis menti.

C

The extent to which the buccal flap is mobilized depends on where the mandible will be sectioned. In this illustration, all but the mental portion of the mandible is to be removed. Accordingly, the masseter muscle is sectioned at its insertion along the lateral inferoposterior aspect of the horizontal ramus of the mandible. If the cancer is situated more posteriorly and laterally, this muscle should be sectioned at a higher level. A stitch of 3-0 chromic catgut through the tip of the tongue is used to manipulate it.

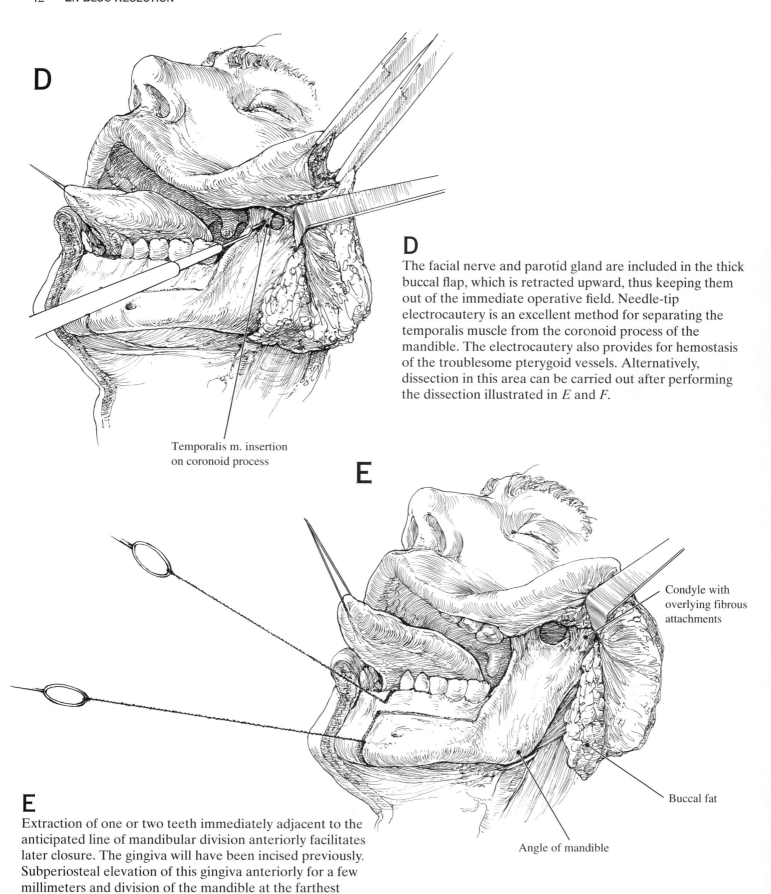

D

D

The facial nerve and parotid gland are included in the thick buccal flap, which is retracted upward, thus keeping them out of the immediate operative field. Needle-tip electrocautery is an excellent method for separating the temporalis muscle from the coronoid process of the mandible. The electrocautery also provides for hemostasis of the troublesome pterygoid vessels. Alternatively, dissection in this area can be carried out after performing the dissection illustrated in *E* and *F*.

Temporalis m. insertion
on coronoid process

E

Condyle with
overlying fibrous
attachments

Buccal fat

Angle of mandible

E

Extraction of one or two teeth immediately adjacent to the anticipated line of mandibular division anteriorly facilitates later closure. The gingiva will have been incised previously. Subperiosteal elevation of this gingiva anteriorly for a few millimeters and division of the mandible at the farthest extent of this subgingival mobilization make gingival tissue available for closure in this critical area. The sharp mandibular edge should be smoothed with a rasp to facilitate a more satisfactory soft tissue closure. Before the mandible is divided with a Gigli saw, the anterior belly of the digastric muscle should be freed. To decrease bleeding, the external carotid artery can be ligated in continuity distal to the origin of the superior thyroid artery.

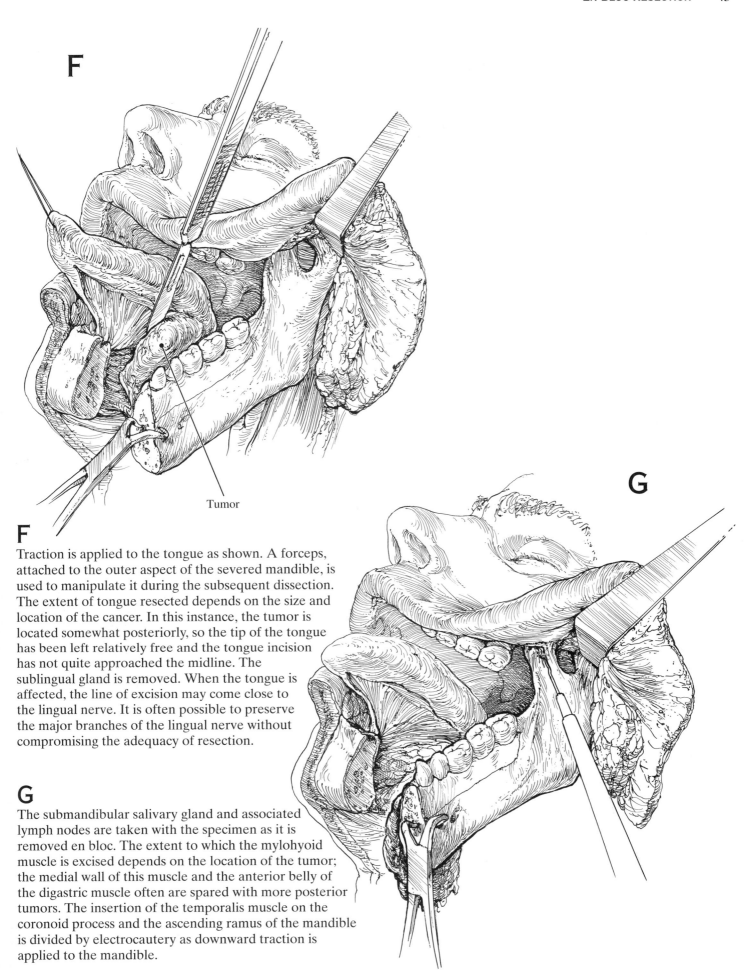

F

Tumor

F

Traction is applied to the tongue as shown. A forceps, attached to the outer aspect of the severed mandible, is used to manipulate it during the subsequent dissection. The extent of tongue resected depends on the size and location of the cancer. In this instance, the tumor is located somewhat posteriorly, so the tip of the tongue has been left relatively free and the tongue incision has not quite approached the midline. The sublingual gland is removed. When the tongue is affected, the line of excision may come close to the lingual nerve. It is often possible to preserve the major branches of the lingual nerve without compromising the adequacy of resection.

G

G

The submandibular salivary gland and associated lymph nodes are taken with the specimen as it is removed en bloc. The extent to which the mylohyoid muscle is excised depends on the location of the tumor; the medial wall of this muscle and the anterior belly of the digastric muscle often are spared with more posterior tumors. The insertion of the temporalis muscle on the coronoid process and the ascending ramus of the mandible is divided by electrocautery as downward traction is applied to the mandible.

Note: Different extents of resection and closure of the resultant defects are discussed in the last part of this chapter.

H

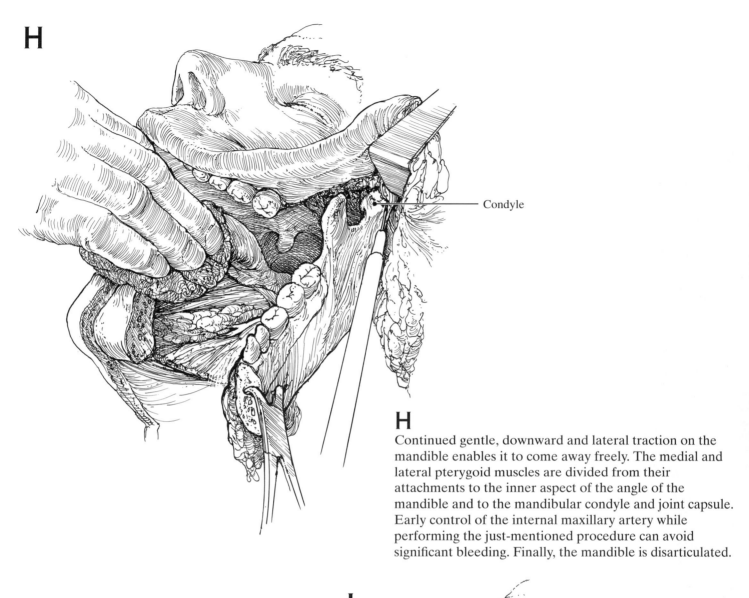

Condyle

H

Continued gentle, downward and lateral traction on the mandible enables it to come away freely. The medial and lateral pterygoid muscles are divided from their attachments to the inner aspect of the angle of the mandible and to the mandibular condyle and joint capsule. Early control of the internal maxillary artery while performing the just-mentioned procedure can avoid significant bleeding. Finally, the mandible is disarticulated.

I

The primary lesion with a portion of the tongue, the floor of the mouth, the mandible, and the contents of a radical neck dissection have been removed en bloc. The contours of the mucosal edges to be approximated vary with the location of the tumor and the extent of its resection. One has to examine the area for a few moments to determine the best way to bring the mucosal edges together so that there is minimal distortion of the soft palate, which is important in deglutition, and of the tip of the tongue, which is important in articulation.

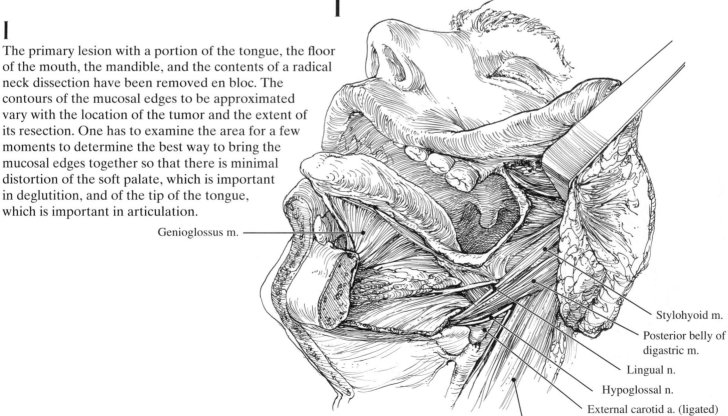

Genioglossus m.

Stylohyoid m.

Posterior belly of digastric m.

Lingual n.

Hypoglossal n.

External carotid a. (ligated)

Sternocleidomastoid m.

J

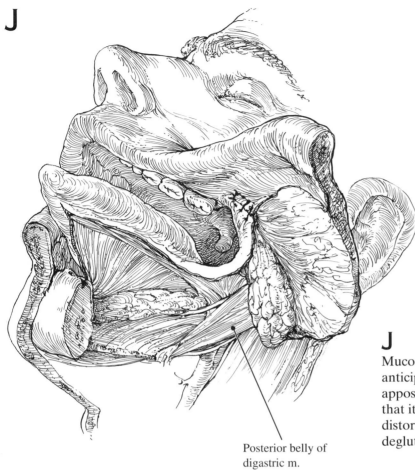

Posterior belly of
digastric m.

J

Mucosal closure is begun posteriorly. Even if there is
anticipated disparity in the lengths of the two edges to be
apposed, priority is given to this posterior area to ensure
that it is closed with minimal tension; avoidance of undue
distortion of tissue in this area minimizes problems with
deglutition postoperatively.

K

The musculature of the tongue is adjusted for optimal
apposition to the raw surface of the buccal flap and then
sutured to it in one layer (sometimes two) with interrupted
stitches of 3-0 absorbable suture. The free mucosal edge of
the tongue is then sutured to the buccal mucosa at the
previous buccogingival sulcus. The stitches are so placed
and tied that the knots reside intraorally in the new
buccogingival sulcus. Inevitably, the buccal, lingual, and
gingival incisions meet. This area resists closure in layers
and is the reason for the attempts early in the operation to
provide some free gingival mucosa. Any disparity in length
between the gingival and lingual mucosal edges has to be
compensated for at this point during the placement of the
stitches.

K

L

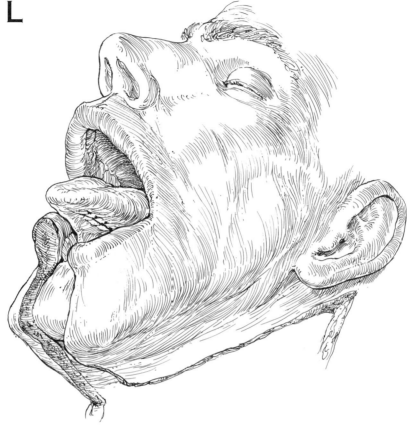

L

Closure of the lip requires reapproximation of the orbicularis oris muscle and the vermilion border. Sometimes removal of a 1- to 2-cm wedge of the resultant excessive lower lip lessens lip drooping and subsequent drooling of saliva; this is not necessary when the anterior portion of the hemimandible remains. Subcutaneous stitches are necessary in the mental area. The wound is closed as in a standard radical neck dissection, and closed suction drainage is instituted.

If it was not done at the beginning of the operation, a tracheostomy is routinely performed before removal of the endotracheal tube. So that the tracheostomy can be performed through a separate incision that has no communication with the neck wound dissection, the radical neck incision and dissection should be kept slightly away from the midline in its lower extent.

Resecting the hemimandible is not a routine component of the en bloc operation. Lesser extents of mandibular involvement permit limited resections. Although such limited resection of the mandible permits maintanance of its continuity, the defect should not be closed by suturing the tongue to the inner aspect of the intact mandible; the suture line is under tension and is likely to undergo dehiscence. If the suture line heals, then the tongue remains tethered, interfering with swallowing, articulation, and dental restoration.

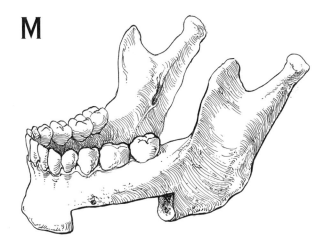

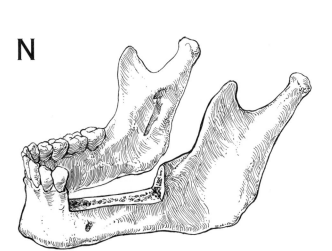

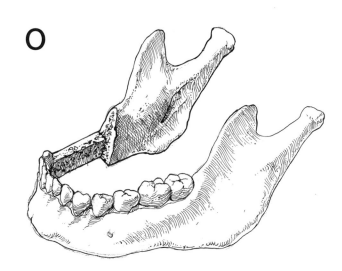

M, N, O

This trio of illustrations shows some of the ways a marginal resection of the mandible can be performed. An air-driven oscillating saw permits fine cutting on the diseased bone.

PECTORALIS MAJOR MYOCUTANEOUS FLAP

A

If the tongue, resected at its lateral border along with the floor of mouth, is not to be so tethered on closure, then a pedicle flap must be used as the intermediary tissue. The pectoralis major myocutaneous flap is the workhorse in such settings. It has the virtue of permitting the transfer of a vascularized flap of both muscle and skin and can be used in the vast majority of defects requiring a significant amount of soft tissue. The upper fibers of the pectoralis major muscle run in a transverse direction and must be transected when fashioning the pedicle. The lower ones run longitudinally and can be split at the lateral edge of the muscle.

B

The pectoral branch of the thoracoacromial artery, a branch of the axillary artery (itself a continuation of the subclavian artery), is the main source of blood for this flap. The axillary artery has three divisions: (1) above the upper border of the pectoralis minor muscle, (2) behind the pectoralis minor muscle, and (3) the lower border of the muscle. The thoracicoacromial artery arises from the first division.

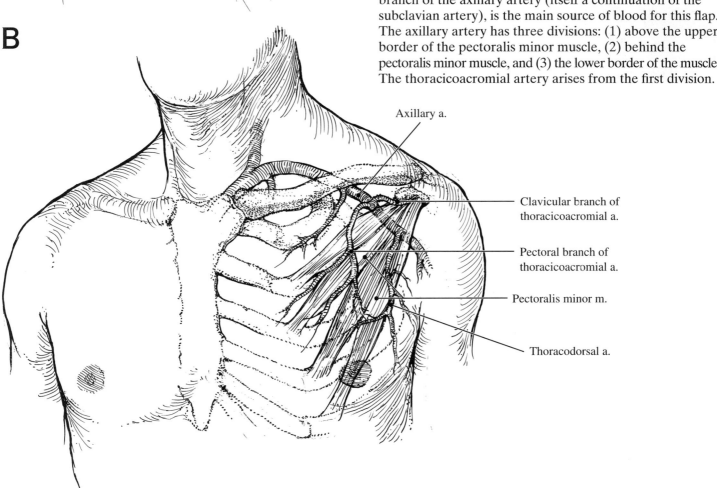

A

— Deltoid m.

— Pectoralis major m.

B

Axillary a.

Clavicular branch of thoracicoacromial a.

Pectoral branch of thoracicoacromial a.

Pectoralis minor m.

Thoracodorsal a.

C

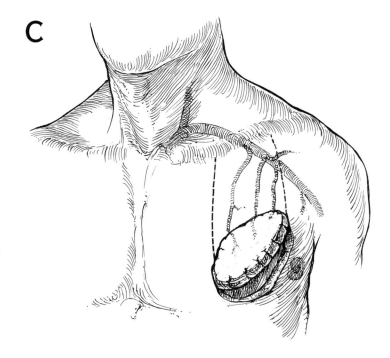

The course of the pectoral branch of the thoracoacromial artery is drawn with a water-soluble pen, as is the size of the desired island of skin. The skin incision is made along this line, and its inferior, lateral, and medial borders are carried down through the pectoralis major muscle to the pectoralis minor muscle. The pectoralis major muscle fibers on the superior border are not affected by this cut, as they anchor and nourish the transferred pedicle of skin and muscle. The pectoralis major muscle is raised at its lateral border, and its underside is examined to be certain the thoracoacromial artery, eventually its sole arterial supply, is present and intact. The dermis is sutured to the underlying pectoralis fascia with 3-0 absorbable suture to prevent the skin from sliding and shearing off its blood supply. This being ensured, the flap is mobilized by freeing it from the underlying pectoralis minor muscle, rectus fascia, and costochondral cartilages. The lateral pectoralis major muscle fibers are split if the pedicle appears too wide.

D

The flap has been mobilized to the clavicle and inverted so that now the nutrient vessels can be seen on the exposed surface. The flap is tunneled under the intervening skin, which sometimes needs to be incised a short distance longitudinally at its superior rim to improve visibility and ensure correct passage of the flap. The flap may be too bulky where it courses over the clavicle. Excessive bulk overriding the clavicle increases the risk of vessel compression during skin closure. In such instances, the muscle fibers can be divided with the most meticulous care so that it is mostly vessels without the associated bulky muscle that override the clavicle.

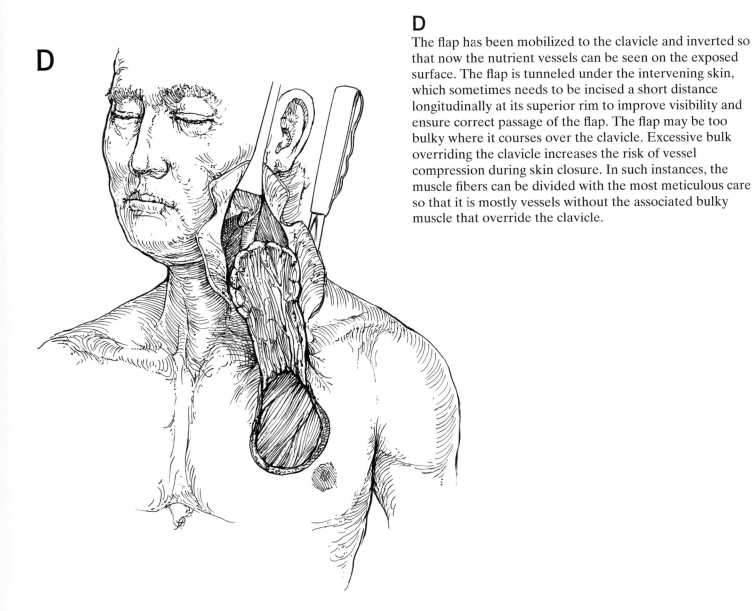

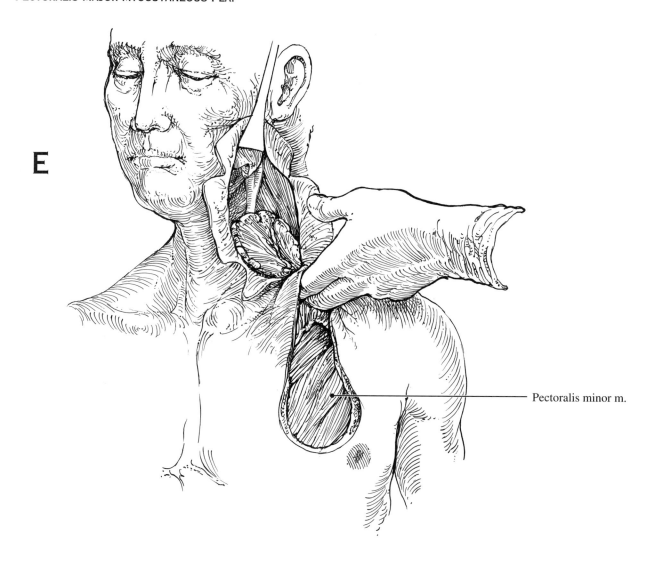

Pectoralis minor m.

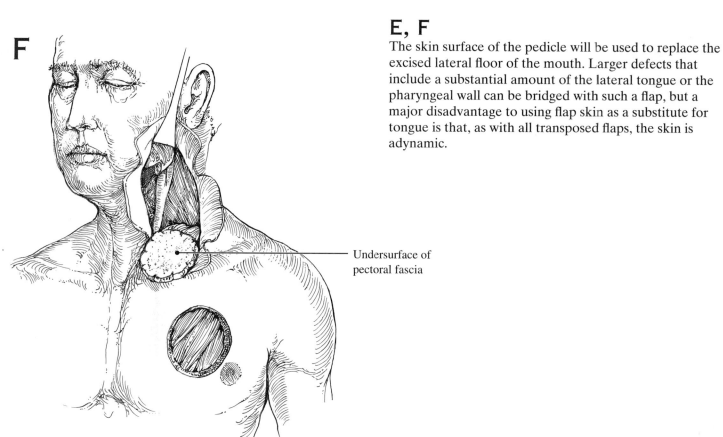

E, F

The skin surface of the pedicle will be used to replace the excised lateral floor of the mouth. Larger defects that include a substantial amount of the lateral tongue or the pharyngeal wall can be bridged with such a flap, but a major disadvantage to using flap skin as a substitute for tongue is that, as with all transposed flaps, the skin is adynamic.

Undersurface of pectoral fascia

G

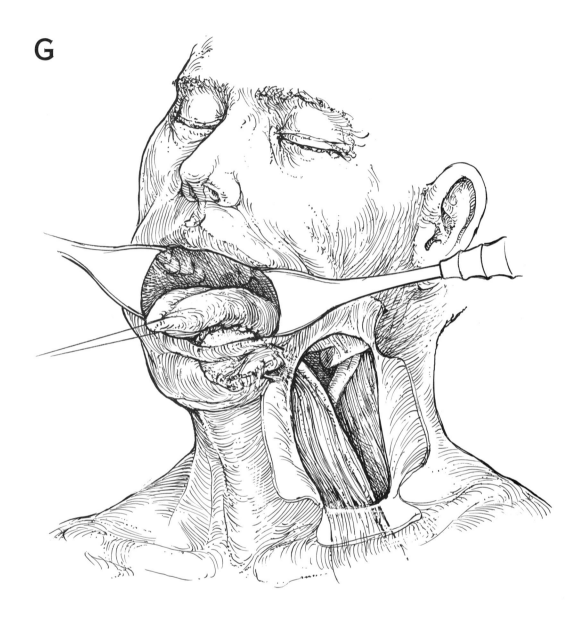

G

The head and neck incision is closed in a routine manner, yet when doing so, critical judgment will determine when a completely closed incision would be too tight and would risk compressing the nutrient vessels; it may be wiser to permit some gaping, which can be closed with a skin graft. Usually the donor sites for the skin and muscle can be closed primarily. Any portion that cannot reasonably be closed is covered with a skin graft.

4

THYROID

A THYROIDECTOMY—STANDARD

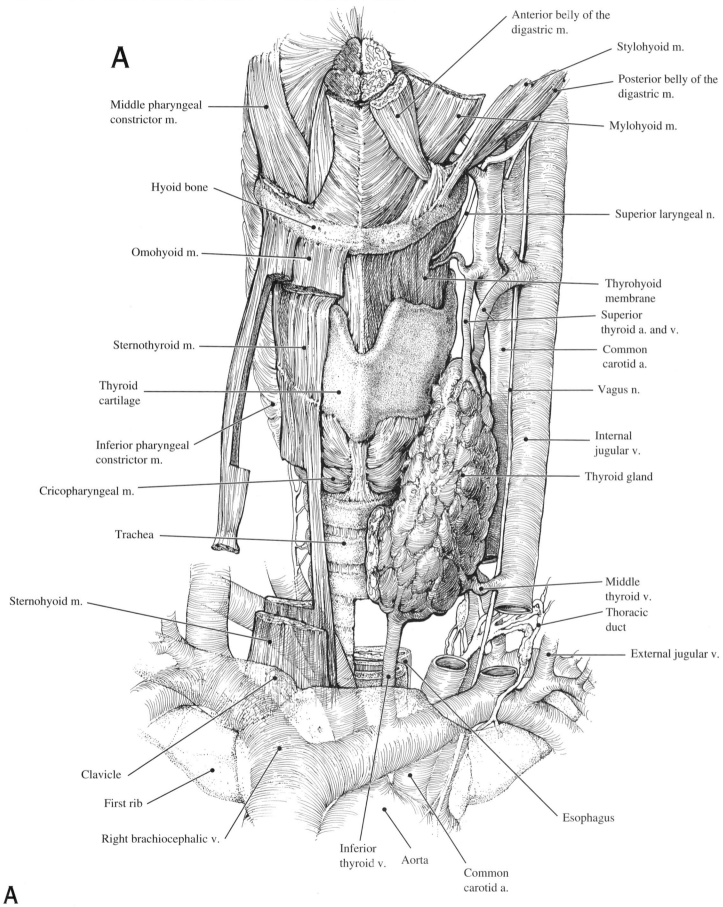

A

Middle pharyngeal constrictor m.

Hyoid bone

Omohyoid m.

Sternothyroid m.

Thyroid cartilage

Inferior pharyngeal constrictor m.

Cricopharyngeal m.

Trachea

Sternohyoid m.

Clavicle

First rib

Right brachiocephalic v.

Inferior thyroid v.

Aorta

Common carotid a.

Anterior belly of the digastric m.

Stylohyoid m.

Posterior belly of the digastric m.

Mylohyoid m.

Superior laryngeal n.

Thyrohyoid membrane

Superior thyroid a. and v.

Common carotid a.

Vagus n.

Internal jugular v.

Thyroid gland

Middle thyroid v.

Thoracic duct

External jugular v.

Esophagus

A

This comprehensive illustration has a wealth of information on the anatomy of the neck and is of value in performing the various operations in this area.

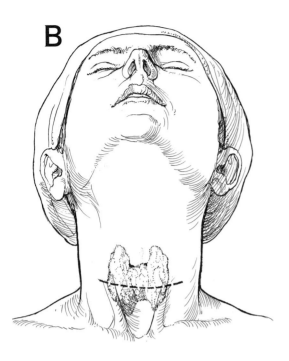

B

B, C

While the patient is still awake and in an upright position, several cervical incisions are traced with a surgical marking pen along the course of skin creases. After the patient is anesthetized, the neck is hyperextended and a small folded blanket or a sandbag is placed between the shoulder blades. The occiput is laid on a foam rubber doughnut-shaped ring, facilitating stability in this position during the operation. One of the marked areas—two fingerbreadths above the sternal notch—is now selected for the cervical incision. Interestingly, a lower incision results in a more conspicuous scar. Several lightly placed crosshatches on the skin ensure an exact realignment when closing. The incision is made in an even, deliberate fashion, with a no. 12 blade. The subcutaneous tissue should be cut with a light sweep of the scalpel; this facilitates seeing and electrocoagulating vessels before they are divid completely. The incision is then continued through the platysma and underlying tissue to the strap muscles.

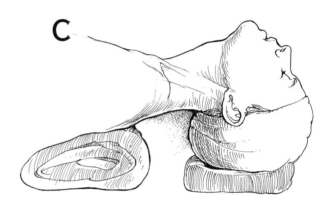

C

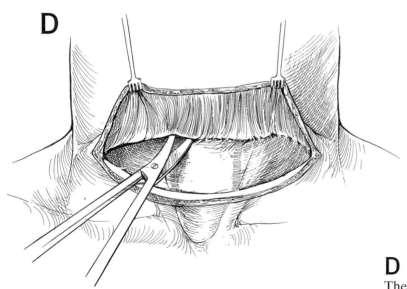

D

D

The upper flaps are developed by exerting firm perpendicular traction with small rakes as the skin and attached platysma are separated from the underlying strap muscles and branches of the anterior jugular vein for several centimeters by sharp scissor dissection. The remainder of the dissection is done with continued upward traction on the flaps and downward firm, steady pressure on the strap muscles with a gauze-wrapped finger.

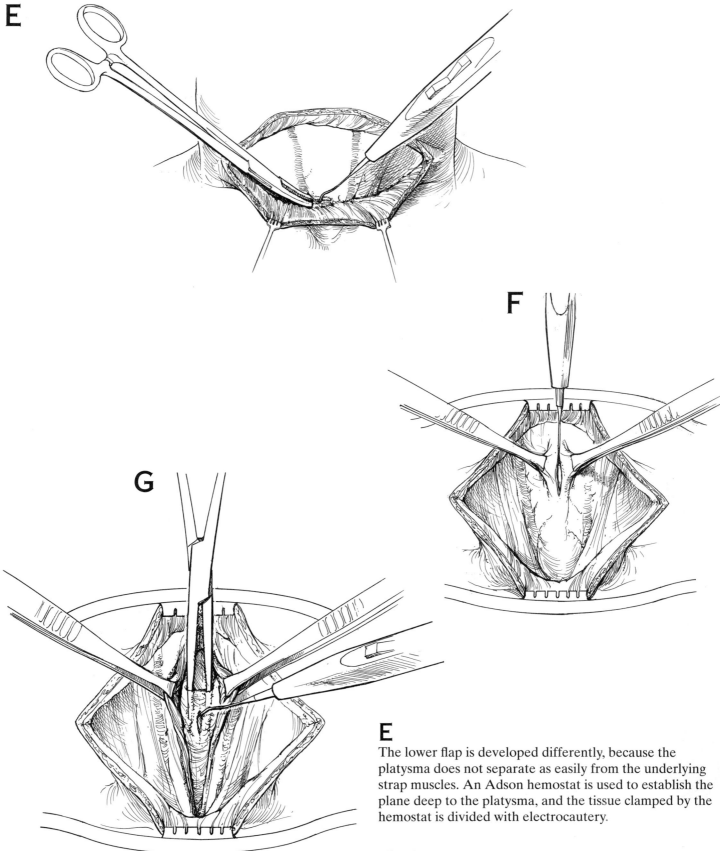

E

The lower flap is developed differently, because the platysma does not separate as easily from the underlying strap muscles. An Adson hemostat is used to establish the plane deep to the platysma, and the tissue clamped by the hemostat is divided with electrocautery.

F, G

A Mahorner retractor is used to retract the skin flaps. If present, the connecting branch of the anterior jugular vein is secured with a 4-0 monofilament suture ligature and divided before separation of the strap muscles is begun. A blunt-needle–tipped electrocautery is used to incise the superficial fascia. The strap muscles are elevated with forceps, and an Adson hemostat is used as a guide to the fine-tipped electrocautery; using this method effectively shields the underlying thyroid from the cautery.

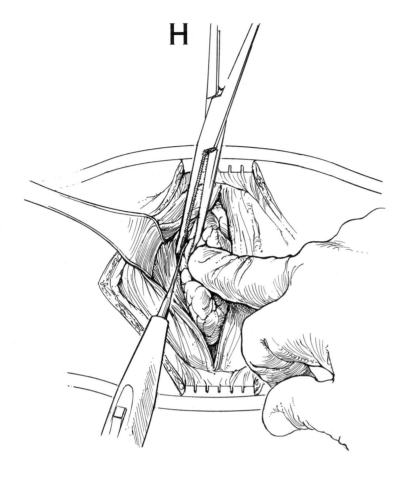

H

A small Richardson retractor is slipped under the strap muscles, retracting them laterally, as a finger (sometimes with gauze under it for better traction) is used to retract the lobe medially. Again, an Adson hemostat is inserted between the strap muscles and the thyroid lobe, and the intervening tissue is divided with a cautery. The strap muscles rarely require division and then only for a very bulky mass.

I

The lobe is now grasped with a Babcock forceps and retracted medially to expose the middle thyroid vein, which is ligated with 3-0 silk and divided; this permits even further mobilization of the lobe from beneath the strap muscles.

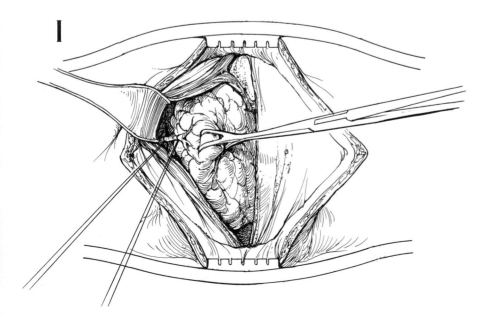

J

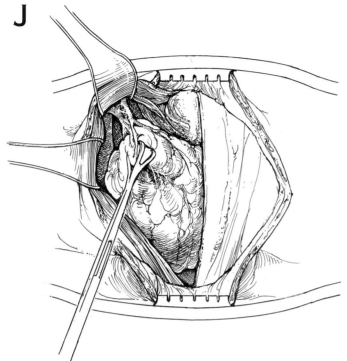

The Richardson retractor should be repositioned medial to the strap muscles and perpendicular to the plane of the superior thyroid vessels. The Babcock clamp may be repositioned on the superior aspect of the lobe. Downward traction on the lobe helps to expose the loose areolar tissue space between the vessels and the underlying thyroid membrane and sternothyroid muscle.

K

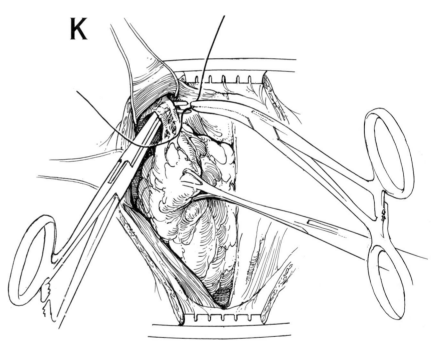

K

A Mixter clamp, which has a thicker, rounder, and longer tip and thus is less likely to puncture vessels, is used to dissect around the superior thyroid artery and vein. The Mixter is insinuated under the superior thyroid vessels and from a medial to a lateral direction close to the gland and the vessels; this lessens the risk of injury to the more superior and medially located superior thyroid nerve. (Here the dissection has been completed.) The superior thyroid artery and vein are tied as one with a double strand of 2-0 silk. This tie is used to retract the vessels caudally as another tie of 2-0 silk is applied 2 mm or so more cephalad. A curved hemostat is applied across the ligated vessels sufficiently close to the gland that on division the resultant stub of ligated vessels is at least 5 mm in length.

L

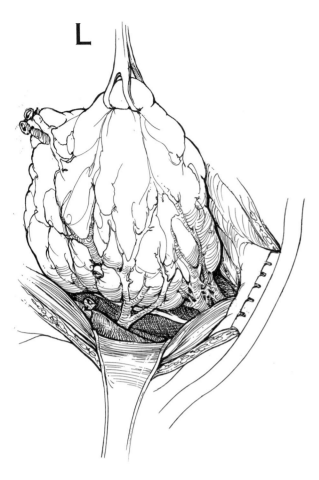

M

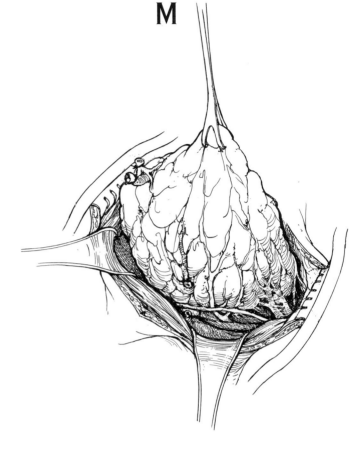

N

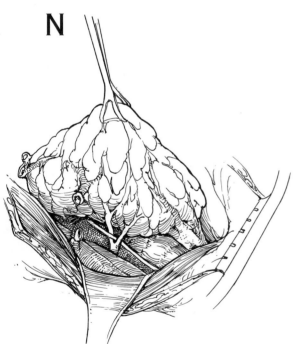

O

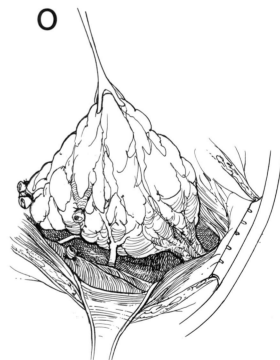

L, M, N, O

The preceding steps allow a full medial rotation of the
gland and facilitate the subsequent search for the recurrent
laryngeal nerve. The lymphoadipose tissue lateral to the
esophagotracheal groove is gently retracted with a blunt
forceps while the tissues in the groove are separated—not
cut—until the glistening nerve is seen. Dissection of the
nerve is done with a blunt hemostat and exposes only as
much as is necessary to safely proceed with the operation.
In this quartet of drawings, *L* shows its most common
course, *M* and *N* variations, and *O* a nonrecurrent (right-
sided only) nerve proceeding directly to the larynx.

P

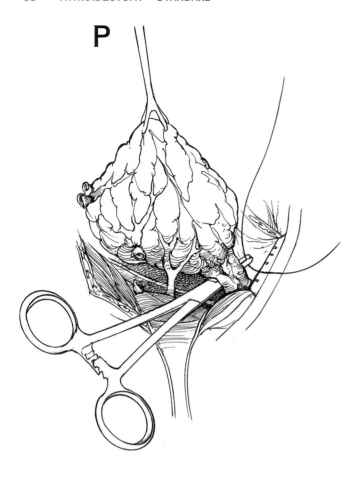

Q

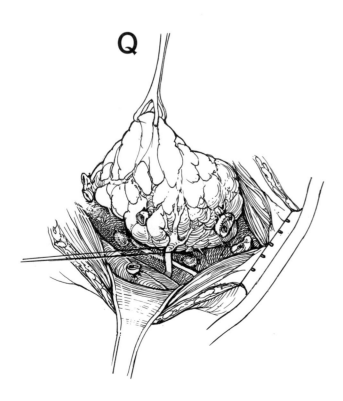

P

With the nerve in direct view, the inferior thyroid veins are isolated and tied doubly with 2-0 silk and divided.

Q

The inferior thyroid artery is tied at the main trunk or, more commonly, at its several branches as it proceeds toward the thyroid. Care is taken to identify the parathyroid glands and leave them undisturbed.

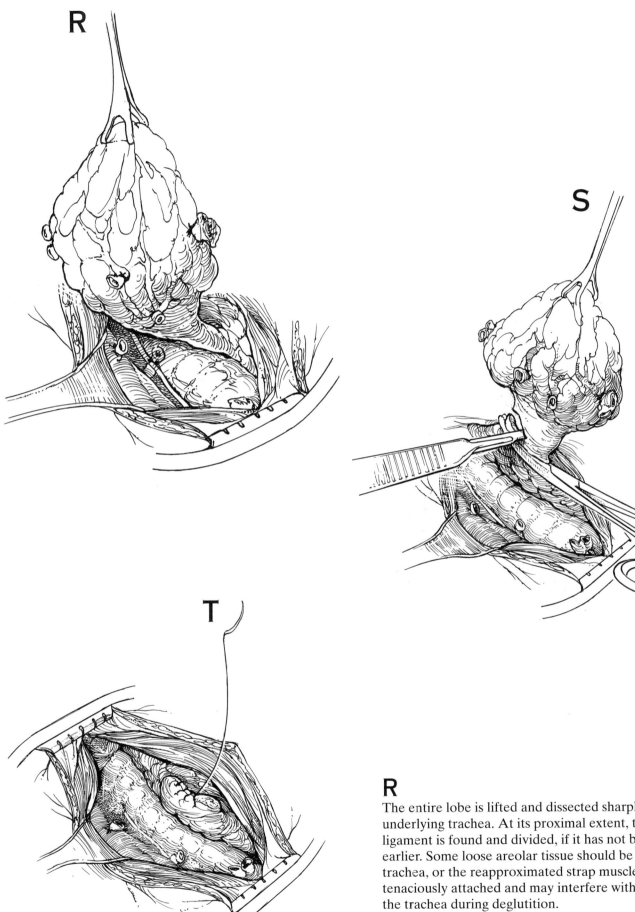

R

The entire lobe is lifted and dissected sharply from the underlying trachea. At its proximal extent, the suspensory ligament is found and divided, if it has not been done earlier. Some loose areolar tissue should be left on the trachea, or the reapproximated strap muscles may become tenaciously attached and may interfere with easy gliding of the trachea during deglutition.

S, T

The contralateral side of the isthmus is cross-clamped, divided, and oversewn with a continuous stitch of 3-0 chromic catgut.

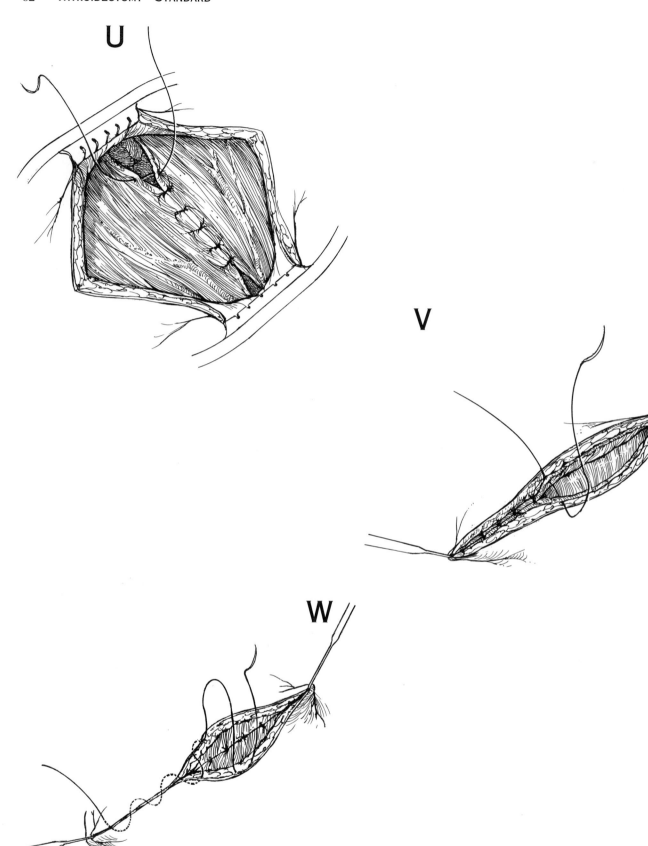

U, V, W

The strap muscles are reapproximated along the midline with an interrupted or continuous stitch of 4-0 chromic catgut; an interrupted technique is used in reapproximating the platysma. The skin is reapproximated with a subcuticular stitch (or interrupted vertical mattress stitch) using 5-0 monofilament suture. A drain is not used routinely, but if it is employed, it is removed the next day.

B THYROIDECTOMY—MODIFIED RADICAL

A

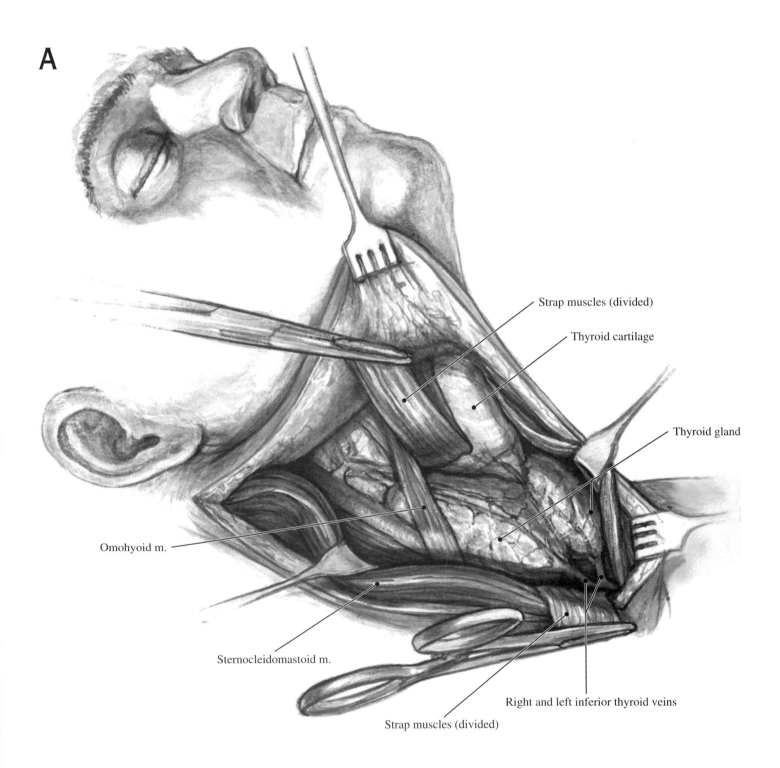

Strap muscles (divided)

Thyroid cartilage

Thyroid gland

Omohyoid m.

Sternocleidomastoid m.

Right and left inferior thyroid veins

Strap muscles (divided)

A

The exposure for this operation is more difficult to establish and maintain by virtue of the incision used and the considerable dissection carried out around the sternocleidomastoid muscle and jugular vein, which are retracted but not resected. A long collar incision, placed 1 or 2 cm more cephalad than usual, offers surprisingly adequate exposure. This is helped by not routinely doing a submandibular triangle resection. Alternatively, a standard incision can be made with a parallel one that is higher and shorter.

The strap muscles are divided at the junction of their middle and lower thirds so that there is minimal disruption of their innervation. The use of a crushing clamp at the point of division eliminates troublesome bleeding during closure, does not appear to affect recovery deleteriously, and is a convenient way to retract the muscles.

B

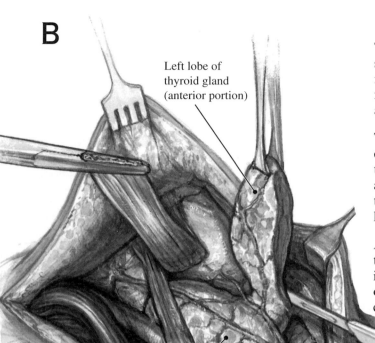

Left lobe of
thyroid gland
(anterior portion)

Right lobe of
thyroid gland

B

The dissection is begun on the lobe opposite the affected
side. The strap muscles on this side are retracted—there is
no need to divide them—so that the thyroid lobe can be
mobilized. The location of the parathyroid glands is noted
at this time.

The lobe is momentarily reflected medially so that the
course of the recurrent laryngeal nerve can be noted. The
thyroid lobe is divided so that the dorsal quarter and the
associated parathyroid glands remain. The dissection within
the posterior capsule minimizes injury to the recurrent
laryngeal nerve and the parathyroid glands.

As the anterior portion of the left thyroid lobe is reflected
toward the right, sharp dissection is used to separate the
isthmus from the trachea. We neither oversew the cut edge
of the thyroid gland nor suture its capsule to the trachea to
cover the cut surface.

C

Unless there is palpable adenopathy, this is the extent of
resection on the left neck. The head is rotated to the left,
and dissection of the right side of the neck is begun in the
right inferolateral area, with the trapezius muscle as the
lateral boundary. The fatty areolar tissue, along with the
associated lymph nodes, is dissected medially. Branches of
the transverse scapular and transverse cervical arteries are
in the tissue in this area and should be clamped before
being divided.

The dissection lateral to the sternocleidomastoid muscle
extends from the supraclavicular area to the mastoid
process. The tissue to be resected is rather scant toward the
upper end. The spinal accessory nerve is preserved;
metastatic tumor deposits in its vicinity are uncommon,
and the incidence of a drop shoulder is sufficiently
disabling that preservation is reasonable for the type of
cancer and extent of involvement being treated.

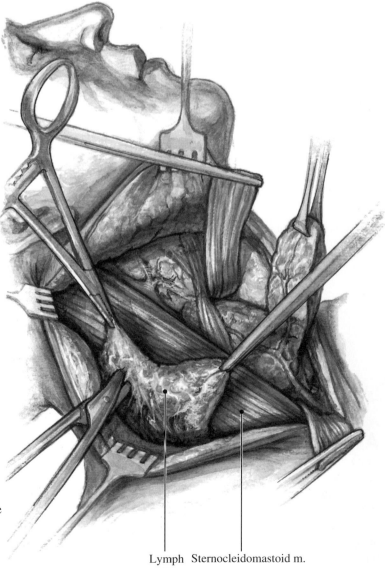

C

Lymph   Sternocleidomastoid m.
nodal
tissue

D

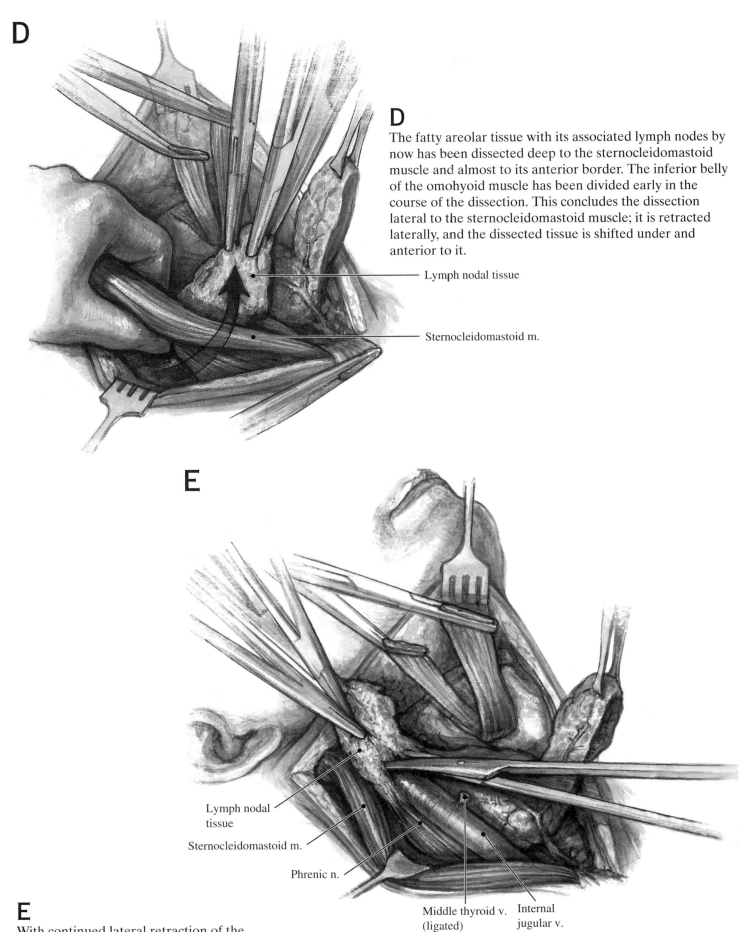

D

The fatty areolar tissue with its associated lymph nodes by now has been dissected deep to the sternocleidomastoid muscle and almost to its anterior border. The inferior belly of the omohyoid muscle has been divided early in the course of the dissection. This concludes the dissection lateral to the sternocleidomastoid muscle; it is retracted laterally, and the dissected tissue is shifted under and anterior to it.

— Lymph nodal tissue

— Sternocleidomastoid m.

E

Lymph nodal tissue

Sternocleidomastoid m.

Phrenic n.

Middle thyroid v. (ligated)   Internal jugular v.

E

With continued lateral retraction of the sternocleidomastoid muscle, the tissue is dissected off the scalene muscles while preserving the phrenic nerve. As the dissection continues along the carotid sheath, care must be taken not to damage the intimately adjacent vagus nerve. The retrotracheal and retroesophageal areas of fatty areolar tissue are next dissected free.

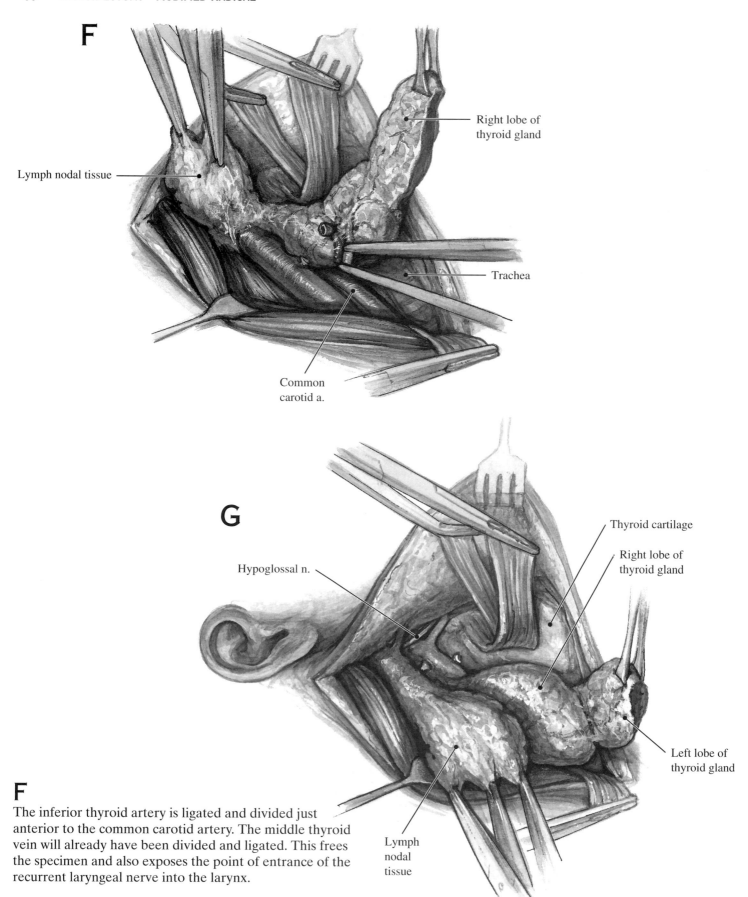

F

Right lobe of thyroid gland

Lymph nodal tissue

Trachea

Common carotid a.

G

Hypoglossal n.

Thyroid cartilage

Right lobe of thyroid gland

Left lobe of thyroid gland

Lymph nodal tissue

F

The inferior thyroid artery is ligated and divided just anterior to the common carotid artery. The middle thyroid vein will already have been divided and ligated. This frees the specimen and also exposes the point of entrance of the recurrent laryngeal nerve into the larynx.

G

The specimen is returned to its normal position, and the superior thyroid artery is ligated with 3-0 silk and divided. There are no other significant vessels that have to be divided. The hypoglossal nerve is identified as it crosses several centimeters cephalad to the carotid bifurcation at about the origin of the lingual artery.

H

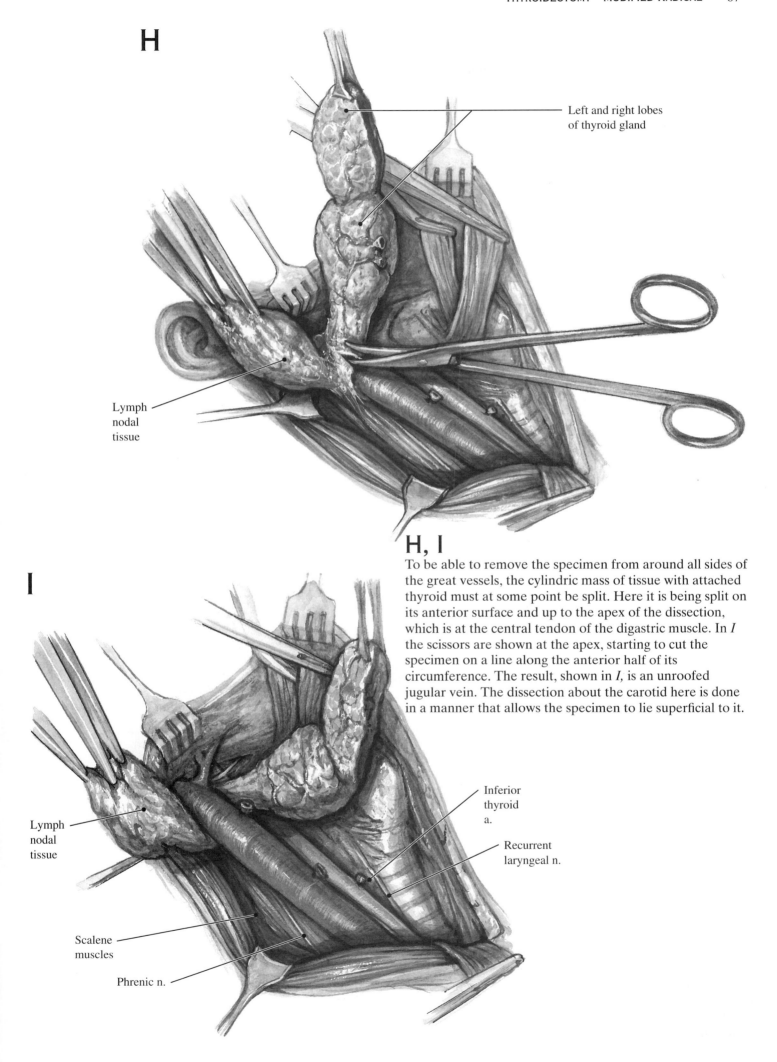

Left and right lobes
of thyroid gland

Lymph
nodal
tissue

I

Lymph
nodal
tissue

Scalene
muscles

Phrenic n.

Inferior
thyroid
a.

Recurrent
laryngeal n.

H, I

To be able to remove the specimen from around all sides of
the great vessels, the cylindric mass of tissue with attached
thyroid must at some point be split. Here it is being split on
its anterior surface and up to the apex of the dissection,
which is at the central tendon of the digastric muscle. In *I*
the scissors are shown at the apex, starting to cut the
specimen on a line along the anterior half of its
circumference. The result, shown in *I*, is an unroofed
jugular vein. The dissection about the carotid here is done
in a manner that allows the specimen to lie superficial to it.

J

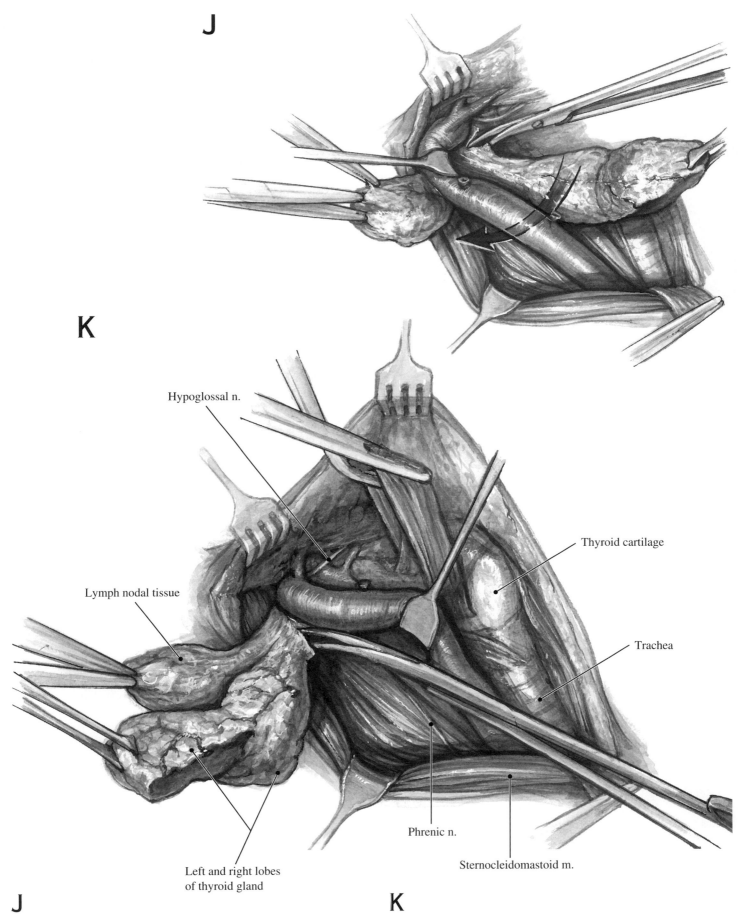

K

Hypoglossal n.

Thyroid cartilage

Lymph nodal tissue

Trachea

Phrenic n.

Sternocleidomastoid m.

Left and right lobes
of thyroid gland

J

The internal jugular vein is retracted laterally so that the specimen may be separated at its posterior circumference. Pharyngeal branches from the jugular vein are immediately adjacent, but traction may empty them of blood, making their detection difficult for the unwary. The medial half of the specimen, which contains the thyroid, is now swung under and lateral to the jugular vein.

K

The jugular vein is now retracted medially at the apex of the dissection, and the specimen is amputated, taking care not to divide the spinal accessory nerve coursing near the vein. A small suction drain is exteriorized through a counterincision. The incision is closed in two layers, the platysma muscle with 4-0 chromic catgut and the skin with 5-0 nylon.

5

PARATHYROID

A PARATHYROIDECTOMY—CERVICAL

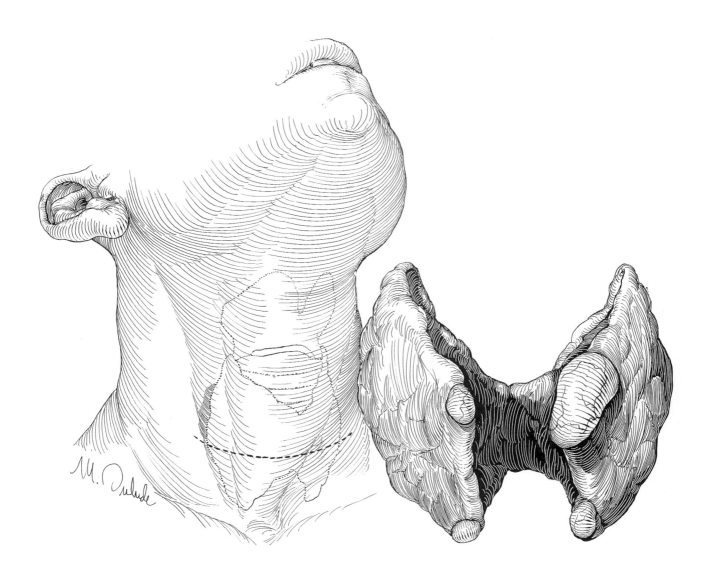

Parathyroidectomy is an endocrine operation for which the diagnosis should be known with virtual certainty preoperatively. It then only remains for the surgeon to excise the often elusive responsible pathologic specimen from its location in a rather fixed space using a combination of technical skill and orderly dissection. Knowledge of the embryologic origin, route, and possible extent of descent of the parathyroids is helpful in achieving success. Failure to find the adenomatous or hyperplastic gland in the neck underscores the reasoning that valid preoperative diagnostic tests and a thorough search within the neck are important determinants of whether to shift the search to the mediastinum.

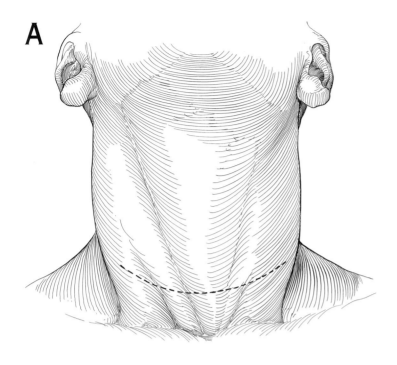

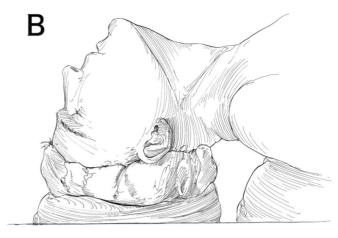

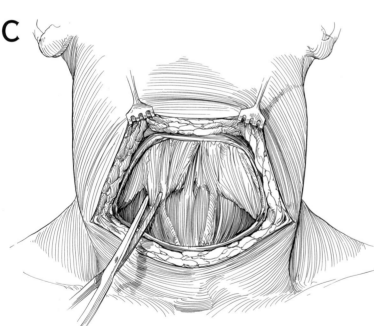

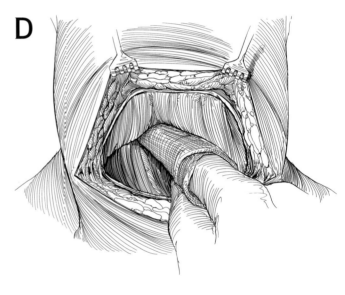

A, B

Several skin creases in the lower neck are marked with a scribe while the patient is still awake and upright. The patient is placed in the supine position. After the patient is anesthetized, the neck is hyperextended by placing a sandbag between the shoulder blades. An approximately 8-cm incision is made 2 to 3 cm above the sternal notch, preferably in one of the marked creases.

C, D

The upper flap is developed by grasping the edges of the incision with two small rakes and exerting upward traction. With countertraction of the tissue below, fine scissors are then used to start the separation just deep to the platysma. This is completed by blunt dissection with a gauze-covered finger. For the inferior flap, the dissection plane is developed by isolating the tissue with an Adson hemostat and dividing it with cautery.

E

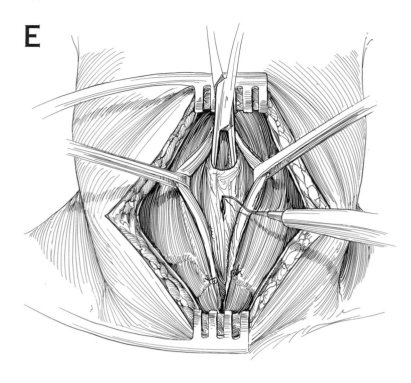

E

The wound retractor is positioned, and any communicating branches of the anterior vein are ligated and divided. The fascia between the strap muscles is separated by using electrocautery to cut tissue between the defining jaws of an Adson hemostat.

F

The middle thyroid vein is ligated with 3-0 silk and divided, facilitating medial rotation the thyroid lobe. A small Richardson retractor may be used to retract the strap muscles laterally.

F

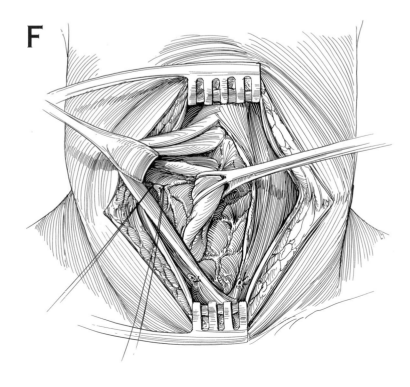

G

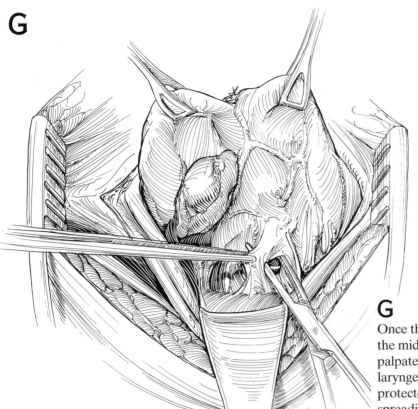

G

Once the thyroid lobe has been mobilized sufficiently toward the midline that the tracheoesophageal groove may be palpated, a careful search can be made for the recurrent laryngeal nerve. This nerve should always be identified and protected from harm. The technique is strictly one of spreading; except in very unusual circumstances, nothing should be divided until the nerve is visualized. Here, a glimpse can be had of the nerve at the tip of the spreading hemostat.

H

The nerve can be identified for its entire cervical length except for where it enters the larynx. The junction between the branches of the inferior thyroid artery and the recurrent nerve should be examined with special attention because the majority of abnormal glands are found in this area. In this case, a suspicious ovoid mass is seen on the dorsal and superior aspect of the thyroid gland. Parathyroid adenomas usually are ovoid, smooth textured, tan to sandy in color, rather soft, and often have a vascular pattern converging to one pole. They bleed easily subcapsularly. By contrast, fat is loose and yellow; thyroid tissue is somewhat coarse and has a reddish tinge; lymph nodes are firmer and appear somewhat edematous. A pledget of gauze is effective in gently teasing the gland away from the thyroid.

H

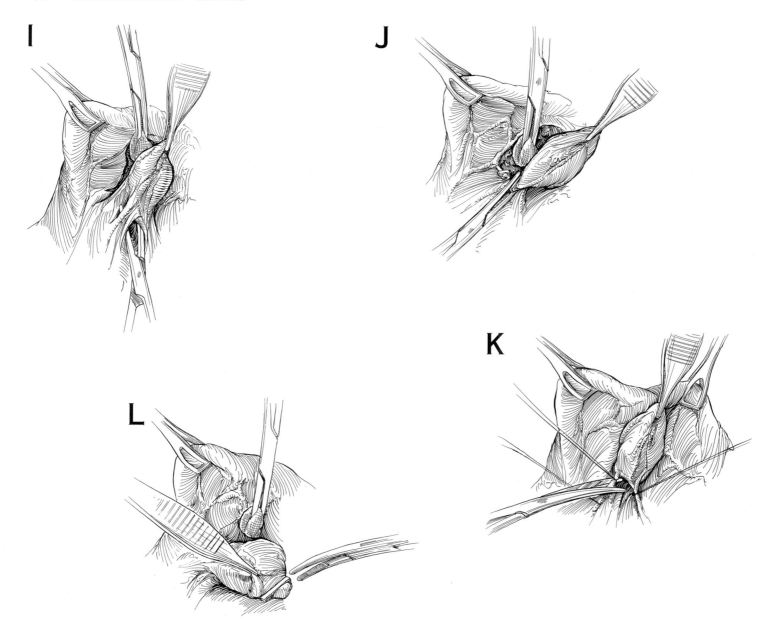

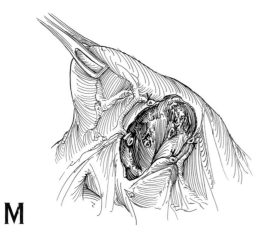

I, J, K, L, M

There are several possibilities to consider regarding how many parathyroid glands are excised, in what sequence, and what intraoperative histologic confirmation is advisable. Important determinants are the clinical history, laboratory information, and operative findings. Here, the focus is narrowed to one gland. Its vascular supply is isolated (*I*) and secured with clips (*J*) or ties (*K*), and the gland is amputated. Or, if histologic confirmation is desired, a clip is placed across the tip of the gland for hemostasis (*L*) and a small fragment sent to the laboratory. On confirmation, the gland is amputated (*M*). Having identified one probable adenoma, it is reasonable to explore both sides of the neck to identify all four glands to avoid missing the 3 to 5% possibility of occurrence of more than one adenoma. Care should be taken, particularly in this circumstance, to avoid an overzealous exploration with possible inadvertent injury to the remaining parathyroid glands.

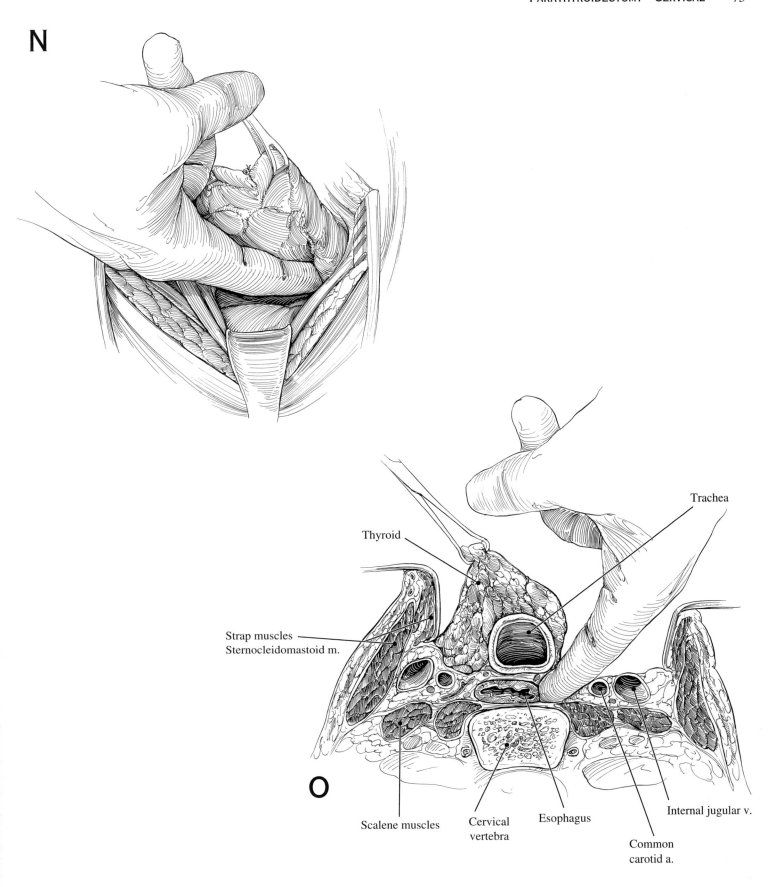

N

O

Thyroid

Trachea

Strap muscles
Sternocleidomastoid m.

Scalene muscles

Cervical
vertebra

Esophagus

Common
carotid a.

Internal jugular v.

N, O

Should a thorough exploration to this point prove fruitless, a mass can be sought in the superior mediastinum by the palpating finger. By hugging the tracheoesophageal groove while developing this area, the risk of injury to blood vessels is lessened.

P

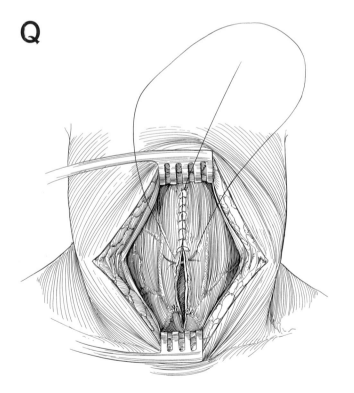

P

A tongue of the thymus is often seen at the sternal notch. It is grasped and as much of it excised as possible; clips should be placed across any vessels before dividing the tissue.

Q

R

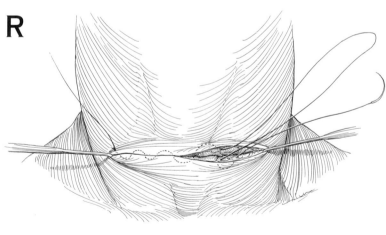

Q, R

If none of these procedures yields an abnormal gland, the wound is closed; exploration of the mediastinum is a later issue. No drain is used. The strap muscles are reapproximated with continuous 4-0 chromic catgut, the platysma with interrupted stitches of 4-0 chromic catgut, and the skin with interrupted vertical mattress stitches using 5-0 monofilament suture.

B PARATHYROIDECTOMY—SUBSTERNAL

A

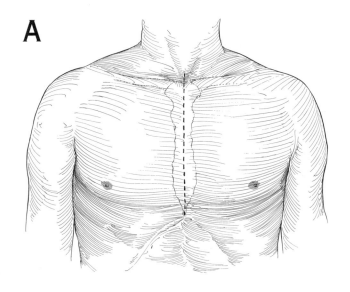

A

It has been concluded that the abnormal glands responsible for this patient's hyperparathyroidism are not in the neck and that a mediastinal exploration is warranted. In this illustration, the dashed line indicates that the full length of the sternum is being incised, the method we prefer. Transverse cuts along an interspace may seem appealing but have the disadvantages of more limited exposure, an awkward cut of the sternum should a longitudinal extension be necessary after all, less secure closure, and sometimes more prolonged healing.

B

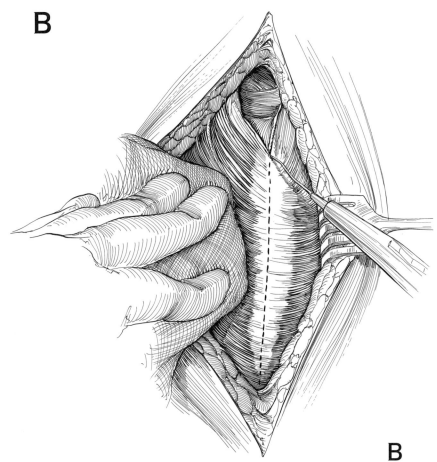

B

Electrocautery is used to divide the tough fascia anterior to and behind the sternal notch so that the sternal saw blade can be introduced. The cautery is carried the full length of the sternum down to bone, both dividing the fascial soft tissue and providing hemostasis.

C

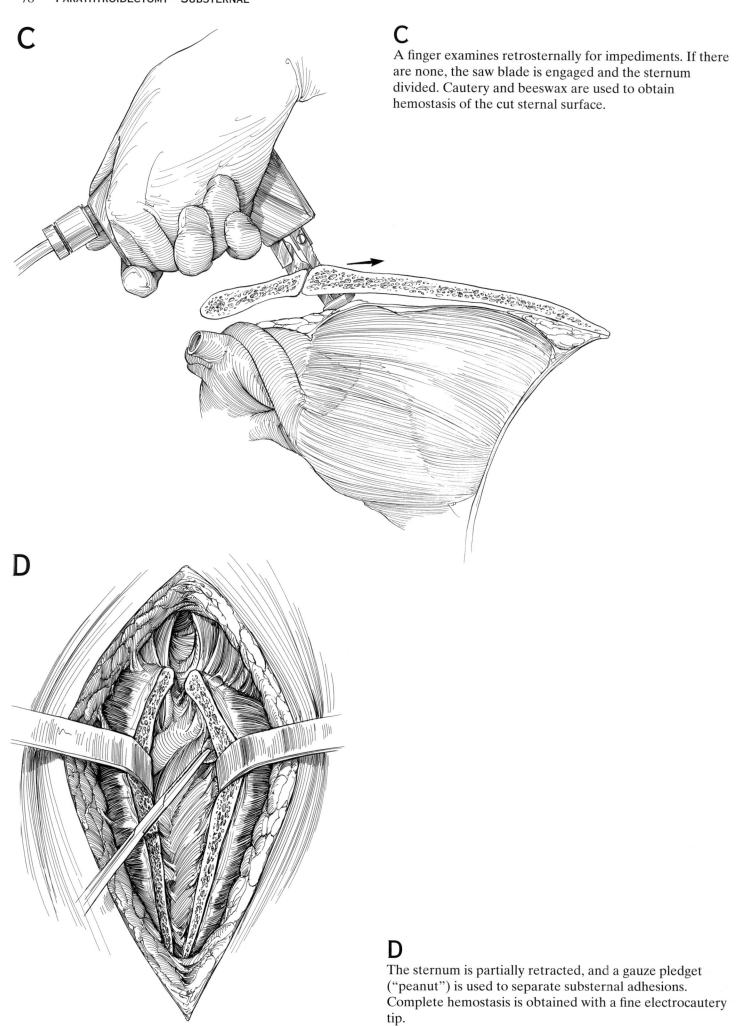

C

A finger examines retrosternally for impediments. If there are none, the saw blade is engaged and the sternum divided. Cautery and beeswax are used to obtain hemostasis of the cut sternal surface.

D

D

The sternum is partially retracted, and a gauze pledget ("peanut") is used to separate substernal adhesions. Complete hemostasis is obtained with a fine electrocautery tip.

E

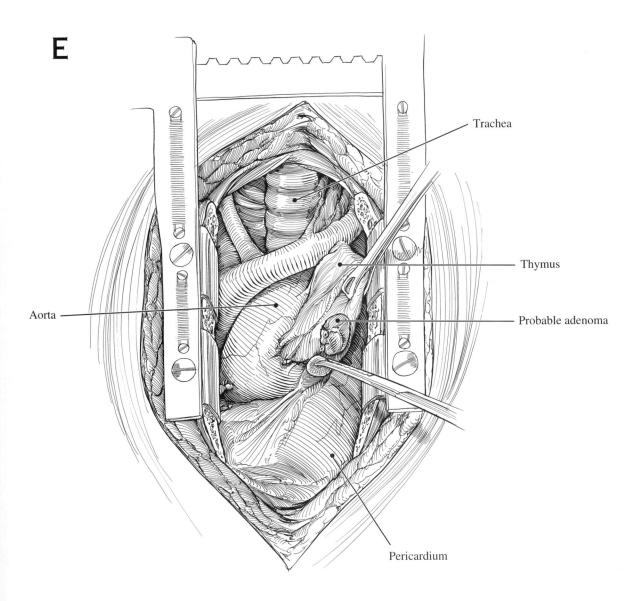

Trachea

Thymus

Probable adenoma

Aorta

Pericardium

E

The area has been cleared sufficiently of restrictions so that
the sternal retractor may be inserted and slowly spread. In
approximately 75% of cases, the adenoma is found within
the thymus. The other 25% of adenomas are in the vicinity,
but a few may be difficult to locate and will be missed
unless there is a determined search. Sternal closure can be
by one of several satisfactory methods.

Chapter

6

LARYNX

A LARYNGECTOMY—RADICAL

Laryngectomy and radical neck dissection are performed concomitantly in instances of probable or certain cervical lymph node involvement.

A

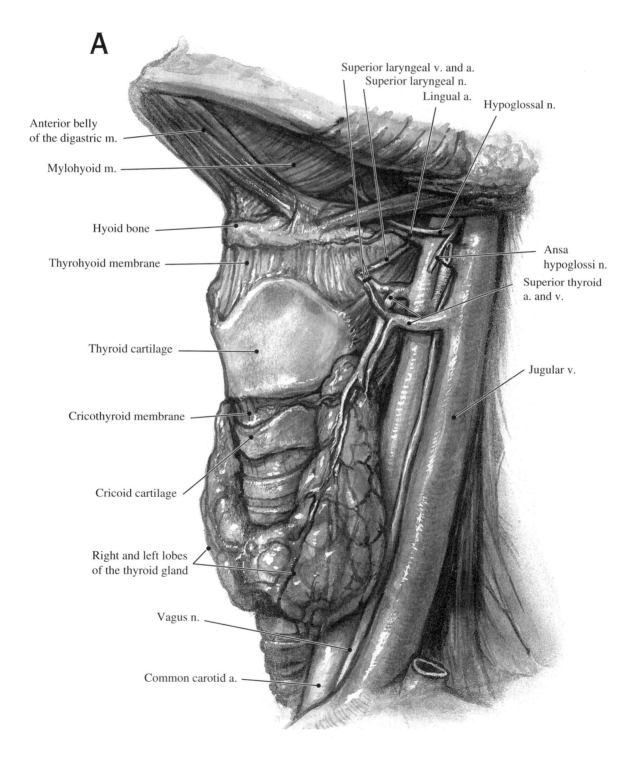

Superior laryngeal v. and a.
Superior laryngeal n.
Lingual a.
Hypoglossal n.

Anterior belly of the digastric m.

Mylohyoid m.

Hyoid bone

Thyrohyoid membrane

Ansa hypoglossi n.

Superior thyroid a. and v.

Thyroid cartilage

Jugular v.

Cricothyroid membrane

Cricoid cartilage

Right and left lobes of the thyroid gland

Vagus n.

Common carotid a.

A

There are so many anatomic structures in this area that a thorough knowledge of their relationships is essential. The larynx is situated between the base of the tongue and the upper trachea. Its blood supply is derived from the superior and inferior thyroid arteries and veins.

The hyoid bone is removed in its entirety. Notice the considerable number of muscles that have to be separated from its superior surface. The hypoglossal nerve starts its anterior swing at about the level the lingual artery branches from the external carotid artery and goes deep to the digastric and stylohyoid muscles.

B

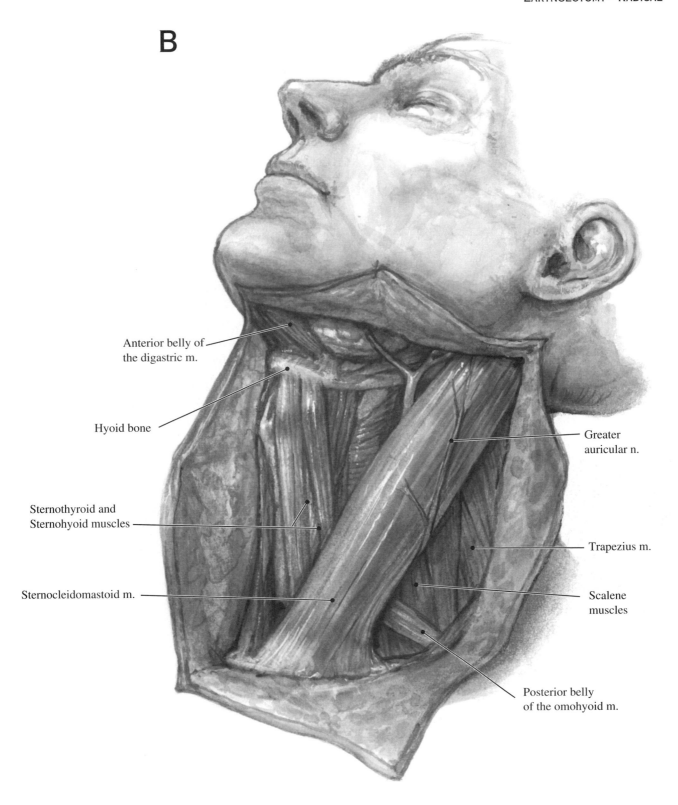

Anterior belly of
the digastric m.

Hyoid bone

Sternothyroid and
Sternohyoid muscles

Sternocleidomastoid m.

Greater
auricular n.

Trapezius m.

Scalene
muscles

Posterior belly
of the omohyoid m.

B

The patient is positioned as for a radical neck dissection.
Routine endotracheal anesthesia is administered, with a
provision for exchange toward the end of the procedure of
the orotracheal tube for a longer cuffed tube directly into
the tracheostomy. The skin flaps are fashioned as in a
radical neck dissection. It is desirable to have the
inferomedial arm of the double trifurcate incision fall short
of the sternal notch so that the eventual tracheal stoma can
be positioned in the medial flap and separated from the
major operative field.

C

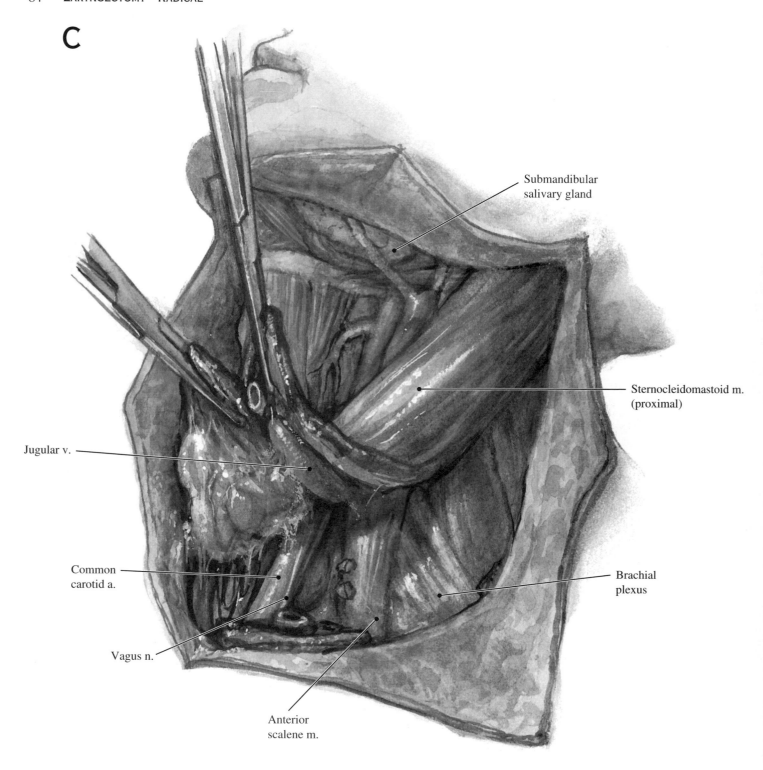

Submandibular
salivary gland

Sternocleidomastoid m.
(proximal)

Jugular v.

Common
carotid a.

Brachial
plexus

Vagus n.

Anterior
scalene m.

C

The radical neck dissection is begun on the affected side, with the eventual pharyngeal entry being on the unaffected or less affected side. The procedure is begun by dissecting the fatty areolar tissue in the inferolateral area, dividing the inferior belly of the omohyoid muscle, and proceeding cephalad along the anterior border of the trapezius muscle. The spinal accessory nerve is found on the deep anterior surface of the junction of the middle and lower thirds of the trapezius muscle and usually is preserved if at all possible. Because some of the fibers of the sternocleidomastoid muscle are intimately attached to the skin in the upper neck, it is reasonable to leave some

behind rather than to try to remove all of them and make the skin flap too thin in this area. Furthermore, this is rarely the area of cancerous deposits, and these need not be skirted widely. As the dissection in the lower neck progresses medially, the transverse scapular and cervical arteries are encountered and divided. The brachial plexus lies deep to this area.

The sternocleidomastoid muscle is divided about 1 cm from its insertions. The sternohyoid and sternothyroid muscles are also divided at their lower ends. The carotid sheath is entered and the jugular vein encircled with the help of a right angle clamp.

D

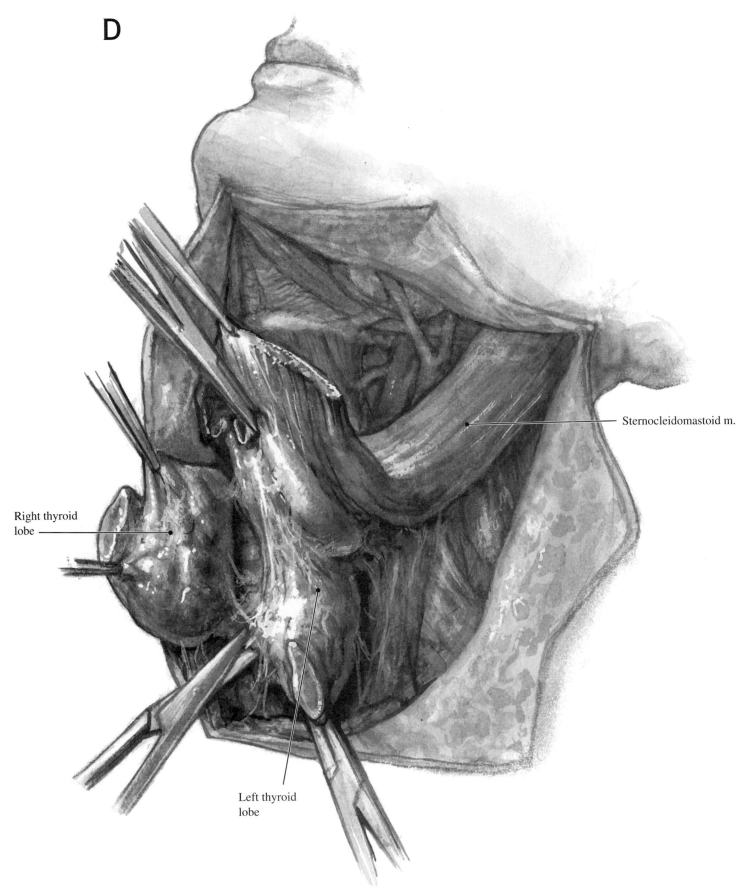

Sternocleidomastoid m.

Right thyroid
lobe

Left thyroid
lobe

D

The thyroid lobe on the affected side is to be removed with
the major specimen. The inferior thyroid vein and artery
on the affected side are ligated and divided. The thyroid
lobe is dissected off the trachea to the first ring. The
isthmus is divided on the far side and oversewn with a
continuous stitch of 4-0 Maxon.

E

The deep plane of the dissection remains just superficial to the deep cervical fascia, as the specimen is dissected in a medial and cephalad direction, remaining superficial to the scalene muscles and sparing the phrenic nerve. The specimen has now been freed to just beyond the carotid bifurcation, at which location the hypoglossal nerve is sought for and preserved. Next, the remainder of the sternocleidomastoid muscle is detached from its origin if this had not been done completely earlier. As the dissection continues in an anterior direction, the lower portion of the parotid gland is severed on a plane parallel to the horizontal ramus of the mandible. This plane of division minimizes the risk of severing the mandibular branch of the facial nerve near its origin. The ansa hypoglossi nerve is severed at its origin and allowed to remain with the strap muscles, which are sacrificed.

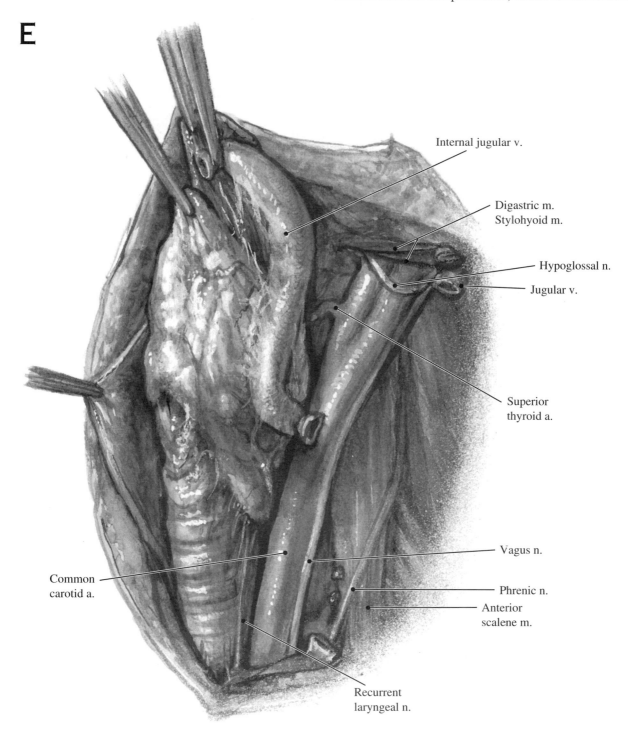

E

Internal jugular v.

Digastric m.
Stylohyoid m.

Hypoglossal n.

Jugular v.

Superior
thyroid a.

Vagus n.

Common
carotid a.

Phrenic n.

Anterior
scalene m.

Recurrent
laryngeal n.

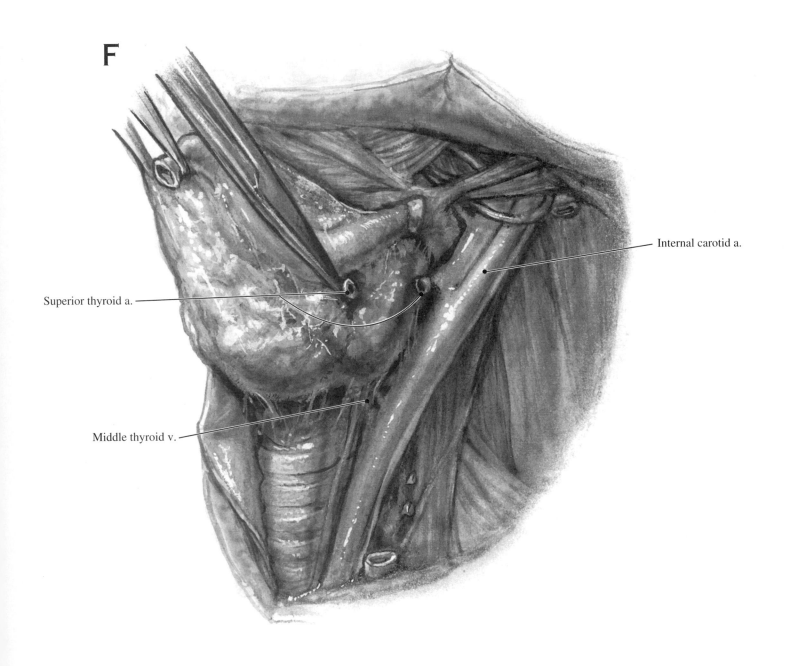

F

Superior thyroid a.

Internal carotid a.

Middle thyroid v.

F

The middle thyroid vein is ligated and divided. The superior thyroid artery and vein are divided at their origins and ligated with 2-0 silk. This releases the specimen considerably and substantially completes the radical neck dissection.

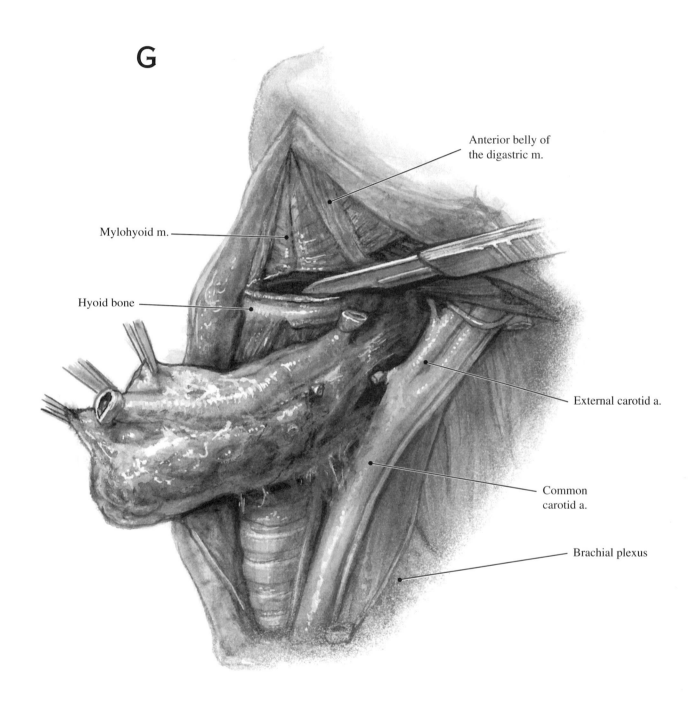

G

Anterior belly of
the digastric m.

Mylohyoid m.

Hyoid bone

External carotid a.

Common
carotid a.

Brachial plexus

G

Removal of the hyoid bone, although not essential to an
adequate cancer operation, results in less tension on the
suture line during the subsequent pharyngeal closure. With
downward traction on the specimen so that the suprahyoid
muscles are made taut, they are separated from the
superior border of the hyoid bone with the scalpel.

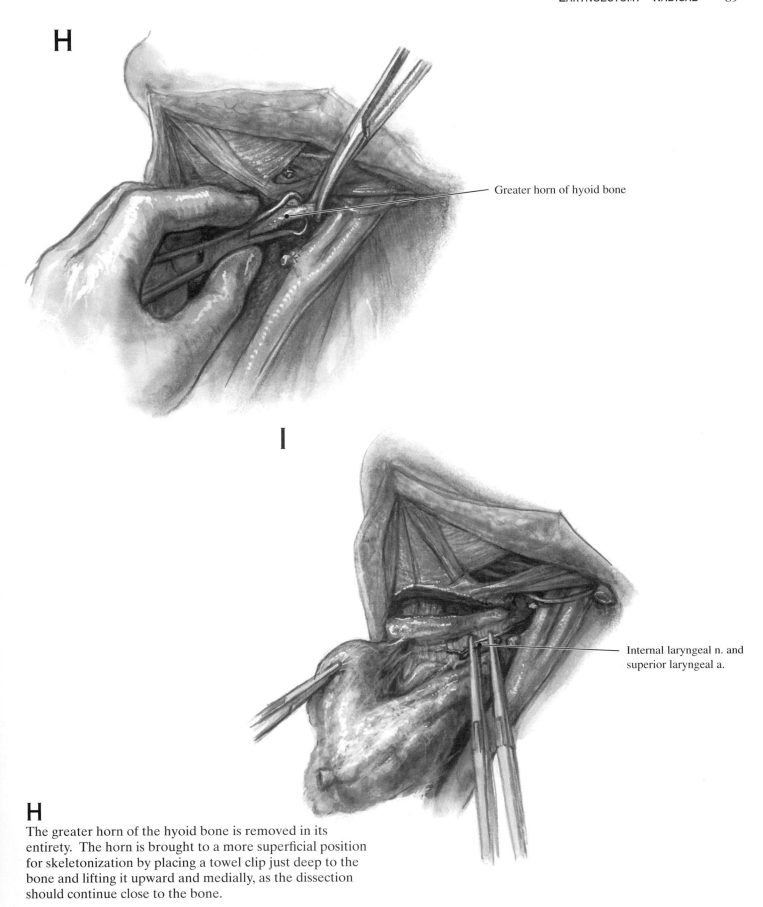

Greater horn of hyoid bone

Internal laryngeal n. and
superior laryngeal a.

H

The greater horn of the hyoid bone is removed in its
entirety. The horn is brought to a more superficial position
for skeletonization by placing a towel clip just deep to the
bone and lifting it upward and medially, as the dissection
should continue close to the bone.

I

The larynx is allowed to fall back into place, and the
superior laryngeal artery and internal laryngeal nerve (a
branch of the superior laryngeal nerve) are clamped, cut,
and ligated; this procedure is then performed on the
contralateral side.

J
The specimen is shifted to expose the side of the larynx less affected by cancer. If the surgeon prefers, the strap muscles can be disengaged from the larynx or left attached to be excised with the specimen. The paratracheal tissues to the cricoid cartilage are removed, and the thyroid lobe is disengaged from the trachea and reflected laterally.

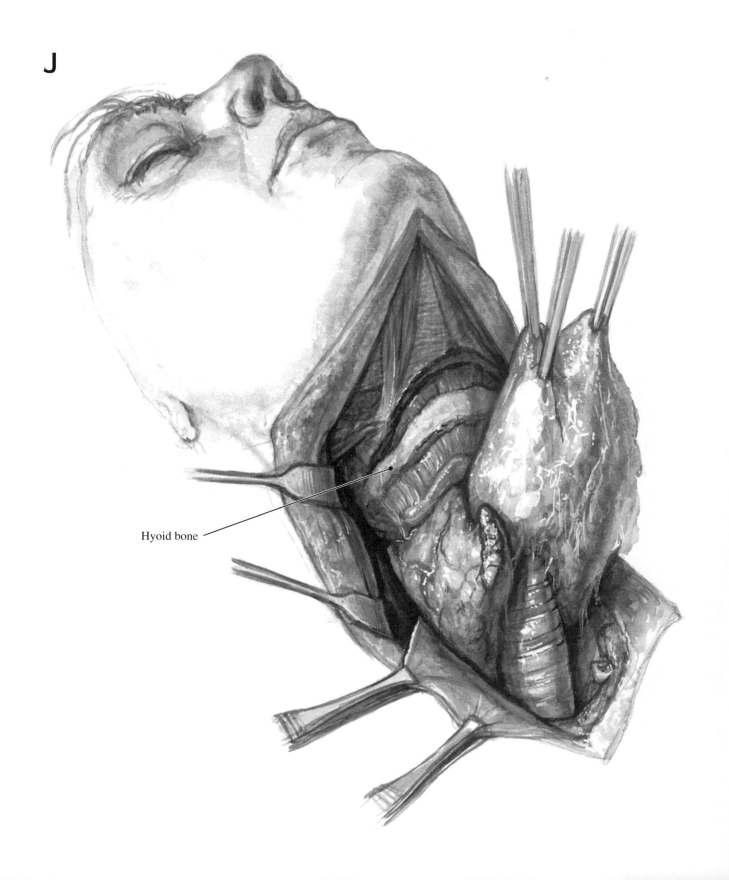

J

Hyoid bone

K

This view of the laryngopharynx (as it appears when entered) is so different from that seen during laryngoscopy that even the experienced observer needs a moment for orientation. The greater horn of the hyoid bone is immediately deep to the submucosa, justifying the need to skeletonize the greater horn during its mobilization if a "buttonhole" in the mucosa is to be prevented; the line of mucosal incision for the laryngectomy depends on the location and extent of the cancer and can be mapped out now.

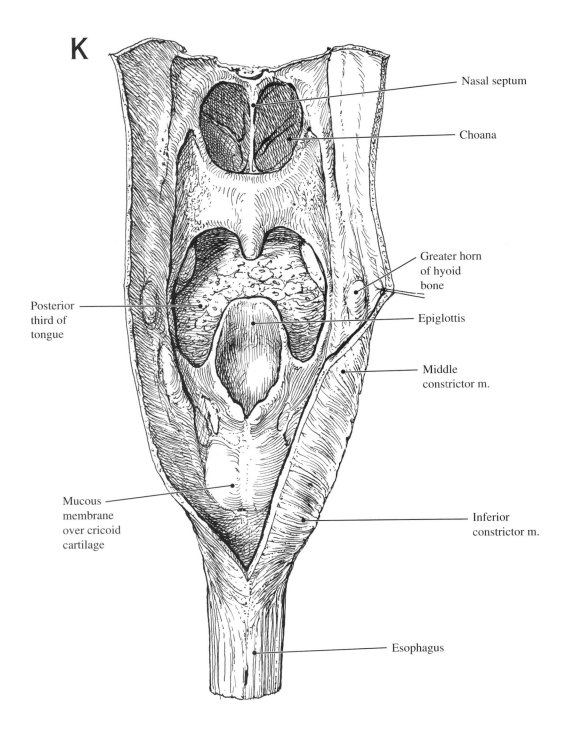

K

Nasal septum

Choana

Greater horn of hyoid bone

Posterior third of tongue

Epiglottis

Middle constrictor m.

Mucous membrane over cricoid cartilage

Inferior constrictor m.

Esophagus

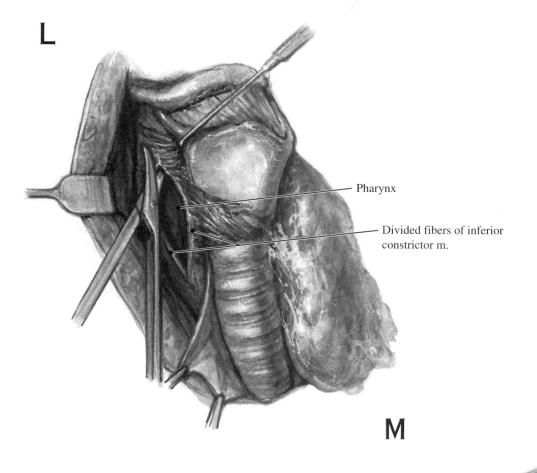

L

Pharynx

Divided fibers of inferior
constrictor m.

M

Thyroid
cartilage

Epiglottis

L, M

Entry into the larynx is on the side of lesser involvement.
The tracheal cartilage is secured with a tracheal hook and
is rotated rather severely in a direction opposite that of the
surgeon. An incision is made lightly over the inferior
constrictor muscle just posterior to the thyroid cartilage.
The pharyngeal mucosa, which then pushes through this
incision, is grasped with thumb forceps and incised for
entry into the pharynx.

N

The tracheal hook is reapplied so that the larynx can be rotated to the right. The division of the constrictor muscles proceeds downwardly with the mucosal incision as a guide, preserving as much mucosa as possible for closure.

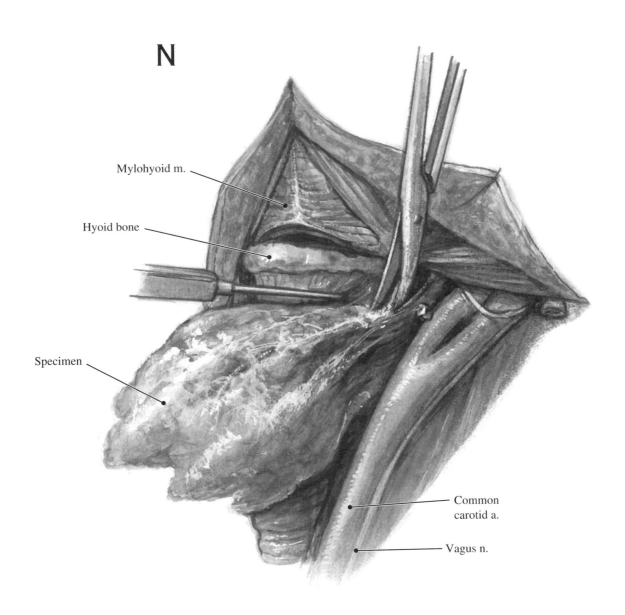

N

Mylohyoid m.

Hyoid bone

Specimen

Common carotid a.

Vagus n.

O

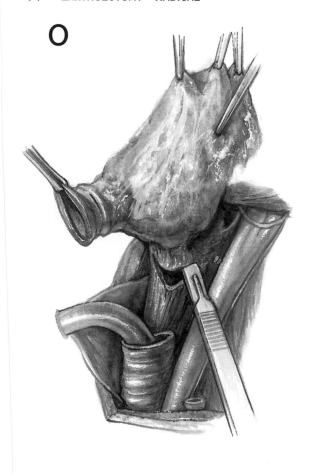

P

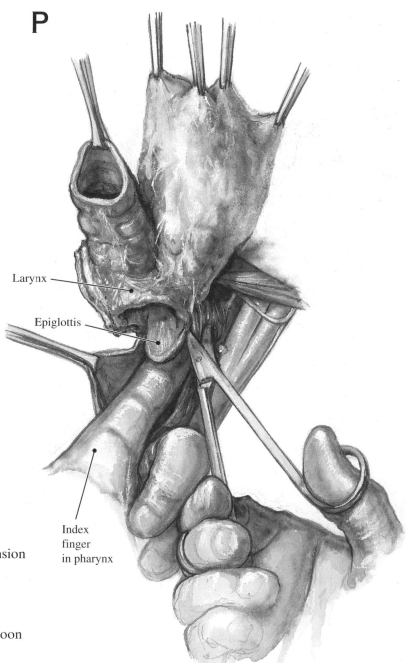

Larynx

Epiglottis

Index
finger
in pharynx

O

The trachea is now divided between tracheal rings; it
should not be so high as to cut into any subglottic extension
of the tumor. An excessive length of trachea can be
trimmed later. A long endotracheal tube is held in
readiness. When the trachea is incised sufficiently, the
current endotracheal tube is removed, the new one in
readiness is inserted through the tracheostomy, the balloon
is inflated, and the proximal end is promptly passed
underneath the drapes to the anesthesiologist.

The trachea is incised to its membranous portion; it is
critical that the esophagus not be entered at this low point.
The pharynx is entered near the postcricoid area or at a
lower point if dictated by the proximity of cancer.

P

If all the fibers of the constrictor muscles have not been
divided, this can now be done. The finger can be inserted
into the pharynx to steady the tissue. Again, the mucosal
incision inside can be followed.

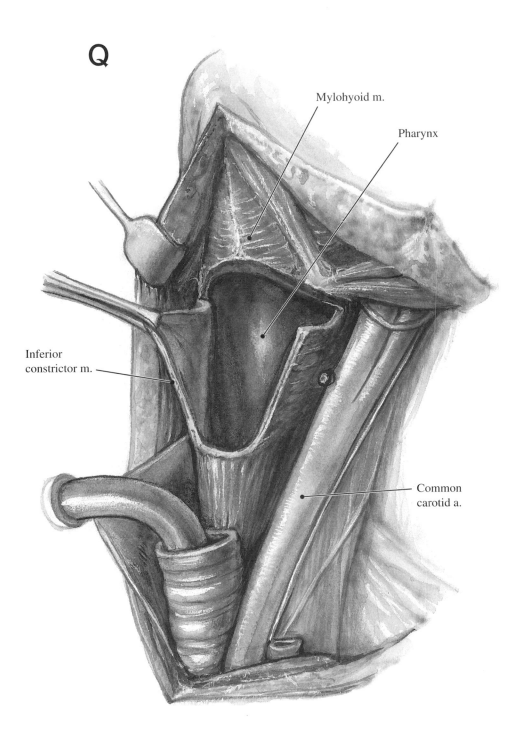

Q

Mylohyoid m.

Pharynx

Inferior
constrictor m.

Common
carotid a.

Q

The specimen has been removed with a resultant defect
that usually but not always is T shaped. This is the time to
examine the cut edges carefully and to order a histologic
examination of sections from suspicious margins. At this
point, a cricopharyngeal myotomy can easily be performed
(not shown) to aid in postoperative swallowing. A
nasogastric tube is introduced through the nose and
directed distally down the esophagus under direct vision.

R

R

Pharyngocutaneous fistula is one of the most serious postoperative complications, and care in closure is important in its prevention. The mucosa must be coapted adequately and with care that the stitches are not tied so tightly that they will cause necrosis of the intervening tissue. The primary closure is in two layers. The first layer is with a horizontal mattress stitch using 3-0 Vicryl; the second layer is with interrupted stitches of 4-0 Vicryl. A critical point in the closure is at the meeting of the trifurcate lines. The strap muscles and other adjacent muscles or tissue are deliberately placed over the suture line to buttress the area where the trifurcate lines meet. Often, the pharyngeal defect can be closed in a straight manner, obviating the need for the less optimal trifurcate configuration.

S

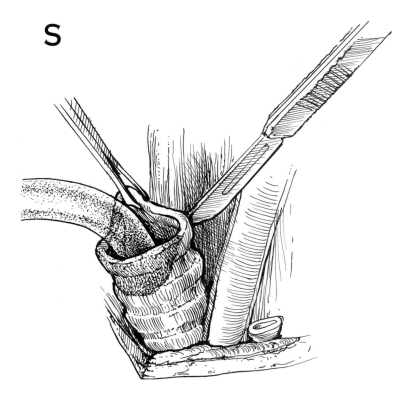

T

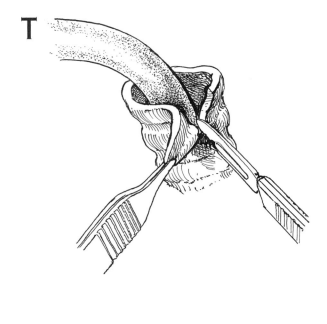

U

S, T, U

It usually is necessary to further mobilize the trachea from the esophagus so that the trachea can arch forward toward the skin surface easily. The trachea also has to be beveled so that it meets the skin comfortably and at a right angle. The stippled area shows the portion of trachea that will be discarded.

As was mentioned in the description of the development of the skin flaps, the inferomedial arm of the incision may be held short so that it ends over the medial third of the clavicle, making it possible for the tracheostomy to end outside the major operative field. A button of skin similar in diameter to that of the trachea is excised. The endotracheal tube is removed briefly so that the trachea can be pulled through the skin opening. The trachea is sutured to the skin with quadratically placed interrupted stitches of 3-0 nylon with additional stitches placed as needed. The trachea can exit at the medial entrance of the lower incision if it is unavoidable (see X).

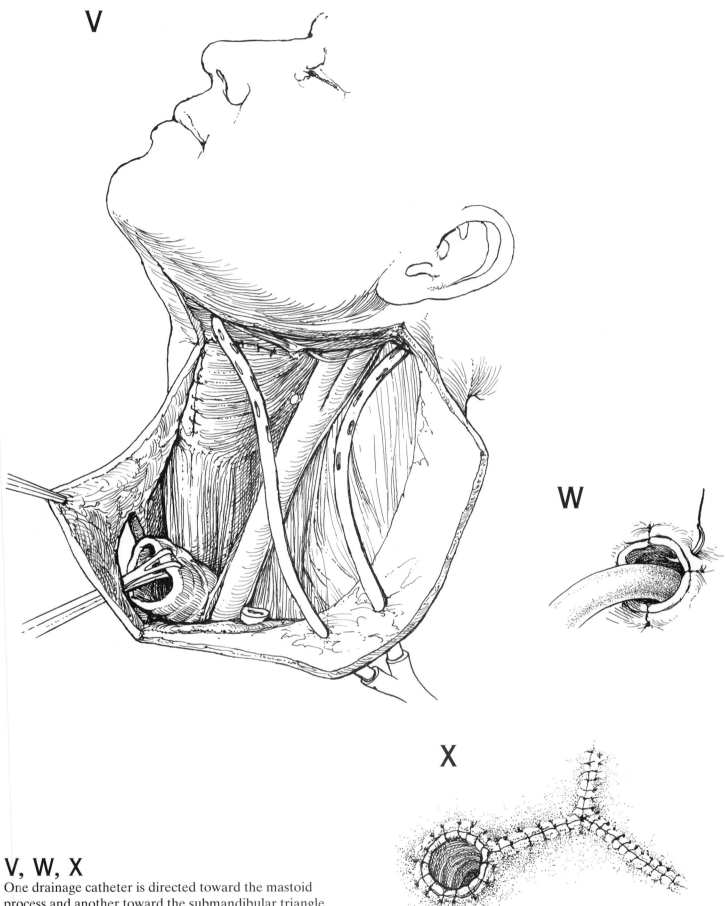

V, W, X

One drainage catheter is directed toward the mastoid process and another toward the submandibular triangle. They are exteriorized through separate tight counterincisions and placed on suction. The skin and platysma are closed as one layer with vertical mattress stitches of 4-0 nylon or with subcutaneous absorbable sutures and skin clips. A laryngectomy tube is inserted. A light dressing is applied, and the patient is transferred to a bed maintained at a 30-degree head elevation.

A MAJOR DUCT EXCISION

Major duct excision is not commonly performed. Yet, when the need for it arises, it must be done with precision and superior hemostasis. If, for example, the intent is to excise a papilloma, the procedure can be terminated once that lesion is found. Sometimes, however, the lesion is not found, and the central ductal system must be excised for a depth of 3 cm or so.

A

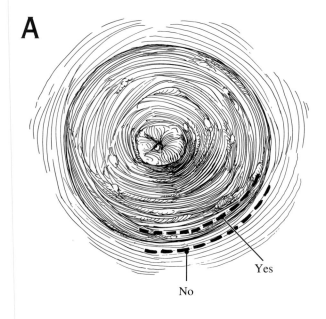

No

Yes

B

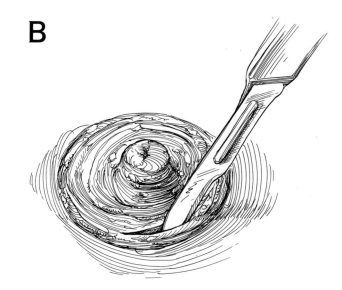

C

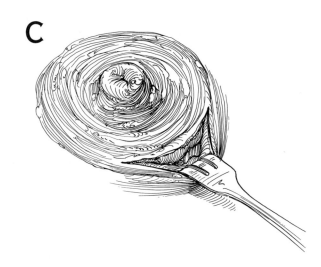

A, B, C

The skin is prepared in the usual manner. The nipple should be cleansed with special care to remove plugs of keratin or dehydrated ductal content that may drop into the wound during the procedure. A few light cross-hatches across the incision will help later with accurate realignment of this wrinkled tissue during closure.

The incision should be 1 to 2 mm inside the areolar border. The resulting scar is less obvious than one just outside the areolar border.

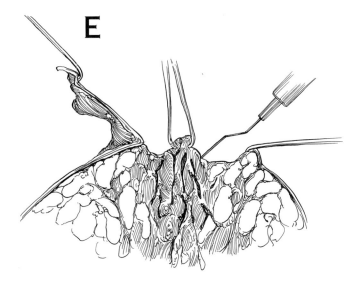

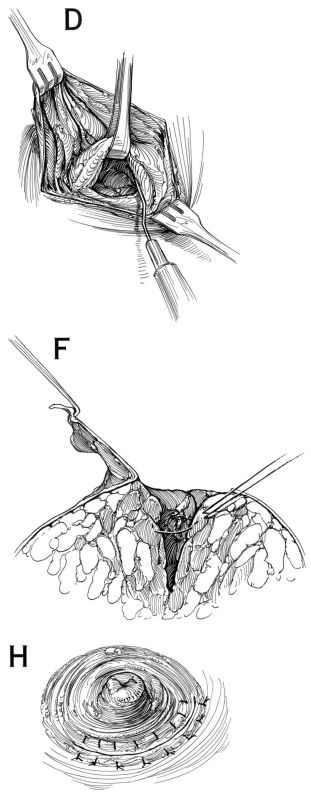

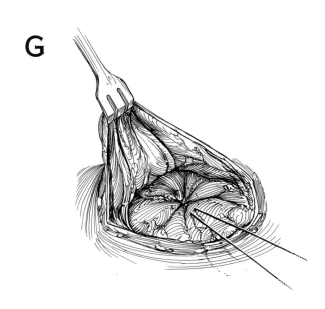

intent here is to excise breast ducts—obviously not all of them—but to leave all other irrelevant tissue intact. The resection, therefore, results in a somewhat conical specimen and a similarly shaped defect.

F, G

Simply closing the skin without an underlying base allows the nipple–areolar complex to sink within this defect, producing a poor cosmetic result that can be prevented. One or two purse-string stitches of 3-0 chromic catgut effectively bring together the sides of this conical defect and provide the base on which the areola can lie.

H

The subcutaneous fatty tissue is reapproximated with stitches of 4-0 chromic catgut applied in an inverted fashion so that the knots and cut ends point into the deeper tissue; otherwise, the catgut lies too close to the skin surface.

The skin should be closed with vertical mattress stitches of 5-0 nylon with the far bite no fewer than 5 mm from the cut edge. The stitches should coapt this soft tissue rather than squeeze it together.

D, E

Very fine rake and manicure scissors are preferred for the initial dissection and electrocautery for the deeper area. The small amount of fat under the areola should be left as is. The dissection continues to the nipple, at which point the amount of tissue that is excised from inside the nipple depends on the surgeon's clinical judgment that the abnormality lies within it rather than deeper in the central breast. If the very terminal portion of the duct needs to be excised, then the central portion of the nipple can be removed, leaving the sides intact. When the nipple is closed, it is somewhat more pointed. Keep in mind that the

B BIOPSY—ROUTINE

A

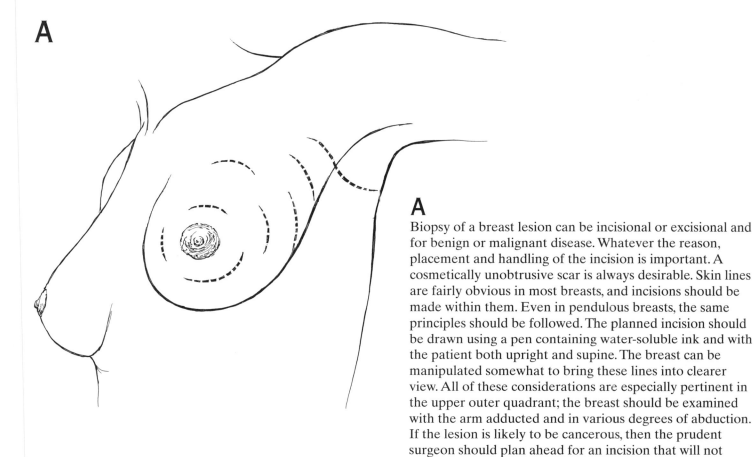

A

Biopsy of a breast lesion can be incisional or excisional and for benign or malignant disease. Whatever the reason, placement and handling of the incision is important. A cosmetically unobtrusive scar is always desirable. Skin lines are fairly obvious in most breasts, and incisions should be made within them. Even in pendulous breasts, the same principles should be followed. The planned incision should be drawn using a pen containing water-soluble ink and with the patient both upright and supine. The breast can be manipulated somewhat to bring these lines into clearer view. All of these considerations are especially pertinent in the upper outer quadrant; the breast should be examined with the arm adducted and in various degrees of abduction. If the lesion is likely to be cancerous, then the prudent surgeon should plan ahead for an incision that will not compromise subsequent work in the area.

B

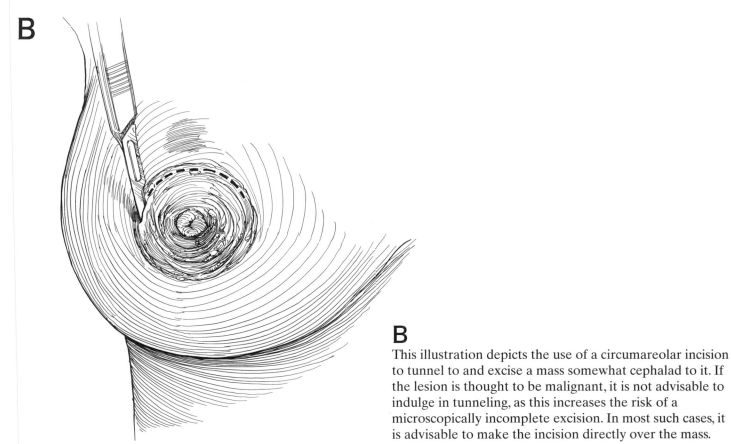

B

This illustration depicts the use of a circumareolar incision to tunnel to and excise a mass somewhat cephalad to it. If the lesion is thought to be malignant, it is not advisable to indulge in tunneling, as this increases the risk of a microscopically incomplete excision. In most such cases, it is advisable to make the incision directly over the mass.

C

D

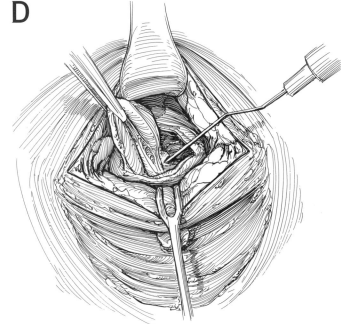

E

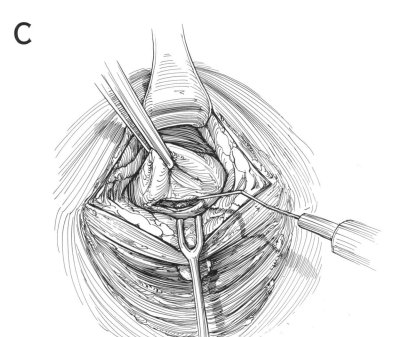

C, D, E

A breast incision made for purposes of biopsy does not constitute the beginning of flap development, as in a mastectomy. Such an incision, therefore, should be carried down toward the tumor itself (*E*). Just before the mass is reached, the normal tissue surrounding it is grasped with a hemostat and its excision begun. The mass is placed under gentle traction while countertraction is applied by the assistant. A scalpel or a fine-tipped electrocautery unit in the cutting mode is used for the dissection; switching to the coagulation mode is effective in obtaining hemostasis.

The biopsy cavity is not obliterated, nor is a drain used. The subcutaneous tissue is reapproximated with interrupted simple stitches of 4-0 chromic catgut. Whenever possible, the skin is closed with a subcuticular stitch of 3-0 or 4-0 monofilament suture material. Loose or flabby tissue is best closed with vertical mattress stitches.

F, G, H, I

F, G, H, and *I* depict the excision of a mass that is located in the inferior hemisphere of the breast close to the inframammary crease. A thoracomammary approach is desirable, especially if the clinical impression is that of a benign lesion.

F

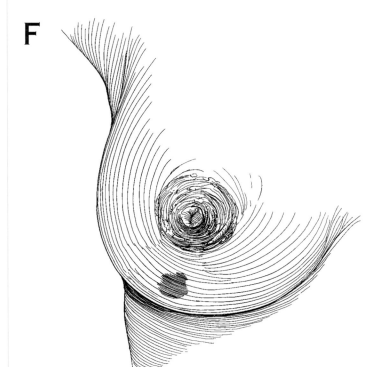

G

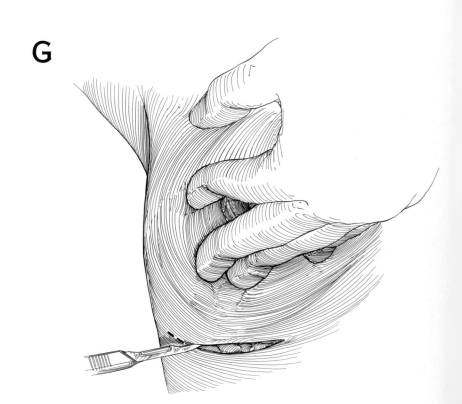

H

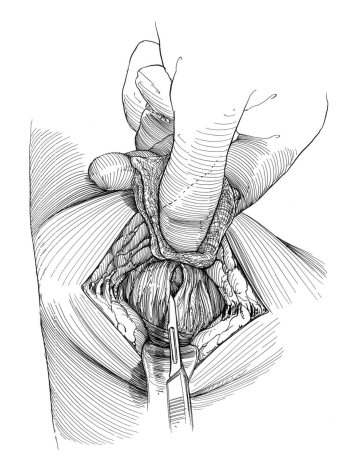

Once the posterior of the breast has been exposed, the upper flap is held by the thumb with a gauze to help prevent slippage, and the breast tissue is pushed forward to bring and hold an otherwise mobile mass into the path of the cutting blade. As soon as the lesion is felt, the tissue around it is grasped with a forceps and excised along with surrounding normal tissue. Transected vessels are electrocoagulated. Subcutaneous closure is accomplished with interrupted 4-0 chromic catgut and skin closure with a subcuticular stitch of 4-0 monofilament suture.

I

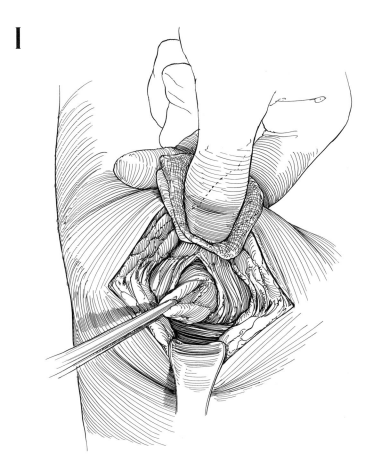

C WIDE LOCAL EXCISION

A

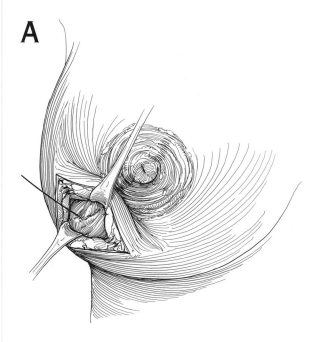

B

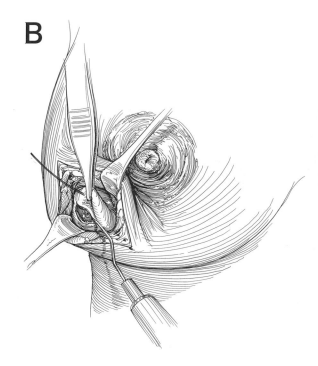

C

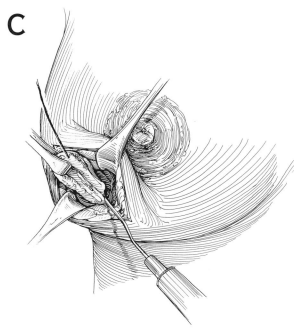

Wide local excision in anticipation of coupling it with an axillary lymph node dissection requires the excision of enough tissue to completely encompass both the palpable mass and the associated mammographically visible but nonpalpable microcalcifications. Preoperative radiologic needle localization will guide the surgeon on the extent of resection necessary to achieve a histologically clear margin.

Again, the surgeon should make the initial incision with a plan as to how it will be incorporated with an axillary incision, namely, whether one or two incisions will be necessary for both fields initially, and whether they will be made synchronously or in two sittings after the diagnosis of cancer has been confirmed. Generally, excising the primary tumor and the axillary lymph nodes through one incision places a stricter responsibility on the surgeon to be certain that the primary tumor is completely encompassed the first time, because cutting across the cancerous primary tumor may contaminate the axillary field with cancer cells. Generally, en bloc resection of the primary tumor and axillary lymph nodes is performed for tumors in the upper outer quadrant of the breast near or within the low axillary tissue.

A, B, C

The localization wire is used to indicate both the location of the tumor and the approach to it. Keep in mind that the point of entry of the localization needle is not necessarily the exact location of the tumor within the underlying breast; careful evaluation of the mammogram and the relationship of the needle tip to the tumor mass are important if one is to avoid unnecessary dissection.

D

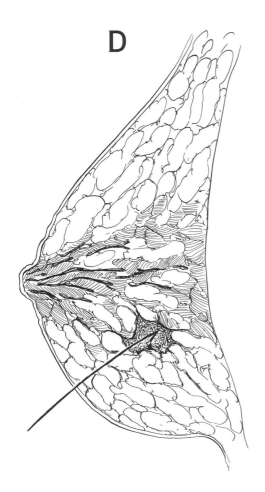

D

It is common practice when performing the needle localization to deposit several drops of methylene blue dye at the center of the lesion. It is helpful to use this stained area as a guide regarding the amount of tissue to excise. Hemostasis should be absolute, as there is minimal tamponade effect in the breast against even minute oozing vessels.

E

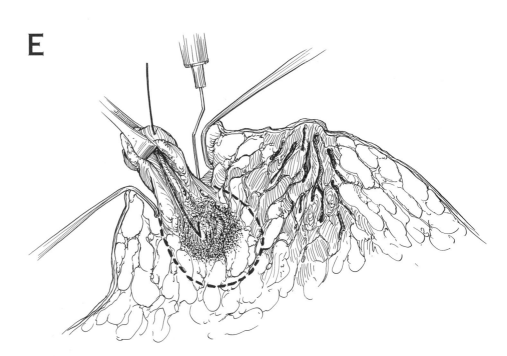

E

Once the lesion is reached, tissue around it that appears normal is grasped with an Allis forceps and, using traction, is excised by electrocautery with a gross clearance of at least 1 cm around the mass.

For the benefit of the pathologist, always orient the specimen and have the margins inked so it can be examined for "clean" margins.

F

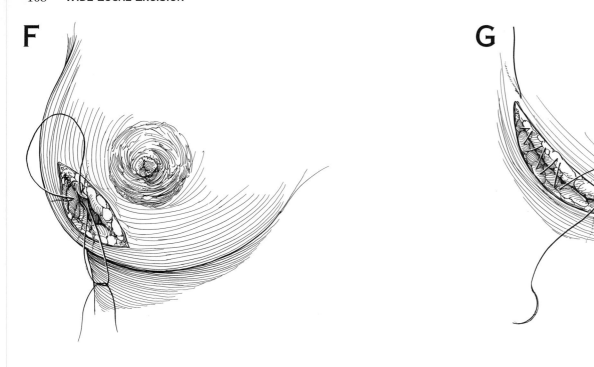

G

H

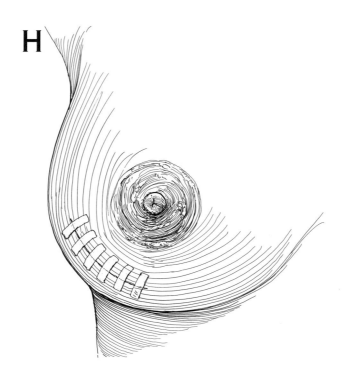

F, G, H

The deep tissue is not reapproximated. The subcutaneous layer is closed with interrupted simple stitches of 4-0 chromic catgut, and the skin is closed with a subcuticular stitch of 4-0 or 3-0 monofilament suture material. The hairline incision is supported with strips of tape.

If a considerable amount of tissue has been resected and there is obvious cavitation of the overlying skin at the completion of the closure, it often is helpful to fill the cavity with an equivalent amount of preservative-free saline solution. Apparently, the slow absorption of the saline allows a better reconfiguration of the surrounding breast tissue, leading to improved short-term and long-term cosmetic results.

D MODIFIED RADICAL MASTECTOMY

Modified radical mastectomy continues, for the present, to be the most widely performed operation for cancer of the breast and is featured in this chapter.

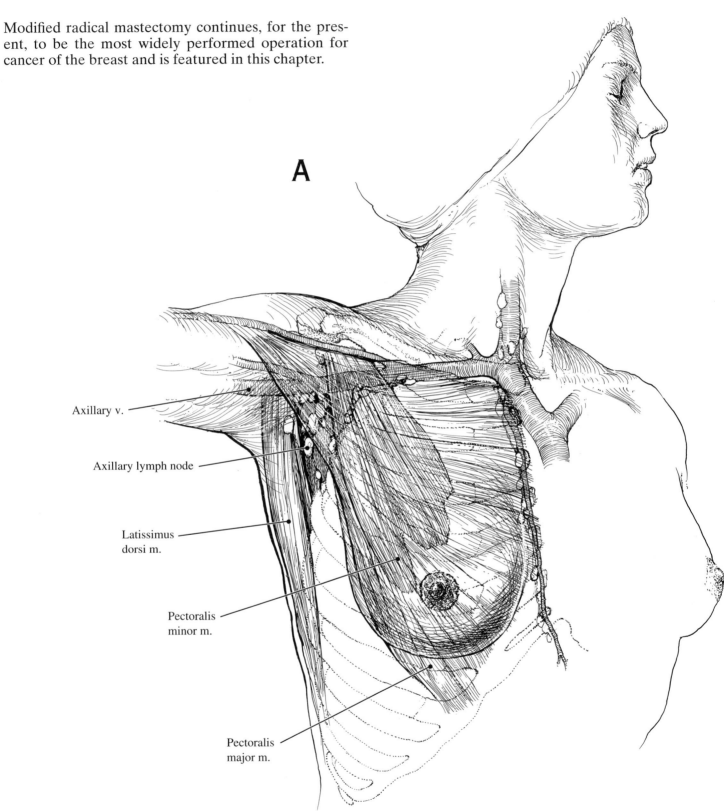

A

Axillary v.

Axillary lymph node

Latissimus dorsi m.

Pectoralis minor m.

Pectoralis major m.

A, B, C

This trio of panoramic views show the muscles and vascular structures the surgeon must work with or know about in performing breast surgery. The breast lies mainly on the pectoralis major muscle. The excision of this muscle and the underlying pectoralis minor muscle is the only major difference that distinguishes a radical from a modified radical mastectomy. The peripheral boundaries of a modified radical mastectomy are the axillary vein, the infraclavicular area, the midline, the anterior border of the latissimus dorsi muscle, and the inferior border of the breast as the tissue blends with the fascia of the rectus abdominis muscle.

B

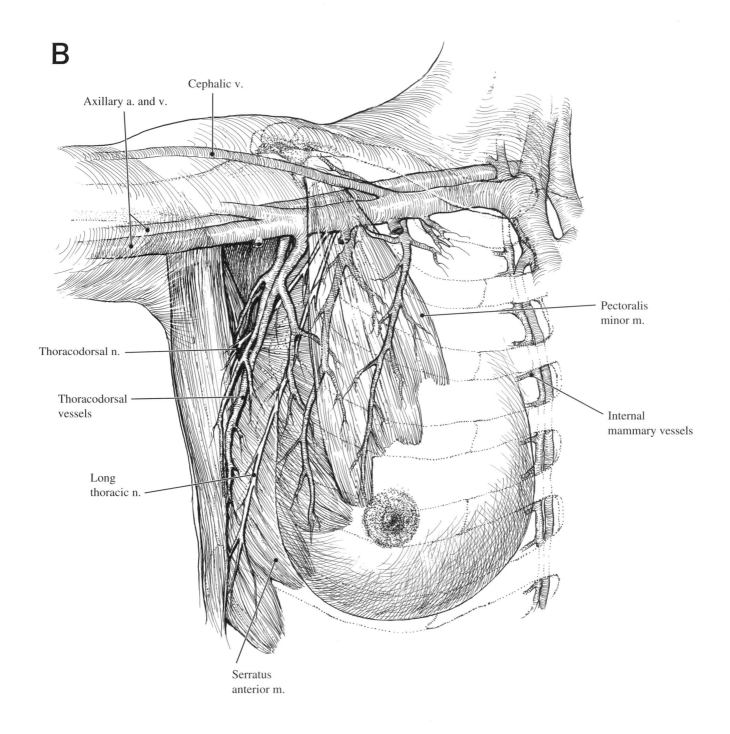

Cephalic v.

Axillary a. and v.

Thoracodorsal n.

Thoracodorsal
vessels

Long
thoracic n.

Serratus
anterior m.

Pectoralis
minor m.

Internal
mammary vessels

The relevant nerves are as follows: the thoracodorsal nerve to the latissimus dorsi muscle; damage to it results in minimal disability. The long thoracic nerve to the serratus anterior muscle deserves special vigilance during the dissection because the winged scapula resulting from injury to it can be very troublesome. The medial and lateral pectoral nerves should be spared unless the presence of cancer mandates their resection. Damage to these nerves while dissecting in the medial aspect of the axilla produces no early effect, but the pectoralis muscles later atrophy,

which can lead to an obvious cavitation in this area. The intercostobrachial nerve usually is sacrificed and results in hypesthesia to the inner aspect of the upper arm. This ameliorates with time. Sometimes it is spared if the tumor is very small and if no suspicious lymph nodes are seen during the axillary dissection.

The locoregional drainage is primarily to the axillary lymph nodes and secondarily to those in the supraclavicular fossa and internal mammary chain.

B1

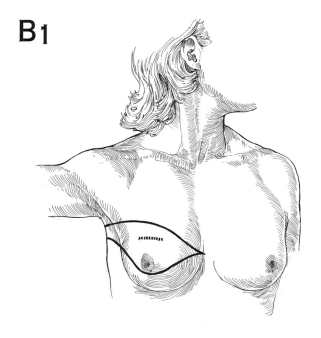

B2

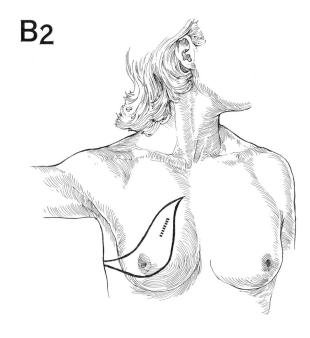

B3

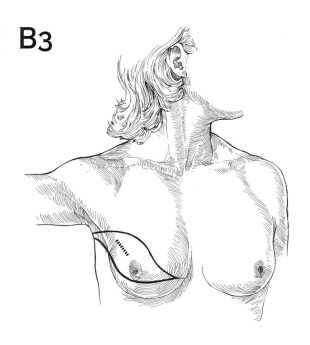

B4

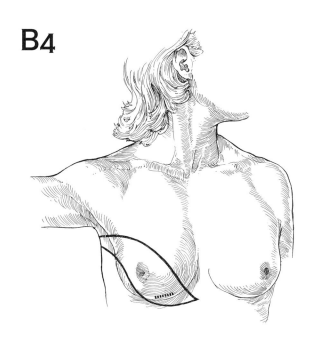

B5

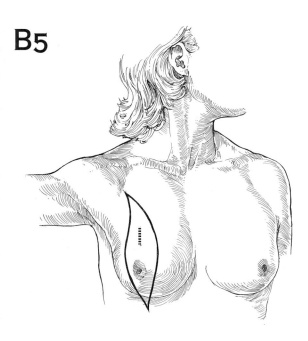

B₁, 2, 3, 4, 5

The incision used depends largely on the site of the tumor and the orientation and length of the open biopsy incision. Of note: a transverse incision is preferable to a vertical one both cosmetically and anatomically; the lateral extent of the incision should be cephalad enough that the axilla can be reached with ease; the incision should avoid the hollow of the axilla and certainly not be made perpendicular to the skin lines when within it. This constellation of illustrations shows incisions that can accommodate the requirements mentioned.

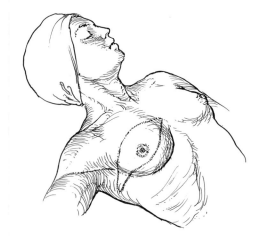

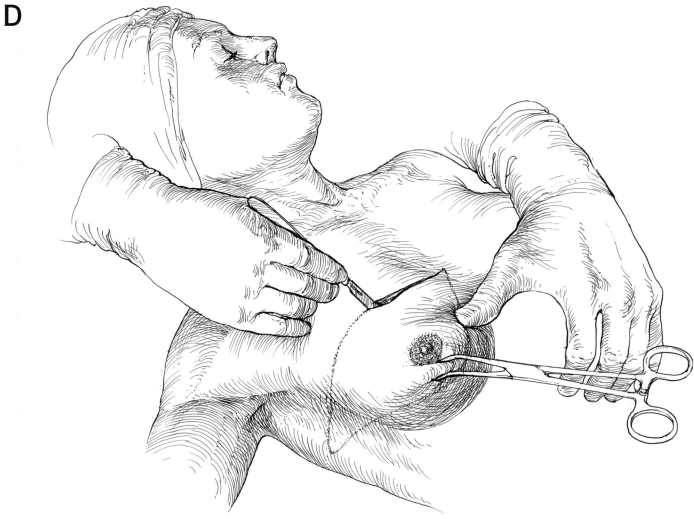

C

A modified radical mastectomy is performed under general anesthesia with the patient supine and the arm abducted at a right angle. We do not drape the arm so that it can be mobile during the operation; it is not necessary from an operative standpoint.

D

A towel clip placed in a non–tumor-bearing area of the breast helps reposition it as the operation progresses. The entire skin incision can be made at this time and hemostasis achieved with fine-tipped electrocoagulation.

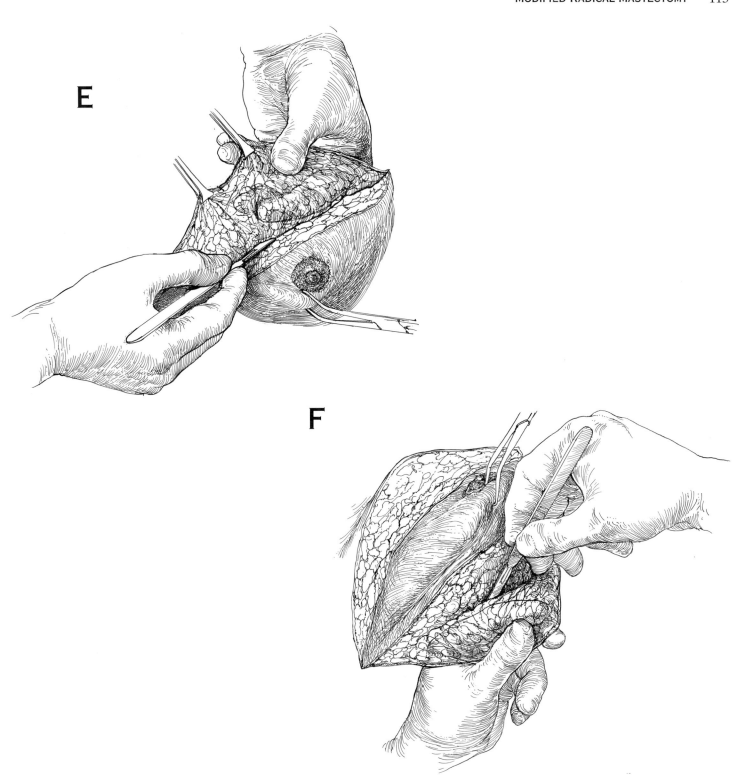

E

F

E, F

These illustrations show a thin-flap technique. Whatever merits thin flaps may have, they carry with them some special needs: meticulous technique during their development; care not to "buttonhole" the skin; pinpoint thermocoagulation; extra gentleness in handling the tissue. One way to maintain an awareness of the thickness of the flap is for the surgeon to stand behind the flap being developed. During dissection, several of the fingers retracting the flaps are placed on the skin side. Concurrently, the first assistant applies traction on the specimen. Our practice is to make the flaps progressively and modestly thicker as the periphery of the resection is approached. If the flaps need to be mobilized for easier closure, the available tissue usually is from the lower margins, with flap dissection continued as full thickness.

In experienced hands, cautery or scissors are equally effective in creating the flaps. When using the cautery, "cooking" the tissue is a common error. Dissecting with a cutting current and not lingering at any one spot are imperative. Hemostasis is achieved with a fine tip and with the unit on a coagulation setting to avoid charring the tissue.

G

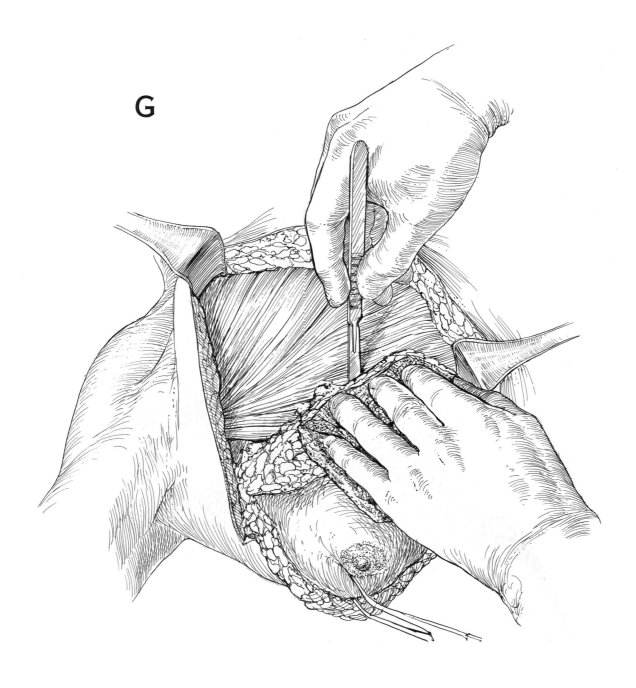

G

With the flaps developed, the breast is so positioned that it hangs over the side and functions as its own retractor. If a scalpel is used to dissect the breast from the pectoral muscles, an Adson clamp is used to grasp the vessels that are emanating from it and that will be coagulated first before dividing them. If the dissection is done with electrocautery, both the cutting and the coagulation settings are reduced or the electrocautery tip will easily cut into the muscle. The direction of dissection, whether by cautery or scalpel, should be parallel to the muscle fiber; this reduces the likelihood that muscle fibers will be divided.

H

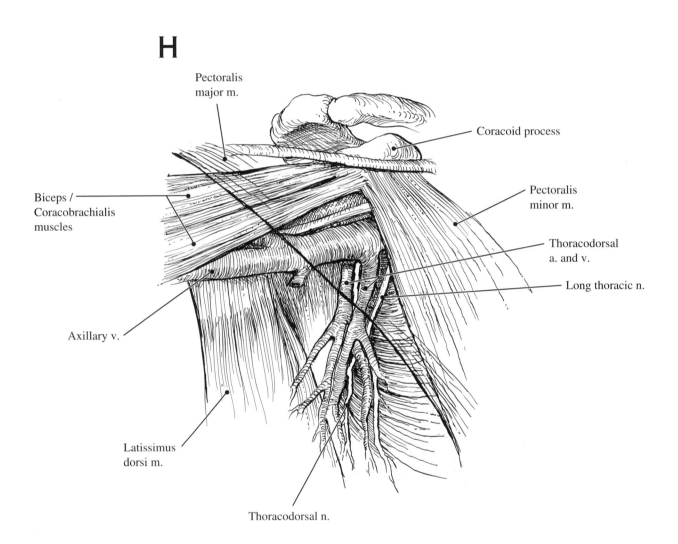

Pectoralis
major m.

Coracoid process

Biceps /
Coracobrachialis
muscles

Pectoralis
minor m.

Thoracodorsal
a. and v.

Long thoracic n.

Axillary v.

Latissimus
dorsi m.

Thoracodorsal n.

H

Anatomic structures in the axilla. Except for the breast and
axillary lymph nodal tissue, most other structures will be
retained.

I

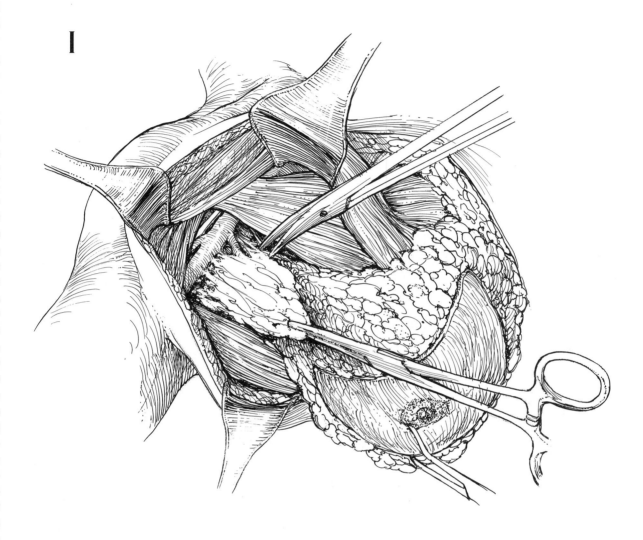

I

The dissection is continued to the lateral border of the pectoralis major muscle, which is retracted medially to expose the pectoralis minor muscle. The axillary dissection is now begun. For purposes of improved anatomic clarity the dissection is shown cephalad to the axillary vein. This is contrary to our actual practice, the feeling being that cancer that has metastasized cephalad to the vein is unlikely to be cured by aggressive dissection at this high level. The axillary dissection can be carried out with a fine scissors as shown. Encountered blood vessels are secured with clips or 3-0 silk. A method that is swift and logically associated with less postoperative lymphorrhea is to segment sections of the lymphoareolar tissue that does not contain sizable vessels with an Adson clamp and divide it by electrocoagulation.

J

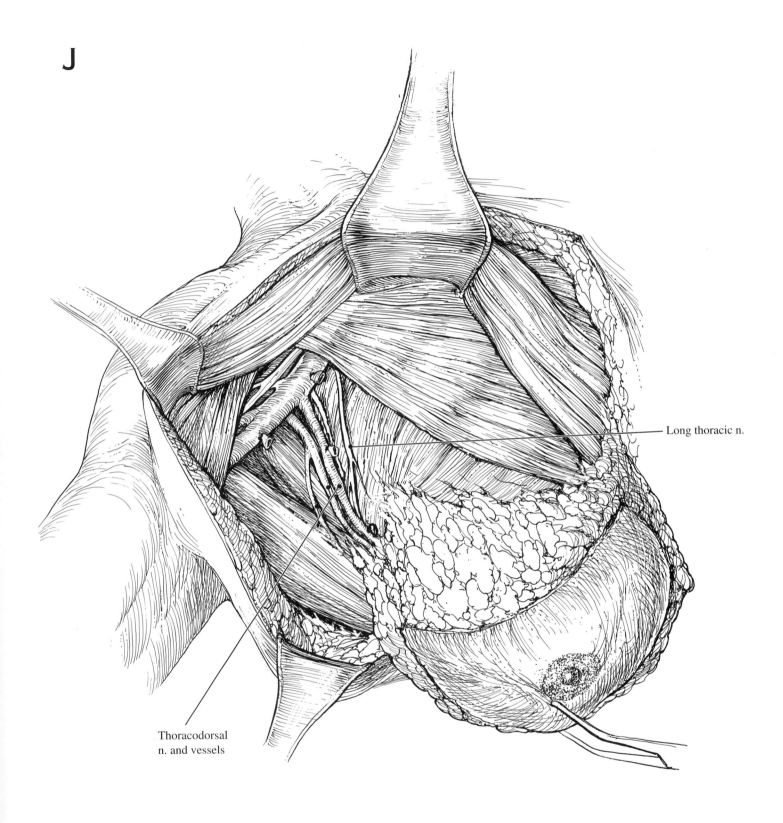

Long thoracic n.

Thoracodorsal
n. and vessels

J

At the completion of the dissection about the axillary vein,
the long thoracic nerve is identified as it hugs the serratus
muscle. Sometimes it is flaccid and can be pulled away
from the chest wall by the hanging breast specimen. It
should be sought in this tissue; cutting should not proceed
until the nerve is visualized. The thoracodorsal nerve is
sought as it courses medial or posterior to the subscapular
artery and vein.

K

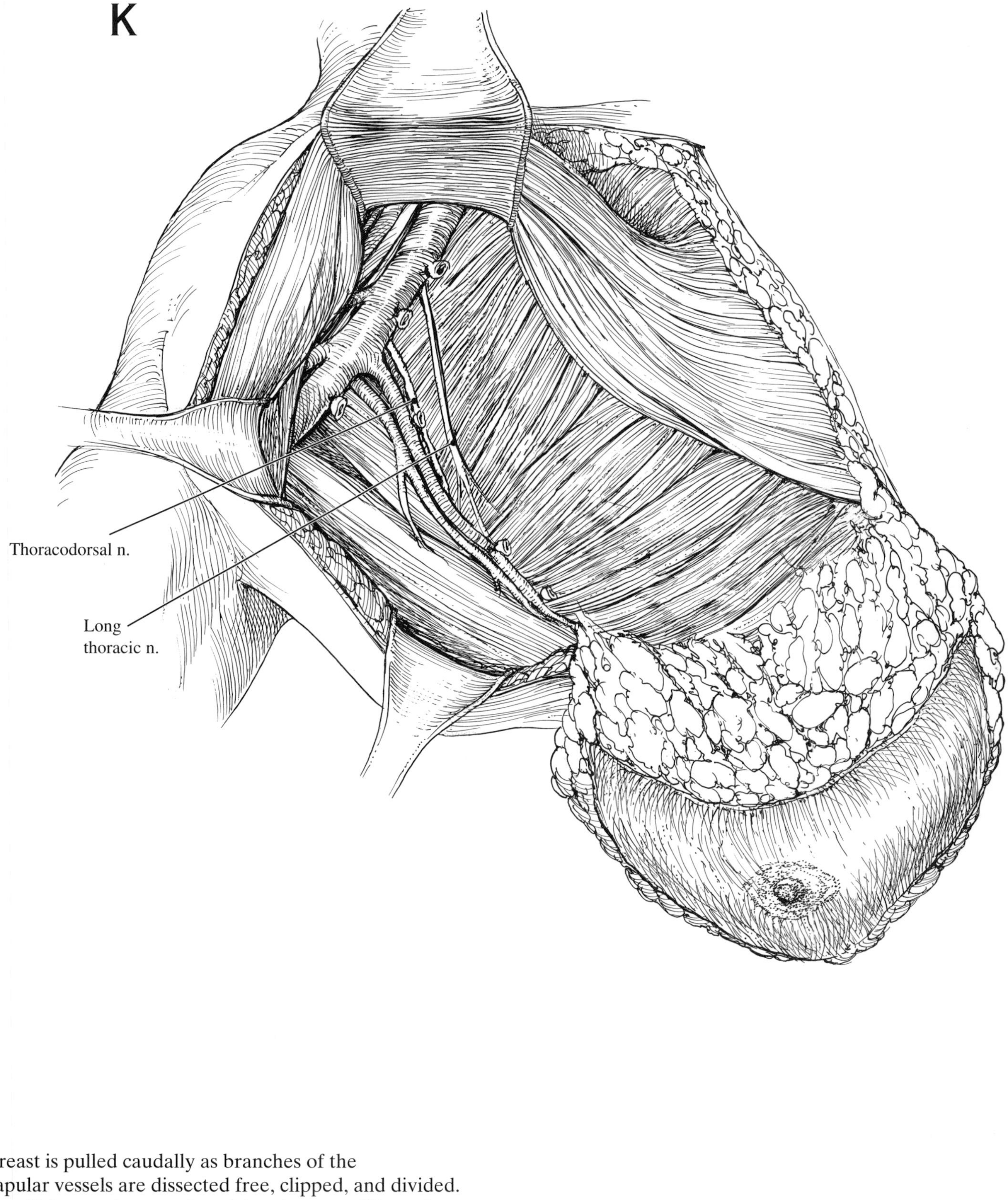

Thoracodorsal n.

Long
thoracic n.

K

The breast is pulled caudally as branches of the
subscapular vessels are dissected free, clipped, and divided.
Pulling off the specimen and avulsing these small branches
is not really necessary. Nor is it beneficial to sweep the
tissue off the subscapularis muscle until it is "squeaky
clean." Indeed, this may impede tissue gliding in the area
and delay restoration of shoulder motion postoperatively.

L

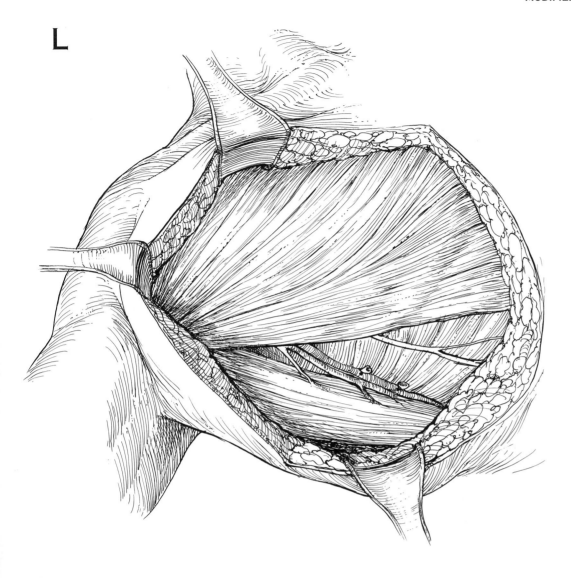

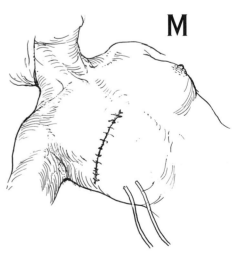

M

L

Once resection is completed, the area is inspected for hemostasis, and bleeding points are electrocoagulated. The wound is rinsed with physiologic saline solution to rid it of fine debris.

M

Two drains, both positioned in the axillary area (the skin over the pectoral muscles is invariably tight and inhibits fluid collection), are exited through counterincisions. The lateral extremes of the incision are accurately coapted with simple interrupted stitches set about 5 mm from the wound edge and as far apart as is necessary. Any disparity in the length of the remaining portions of the flaps is rectified at this time. If there is only minimal tension, most of the incision can be closed with a simple running stitch of monofilament suture. A large dressing is used to cover—not bind—the incision.

8

ESOPHAGUS

A ESOPHAGECTOMY

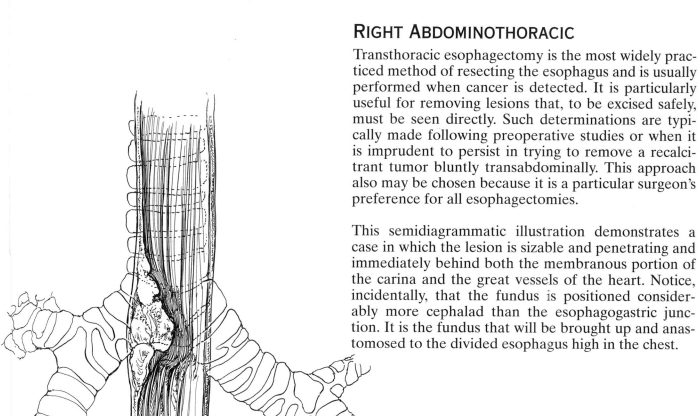

RIGHT ABDOMINOTHORACIC

Transthoracic esophagectomy is the most widely practiced method of resecting the esophagus and is usually performed when cancer is detected. It is particularly useful for removing lesions that, to be excised safely, must be seen directly. Such determinations are typically made following preoperative studies or when it is imprudent to persist in trying to remove a recalcitrant tumor bluntly transabdominally. This approach also may be chosen because it is a particular surgeon's preference for all esophagectomies.

This semidiagrammatic illustration demonstrates a case in which the lesion is sizable and penetrating and immediately behind both the membranous portion of the carina and the great vessels of the heart. Notice, incidentally, that the fundus is positioned considerably more cephalad than the esophagogastric junction. It is the fundus that will be brought up and anastomosed to the divided esophagus high in the chest.

A

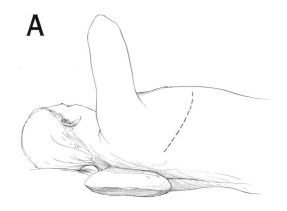

A

The patient is intubated orotracheally with a double-cuffed tube and placed supine on the table but with the right side elevated 45 or 90 degrees, depending on the surgeon's preference. Both the abdomen and thorax should be accessible.

The stomach will have been mobilized transabdominally as has been illustrated in several other procedures, which will not be repeated here. The stomach must be sufficiently mobilized, however, that it can be transposed high in the chest.

B

The chest is entered through the fifth intercostal space, and the rib spreader is inserted and gently cranked open. The inferior pulmonary ligament is divided so that the lung can be covered with a lap pad and retracted medially for the remainder of this procedure.

B

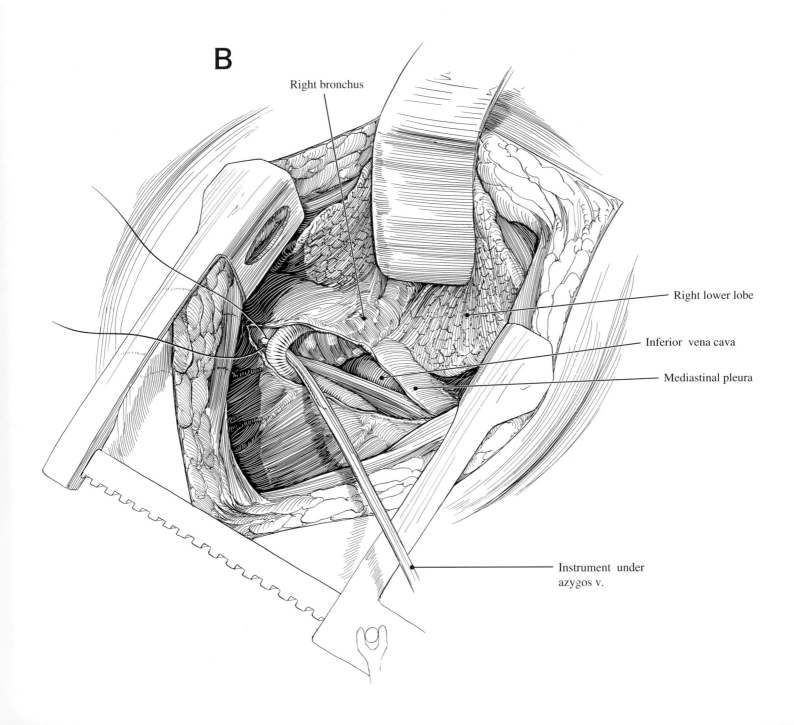

Right bronchus

Right lower lobe

Inferior vena cava

Mediastinal pleura

Instrument under azygos v.

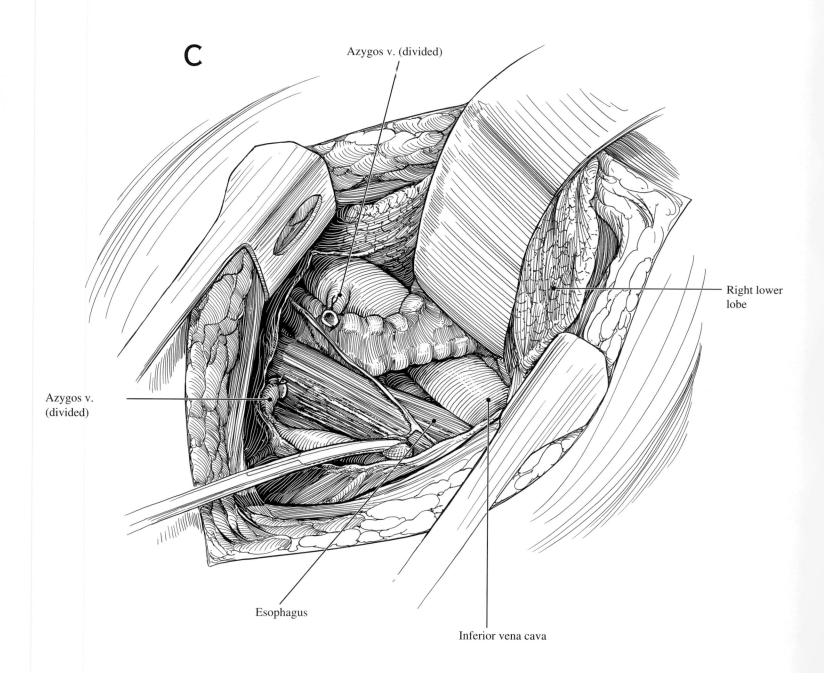

C

Azygos v. (divided)

Right lower lobe

Azygos v. (divided)

Esophagus

Inferior vena cava

C

The upper part of the mediastinal pleura is incised, exposing the vena cava, esophagus, carina, and azygos vein. The latter is suture ligated doubly with 2-0 silk before division.

D

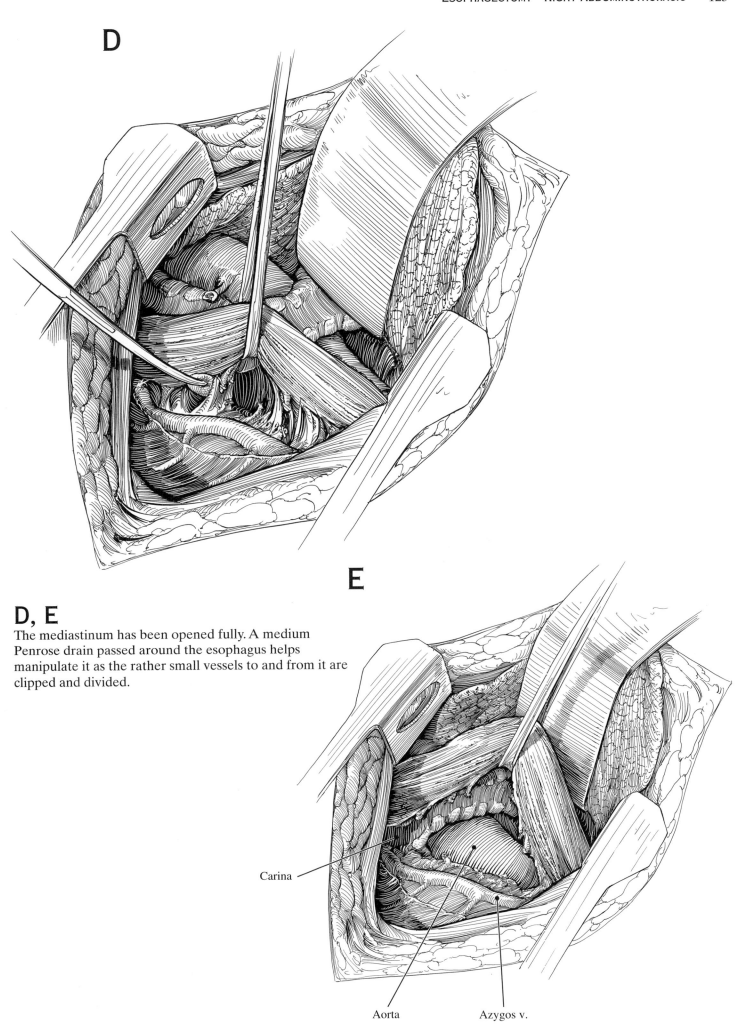

D, E

The mediastinum has been opened fully. A medium Penrose drain passed around the esophagus helps manipulate it as the rather small vessels to and from it are clipped and divided.

E

Carina

Aorta   Azygos v.

F

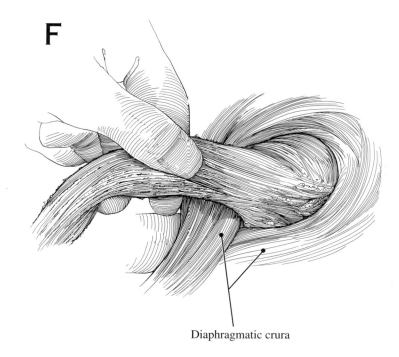

Diaphragmatic crura

G

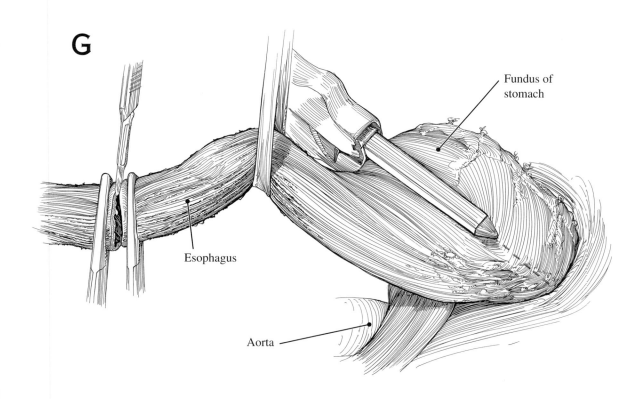

Fundus of
stomach

Esophagus

Aorta

F, G

When this part of the dissection has been completed, the crura are divided enough anteriorly so that half of the mobilized stomach can be delivered into the chest. The stomach should be kept properly oriented at all times.

The GIA-60 stapler is placed across the upper part of the stomach with the lymph node–bearing area along the lesser curvature included in the area to be amputated. Multiple applications of the stapler may be necessary to complete the transaction. In some instances it is easier to perform this step from the abdominal side.

H

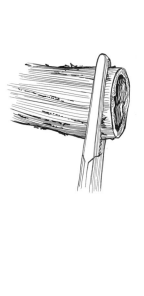

Fundus of stomach

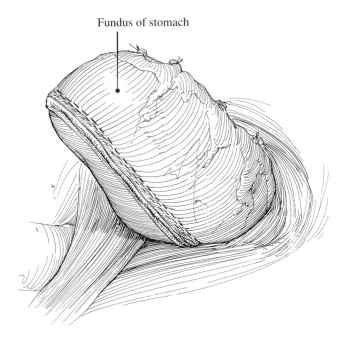

I

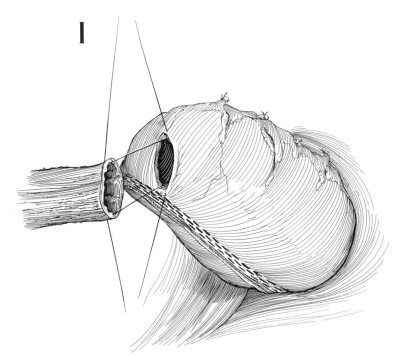

J

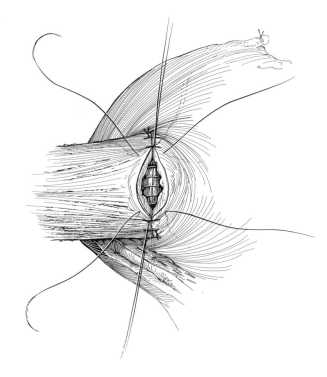

H

The specimen is shown dissected free as well as transected at both ends in readiness for the esophagogastric anastomosis. If there is any question about the viability of the staple line, it can be reinforced with interrupted stitches of 3-0 silk.

I

A spot is selected on the anterior face of the stomach just short of its apex and adjacent to the transected esophagus. An incision is made that will open to a diameter equal to that of the esophagus.

J

Traction stitches are placed at each extreme of the esophagus and stomach as they are coapted in readiness for the anastomosis. The anastomosis is executed in one layer using 4-0 Maxon sutures. The posterior anastomosis is accomplished using a continuous simple stitch, the anterior one using interrupted simple stitches. Buttressing stitches can be added if necessary.

K

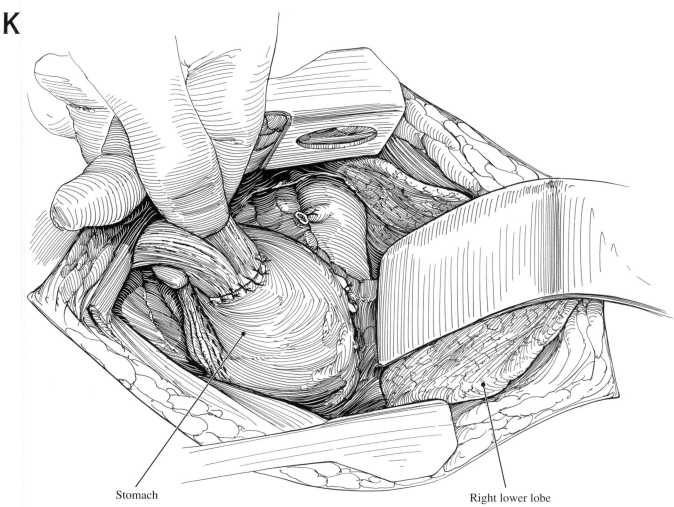

Stomach

Right lower lobe

K

The complete anastomosis is shown. The stomach is anchored to the surrounding tissue with interrupted stitches. A chest tube is brought out through a counterincision and the chest closed in the customary manner. The abdomen is given a final examination and closed in a preferred manner.

TRANSABDOMINAL (BLUNT)
Gastric Pull-up

A

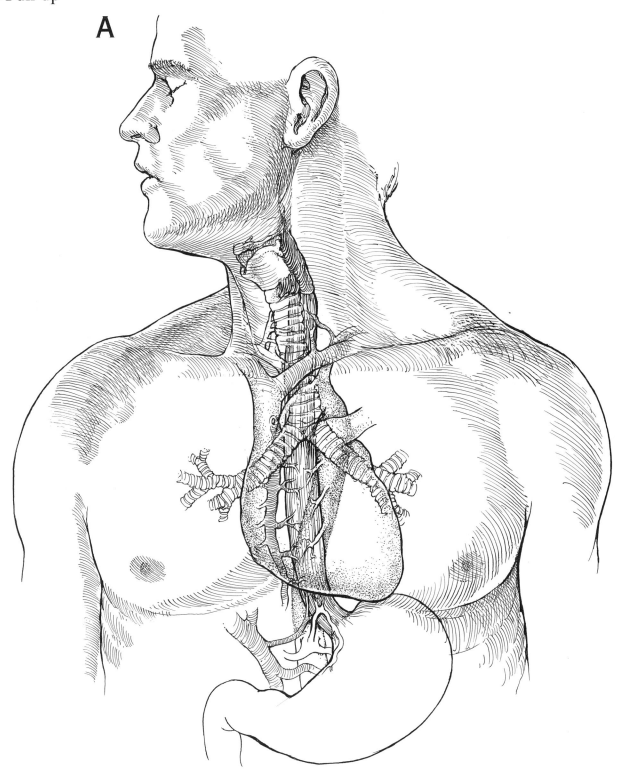

A

This panoramic illustration demonstrates the varied structures that must be dealt with in the three distinct anatomic areas—abdomen, thorax, and neck—in the course of performing a transabdominal, blunt thoracic esophagectomy with gastric pull-up.

B

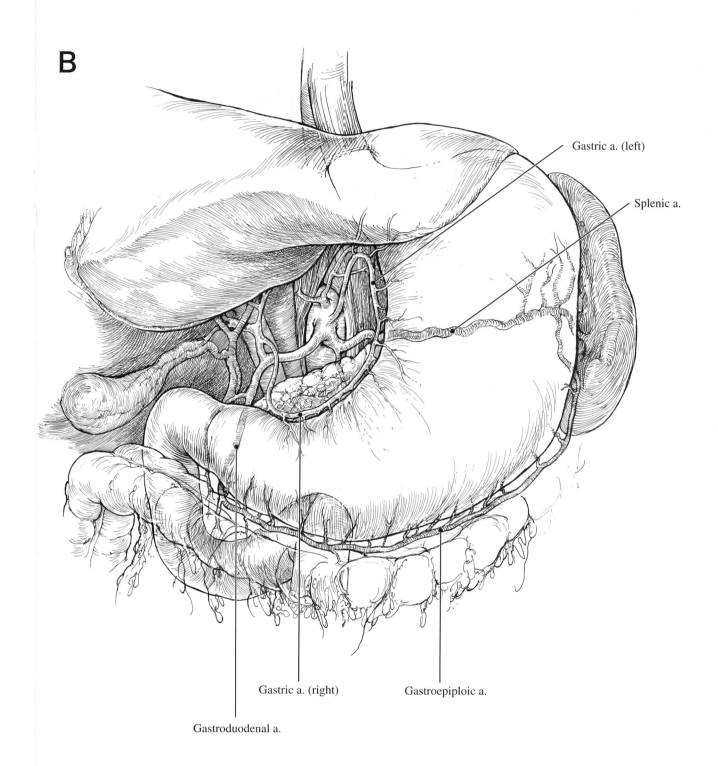

Gastric a. (left)

Splenic a.

Gastric a. (right)

Gastroepiploic a.

Gastroduodenal a.

B

The illustration emphasizes the important role played by
the stomach and the need to be thoroughly acquainted with
the anatomy of this area. A pull-up under tension invites
anastomotic disruption; careless mobilization of the
stomach and loss of its viability is a serious setback.

C

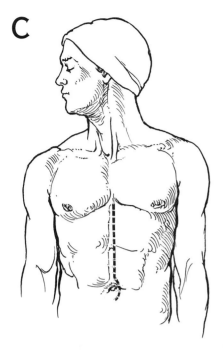

D

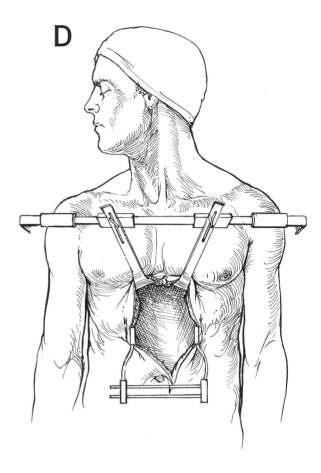

C

The patient should be in the supine position with the neck slightly extended and the head rotated to the right. A longitudinal incision is best because it can be extended cephalad at the midline; often the xiphoid process is excised for additional exposure.

D

Firm cephalad and slightly ventral retraction is essential to making this operation easier and safer. This is best achieved by attaching a retractor to the table with a crossbar about 15 cm cephalad to the upper end of the incision and about 5 cm above the surface of the thorax. Each of the two blades of the retractor are positioned on one side of the xiphoid.

The abdominal cavity is examined for metastasis beyond the regional lymph nodes, involvement that probably does not warrant resection even for purposes of palliation only. Metastatic deposits in the celiac axis, which cannot be excised but can be freed from the stomach, do not preclude performance of this operation. Such an aggressive stance has evolved following the realization that most patients who appear to be cured nonetheless later manifest recurrence. This being the case, dissection is not confined only to those who have cancers with local involvement. Rather, it is offered to patients who are able to tolerate the operation physiologically and in whom the amount or location of cancer, or both, would not prevent them from living long enough to enjoy any resultant palliation.

E

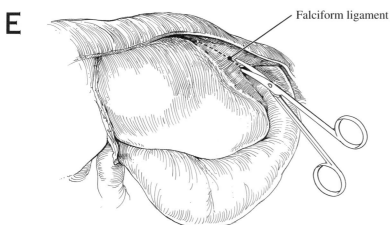

Falciform ligament

F

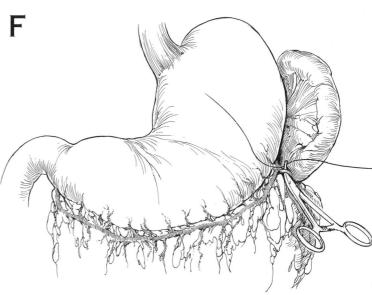

G

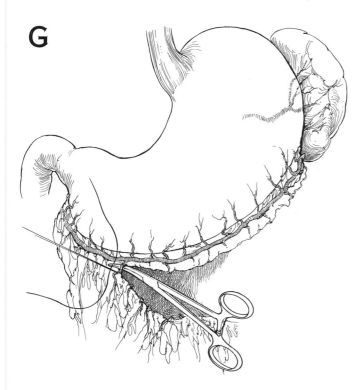

E

If the left lobe needs to be retracted to the patient's right for optimal exposure of the esophageal hiatus, the falciform ligament is divided using scissors or a fine-tipped electrocautery unit.

F, G

The right gastroepiploic artery is divided at its left extreme as it enters the stomach, as are other branches (here to the spleen) that would prevent full mobilization of the stomach. Progressing toward the patient's right, the omentum is separated from the gastroepiploic artery, being careful that the artery, so important to survival of the mobilized stomach, is not injured. This dissection is carried just short of where the gastroepiploic artery appears from the dorsal side of the stomach. The dorsal portion of the stomach can be separated from the avascular tissue on which it rests with a light sweep of the fingers. In addition, this facilitates manipulation of the greater curvature of the stomach to gain easier and more certain exposure of the short gastric vessels as they are ligated with 3-0 silk and divided.

H

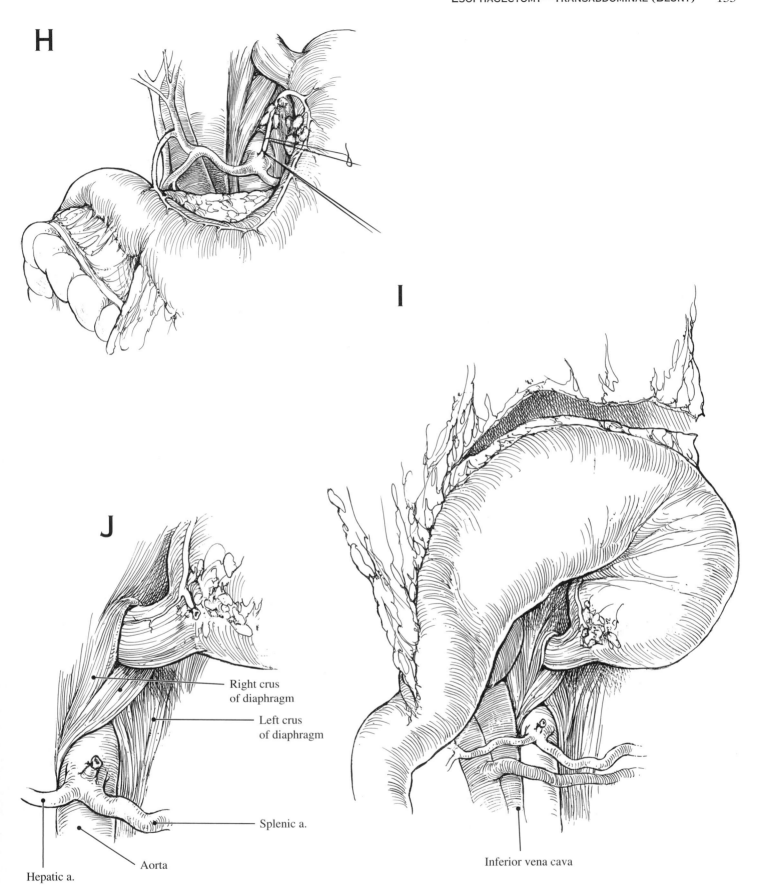

I

J

Right crus
of diaphragm

Left crus
of diaphragm

Splenic a.

Hepatic a.

Aorta

Inferior vena cava

H, I, J

The left gastric artery is divided as close as possible to its origin; for the sake of anatomic clarity, it is shown skeletonized here. In practice, lymph nodes of the celiac axis are included on the gastric side of the vessel; shortly they will be part of the specimen when the upper part of the stomach is removed.

K

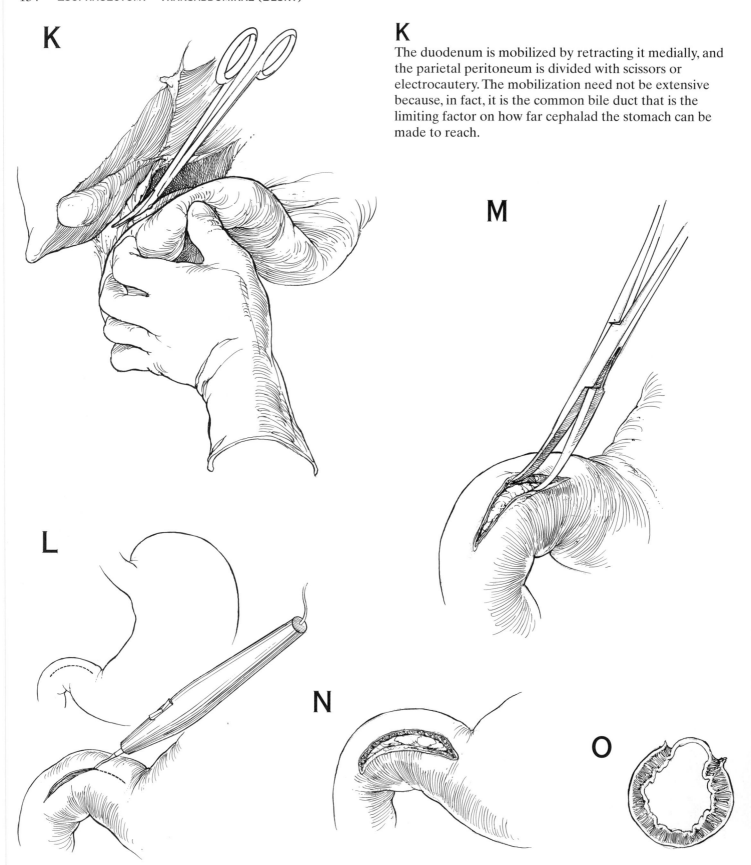

K

The duodenum is mobilized by retracting it medially, and the parietal peritoneum is divided with scissors or electrocautery. The mobilization need not be extensive because, in fact, it is the common bile duct that is the limiting factor on how far cephalad the stomach can be made to reach.

L, M, N, O

A pyloromyotomy is performed. The serosa of the area to be worked on is lightly scored with electrocautery and the muscle fibers gently spread with the convex side of a curved hemostat until they are disrupted. When this step is completed, the submucosa pouts and is at a level flush with the serosa.

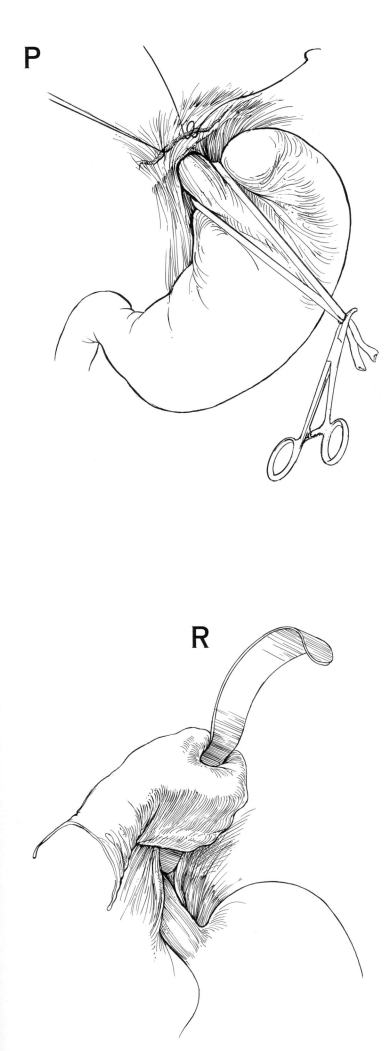

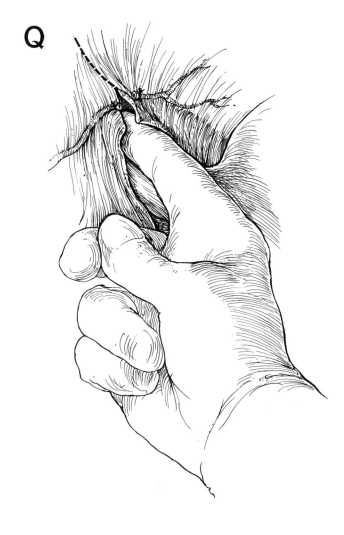

P, Q

The esophagus is looped with a small Penrose drain to facilitate placing traction on it. The esophageal hiatus needs to be enlarged to facilitate the esophageal dissection. In preparation for this, the moderately sized inferior phrenic vein is secured with a suture ligature on either side of the cut that will be made in line with the diaphragmatic fibers.

R

The acutely curved end of the handle of the Deaver retractor is hooked under the cut edge of the enlarged hiatus, a step that, when firm traction is used, provides ample exposure of the terminal esophagus, which can be dissected free.

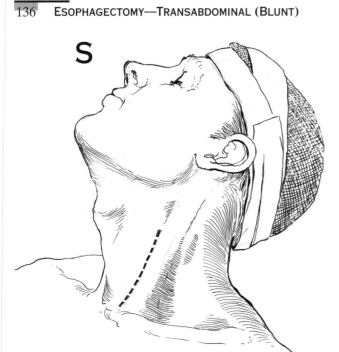

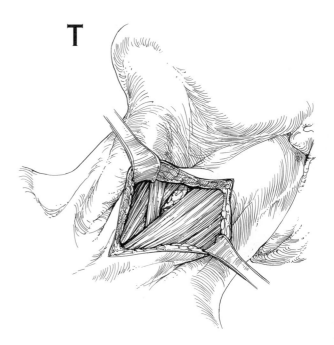

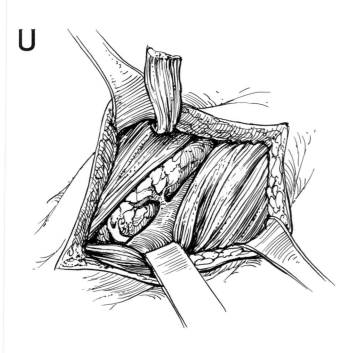

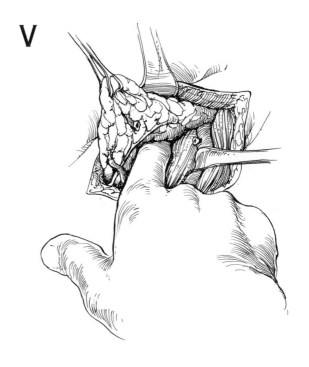

S, T

The abdominal field is temporarily abandoned, and attention is focused on mobilizing the cervical esophagus. A longitudinal incision is made along the anterior border of the lower two thirds of the sternocleidomastoid muscle and carried down to the internal jugular vein.

U

The middle thyroid vein is ligated with 3-0 silk and divided.

V

The thyroid gland is grasped with a Babcock forceps and retracted toward the right side; the index finger is used to free the esophagus from the prevertebral fascia. The anterior surface of the esophagus is freed next, making certain throughout that the recurrent laryngeal nerve is in view and is not injured.

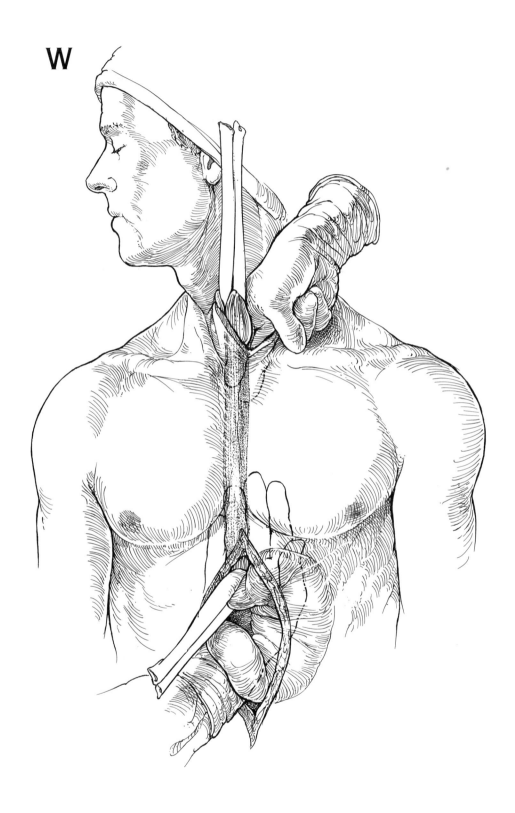

W, X, Y

In this series of illustrations, the fingers and hand are used to dissect; they will need to be in almost every position to get the job done. They are more effective, however, if their palmar surfaces face the esophagus whenever possible.

X

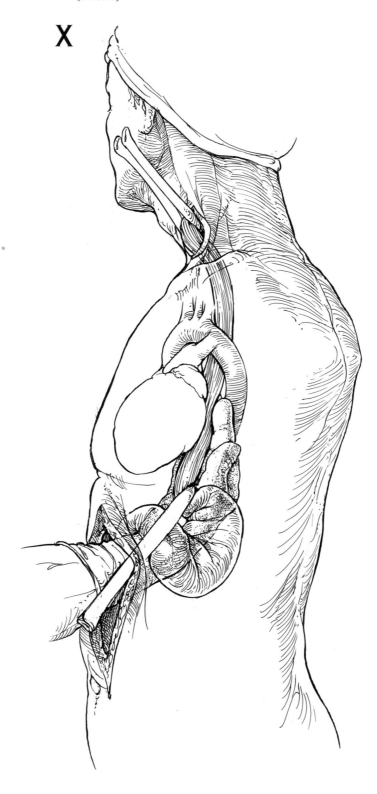

X

A large Penrose drain is looped around the cervical esophagus and is used for traction during the upper esophageal dissection. A similar drain is looped around the esophagus at the esophagogastric junction during the dissection in this area. The bulky stomach can get in the way during the low dissection, so one can divide the stomach at the anticipated point now to get it out of the way; the looped Penrose drain will not slip off.

The posterior aspect of the esophagus is approached. The entire hand (or just four fingers) can be insinuated through the enlarged esophageal hiatus.

Y

As to the thoracic inlet, usually only two fingers will fit into it. A tightly folded sponge on a ring forceps can help with the deeper areas of the dissection from above.

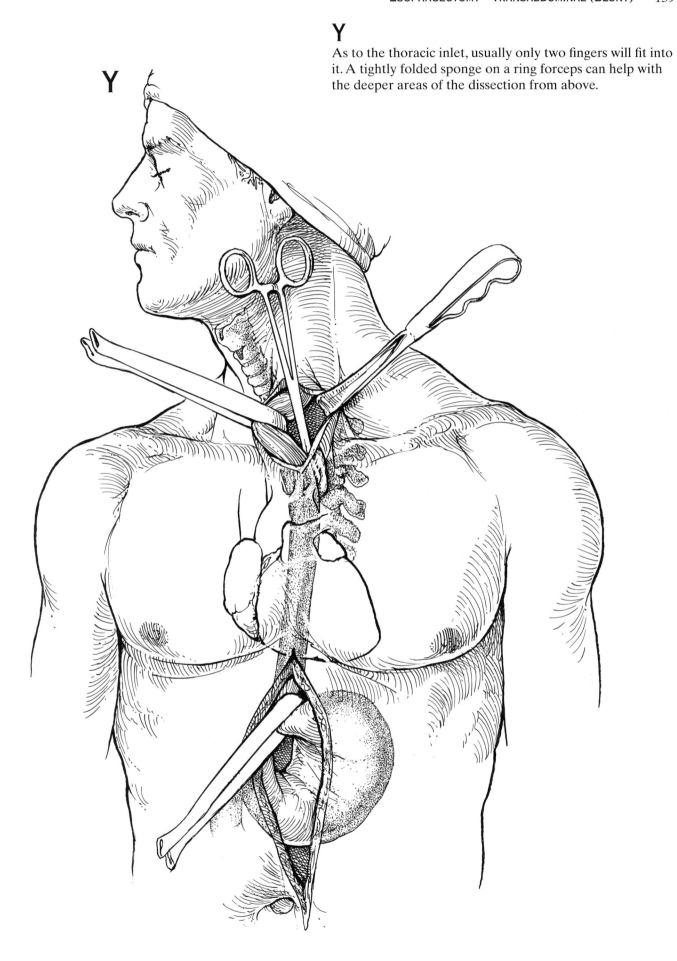

Y

Z

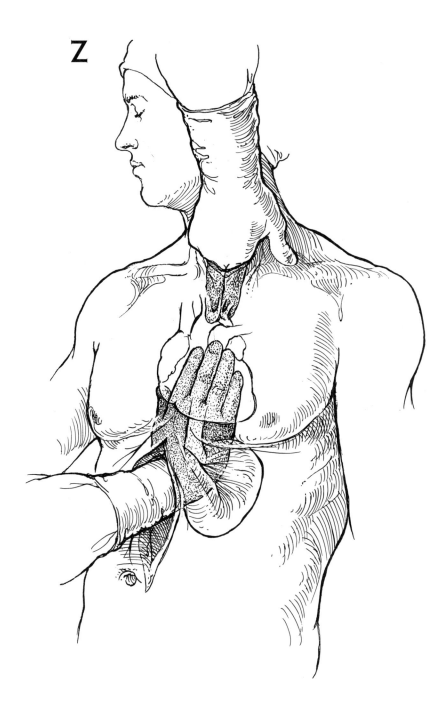

Z

After the dorsal surface of the esophagus is fixed, the hands are rotated and dissection of the ventral surface of the esophagus is begun.

AA

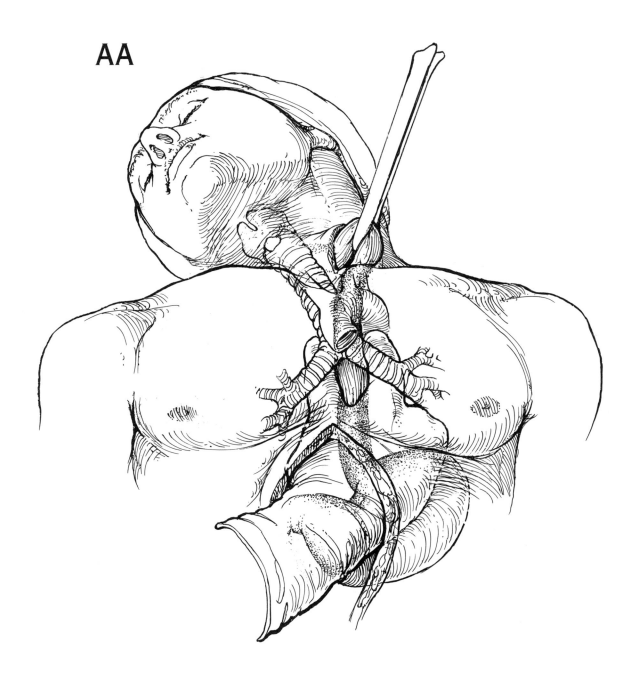

AA

The carina needs special attention if its membranous portion is not to be torn during the dissection at this level; this is especially so when the cancer is opposite the carina. The entire hand can now be inserted from below.

BB, CC

Using two fingers to dissect the esophagus provides the necessary delicate touch and is less likely to lead the surgeon to rely on strength to accomplish the task. Ideally, simple spreading of the index and middle fingers or sweeping them side to side will suffice. Or the fingers can straddle the esophagus and perform both a sweep and pull motion. On occasion, the thumb and index finger need to be used to "squeeze" the tissue apart.

BB

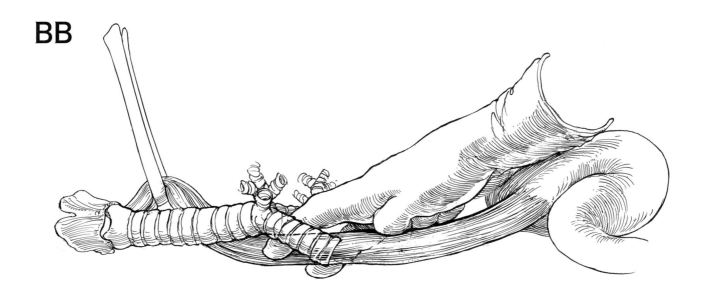

CC

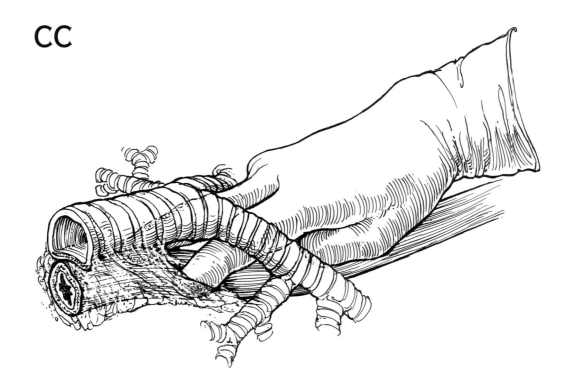

DD

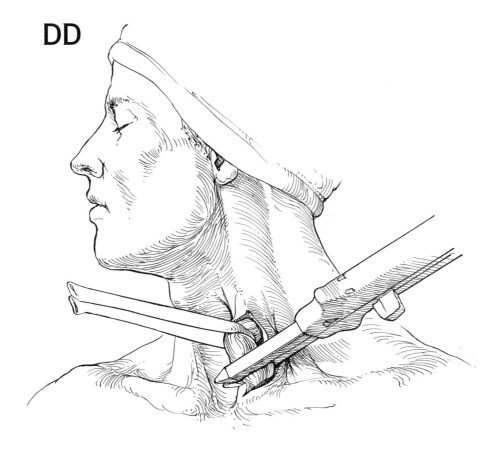

DD

With the stomach and esophagus mobilized, upward traction is applied to the cervical esophagus as it is stapled as low as possible.

EE

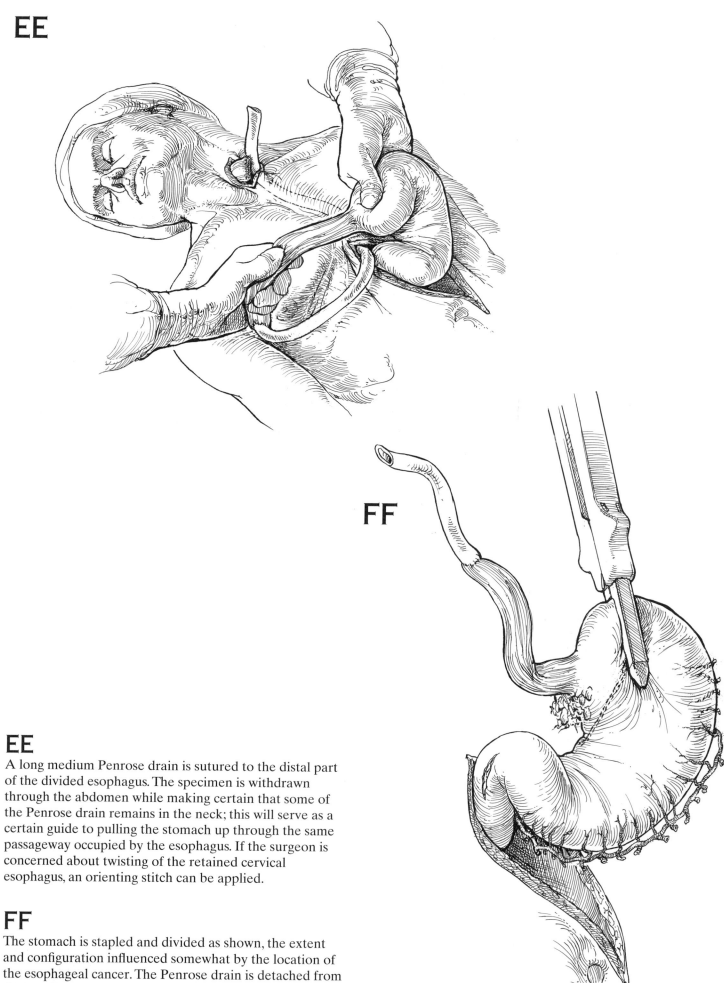

FF

EE

A long medium Penrose drain is sutured to the distal part of the divided esophagus. The specimen is withdrawn through the abdomen while making certain that some of the Penrose drain remains in the neck; this will serve as a certain guide to pulling the stomach up through the same passageway occupied by the esophagus. If the surgeon is concerned about twisting of the retained cervical esophagus, an orienting stitch can be applied.

FF

The stomach is stapled and divided as shown, the extent and configuration influenced somewhat by the location of the esophageal cancer. The Penrose drain is detached from the esophagus and reattached to a leading portion of the stomach.

GG

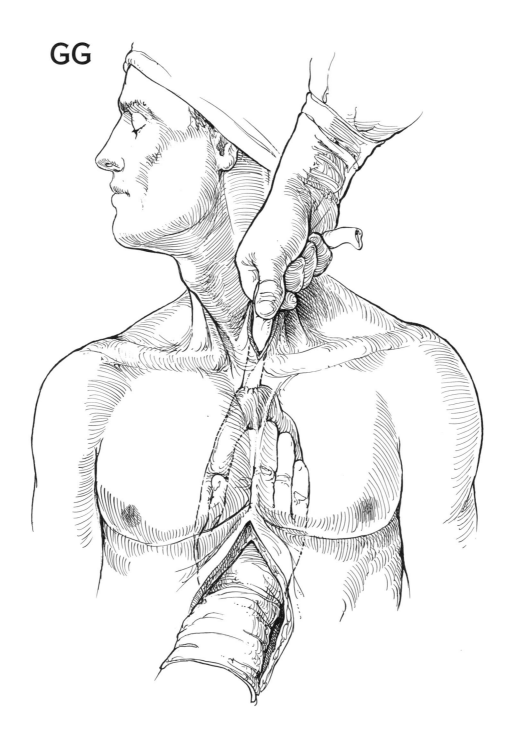

GG

The stomach is kept in its natural anteroposterior orientation as it is gently pushed through the chest by the full hand from below and pulled and guided by the Penrose drain from above.

HH

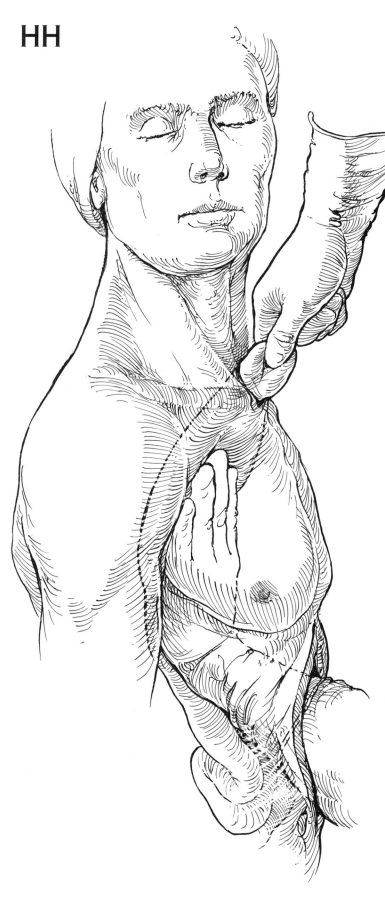

HH

As the stomach appears at the thoracic inlet, the presenting portion is grasped with index finger and thumb, and enough of it is brought into the neck to effect the anastomosis.

II

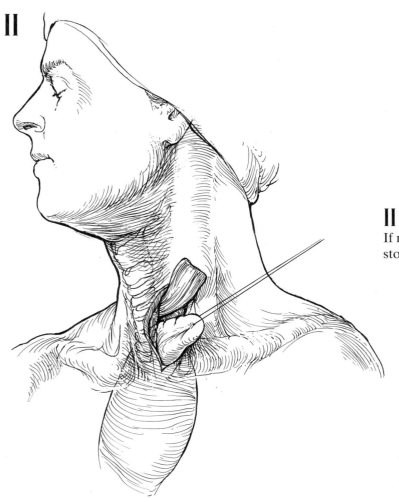

II

If needed, a traction stitch can be used to maintain the stomach in position.

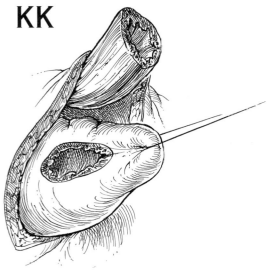

KK

JJ

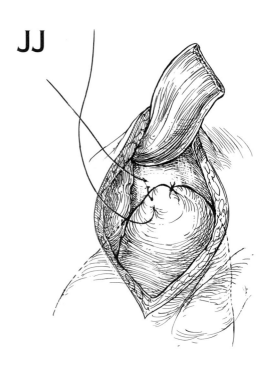

JJ

An area of the dorsal surface of the stomach, several centimeters caudal to the intended area of anastomosis, is chosen to anchor the stomach to the prevertebral fascia with two or three stitches of 2-0 silk.

KK

An opening is made in the stomach that is equal in diameter to that in the esophagus.

LL

MM

NN

OO

PP

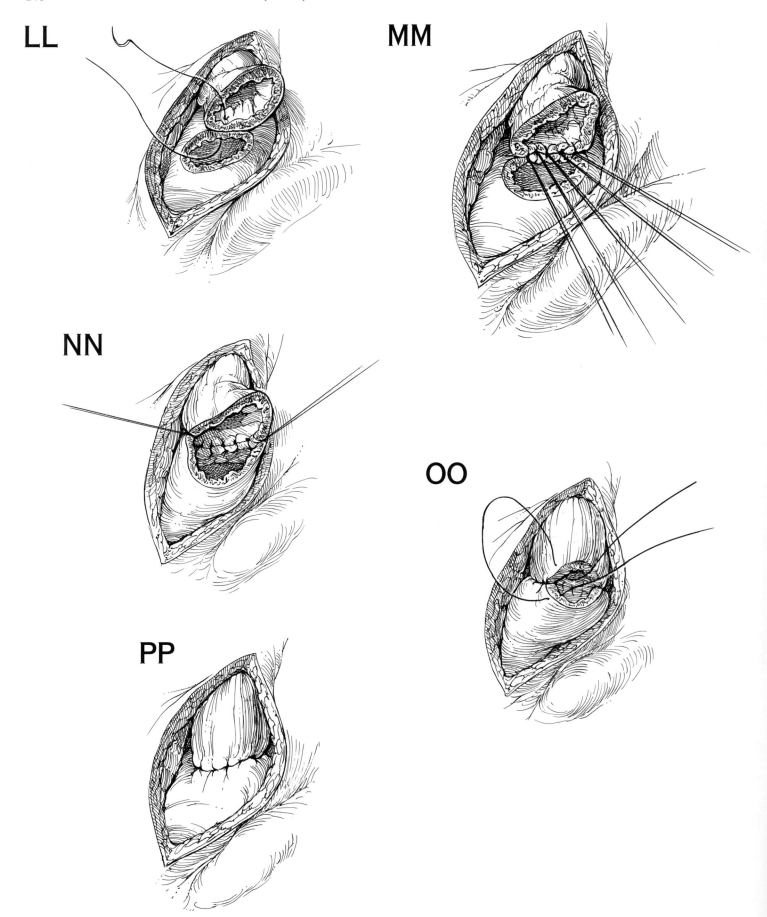

LL, MM, NN, OO, PP

The stitching is simple and interrupted with nonabsorbable material. The stitches are so placed that the knots and cut suture ends lie in the lumen of the esophagogastric anastomosis rather than within the interphase between esophagus and stomach.

QQ

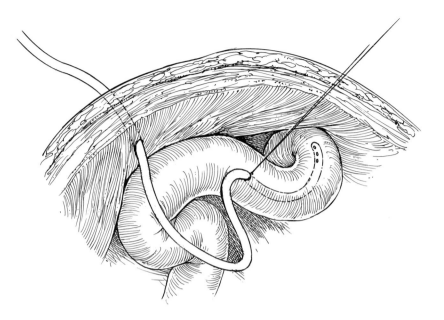

QQ, RR, SS
A jejunostomy is performed. Notice that the tube is "tunneled" in the area it enters the jejunum.

RR

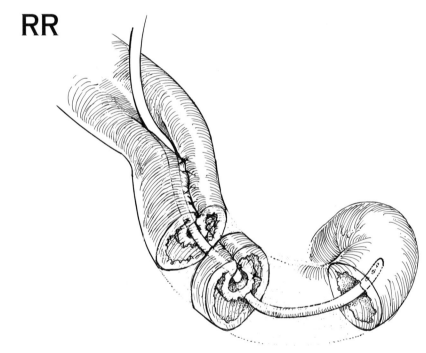

SS

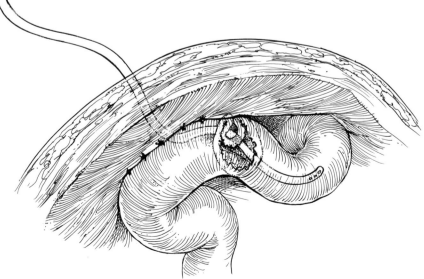

TT

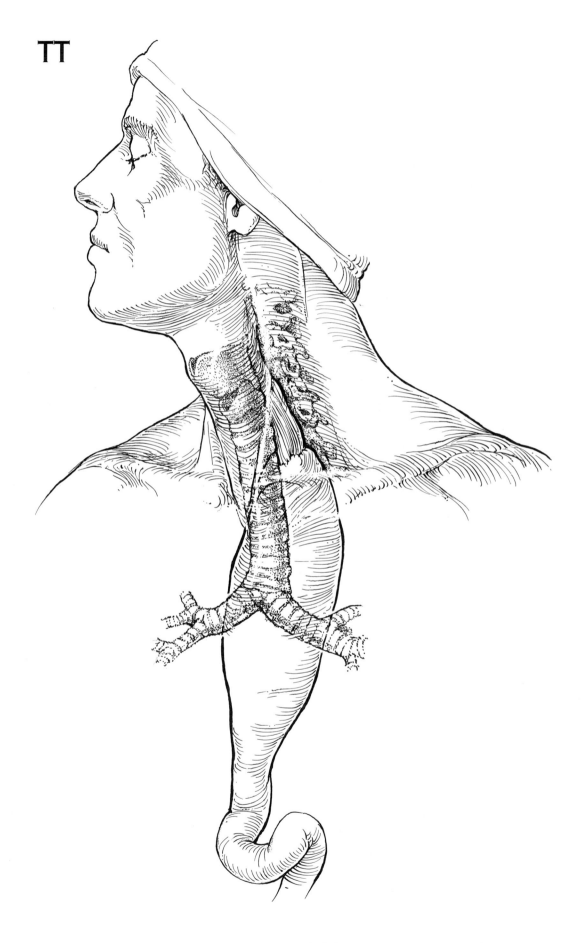

TT

The abdominal cavity is given a final examination, and closure is performed in a preferred manner.

COLON INTERPOSITION—ANTIPERISTALTIC

Blunt esophagectomy with gastric pull-up is swiftly becoming the favored operation for esophageal cancer. Sometimes, however, clinical and operative constraints do not permit this approach, nor for that matter the Ivor-Lewis intrathoracic esophagectomy with primary anastomosis. In such instances, one can interpose the colon as an esophageal substitute.

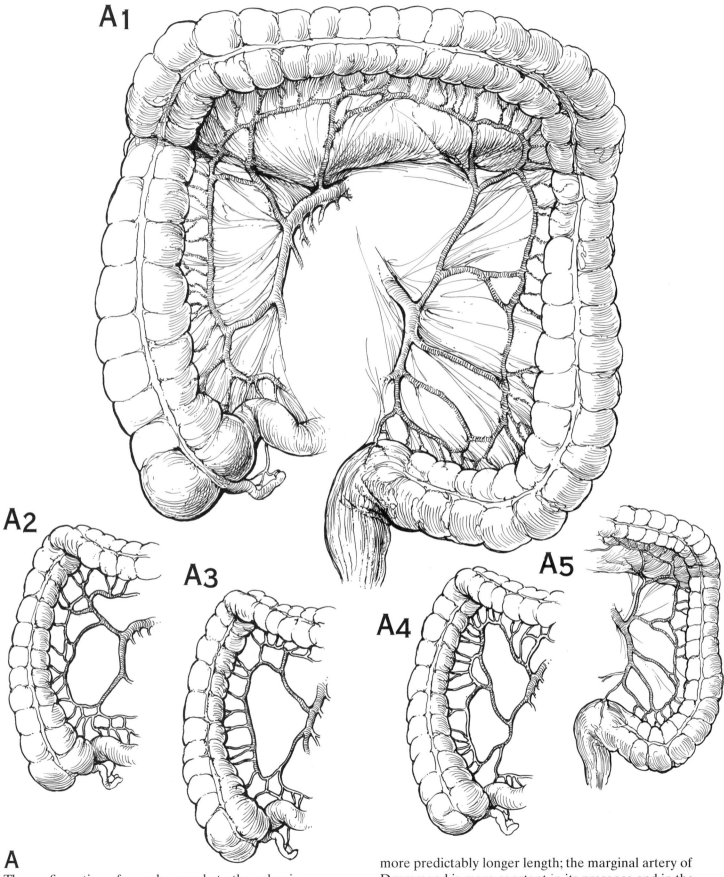

A1

A2

A3

A4

A5

A

The configuration of vascular supply to the colon is sufficiently varied that it must be examined carefully before deciding which segment of the colon to use. One of the advantages of using the left segment of the colon is its more predictably longer length; the marginal artery of Drummond is more constant in its presence and in the adequacy of its vascular pattern. In addition, it is more nearly the diameter of the esophagus to which it will be anastomosed.

B

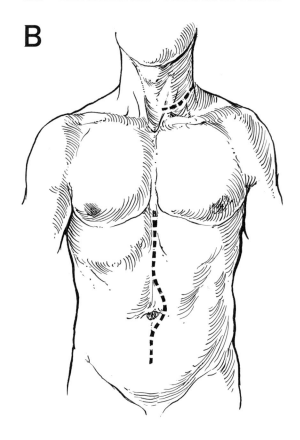

B

The incision extends the full length of the abdomen.

C

The abdominal cavity is examined for metastasis that might preclude performing the operation. The omentum is excised. The left lateral peritoneal reflection is cut with a fine-tipped cautery from the splenic fixture to the first part of the sigmoid colon. The transverse colon is mobilized to the right of the middle colic artery and vein while staying inside the gastroepiploic vessels.

C

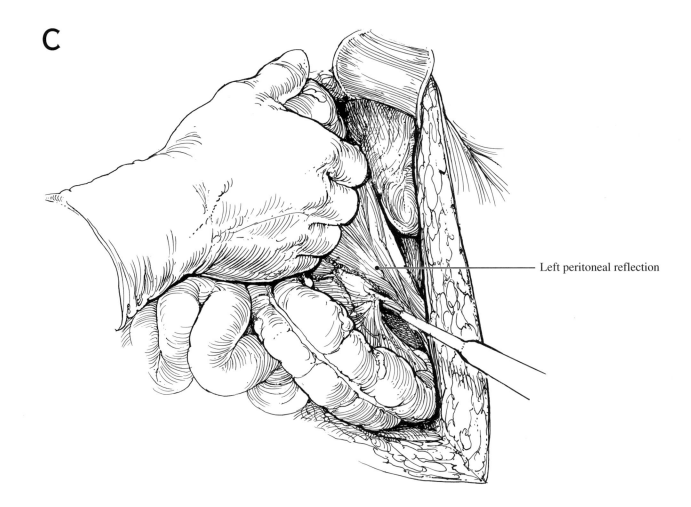

Left peritoneal reflection

D

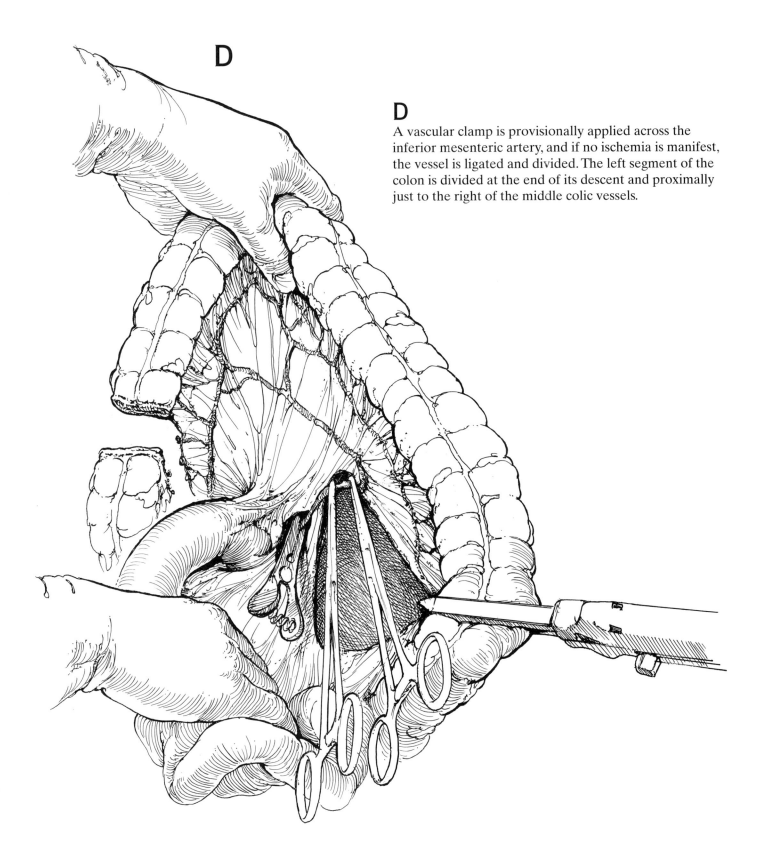

D

A vascular clamp is provisionally applied across the inferior mesenteric artery, and if no ischemia is manifest, the vessel is ligated and divided. The left segment of the colon is divided at the end of its descent and proximally just to the right of the middle colic vessels.

E

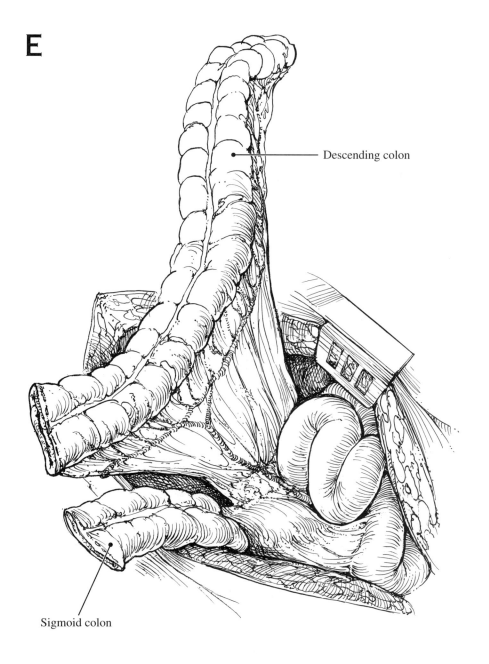

Descending colon

Sigmoid colon

E

The divided end of the sigmoid colon is swung cephalad to see if it reaches the neck easily.

F

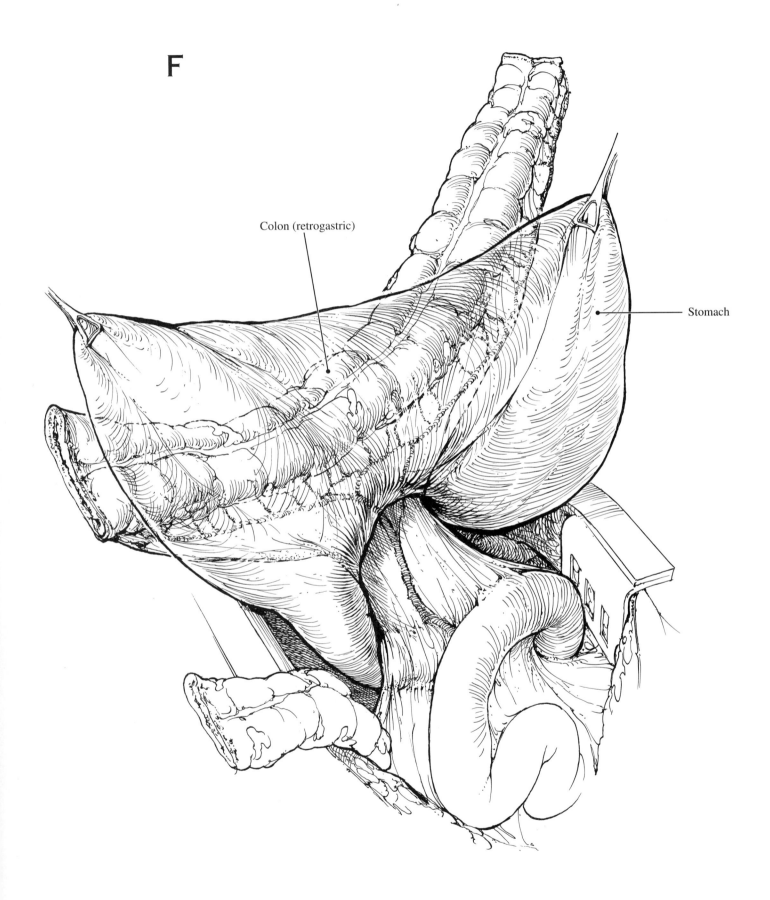

Colon (retrogastric)

Stomach

F

An opening in the avascular area of the gastrohepatic
omentum is made and the colon segment passed through it.

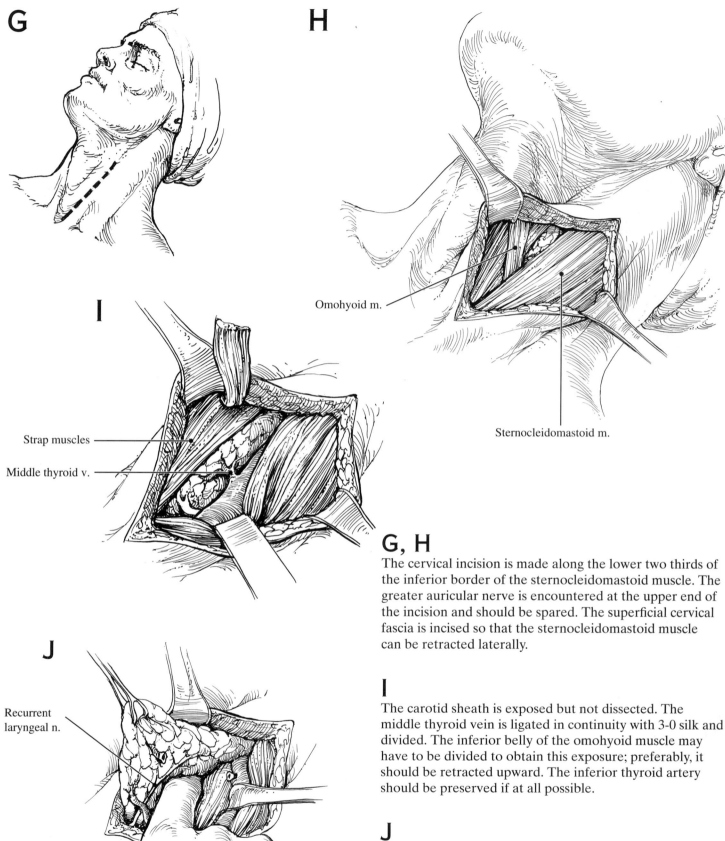

G

H

Omohyoid m.

Sternocleidomastoid m.

I

Strap muscles

Middle thyroid v.

J

Recurrent
laryngeal n.

G, H

The cervical incision is made along the lower two thirds of
the inferior border of the sternocleidomastoid muscle. The
greater auricular nerve is encountered at the upper end of
the incision and should be spared. The superficial cervical
fascia is incised so that the sternocleidomastoid muscle
can be retracted laterally.

I

The carotid sheath is exposed but not dissected. The
middle thyroid vein is ligated in continuity with 3-0 silk and
divided. The inferior belly of the omohyoid muscle may
have to be divided to obtain this exposure; preferably, it
should be retracted upward. The inferior thyroid artery
should be preserved if at all possible.

J

The thyroid gland can now be rotated medially, exposing
the recurrent laryngeal nerve, which is protected from
harm. The finger is placed on the cervical prevertebral
fascia, and the esophagus is dissected away from it. The
overlying trachea is gently separated from the cervical
esophagus. The vessels through this portion of the
esophagus come from the inferior thyroid artery and
usually do not require ligation. Because the esophagus
lacks a serosa, it is more fragile than the intestine and
should be handled gently.

K

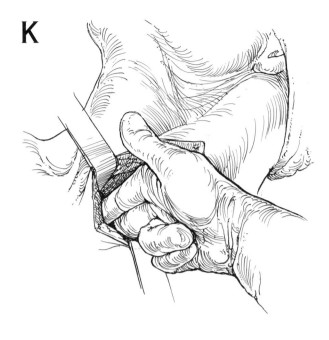

K

The finger is used to dissect the esophagus free at the thoracic inlet so that the fullest length will be available later.

L

The cervical esophagus is stapled and divided as low as possible and the distal end allowed to fall back into the thorax. The proximal side is trimmed of staples and oriented with an anteriorly placed stitch.

L

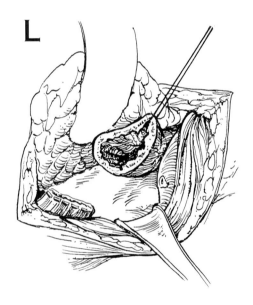

M

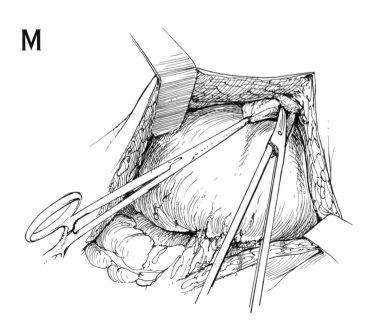

M

Attention is again directed to the upper abdomen, where the xiphoid process is excised for the several centimeters of additional exposure it provides and as a prelude to the substernal dissection.

N

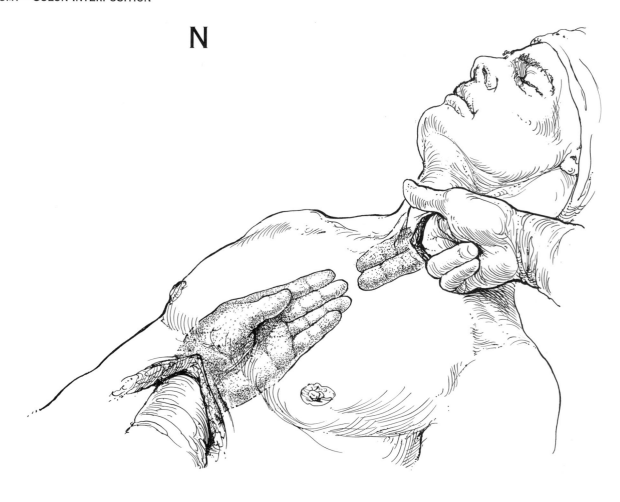

N, O

The retrosternal tunnel is now developed entirely by fingers and then the hand. From above one should strive for at least a three-finger opening if possible; from below, it is desirable to develop an opening large enough for entry of the entire hand. The sagittal view shows how the fingers work toward each other in establishing the substernal tunnel. For the hand progressing upward from below, both fingers and thumb need to be held together tightly if it is to fit into this confined space.

O

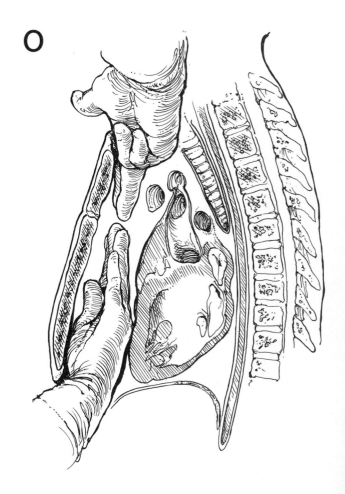

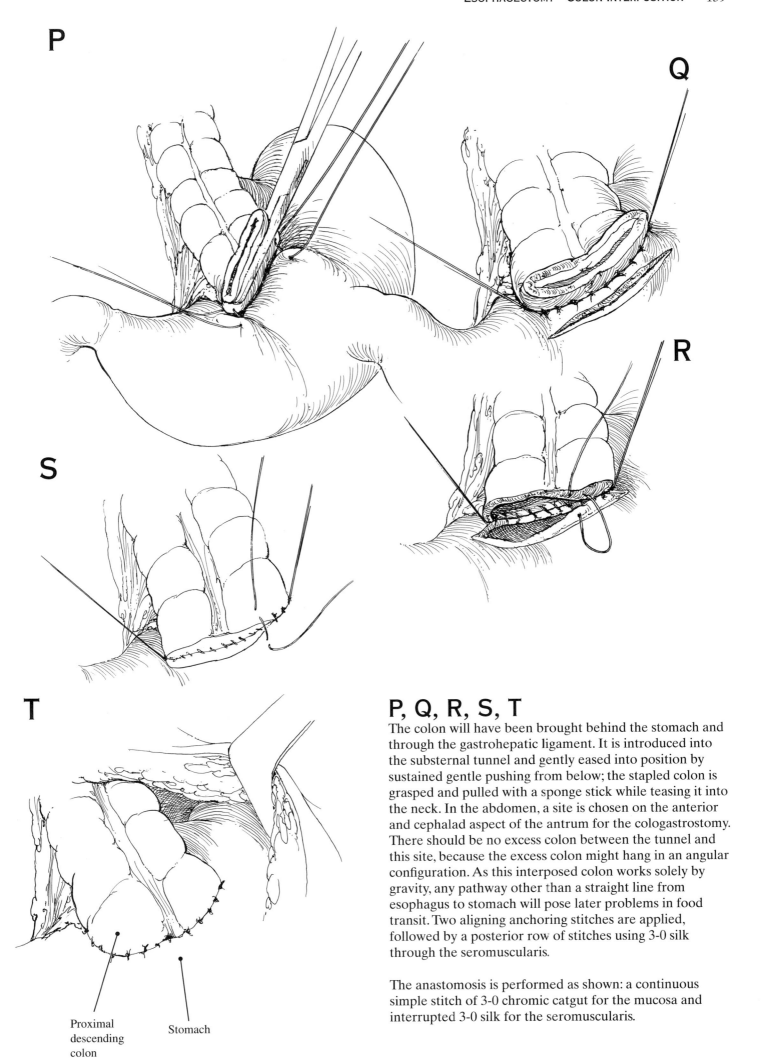

P

Q

R

S

T

Proximal
descending
colon

Stomach

P, Q, R, S, T

The colon will have been brought behind the stomach and through the gastrohepatic ligament. It is introduced into the substernal tunnel and gently eased into position by sustained gentle pushing from below; the stapled colon is grasped and pulled with a sponge stick while teasing it into the neck. In the abdomen, a site is chosen on the anterior and cephalad aspect of the antrum for the cologastrostomy. There should be no excess colon between the tunnel and this site, because the excess colon might hang in an angular configuration. As this interposed colon works solely by gravity, any pathway other than a straight line from esophagus to stomach will pose later problems in food transit. Two aligning anchoring stitches are applied, followed by a posterior row of stitches using 3-0 silk through the seromuscularis.

The anastomosis is performed as shown: a continuous simple stitch of 3-0 chromic catgut for the mucosa and interrupted 3-0 silk for the seromuscularis.

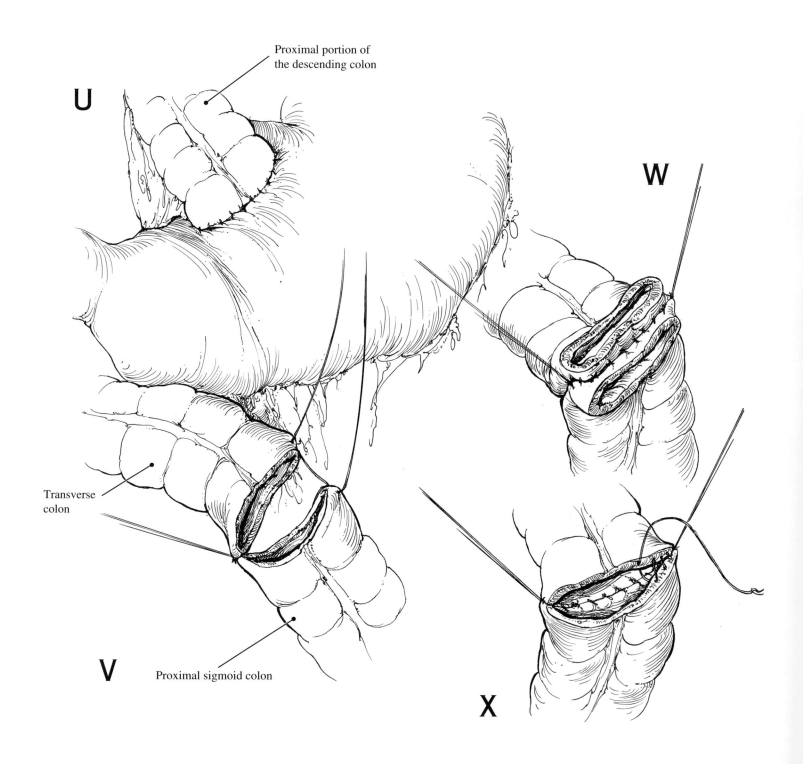

U

Proximal portion of
the descending colon

W

Transverse
colon

V

Proximal sigmoid colon

X

U, V, W, X

The colocolostomic anastomosis is performed in a similar
manner: a continuous simple stitch of 3-0 chromic catgut
for the mucosa and interrupted simple stitches of 3-0 silk
for the seromuscularis.

Y

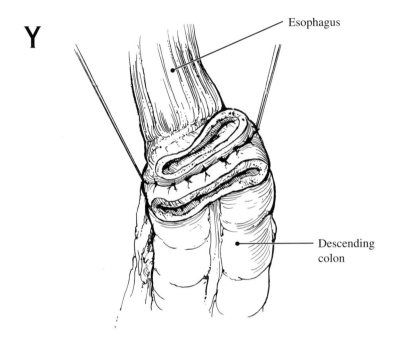

Esophagus

Descending
colon

Z

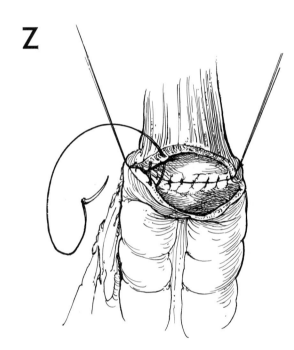

AA

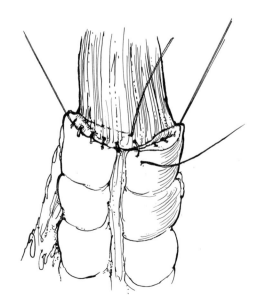

Y, Z, AA

The esophagocolic anastomosis in the neck is closed
similarly. The esophagus, lacking a serosa, can be cut
through easily by stitches that are tied too snugly. The
longitudinal direction of the outer muscular layer of the
esophagus allows stitches to cut through readily with even
slight tension. Having the needle go through the
esophageal bite on a bias, offers some improvement in
holding power. Occasionally the manubrium needs to be
resected so that venous congestion of the colonic segment
in the neck does not occur.

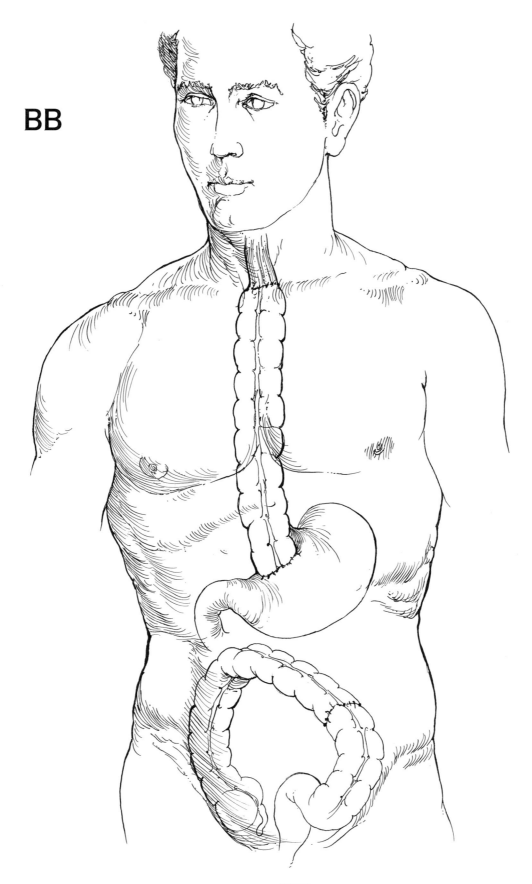

BB

A Stamm gastrostomy is performed with care so that it does not distort the stomach. A small Penrose drain is placed at the esophagocolic anastomosis and brought out through a counterincision. The neck wound is closed in one layer with 5-0 nylon. A Jackson-Pratt drain is placed at the cologastrostomy and brought out through a counterincision. The abdomen is closed in a preferred manner.

B ZENKER'S DIVERTICULECTOMY

A

Zenker's diverticulum, the most commonly occurring pulsion diverticulum, manifests at the superior transverse fibers of the cricopharyngeal muscle and inferior to the oblique fibers of the inferior pharyngeal constrictor muscle. The other types, hypopharyngeal and cervical, are both uncommon. It is believed that the diverticulum is related to incoordination of relaxation and retraction of the cricopharyngeal muscle. Diverticula smaller than 1.5 cm can be treated simply by a cricopharyngeal myotomy. Larger ones are excised, sometimes in combination with a myotomy.

This dorsal view demonstrates the anatomy pertinent to a Zenker's diverticulum.

B

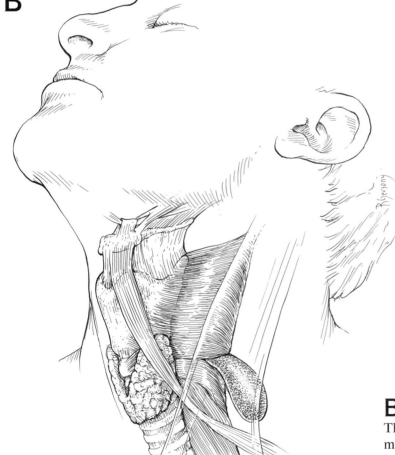

 A

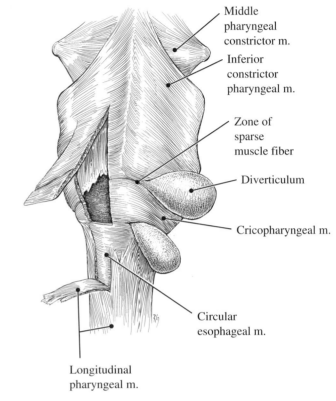

Middle pharyngeal constrictor m.

Inferior constrictor pharyngeal m.

Zone of sparse muscle fiber

Diverticulum

Cricopharyngeal m.

Circular esophageal m.

Longitudinal pharyngeal m.

B

This oblique frontal view highlights the structures that must be dissected to reach and resect the diverticulum. The incision is made along a transverse skin crease and through the platysma to the superficial cervical fascia.

The anterior border of the middle one third of the sternocleidomastoid muscle is mobilized and retracted dorsally. The omohyoid muscle is in the field and should be dissected free and retracted; if necessary, it can be cut with near impunity. The thyroid gland should be rotated or retracted medially for more exact visualization of the neck of the diverticulum and of the recurrent laryngeal nerve that needs to be protected from harm.

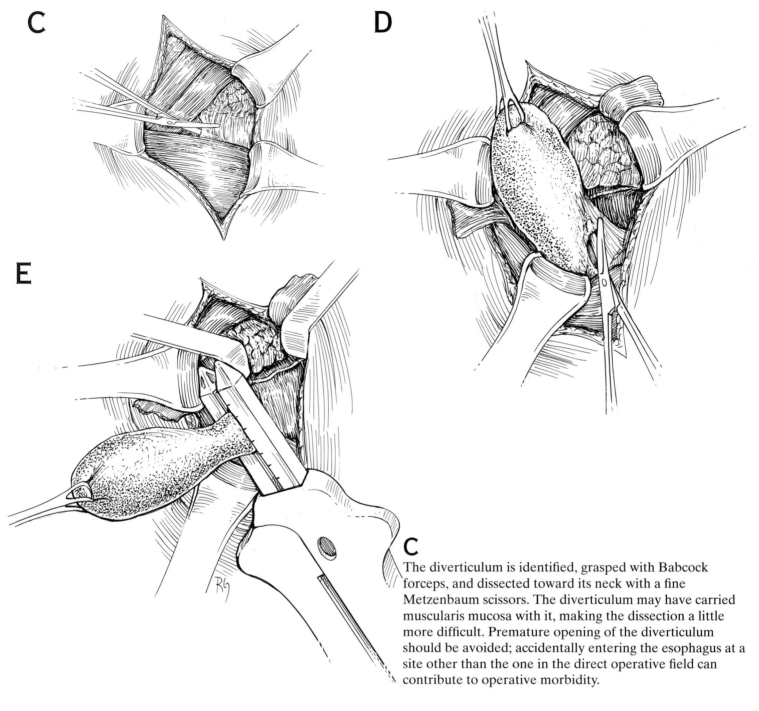

C

The diverticulum is identified, grasped with Babcock forceps, and dissected toward its neck with a fine Metzenbaum scissors. The diverticulum may have carried muscularis mucosa with it, making the dissection a little more difficult. Premature opening of the diverticulum should be avoided; accidentally entering the esophagus at a site other than the one in the direct operative field can contribute to operative morbidity.

D

The diverticulum has been freed; accurate delineation of the junction of the neck and esophagus is important.

E

A GIA stapler is applied across the neck of the diverticulum and fired with care that the size of the esophageal lumen is not compromised and the amputation stump left behind is not unduly long.

The wound is examined for bleeding or leak and proper placement of staples. A small suction drain is positioned adjacent to the staple line and brought out through a counterincision. Alternatively, a small Penrose drain can be brought to the outside through the incision. The platysma and skin are closed as one layer with vertical mattress stitches of 5-0 nylon.

Chapter

9

ESOPHAGEAL HIATAL HERNIA

Ā HIATAL HERNIORRHAPHY

TRANSABDOMINAL (WITH NISSEN FUNDOPLICATION)

Esophageal hiatal hernia is the commonest of all diaphragmatic hernias and is seen more often in older patients. It is a sliding hernia, in that the cardia and stomach slide posteriorly and retroperitoneally up into the chest in such fashion that the anterior part of the hernia is invested with a hernial sac. Most of these hernias do not produce sufficient discomfort to warrant surgical correction. The operative approach for their correction can be abdominal—open or laparoscopic—or it can be performed transthoracically.

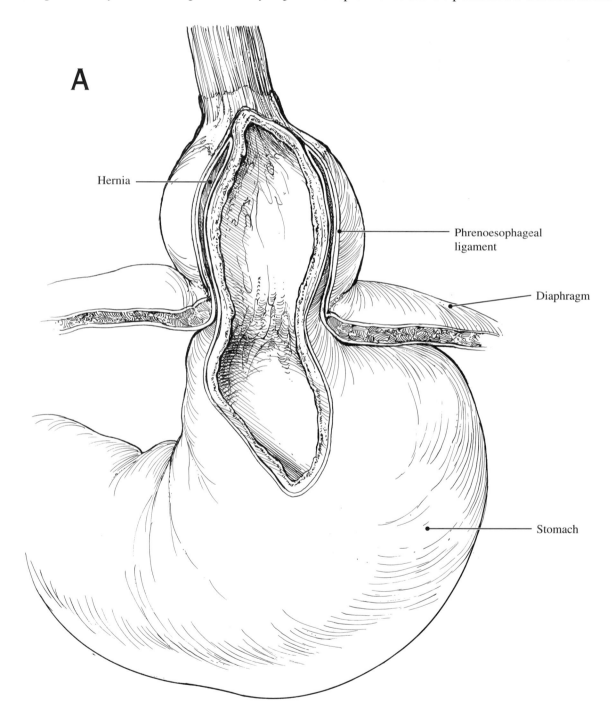

A

A

The pouch of peritoneum that includes an esophageal hiatal hernia is in front and to the right of the stomach; the anterior wall of the cardia of the stomach is the posterior wall of the hernial sac. The esophagogastric junction is located at a variable distance from the esophageal hiatus, just as the latter may be widened minimally or to the point of severe attenuation of the crural fibers. The transversalis fascia of the abdominal cavity and the mediastinal fascia of the thorax fuse at the esophageal hiatus to become the phrenoesophageal ligament, which is attached to the esophagus. Use of this ligament is an integral part of most types of repair.

B

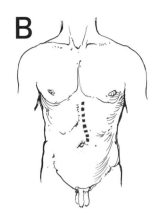

C

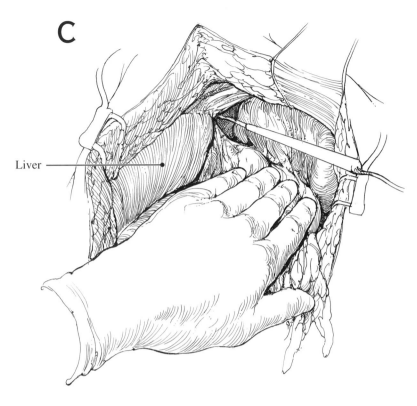

Liver

D

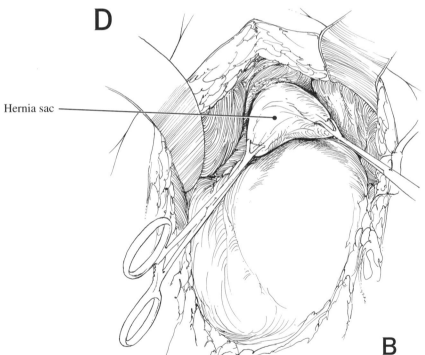

Hernia sac

B

A midline incision is used and carried up to the xiphoid process, which, if large and in the way, can be excised with impunity.

C

The left lobe of the liver is mobilized and retracted toward the patient's right to just short of the inferior vena cava. A laparotomy pad is placed over it and held in this position with a Deaver retractor.

D

With gentle traction on the stomach—here facilitated by a Babcock forceps on that portion of it that had been lying intrathoracically—the entire stomach is delivered into the abdominal cavity.

E

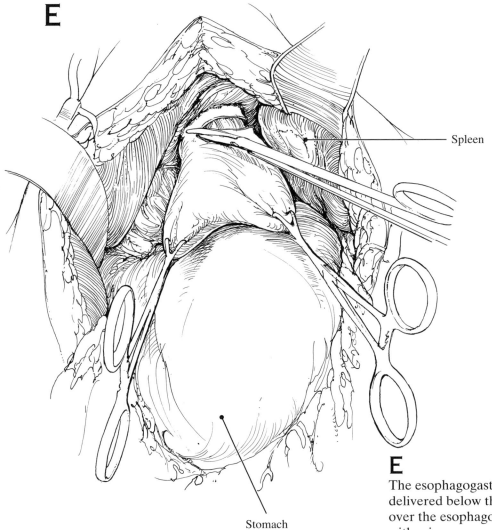

Spleen

Stomach

E

The esophagogastric junction will perforce have been
delivered below the esophageal hiatus. The peritoneum
over the esophagogastric junction is then cut transversely
with scissors.

Esophagus

F

Vagus n.

F

The left index finger is used to encircle the esophagus
and through this opening a small rubber drain is passed
and used for traction. All of any remaining peritoneum is
divided and the traction sustained; the esophagogastric
junction can be made to migrate 3 to 5 cm below the
esophageal hiatus in the diaphragm.

G

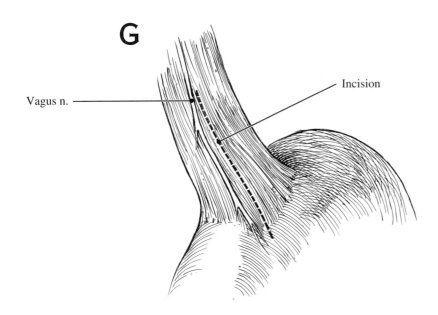

Vagus n.

Incision

H

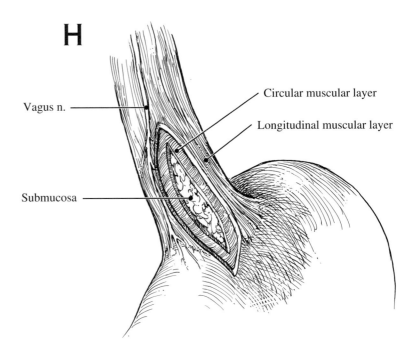

Vagus n.

Circular muscular layer

Longitudinal muscular layer

Submucosa

G, H

If a myotomy is necessary—usually carried out if there is
symptomatic reflux esophagitis—it is a simple matter to
perform one now by making a longitudinal cut through the
longitudinal and circular layer of the esophagus to the
submucosa. This segment of esophagus can be included in
the wraparound.

I

The crura must next be identified and prepared for approximation. In this illustration the operative area is purposely denuded of peritoneum and fatty tissue, and the stomach and liver are omitted. The esophageal hiatus is in the shape of an inverted teardrop. The rounded margin is located anteriorly, with the acutely angled margin located posteriorly; this is the "weak" area wherein the crural fibers must be approximated. The esophageal hiatus is almost always composed of fibers from the right crus, those of the left margin usually being thicker than those of the right. Notice how the muscle fibers of the right crus are arranged in a sling as they form the esophageal hiatus.

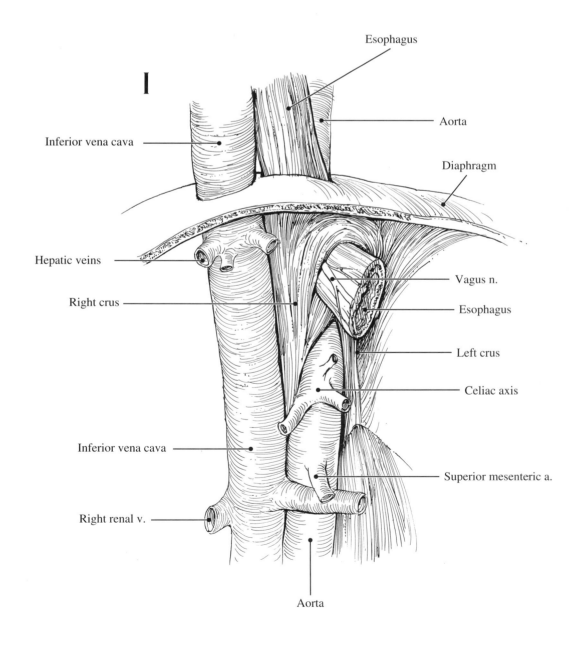

I

Esophagus

Aorta

Inferior vena cava

Diaphragm

Hepatic veins

Vagus n.

Right crus

Esophagus

Left crus

Celiac axis

Inferior vena cava

Superior mesenteric a.

Right renal v.

Aorta

J

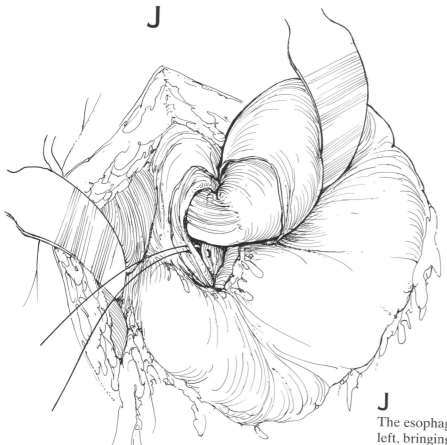

J

The esophagogastric junction is severely displaced to the left, bringing into view the right margin of the hiatus. Sutures readily cut through muscle, especially the thinner right marginal fibers. It is advisable, therefore, not to dissect the crura too thoroughly so that the muscle fibers can be buttressed by the peritoneum, which is included in the bite of the needle.

K

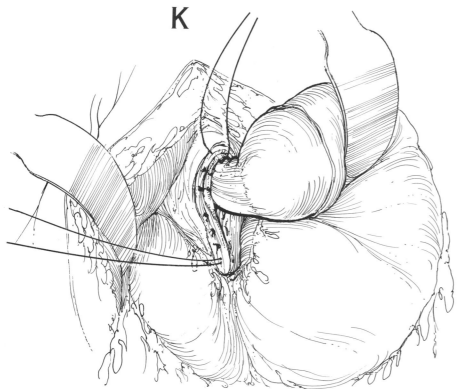

K

Three or four stitches of 1-0 silk are usually sufficient for repair of the hiatus. The surgeon should be cognizant of the nearby inferior vena cava during placement of these stitches.

L

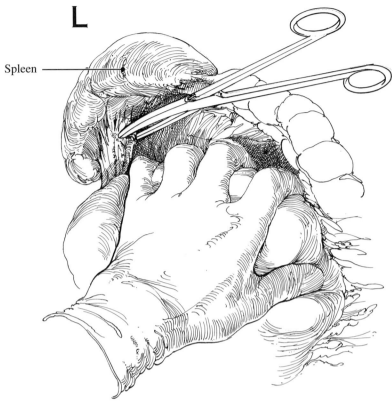

Spleen

M

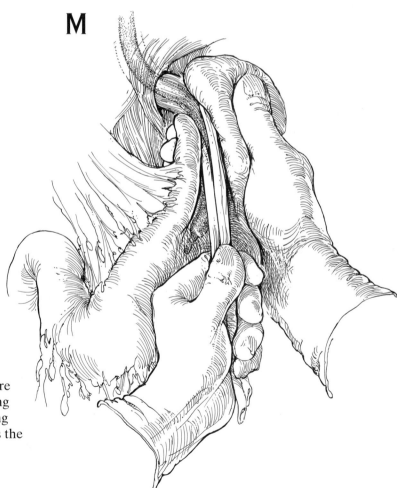

L

For anatomic clarity the fundoplication is illustrated here
without the crural approximation. It is begun by securing
the short gastric vessels with double clips before dividing
them. This facilitates the stomach wrap and also lessens the
risk that one of them might avulse the capsule of the
spleen.

M

Traction is applied on the Penrose drain to bring the
esophagus into the abdominal cavity and have the stomach
wrapped around it. A no. 58 Maloney dilator is placed
down the esophagus and into the stomach; this will ensure
that the wraparound of the esophagus is not too snug.

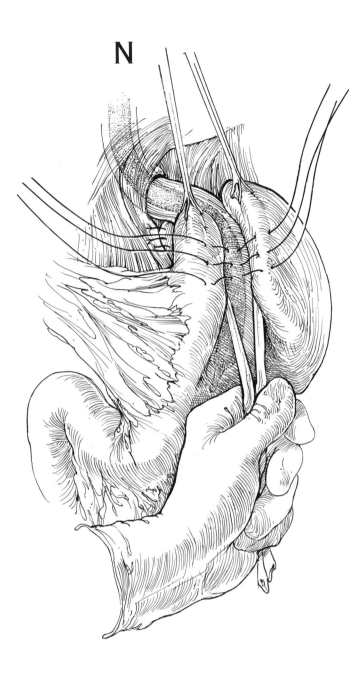

N

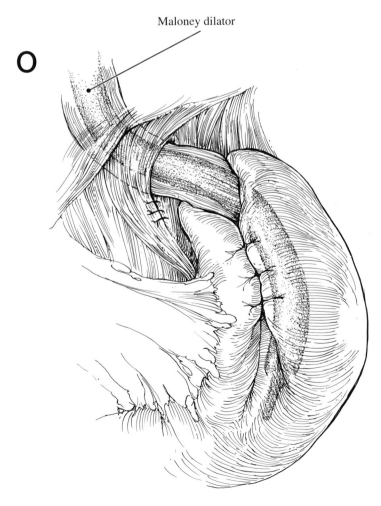

O

Maloney dilator

N, O

Three or four stitches of 1-0 silk are used to bring the
stomach together and hold it in the wraparound position. It
may help stabilize the wrap if the deep bites of the stitches
incorporate some of the longitudinal fibers of the
esophagus.

A

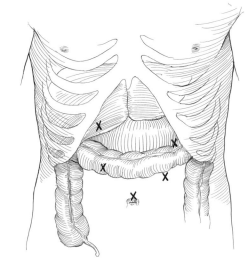

LAPAROSCOPIC (WITH NISSEN FUNDOPLICATION)

A

The port placements (marked by Xs) depend on the position of the operating surgeon. The preferred one is for the patient to be in the lithotomy position with the surgeon standing between the legs, the first assistant to the right of the patient, and the camera person to the left of the patient.

B

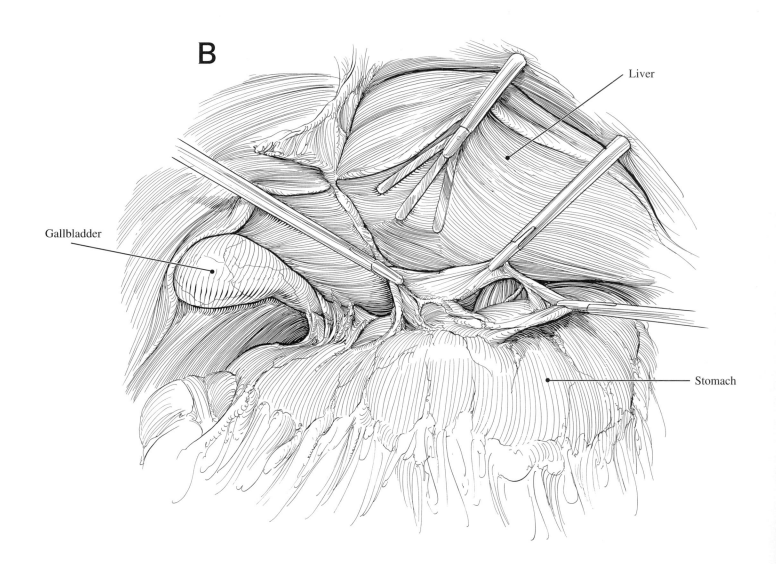

Liver

Gallbladder

Stomach

B

This panoramic view shows substantially more than is viewed through the laparoscope, and it is so rendered for purposes of orientation. Here, the peritoneum is being freed from over the esophagogastric junction. A Babcock forceps introduced through an inferior port and applying caudal traction on the stomach helps with this dissection (see *C*).

C

Esophagus

Vagus n.

Stomach

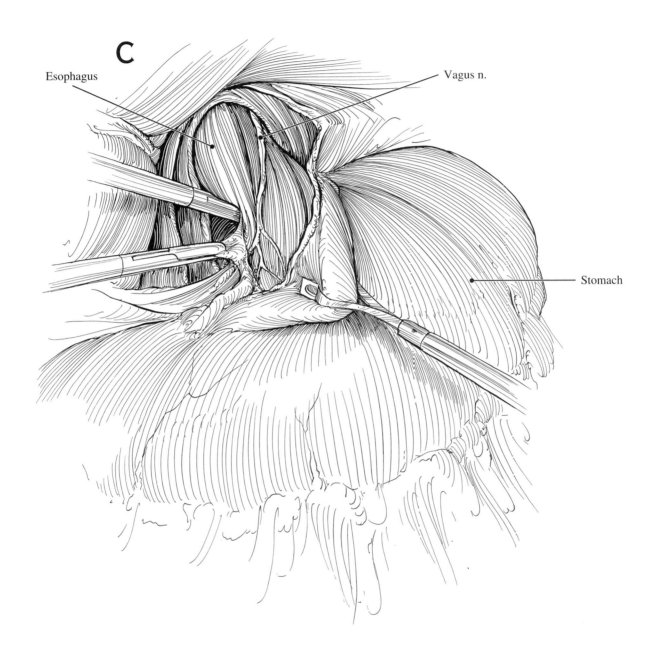

C

The peritoneum in the area of the esophagogastric junction has been dissected, exposing the anterior (left) vagus, which will be included in the wrap. The posterior vagus will not be incorporated within the wrap. The crura are cleaned so that they will be available for apposition. Also, a "window" is created behind the esophagus at its junction with the stomach as a passageway for the wrap.

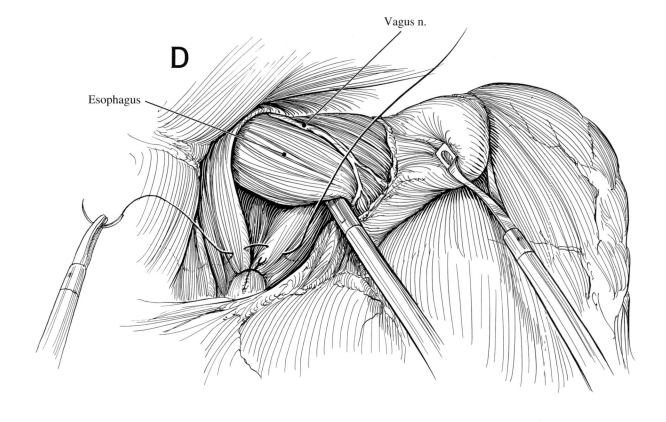

D

The left and right crura are brought together with two or three stitches of 1-0 silk or similarly stout nonabsorbable suture material. The crural closure must not constrict the esophagus. The vagus nerve most commonly is left above the crural closure and out of the wrap. Sometimes it is kept deep to the crura, to surface just below the last crural stitch.

E

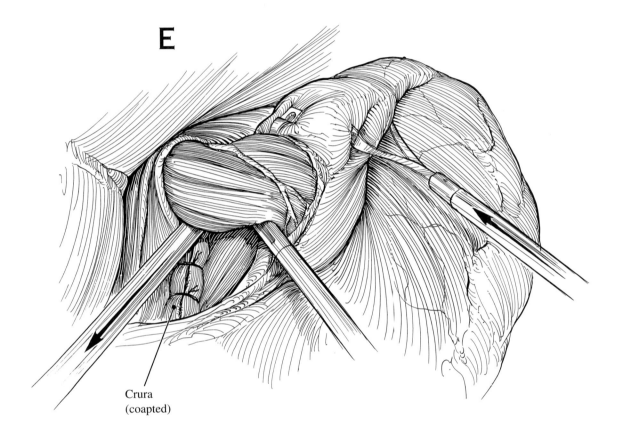

Crura
(coapted)

E

The short gastric vessels have been divided and ligated in the area of the fundus to be involved in the wrap. Not all the short gastric vessels need to be taken, but tension-free mobilization of the fundus must be ensured. One Babcock forceps has been passed through the window to grasp and pull a portion of the stomach fundus to the patient's right. A second Babcock assists by pushing the stomach through the window.

F

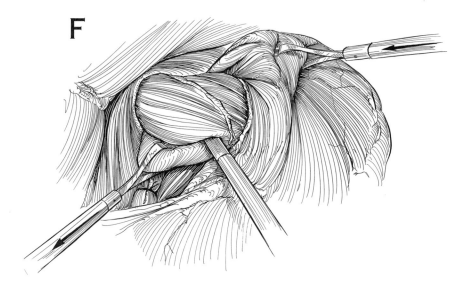

G

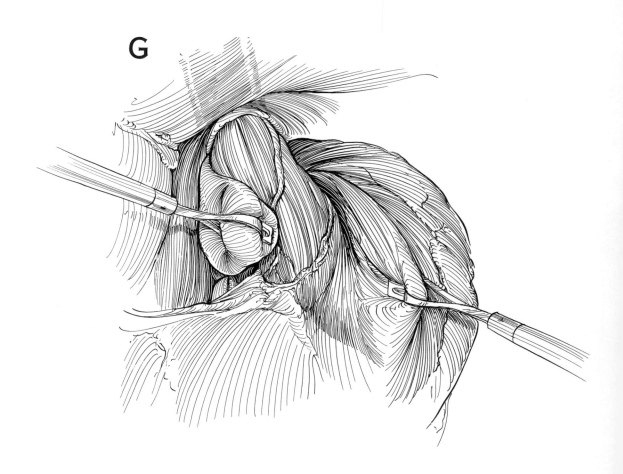

F, G

The fundus has been eased through the window. This
tug-push is gently continued until the surgeon feels there
will not be excessive tension on the stomach tissue when it
is stitched to itself as the wrap. The Maloney dilator, usually
a no. 58 French, has been positioned within the lumen as a
safeguard that the esophagogastric lumen being fashioned
will not be too tight.

Maloney dilator

H

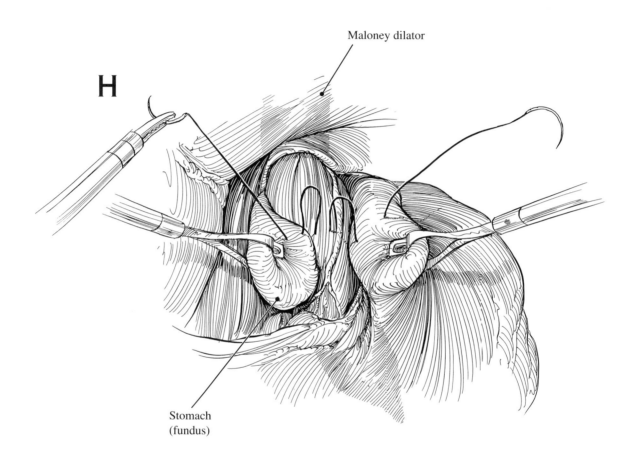

Stomach
(fundus)

H

The fundic tissue is stitched to itself, usually with three 2-0 nonabsorbable sutures placed 1 cm apart. The esophagus is incorporated in each stitch, taking care that the vagus nerve is excluded from it.

I

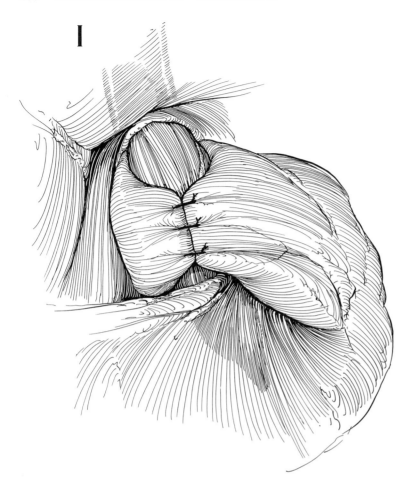

J

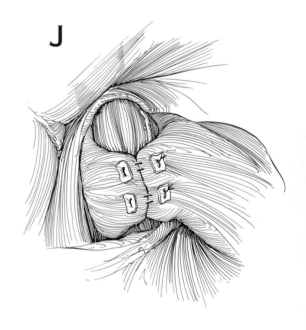

I, J

The stitching has been completed. Notice that the Maloney dilator has been in position all this time. It is removed, and a decompressing nasogastric tube may be placed at the surgeon's discretion. An alternative method of stitch placement is to use bolsters of Teflon with the sutures to lessen the risk of their cutting through the stomach tissue.

K

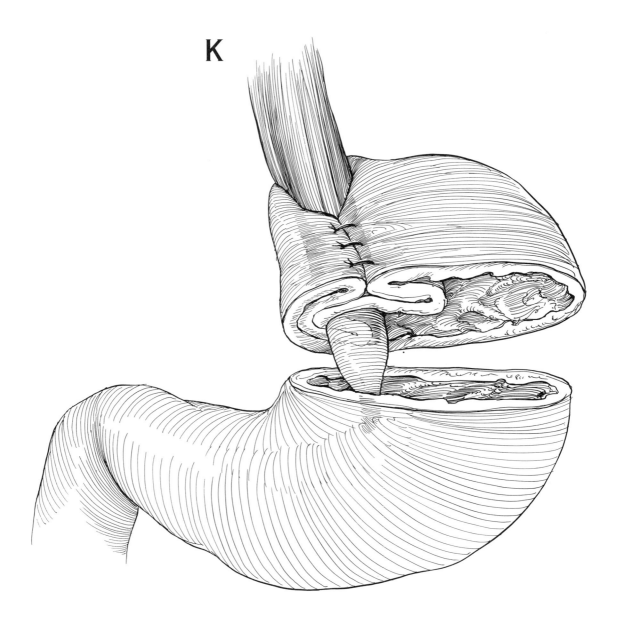

K

This cross-section of the stomach at the completion of the procedure demonstrates the desired effect. A final inspection is made, especially of the splenic area, for any bleeding associated with traction on the short gastric vessels, and the port sites are closed. The operation is completed in a routine manner.

A

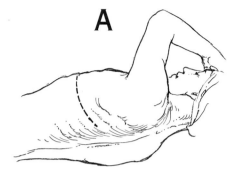

TRANSTHORACIC

The transthoracic approach to repair of an esophageal hiatal hernia consists of freeing the esophagus and herniated stomach and of opening the sac as far around the esophagogastric junction as possible and using this tissue where it joins the esophagus just above the cardia—the phrenoesophageal ligament—to suture to the diaphragmatic hiatus. The esophageal hiatus is tightened by sutures approximating the crura posterior to the cardia with heavy suture material. The reconstructed esophageal hiatus should permit a fingertip to comfortably pass next to the esophagus.

B

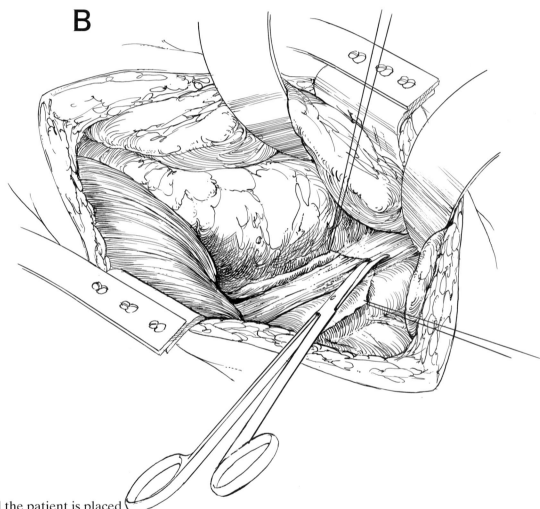

A

General anesthesia is used, and the patient is placed in the right lateral decibutus position. A lateral thoracotomy is made through the seventh intercostal space on the subperiosteally excised eighth rib.

B

When the pleural cavity has been entered, the left lower lobe is gently retracted upward. At its lowermost attachment, the inferior pulmonary ligament is divided with electrocautery and then dissected up to the level of the inferior pulmonary vein. The mediastinal pleura over the lowermost portion of the esophagus is incised. The dissection is continued to free the lateral portion of the lower esophagus for a distance of about 8 to 10 cm. Small arterial branches from the aorta that supply the lower portion of the esophagus are identified, for whatever exposure seems necessary, clipped, and divided.

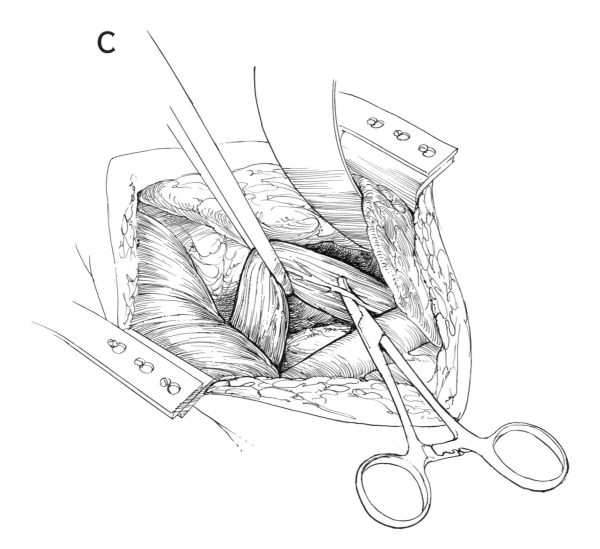

C

The remainder of the lower esophagus is dissected free from the surrounding mediastinal tissues by blunt finger dissection with care that the vagi are left in their normal anatomic positions and the right pleural space is not entered. A Penrose drain placed around the esophagus facilitates further dissection of the sac and the posterior aspects of the crura.

D

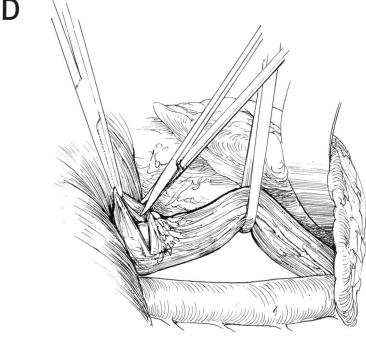

E

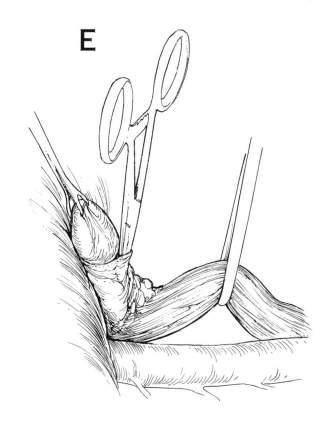

F

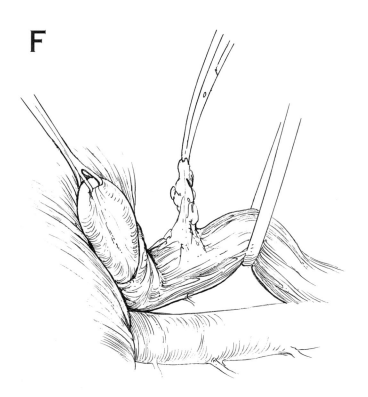

D, E, F

The medial and lateral components of the right crus are now dissected; this is begun with scissors, and the tissue over the crura is pushed away bluntly with a pledget of gauze at the tip of an 8-inch forceps. One must be careful that the lateral component of the crus is not attenuated or destroyed by the dissection because this tissue sometimes is not substantial and if greatly distorted makes repair of the crus most difficult. The medial component of the crus usually has to be freed from the parietal pericardium until a firm fascial component is well delineated. This is readily felt with the thumb and index finger.

The sac is opened and transected so that a cuff of phrenoesophageal ligament remains attached to the esophagus. The hernial sac is cut laterally, anteriorly, and medially; there is no sac posteriorly. This trimming is carried down to the crura. At times we have not trimmed the sac but have used it to sew to the new hiatus.

The posterior aspect of the esophagogastric junction is then dissected free. Care must be taken that all arterial bleeders are ligated, as posterior bleeding can become troublesome. Opening the sac also facilitates further dissection of the medial component of the right crus, and if previous dissection has been inadequate, this can now be accomplished.

G

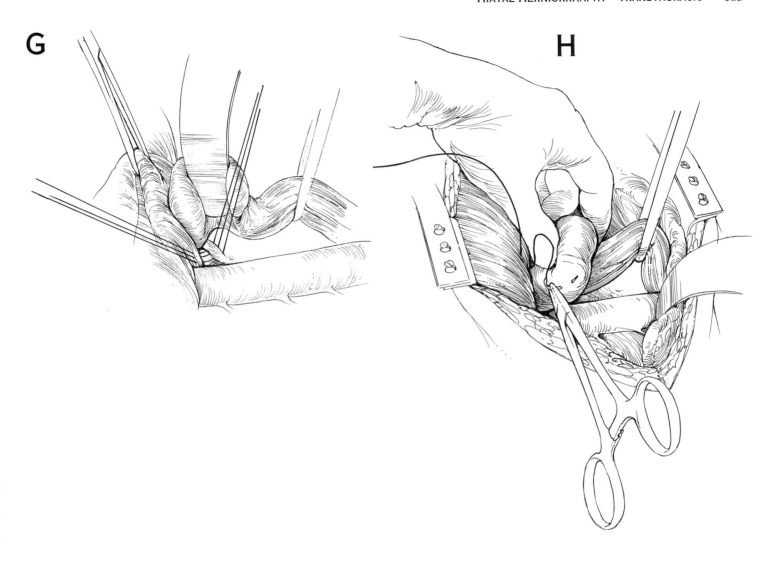

I

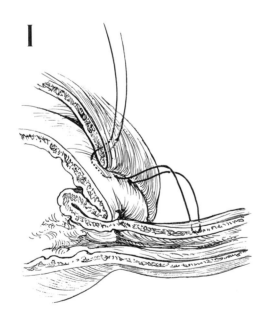

G

Three or four posterior crural stitches of 0 silk are now placed in substantial tissue. The crural fibers should not be cleaned too thoroughly from their esophageal edge so that it is possible during placement of the crural stitches that the needle can include peritoneum and pleura in its bites; this helps to buttress the crural fibers against the shearing effect of the stitches. The crural stitches are allowed to hang free and are not tied until later in the procedure.

H, I

A series of stitches are now so placed that when tied, the phrenoesophageal ligament lies and is anchored to the undersurface of the esophageal crura. These consist of mattress stitches of 2-0 black silk on a double-needle suture. They are first placed through the phrenoesophageal ligament near the esophagus, keeping in mind that a good bite of tissue must be taken during placement of each stitch to ensure that it will hold. The needle is passed through the esophageal hiatus, the tip of the needle engaging the undersurface of the diaphragm approximately 0.5 to 1.0 cm from the crural edge. The other end of the suture strand is brought through the diaphragm 3 to 4 mm from its partner as a mattress stitch.

J

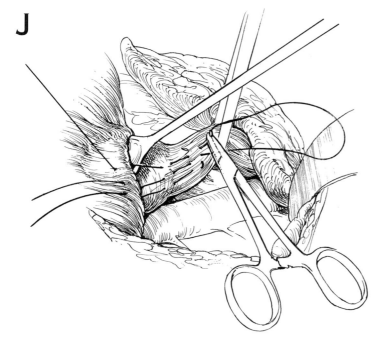

K

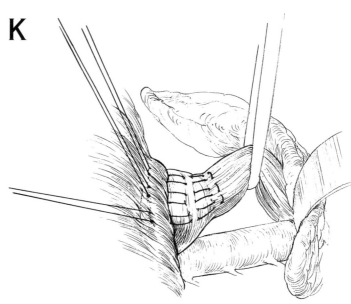

L

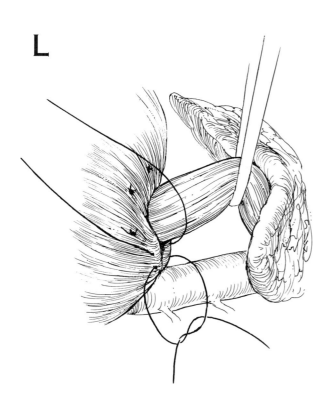

J, K, L

About 8 to 10 of these stitches are placed laterally, anteriorly, and medially. As there is no posterior attachment of the phrenoesophageal ligament and hernial sac, stitches obviously cannot be placed in this small area. The stitches through the phrenoesophageal ligament and diaphragm are now tied securely.

The crural sutures are tied now but not so tightly they cause muscle necrosis and in time cut through the crural fibers. The area of dissection is carefully inspected to make certain all bleeding points have been secured. A single no. 28 chest catheter is introduced intercostally just above the diaphragm and placed so that it lies adjacent to the area of lower esophageal dissection. The chest is closed in an appropriate manner.

Chapter

10

STOMACH

A TOTAL GASTRECTOMY

Total gastrectomy is most commonly performed for cancer of the stomach. The omentum is removed, and the spleen also should be sacrificed for cancers along the greater curvature. Any adherent viscera, such as colon, small intestine, and pancreas, can also be removed en bloc. On the lesser curvature, the celiac axis should be dissected clear. The left gastric and splenic arteries can be removed, but the hepatic artery is spared. The mesentery of the stomach is removed.

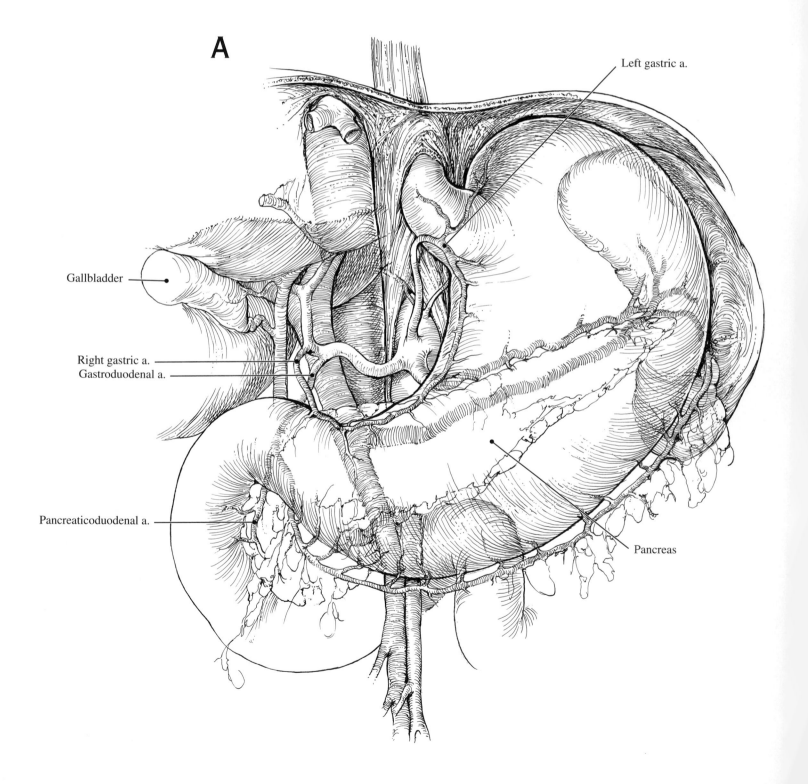

A

Left gastric a.

Gallbladder

Right gastric a.

Gastroduodenal a.

Pancreaticoduodenal a.

Pancreas

B

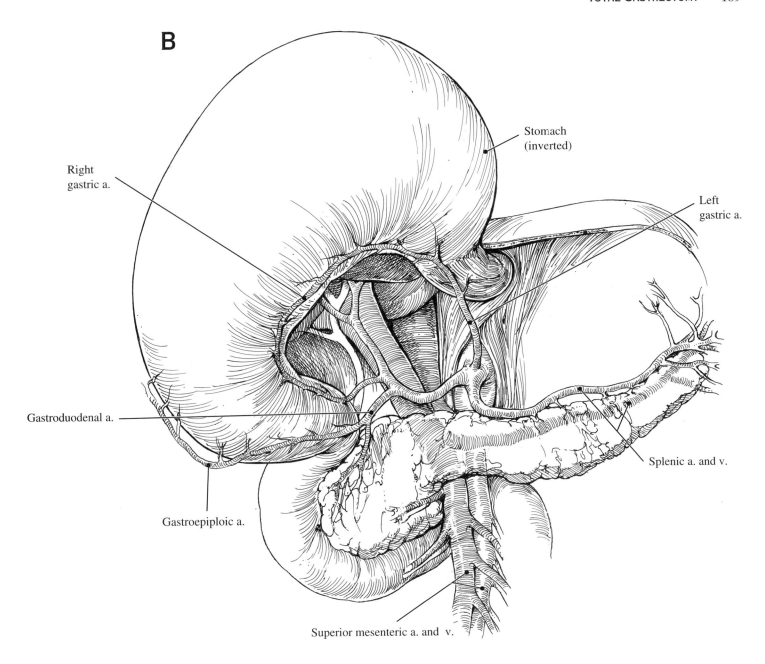

Stomach
(inverted)

Right
gastric a.

Left
gastric a.

Gastroduodenal a.

Gastroepiploic a.

Splenic a. and v.

Superior mesenteric a. and v.

A, B

The blood supply to the stomach is abundant. Lymph nodes also abound in this area in proximity to adjoining organs or to the vessels supplying them. In *A* and *B*, the liver, greater and lesser omenta, and peritoneum have been omitted for better anatomic clarity. The blood supply to the stomach is as follows: From the right gastric artery, which branches off the hepatic artery and courses along the lesser curvature of the stomach to meet the left gastric artery, which branches off at the celiac axis; the right gastroepiploic artery, a branch of the gastroduodenal artery, which courses along the greater curvature of the stomach to meet the left gastroepiploic artery, which is a branch of the splenic artery. In addition, the stomach receives the short gastric branches from the splenic artery. The venous drainage of the stomach is into the portal venous system.

C

General anesthesia is administered by endotracheal intubation, and the patient is placed in the supine position. The entire abdomen and thorax are prepared and draped. A longitudinal or transverse incision can be made depending on the body habitus of the patient and the anticipated magnitude of the operation.

D

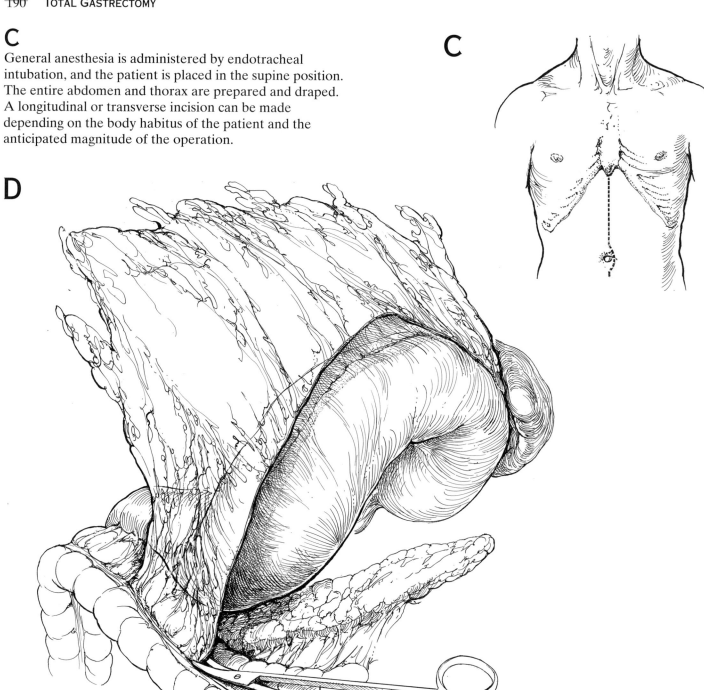

C

D

On opening the peritoneal cavity, a search is made for metastases. Not all metastases, of course, preclude resection of the affected portion of the stomach for present or imminently anticipated symptoms of obstruction.
In the absence of signs of categorical incurability, the omentum is detached from the transverse colon but remains attached to the stomach, with which it will be removed.

When the whole of the greater omentum has been freed, it is swung cephalad. The right gastroepiploic artery is then isolated at its origin from the gastroduodenal artery, clamped, divided, and ligated with 2-0 silk.

E

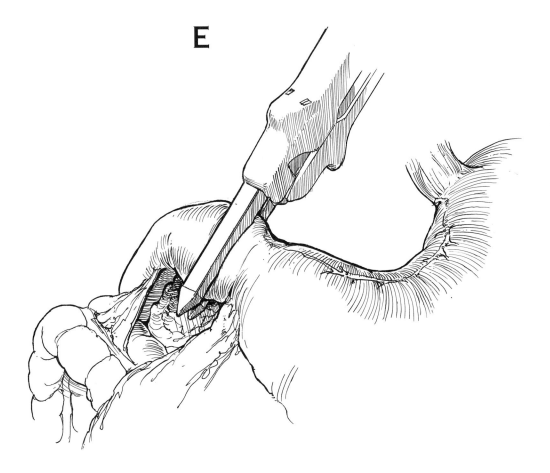

E, F, G

The duodenum is freed from any underlying pancreatic tissue and divided with a GIA stapler. The stapled duodenum can be left as is or oversewn with 3-0 silk.

F

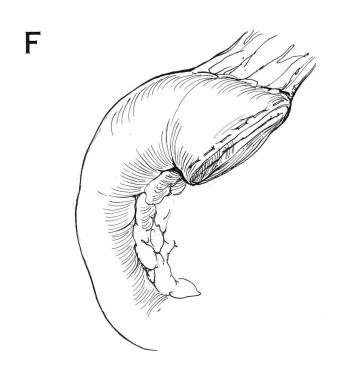

G

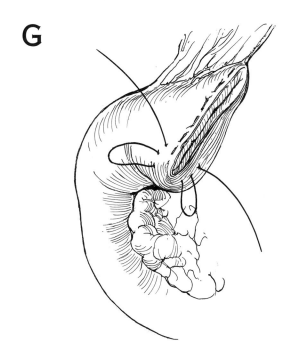

H

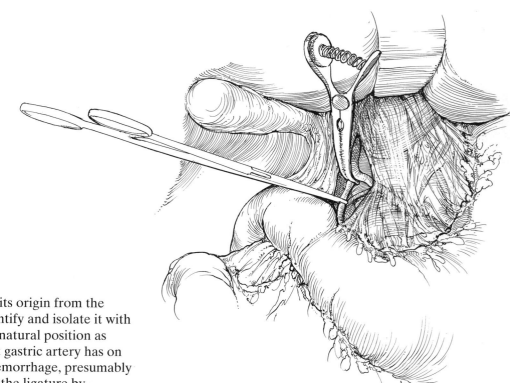

H, I

The right gastric artery is divided at its origin from the hepatic artery. One method is to identify and isolate it with the stomach and duodenum in their natural position as depicted. Simple ligation of the right gastric artery has on several occasions led to secondary hemorrhage, presumably from digestion of the vessel distal to the ligature by pancreatic enzymes in this area, incidental to the retropancreatic and retroduodenal dissection. As a precaution, this artery is occluded with a Potts clamp and oversewn with 5-0 arterial suture. This effectively opens the lesser omental cavity in readiness for the dissection of the gastrohepatic ligament.

I

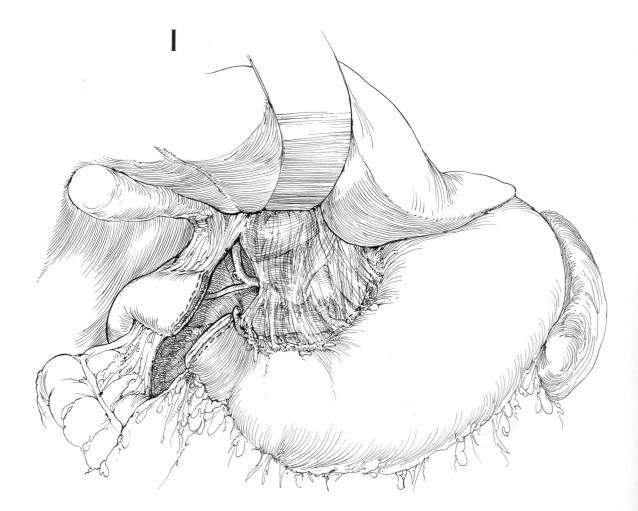

J

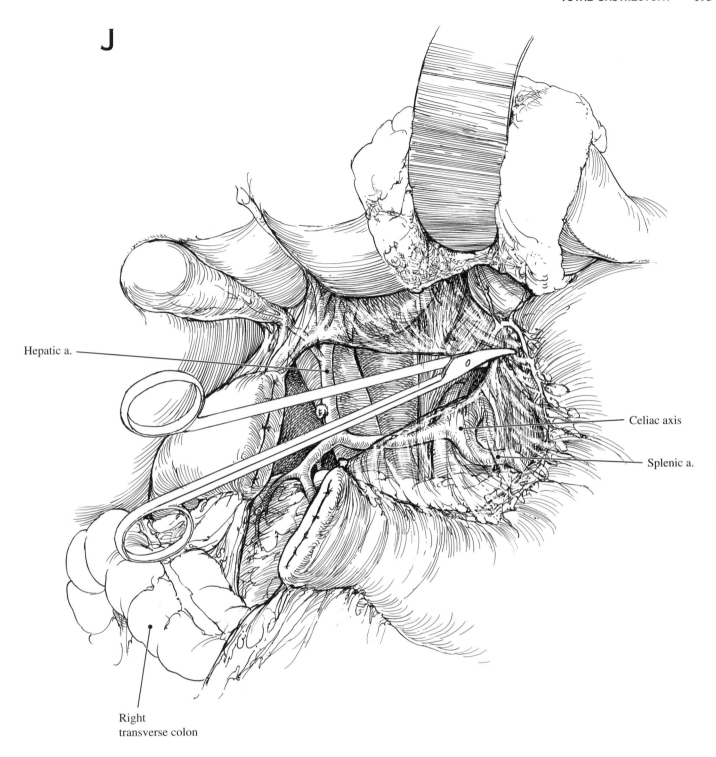

Hepatic a.

Celiac axis

Splenic a.

Right
transverse colon

J

The gastrohepatic omentum and the retropancreatic area
have abundant lymph nodal tissue that can be involved
early with metastases. As such, they warrant a methodical
dissection. The hepatic artery is being cleaned of
surrounding tissue as the dissection proceeds cephalad,
remaining close to the liver and sweeping the tissue
medially.

K

The stomach is reflected cephalad, exposing the origin of
the left gastric artery, which is ligated doubly with 3-0 silk
and divided. The spleen was detached from its blood
supply earlier during mobilization of the stomach.

K

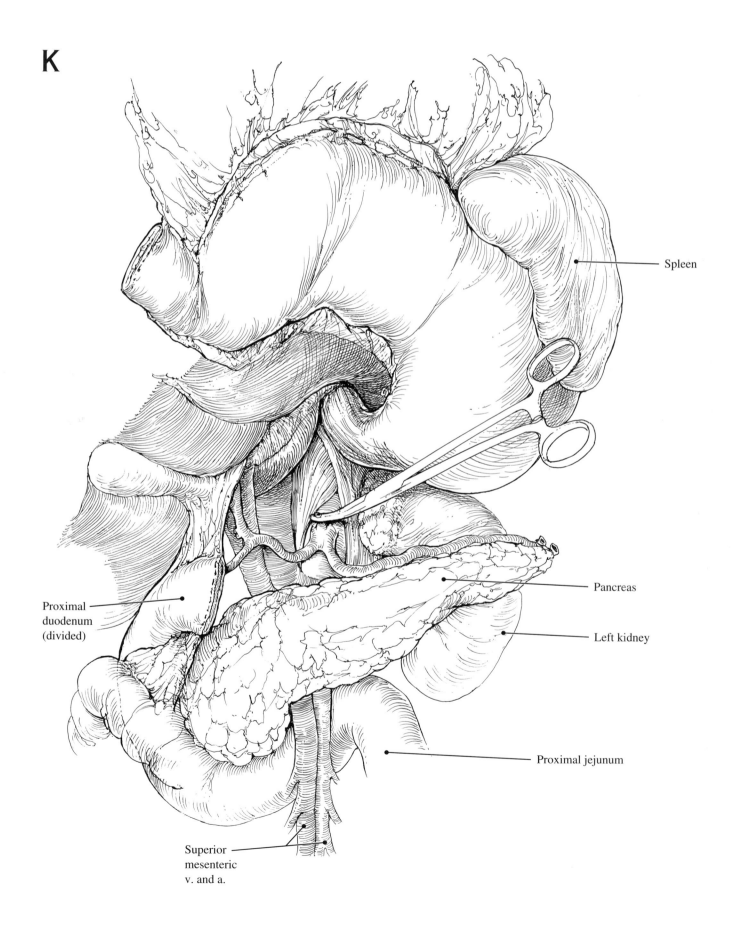

Spleen

Pancreas

Left kidney

Proximal
duodenum
(divided)

Proximal jejunum

Superior
mesenteric
v. and a.

L

The stomach is returned to its natural position. With dissection of the gastrohepatic omentum and celiac axis completed, the stomach remains attached only by the esophagus and is used to orient the esophagus before the anastomosis. The stomach is amputated and removed from the operative field.

L

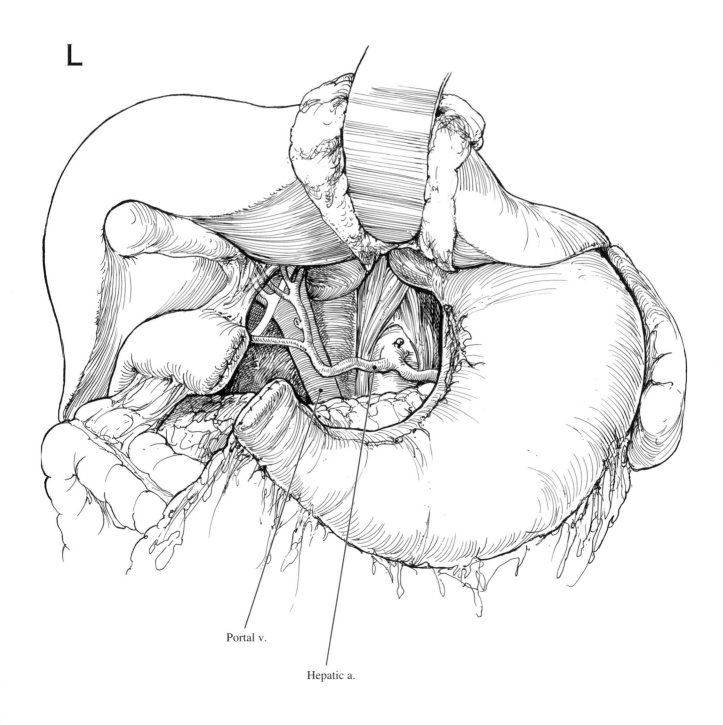

Portal v.

Hepatic a.

M

A window is made in an avascular area of the transverse mesocolon. The jejunum is divided about 15 cm from the ligament of Treitz, and the distal limb is brought through this window as a Roux-en-Y. Two anchoring stitches are placed first.

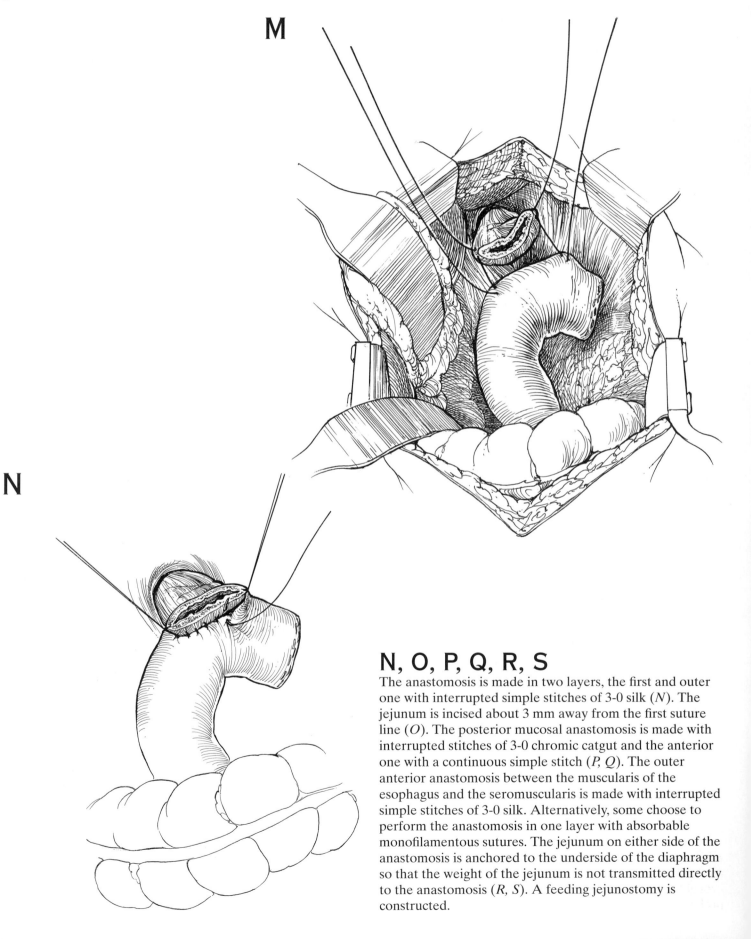

M

N

N, O, P, Q, R, S

The anastomosis is made in two layers, the first and outer one with interrupted simple stitches of 3-0 silk (*N*). The jejunum is incised about 3 mm away from the first suture line (*O*). The posterior mucosal anastomosis is made with interrupted stitches of 3-0 chromic catgut and the anterior one with a continuous simple stitch (*P, Q*). The outer anterior anastomosis between the muscularis of the esophagus and the seromuscularis is made with interrupted simple stitches of 3-0 silk. Alternatively, some choose to perform the anastomosis in one layer with absorbable monofilamentous sutures. The jejunum on either side of the anastomosis is anchored to the underside of the diaphragm so that the weight of the jejunum is not transmitted directly to the anastomosis (*R, S*). A feeding jejunostomy is constructed.

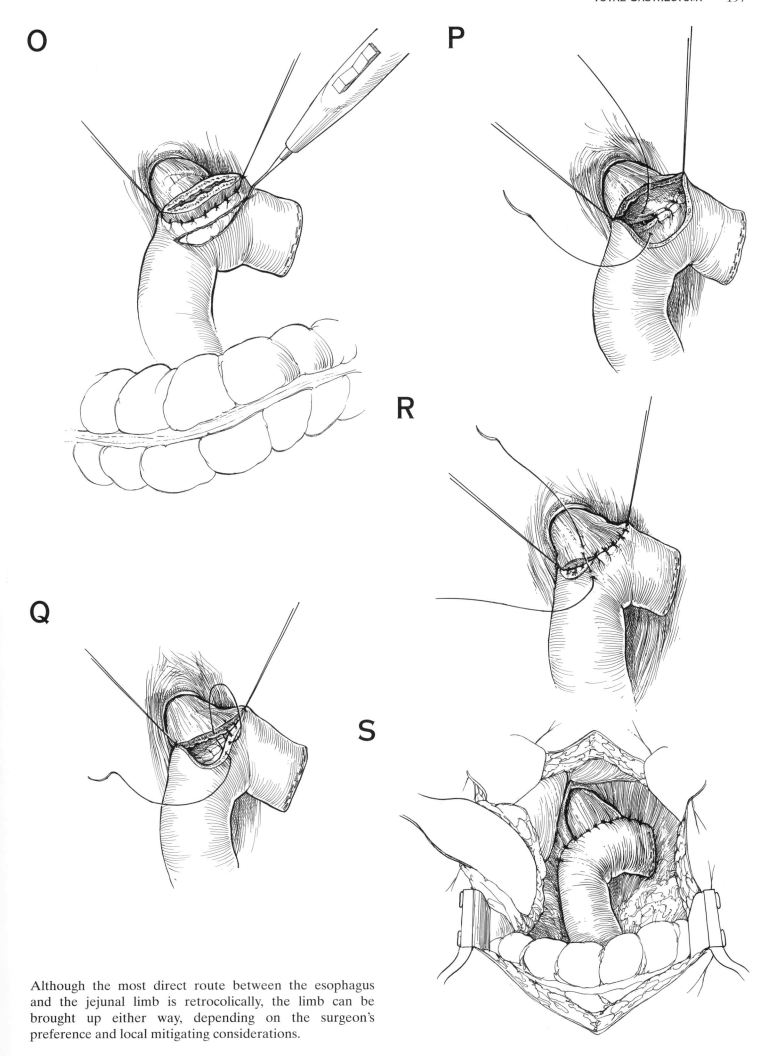

Although the most direct route between the esophagus and the jejunal limb is retrocolically, the limb can be brought up either way, depending on the surgeon's preference and local mitigating considerations.

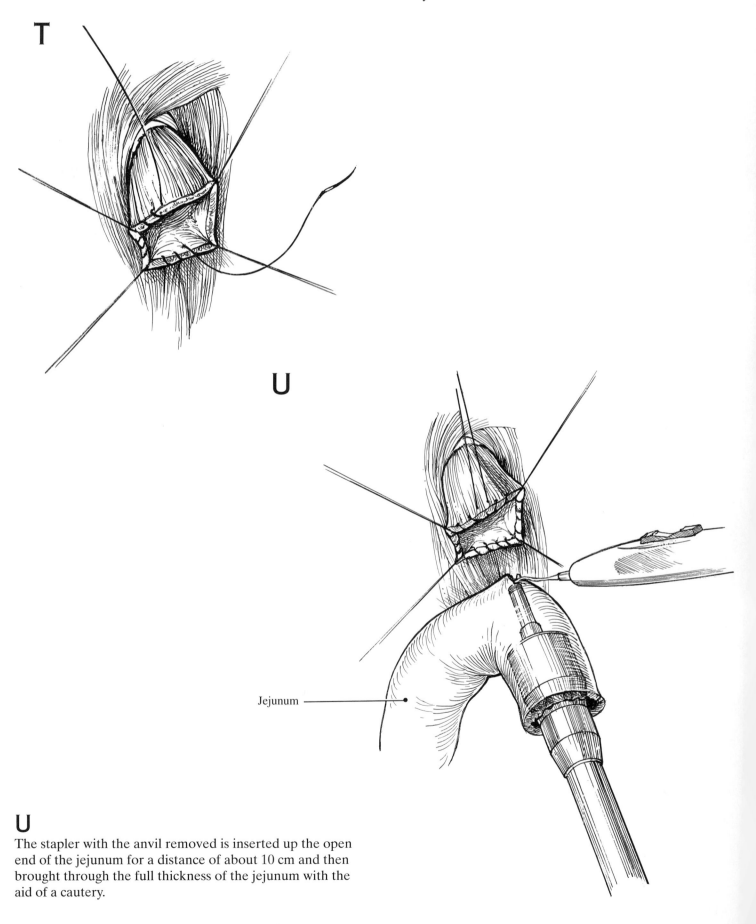

T

A stapled esophagogastric anastomosis is as effective as one sewn by hand yet is easier and faster to perform. Quadratic stitches are positioned, and the edge of the opened esophagus is oversewn with a continuous stitch of 2-0 nylon.

Jejunum

U

The stapler with the anvil removed is inserted up the open end of the jejunum for a distance of about 10 cm and then brought through the full thickness of the jejunum with the aid of a cautery.

V

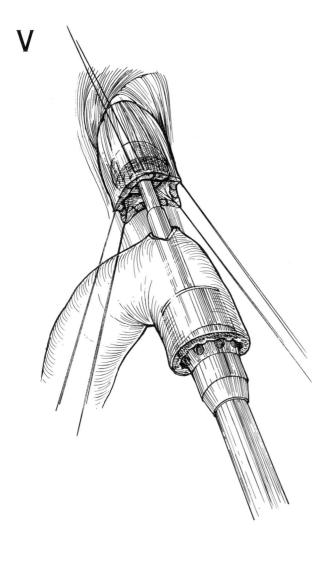

W

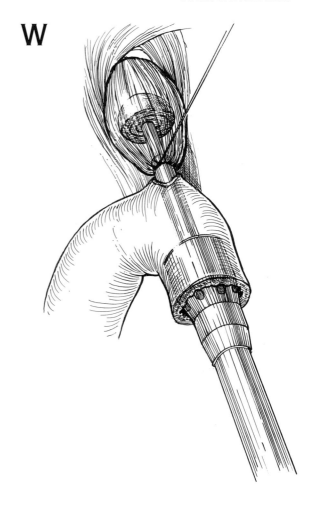

X

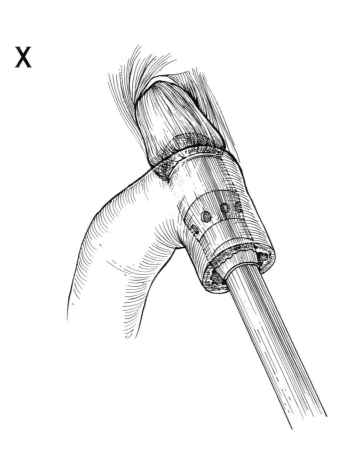

V

The anvil is reattached and placed inside the esophagus, with the shaft still extended.

W, X

The circumferentially placed purse-string suture of nylon on the esophagus is tied down on the shaft very snugly (*W*). The anvil and stapler are approximated and the stapler is fired (*X*).

Y

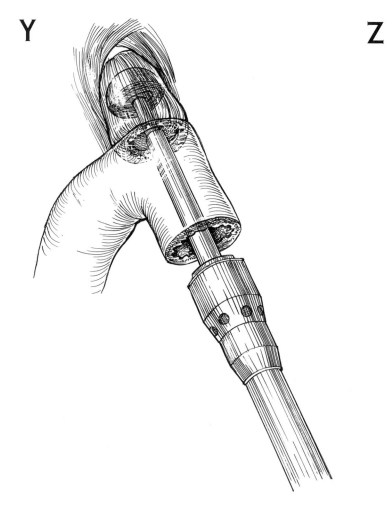

Z

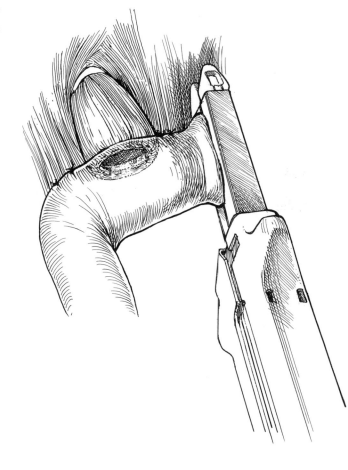

Y

The shaft again is extended and the stapler gently disengaged and withdrawn. The specimen is examined for its physical integrity circumferentially and then sent to the pathologist for histologic examination.

Z

The jejunum is closed by stapling across its open end. The jejunum on either side of the anastomosis is anchored to the diaphragm with 3-0 silk.

One Jackson-Pratt drain is placed adjacent to the esophagojejunal anastomosis and another from the area of the duodenal stump, and each is brought to the outside through separate incisions. The abdomen is closed in a preferred manner.

B SUBTOTAL GASTRECTOMY

BILLROTH I

A

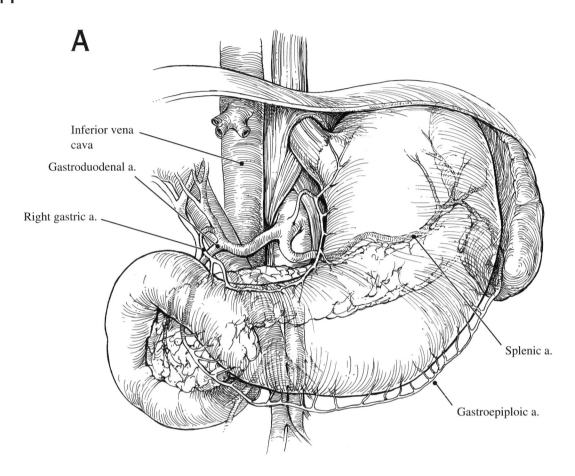

Inferior vena cava

Gastroduodenal a.

Right gastric a.

Splenic a.

Gastroepiploic a.

A

The surgeon who plans to perform a Billroth I gastrectomy should have a thorough knowledge of the anatomy of this area, and should know how to perform alternative operations, as certain conditions that appear at the time of exploration may preclude a Billroth I. The principal contraindications to a Billroth I operation are edema from acute current or recurrent inflammation and scarring and deformation secondary to chronic disease, both of which prevent an adequate or safe dissection of the duodenum and associated tissue.

B

An upper midline incision or a subcostal one skewed somewhat to the right is satisfactory.

On entry, the exploration includes a search for unexpected abnormalities. In their absence, attention is focused on the stomach and duodenum. The dashed line indicates the approximate transection: a line from the lesser curvature slightly proximal to the incisura angularis that extends inferolaterally at a 45-degree angle. This effectively permits removal of approximately 50% of the distal stomach. The omentum can be left in place as shown; if voluminous or heavy and likely to weigh on the anastomosis, it is included in that portion of the stomach to be removed.

B

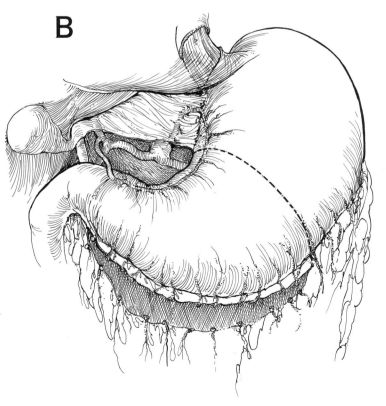

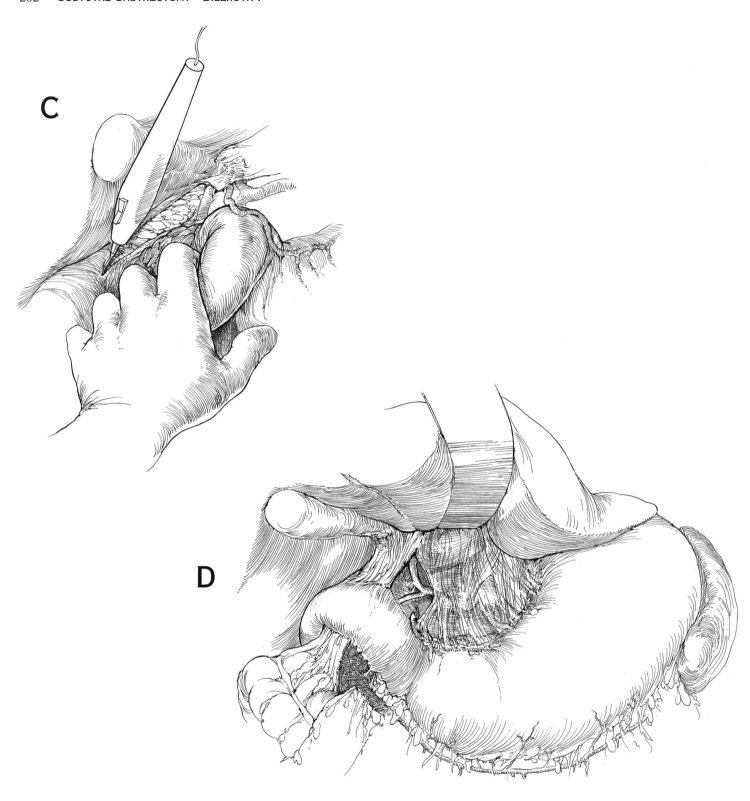

C

The duodenum is mobilized for about 3 cm by dividing the peritoneal fold with a blunt needle–tipped cautery. At this stage a final assessment is made regarding the suitability of a Billroth I procedure.

D

The thin gastrohepatic omentum is divided, not only to prepare for subsequent steps, but also to provide a direct view of the anatomy and of any abnormalities, particularly of the hepatic artery. Hepatic branches of the right vagus nerve should be preserved. The right gastric artery is divided and oversewn.

E

The left gastric artery is ligated close to the stomach, with creation of a free area for later placement of the stapler. The right gastroepiploic vessels are divided. The sizable gastric artery (see *D*) is divided between vascular clamps, and the proximal side is oversewn with vascular suture material; it is thought that this technique reduces the likelihood of a "blowout" should an abscess develop in this anastomotic area. Blunt dissection along a plane of areolar tissue on the dorsal surface of the stomach frees this area in a swift and bloodless manner.

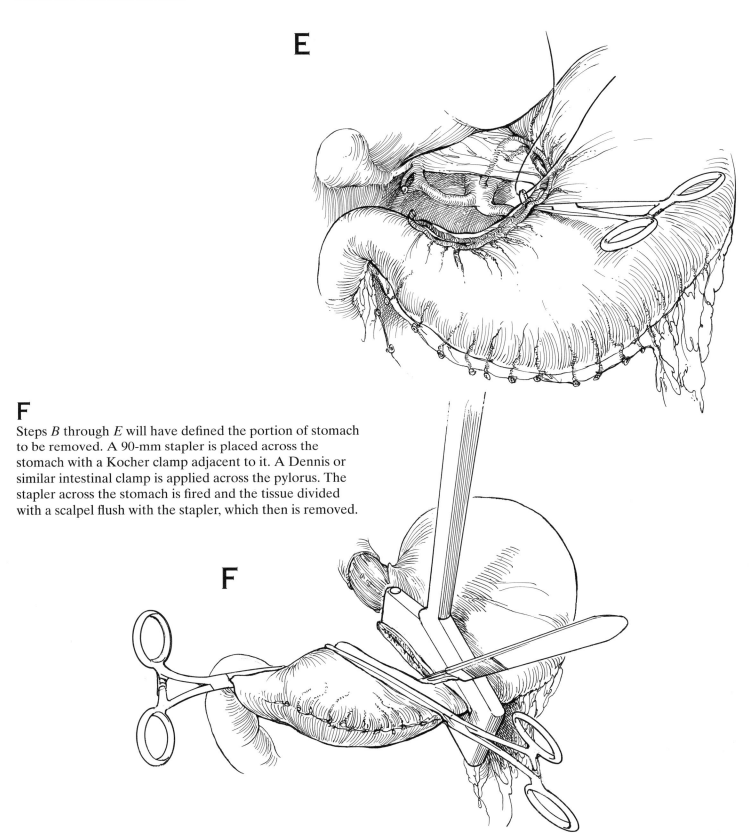

E

F

Steps *B* through *E* will have defined the portion of stomach to be removed. A 90-mm stapler is placed across the stomach with a Kocher clamp adjacent to it. A Dennis or similar intestinal clamp is applied across the pylorus. The stapler across the stomach is fired and the tissue divided with a scalpel flush with the stapler, which then is removed.

F

G

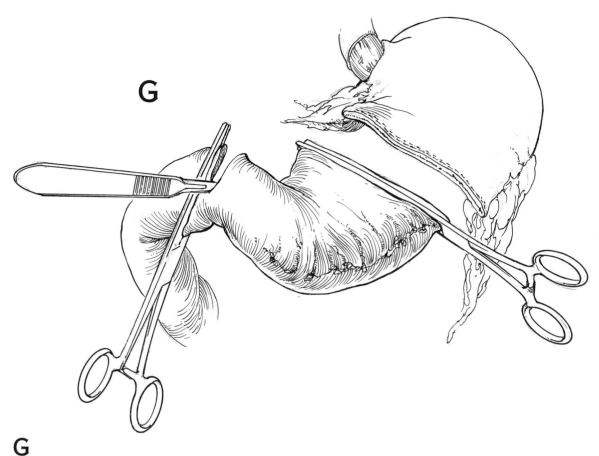

The pylorus is divided with a scalpel very close to the crushing intestinal clamp. The purpose of such a crushing clamp is to prevent bleeding from small vessels in the line of division. The bites of the stitching needle will be immediately inside the crushed tissue; thus, the crushed tissue is incorporated into the anastomosis.

H

The stomach is prepared for anastomosis by excising tissue along the greater curvature to create an opening of dimensions equal to the diameter of the transected duodenum.

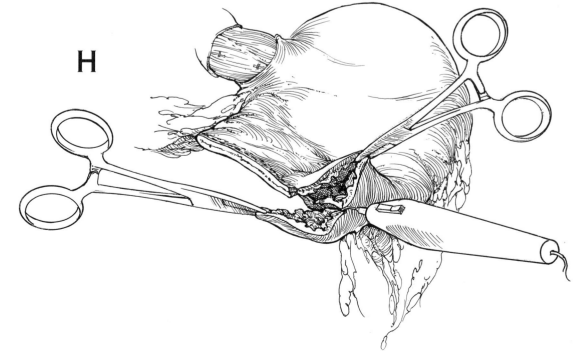

I

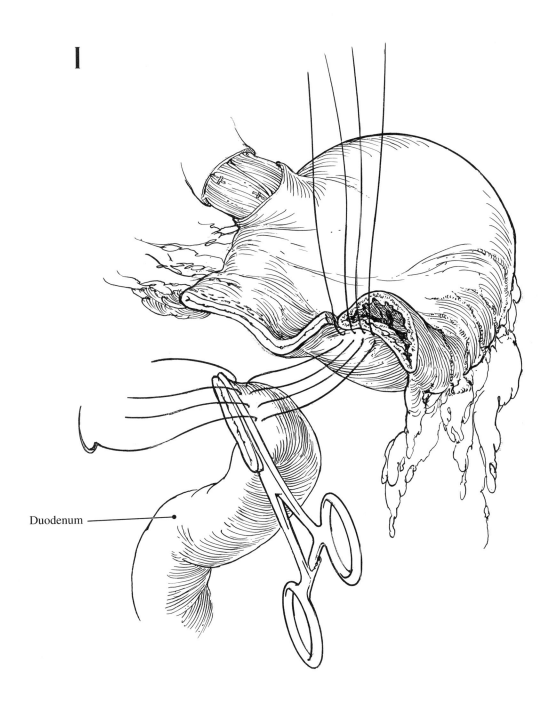

Duodenum

I

The gastroduodenal anastomosis is performed by placing interrupted stitches through the seromuscular tissue with 3-0 nonabsorbable sutures as shown.

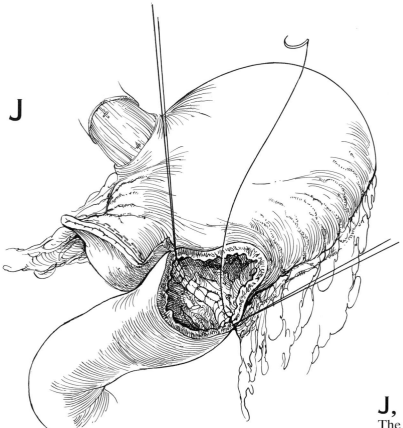

J, K

The two lateral-most seromuscular stitches are left in place and used for traction. The mucosal stitching is done with a continuous absorbable suture; it must not be placed under tension, which can lead to purse-stringing of the anastomosis. The stitching of the mucosa should be through viable tissue immediately inside the crushed tissue; the latter will slough off harmlessly, while in the meantime having served its purpose of hemostasis.

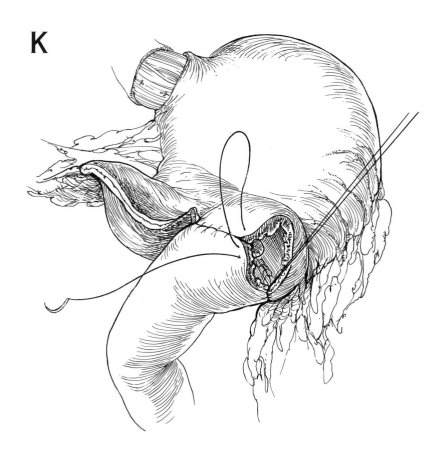

L

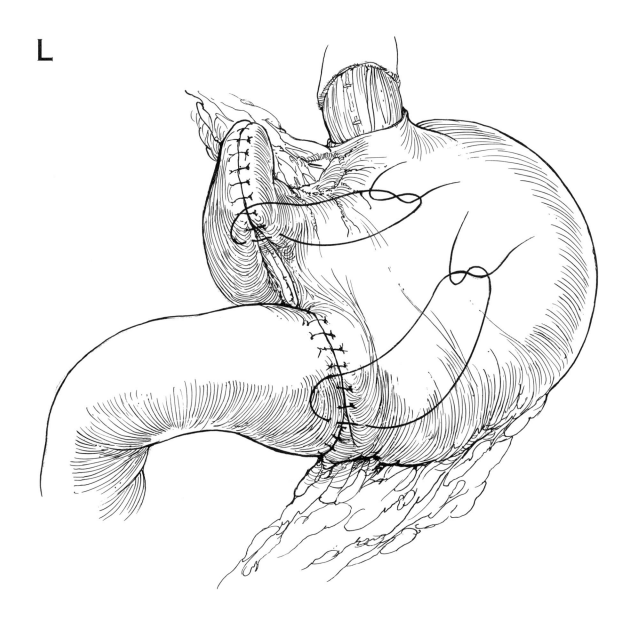

L

The staple line on the stomach is reinforced with interrupted inverting stitches of nonabsorbable material through the seromuscularis. The same is done with the gastroduodenal anastomosis; the tissue here should not be inverted too generously lest the resultant bulk unacceptably narrow the anastomotic lumen.

M

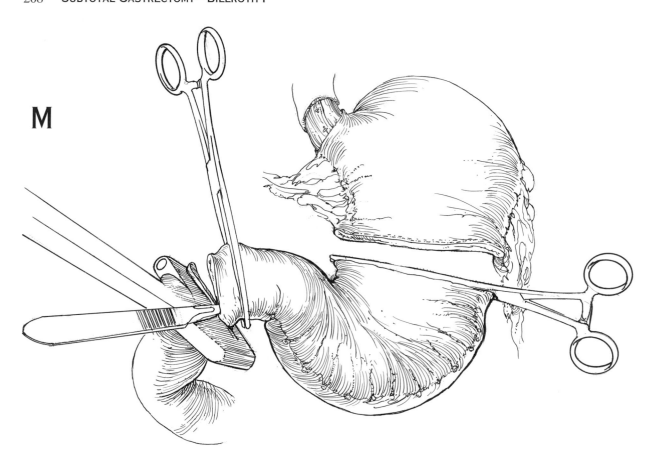

M, N

Alternatively, the gastroduodenal anastomosis can also be
performed with a stapler and in several ways. The stomach
and duodenum are divided as before. A gastrotomy is
made on the anterior surface of the stomach about 3 to
4 cm from the staple line and in an area devoid of large
vessels.

N

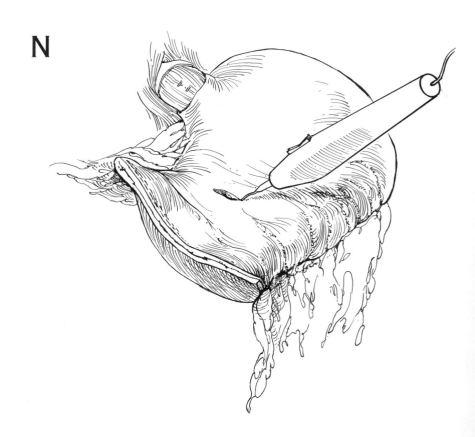

O

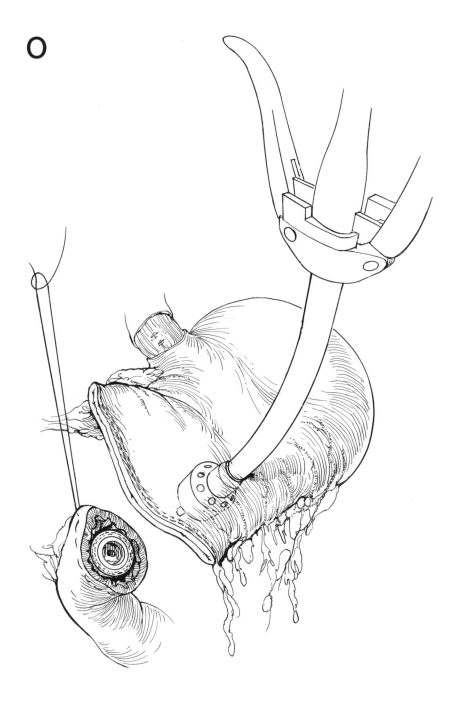

O

The stapling device without the anvil is inserted into the stomach and the center rod pressed against the posterior wall of the stomach, again 3 to 4 cm from the staple line. A blunt-tip cautery applied against the center rod burns a hole, permitting its easy exit. An anvil of appropriate size is inserted into the duodenum, the purse-string suture of 3-0 nylon around the duodenum is tied snugly, and the stapling device and anvil are approximated. The incorporated area should be examined for any extraneous tissue that may have insinuated itself between the anvil and the cartridge. The stapler is fired and the instrument withdrawn. The circular pieces of tissue from the duodenum and the stomach should be inspected to ensure their integrity. The gastrostomy is closed using either a stapler or a traditional technique.

P

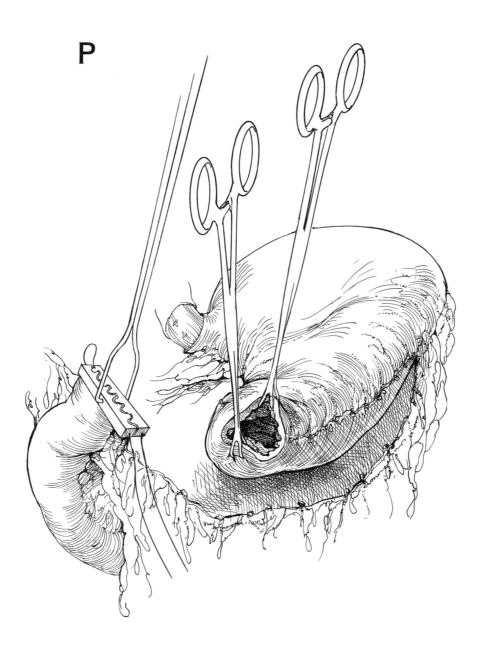

P

An alternative technique that avoids the anterior
gastrostomy is first to mobilize the stomach the necessary
amount. The purse-string instrument is positioned across
the duodenum in the same location as before, and the
tissue is cut with a scalpel flush with this instrument.

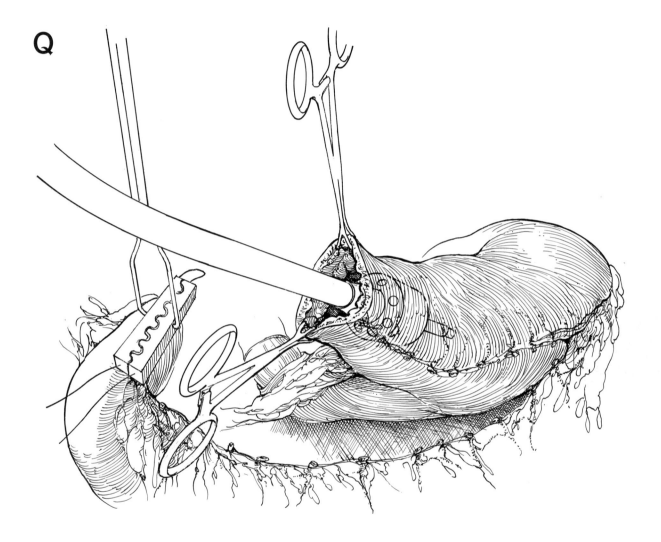

Q

The circular end-to-end stapler without the anvil is introduced into the stomach. At a point 3 to 4 cm proximal to the point of anticipated gastroduodenostomy, the rod is pressed against the posterior surface of the stomach.

R

Electrocautery is applied against the pressure point to
allow easy passage of the rod, which now is reconnected to
the center post.

R

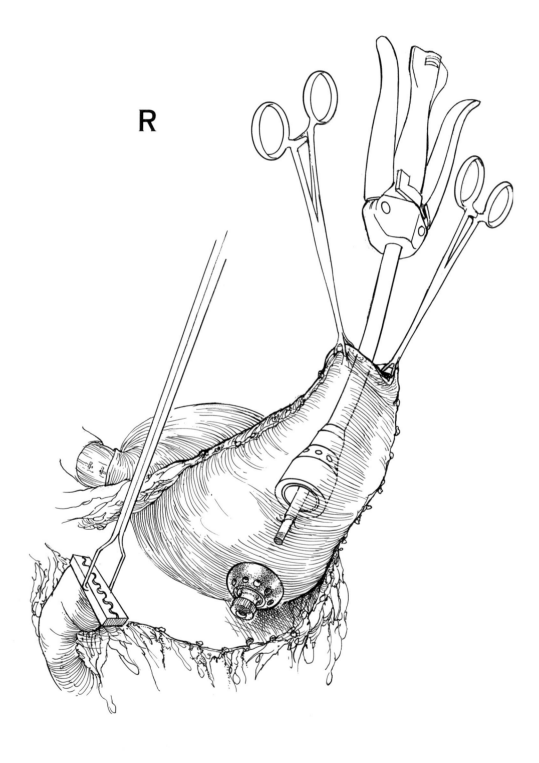

S

T

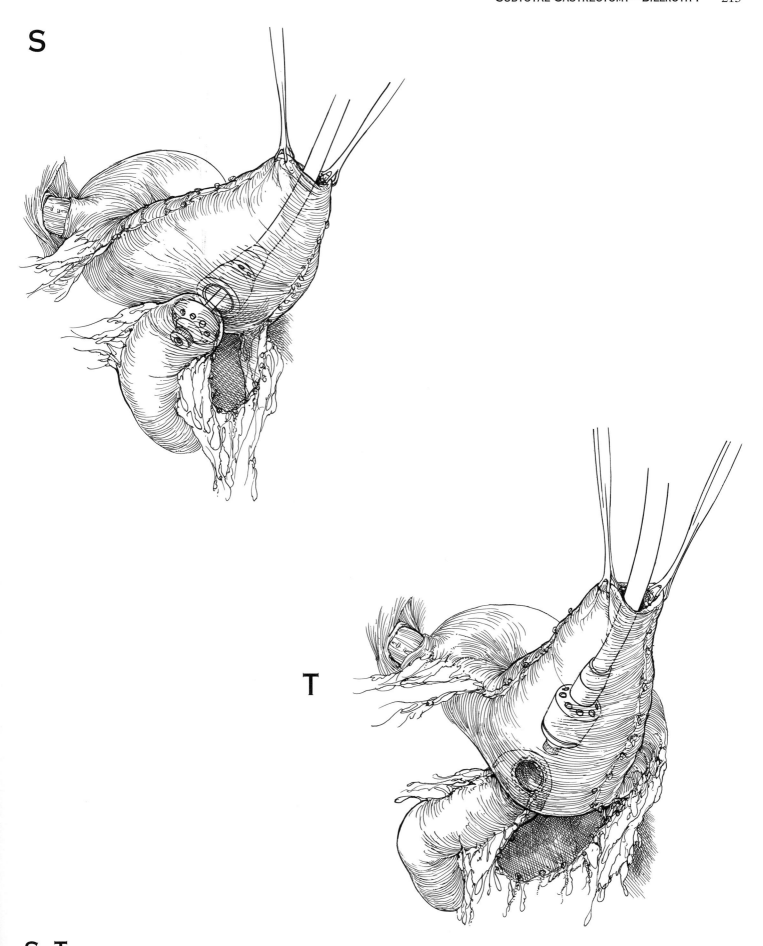

S, T

The purse-string suture on the duodenum is tied, the anvil
and circular stapler approximated, and the instrument
fired. The instrument is withdrawn, and again the rings of
the duodenal and gastric tissue are examined for integrity.

U

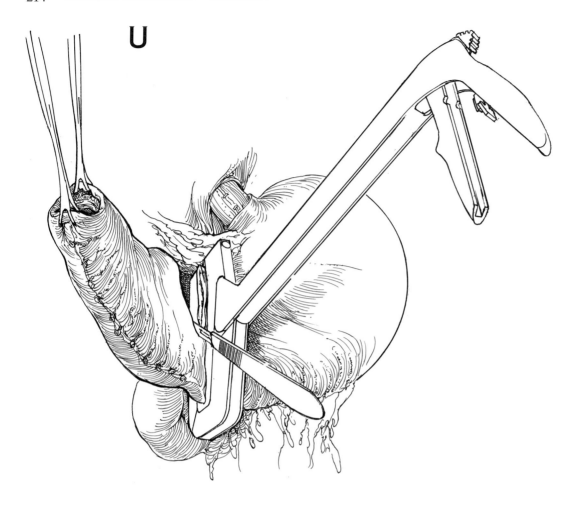

V

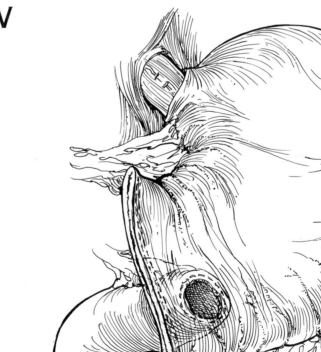

U, V

The 90-mm stapler is positioned across the stomach at a point approximately 3 to 4 cm distal to the gastroduodenostomy and fired.

The abdomen is closed in a preferred manner.

A

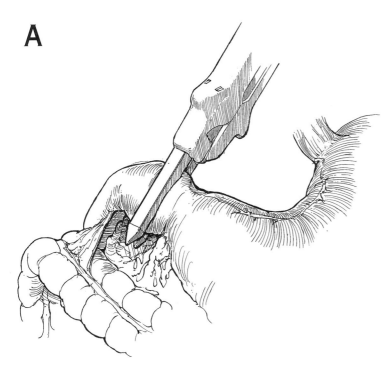

BILLROTH II

Technically, there are few differences between the Billroth I and Billroth II operations, the principal one being that the anastomosis in the former is with continuity between stomach and duodenum and in the latter between stomach and jejunum.

The gastroepiploic artery, a branch of the gastroduodenal artery, is identified as it appears on the undersurface of the greater curvature of the antrum, ligated with 2-0 silk in continuity, and divided. The dissection proceeds toward the patient's left almost to the point at which the artery buries itself into the stomach.

B

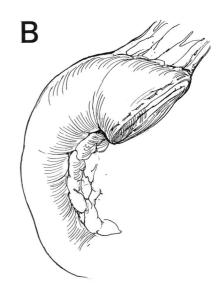

A, B

A finger is used bluntly to encircle the prepyloric area. Small vessels are identified and secured with clips or 3-0 silk. The GIA stapler is applied across the duodenum immediately distal to the pylorus and fired.

C

All vessels in the filmy gastrohepatic omentum are divided with care. The hepatic branch of the vagus nerve is left intact.

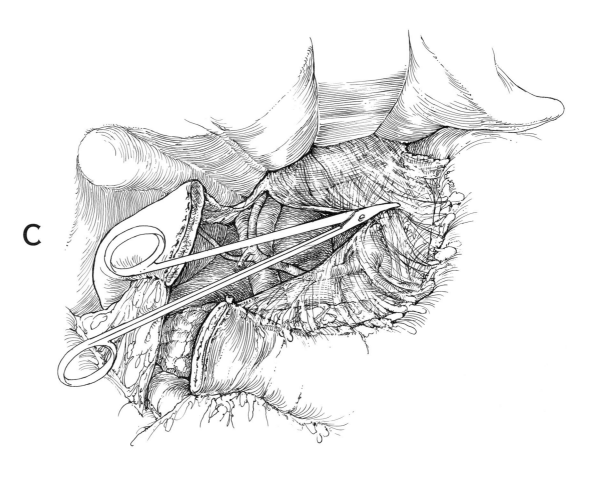

D

The anticipated line of resection is from the incisura angularis gastris proceeding downward at a 45-degree angle toward the greater curvature.

E

The left gastric artery and vein are ligated in continuity with 2-0 silk and divided.

F

The stomach is stapled for its full width and divided by a sweep of the scalpel blade across the stapler jaws.

D

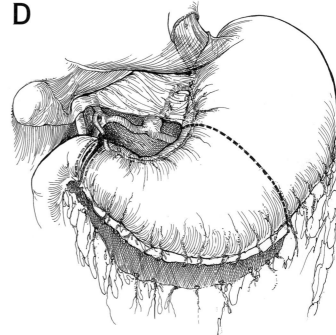

E

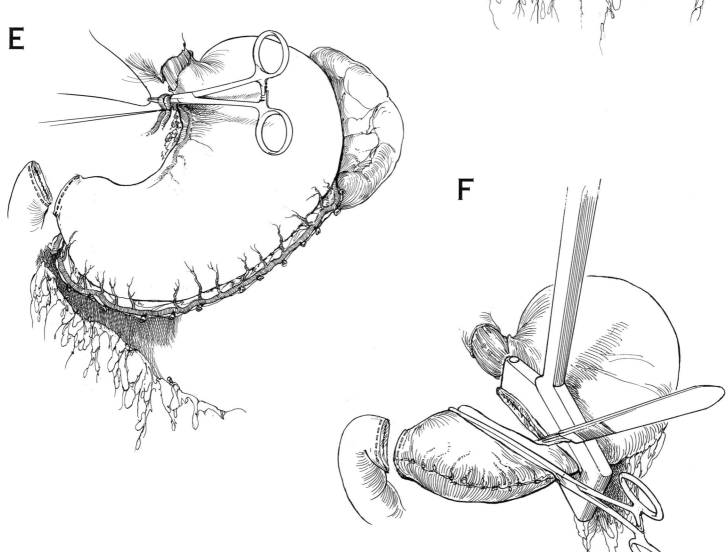

F

G

G

The specimen is removed from the operative field.

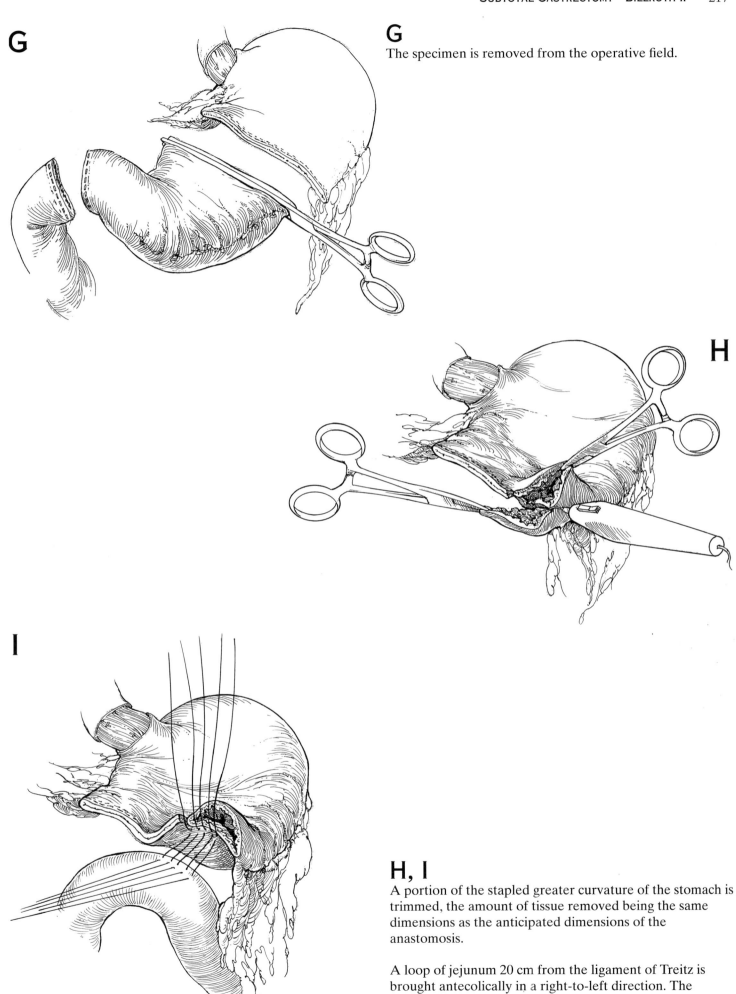

H

I

H, I

A portion of the stapled greater curvature of the stomach is trimmed, the amount of tissue removed being the same dimensions as the anticipated dimensions of the anastomosis.

A loop of jejunum 20 cm from the ligament of Treitz is brought antecolically in a right-to-left direction. The posterior seromuscular anastomosis is made with interrupted simple stitches of 3-0 silk.

J

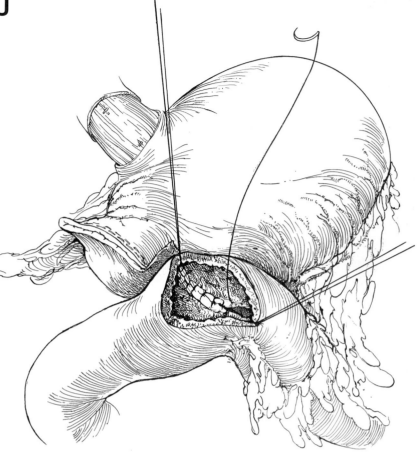

J

The mucosal stitch is continuous and simple with 3-0 chromic catgut.

K

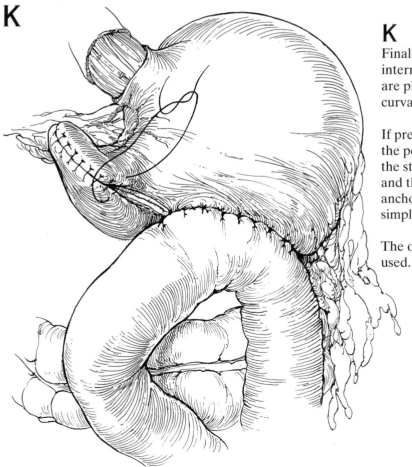

K

Finally, the anterior seromuscular anastomosis is made with interrupted simple stitches of 3-0 silk. Supporting stitches are placed across the anastomosis at the lesser and greater curvatures.

If preferred or necessary, the anastomosis can be seated in the postcolic area, but the surgeon must make certain that the stomach is brought through the transverse mesocolon and that the anastomosis is kept in this location by anchoring it to the transverse mesocolon with interrupted simple stitches of 3-0 silk.

The operative site is given a final examination. No drain is used. The abdomen is closed in the customary manner.

C GASTROJEJUNOSTOMY

POSTCOLIC

Usually, gastrojejunostomy is performed antecolically because the portion of the stomach and jejunum to be anastomosed are directly available to the surgeon. In some instances, the more natural, direct path of a postcolic anastomosis is necessary. This operation is not only somewhat more difficult to perform, but also more difficult to disengage and recreate if this becomes necessary.

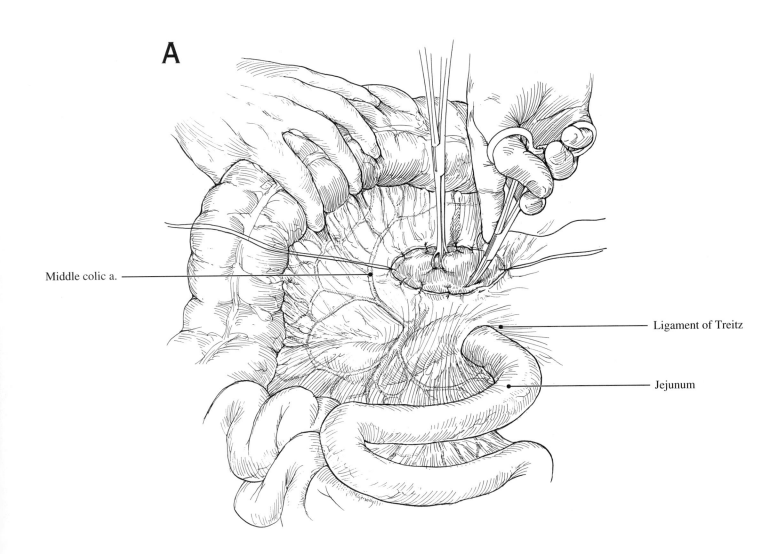

A

Middle colic a.

Ligament of Treitz

Jejunum

A

The transverse colon is lifted out of the abdomen, and the bare area in the mesocolon to the right of the middle colic vessels is identified and opened with cautery. The presenting greater curvature of the stomach is pulled through the opening and is secured in this herniated position with interrupted stitches of 3-0 silk.

B, C

A portion of jejunum about 15 cm from the ligament of Treitz is chosen and laid next to the stomach in preparation for the anastomosis. Unlike the procedure for the Billroth II anastomosis, it appears to make little difference here whether the procedure is conducted left to right (or vice versa) and parallel or transverse to the axis of the stomach. It is, however, essential that the anastomosis be of adequate size and under no tension. An antral location is desirable. Intestinal clamps are applied across either side of the planned anastomosis to reduce the degree of intestinal spillage (*B*). The posterior seromuscular stitch is continuous, using 3-0 silk (*C*).

B

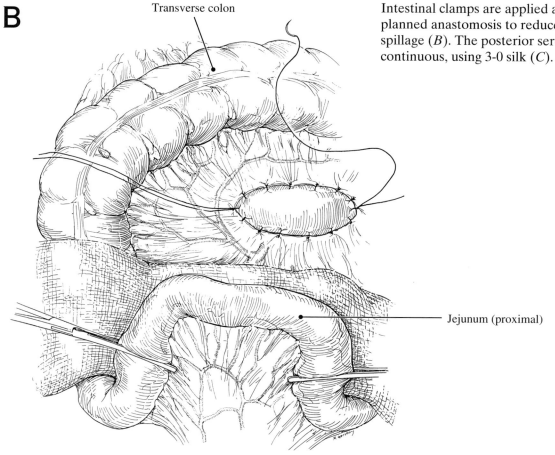

Transverse colon

Jejunum (proximal)

C

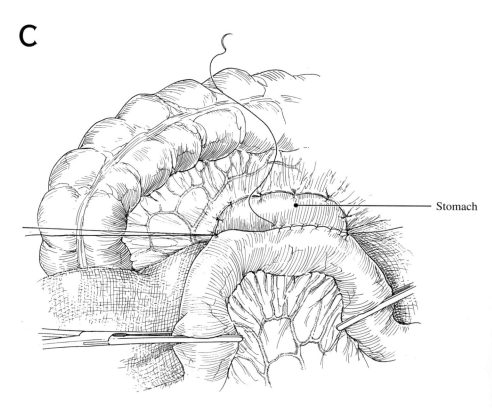

Stomach

D

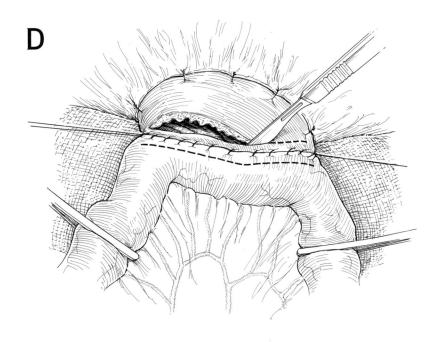

D, E

The jejunum is opened about 5 mm from the posterior suture line (*D*), and the continuous posterior mucosal stitch of 3-0 chromic catgut is begun and continued in both directions (*E*).

E

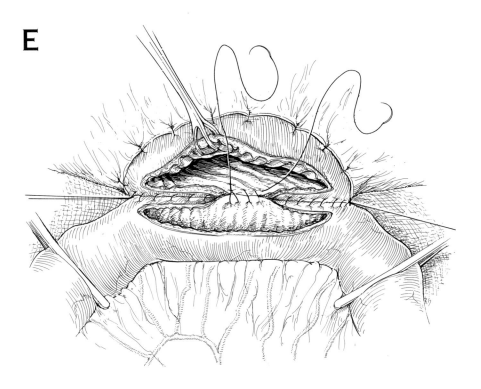

F, G

At the turns, one of the stitches is applied in a Connell fashion. Now the sutures approach each other anteriorly in a more natural fashion so that when tied they will least distort the tissue.

F

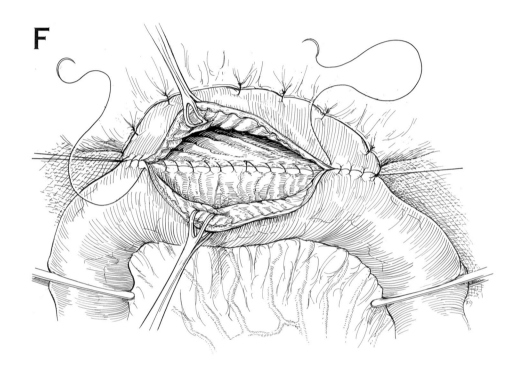

G

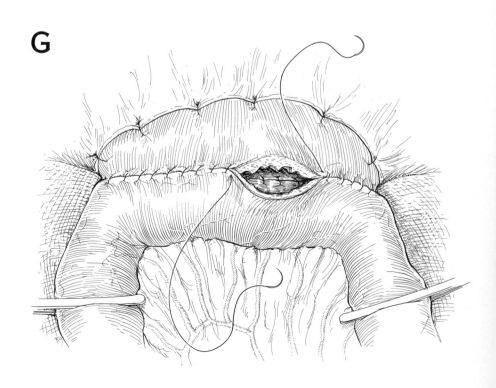

H

The anterior seromuscular layer is closed with 3-0 silk in either a continuous or an interrupted fashion. A continuous stitch takes less time but also requires attention so that each bite of the needle is in the same plane as the previous one if a gradual rolling in and distortion of the suture line is to be avoided. One safeguard is to perform the anastomosis with interrupted stitches, leaving the tissue undisturbed until all stitches are in position before tying.

H

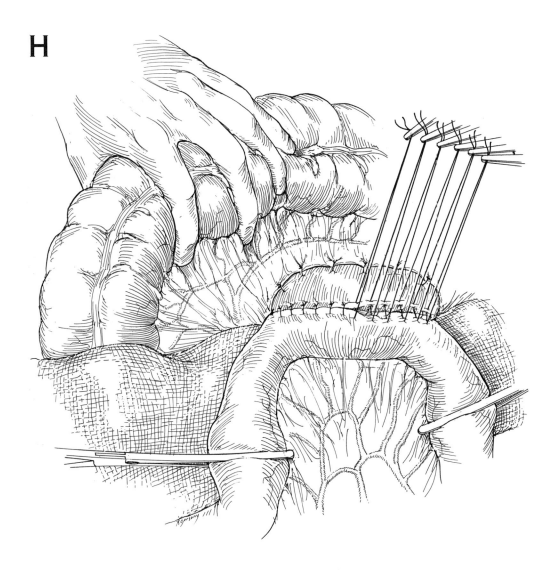

D PYLOROPLASTY

HEINEKE-MIKULICZ

A

The Heineke-Mikulicz pyloroplasty is the one done most commonly because it takes the least amount of time and has a low surgical morbidity and mortality. The pyloric vein runs across the pylorus transverse to the axis of the duodenum and serves to identify the pylorus.

B, C

A 3-cm incision is made equidistant proximal and distal to the pylorus. Two Babcock forceps are placed at the points of the divided pyloric ring. Slight traction aligns the tissue

so that it is now perpendicular to its original axis. Silk sutures can serve as traction equally well. Indeed, traction is not essential; it is simplest to establish visually the incision midpoint and proceed from it.

D, E

A two-layer anastomosis is performed with continuous stitches of 3-0 chromic catgut for the mucosa and interrupted minimally inverting stitches of 3-0 silk for the seromuscularis. If the tissue is edematous and nonyielding, a simple rather than an inverting stitch is advisable.

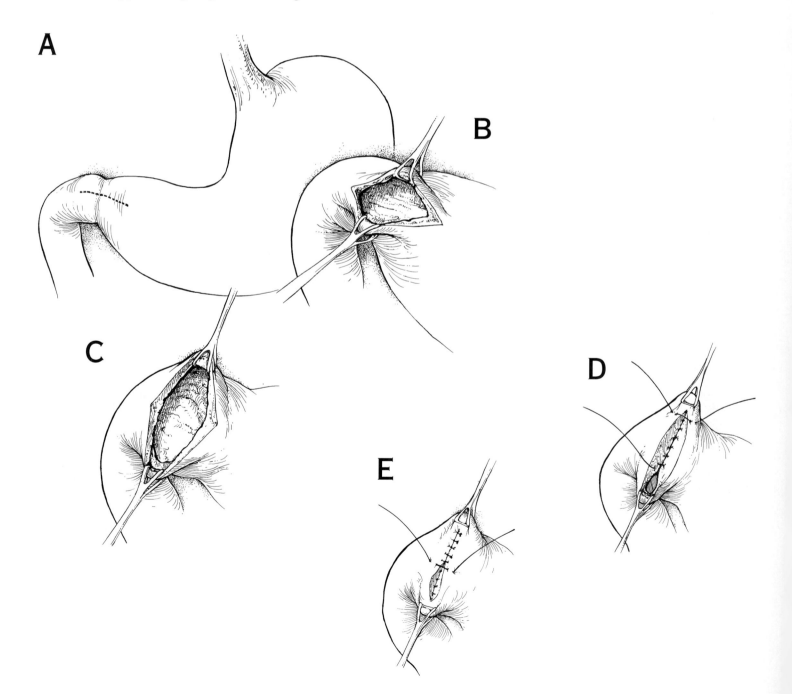

FINNEY

A

A Finney pyloroplasty is a side-to-side anastomosis between antrum and duodenum and includes the pyloric area. The duodenum needs to be mobilized generously with a Kocher maneuver.

B

The midpoint of the pylorus is grasped and lifted with a Babcock forceps, and simple, interrupted stitches of 3-0 silk are used to approximate the antrum and duodenum progressively for a length of about 5 cm. Placing these stitches as posteriorly as possible lessens tension later on the anterior suture line.

C, D

The continuous simple mucosal stitch is with 3-0 chromic catgut.

E

The seromuscular stitch is with interrupted, inverting stitches of 3-0 silk.

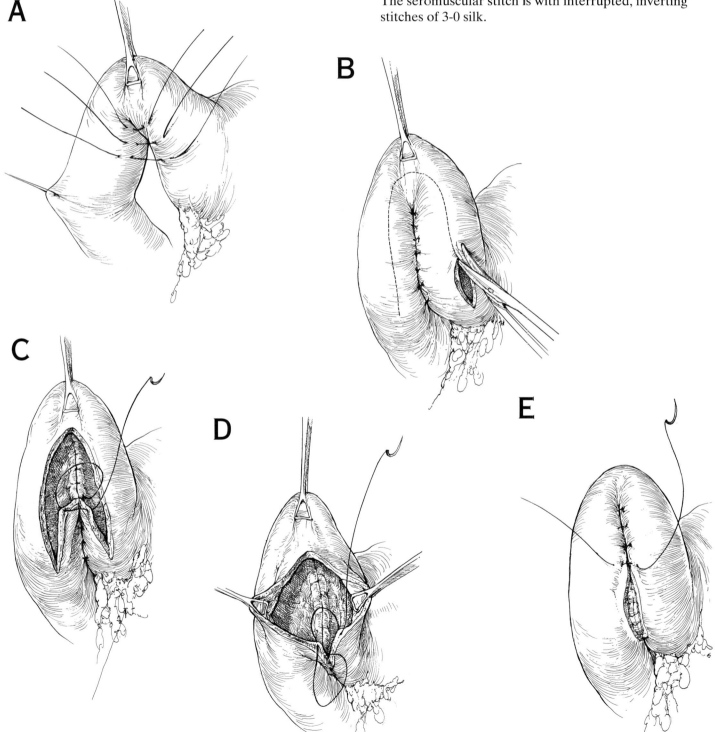

JABOULAY

The Jaboulay procedure is, in reality, a bypass operation that does not directly address the pylorus. It is useful when a chronically scarred ulcer has resulted in firm tissue that is difficult to work with and more likely to present too serious a risk of developing an anastomotic leak.

A, B

The duodenum is mobilized by a very generous Kocher maneuver. The pyloric area is grasped with a Babcock forceps, and a stitch of 3-0 silk is placed about 7 cm from this point to incorporate the antrum and duodenum. The softness of the tissue indicates the point from the ulcer at which the anastomosis can begin. Simple stitches of 3-0 silk are used to appose the antrum and duodenum progressively.

C

The stitches are continued for a distance of approximately 5 cm. The seromuscularis is incised down to the mucosa, and bleeding points are electrocoagulated with a fine-tipped instrument.

D

Electrocautery is used to incise the mucosa and coagulate fine vessels. Here, a scissors is being used to open the duodenum.

A

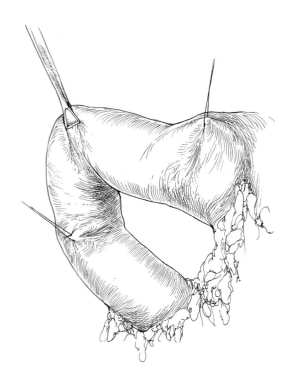

C

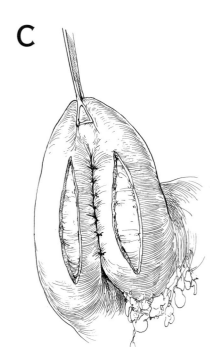

B

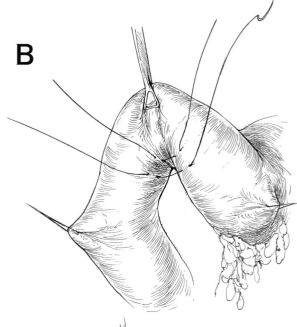

D

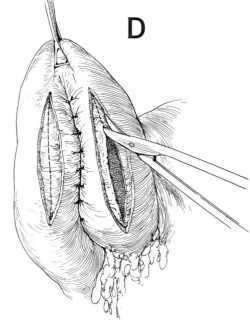

E, F

The mucosa is approximated with a continuous simple stitch of 3-0 chromic catgut. It is started at the lower or upper end posteriorly and is progressively brought anteriorly.

G

The seromuscularis is approximated with interrupted simple or inverting stitches of 3-0 silk.

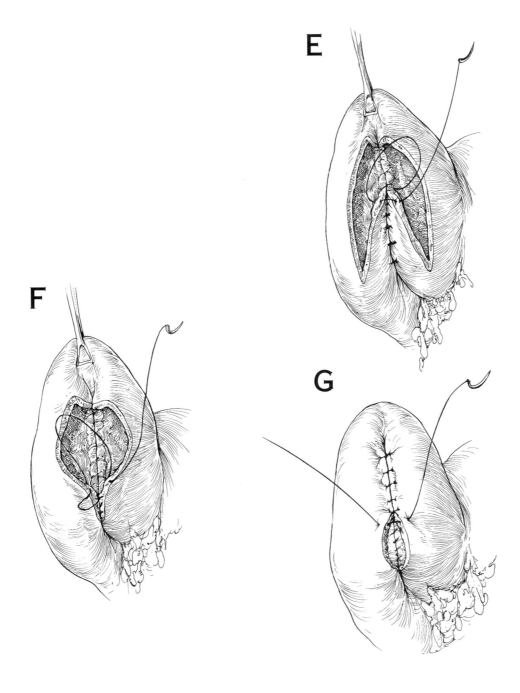

Ē VAGOTOMY

TRUNCAL

Division of the vagus nerves is a key component in any operation whose aim is to control the acid factor in gastric secretion. Affected normally are the right and left vagi, whose pathways may be interrupted intra-abdominally by one of three main operations: (1) Truncal vagotomy: The two trunks are divided 5 to 7 cm cephalad to the esophagogastric junction. (2) Selective vagotomy: The vagal branches are divided distal to the celiac and hepatic branches. This operation is not commonly used at present. (3) Highly selective vagotomy: The celiac and hepatic branches are retained, as is the innervation to the distal antrum. In this operation only the proximal two thirds of the stomach is denervated.

A

This view demonstrates the general anatomy of the stomach. The right (posterior) vagus is ghosted in. Several hepatic branches rather than the usual one are shown. Only the anterior branches of the nerve of Latarjet are visible.

A

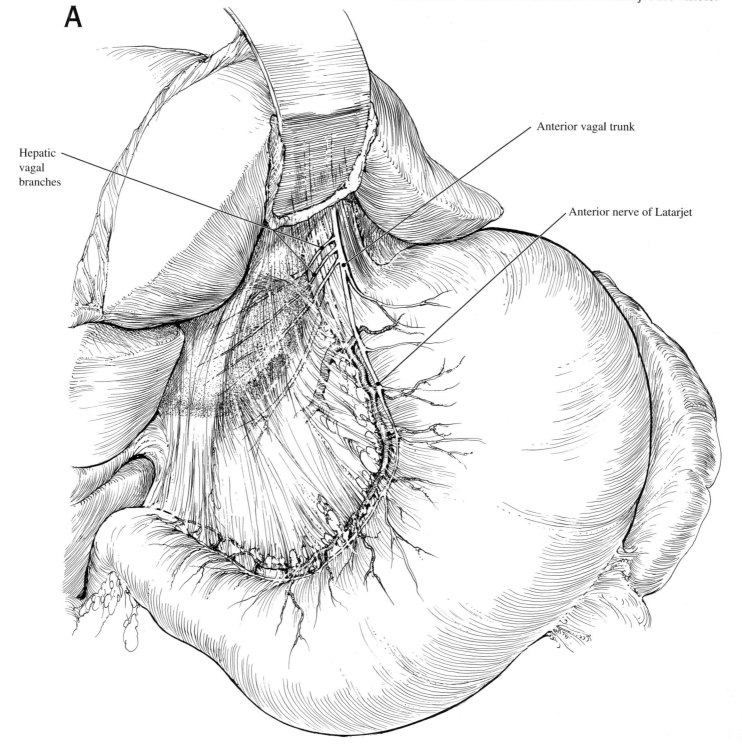

Hepatic vagal branches

Anterior vagal trunk

Anterior nerve of Latarjet

B

The midline incision is best for patients with a narrow costal angle; a transverse subcostal or midline one will do for all others. The abdomen is explored for associated pathology before focusing on the vagotomy. The left lobe of the liver is protected with a large lap pad as it is lifted slightly and retracted to the patient's right. In some patients, the left triangular ligament may need to be divided for adequate mobilization of the left lobe and exposure of the esophagus.

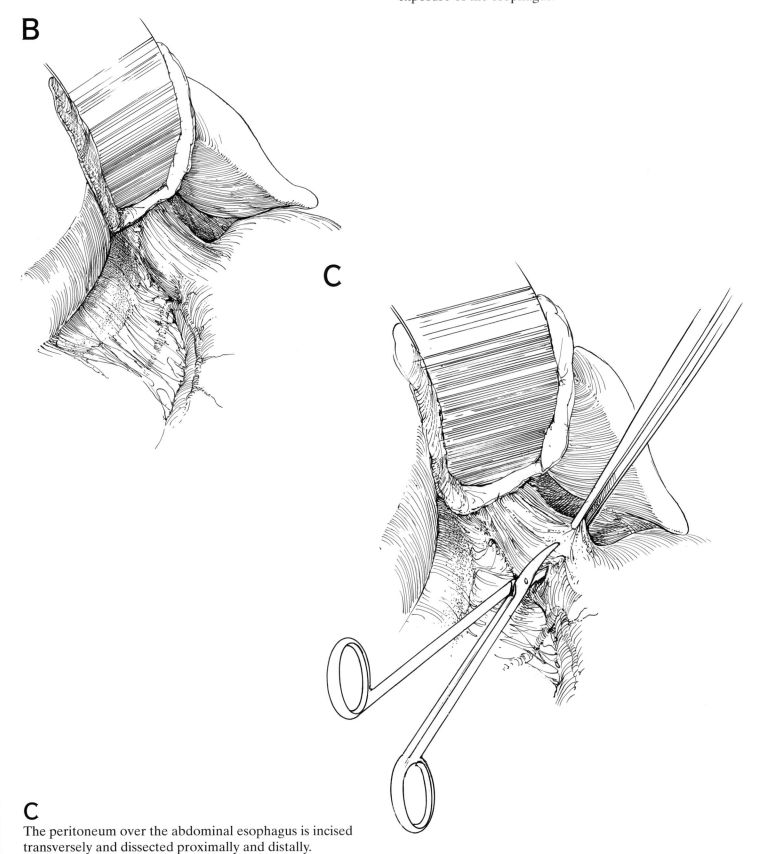

B

C

C

The peritoneum over the abdominal esophagus is incised transversely and dissected proximally and distally.

D

The right index finger is insinuated fully around the
esophagus and associated tissue. If the finger is kept too
close to the esophagus, the posterior vagus likely will not
be in the tissue being mobilized in preparation for
vagotomy. A pledget of gauze on a 6-inch forceps (a
"peanut") applied anterior to the esophagus enables some
fixation and easier dissection with the index finger.

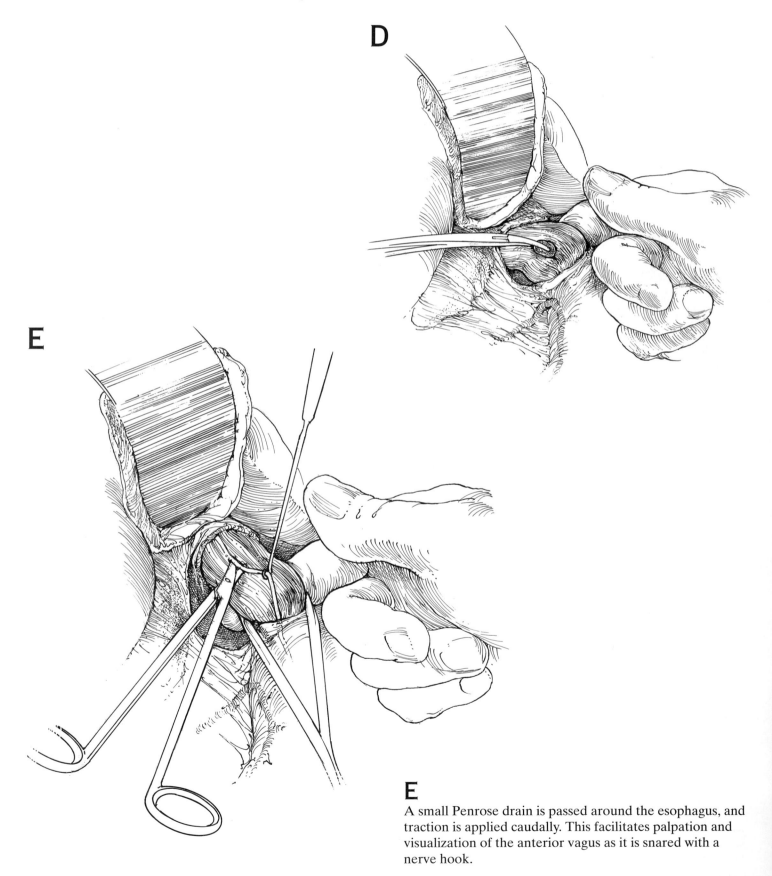

D

E

E

A small Penrose drain is passed around the esophagus, and
traction is applied caudally. This facilitates palpation and
visualization of the anterior vagus as it is snared with a
nerve hook.

F

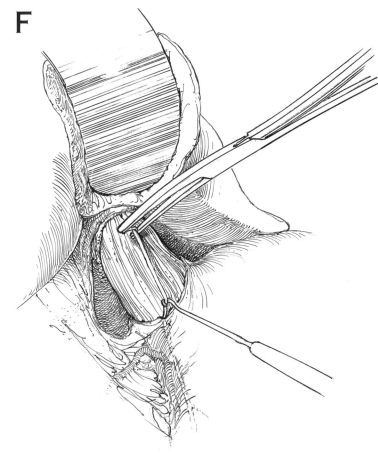

G

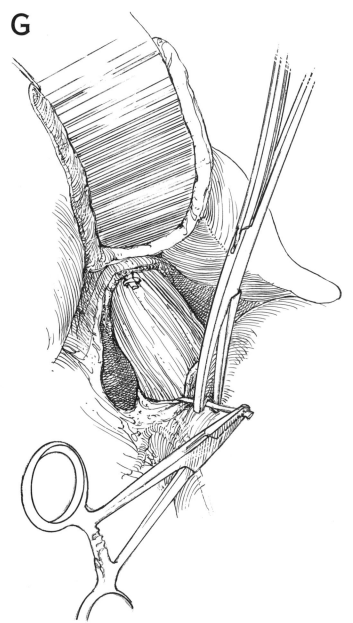

F, G

The nerve is pulled taut, clipped proximally and divided. It is swung downward and handled similarly at its distal part. A portion of it is removed and sent to the pathologist for histologic confirmation.

H, I

If the posterior vagus is not found in the retracted tissue, it is sought in the tissue dorsal to this. It, too, is cleared proximally and distally before a 1-cm length is removed for histologic confirmation.

H

I

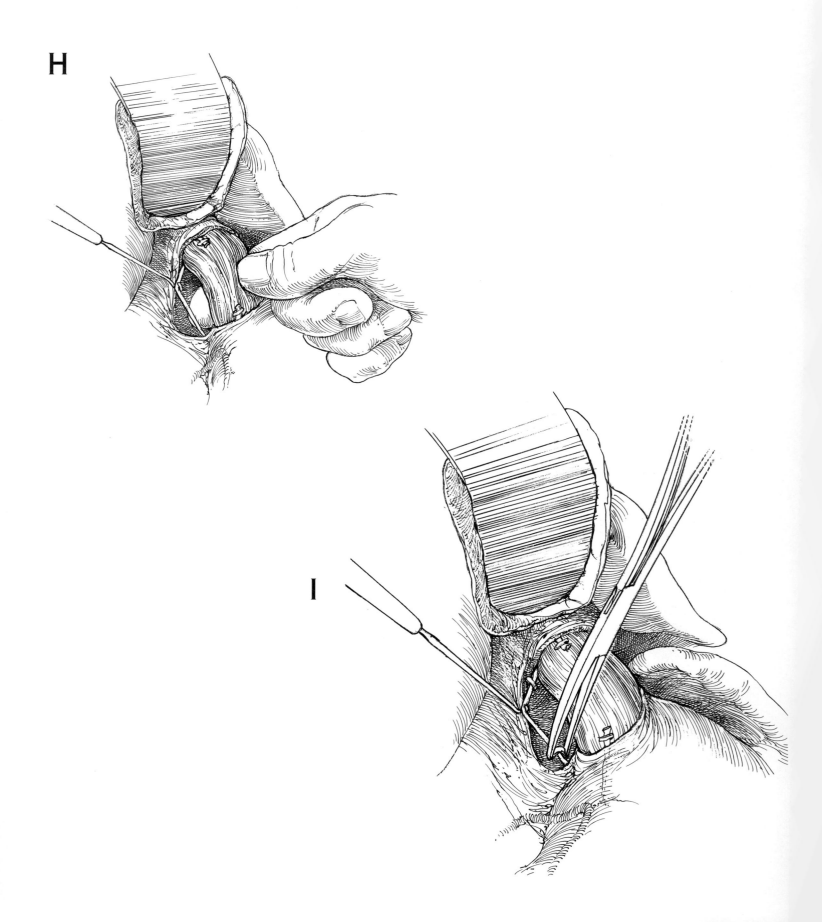

SELECTIVE

A

Selective vagotomy is performed in an attempt to lessen the problems of postprandial diarrhea and the formation of gallstones. This procedure entails division of the anterior vagus nerve just after it gives off a branch (or branches) to the liver and of the celiac branch of the posterior trunk.

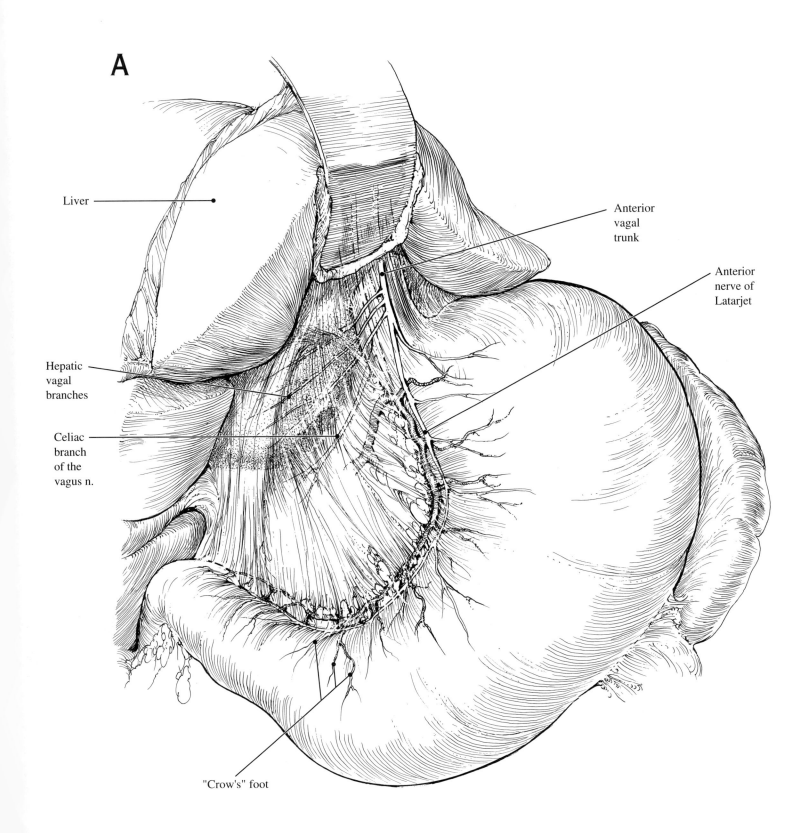

A

Liver

Anterior
vagal
trunk

Anterior
nerve of
Latarjet

Hepatic
vagal
branches

Celiac
branch
of the
vagus n.

"Crow's" foot

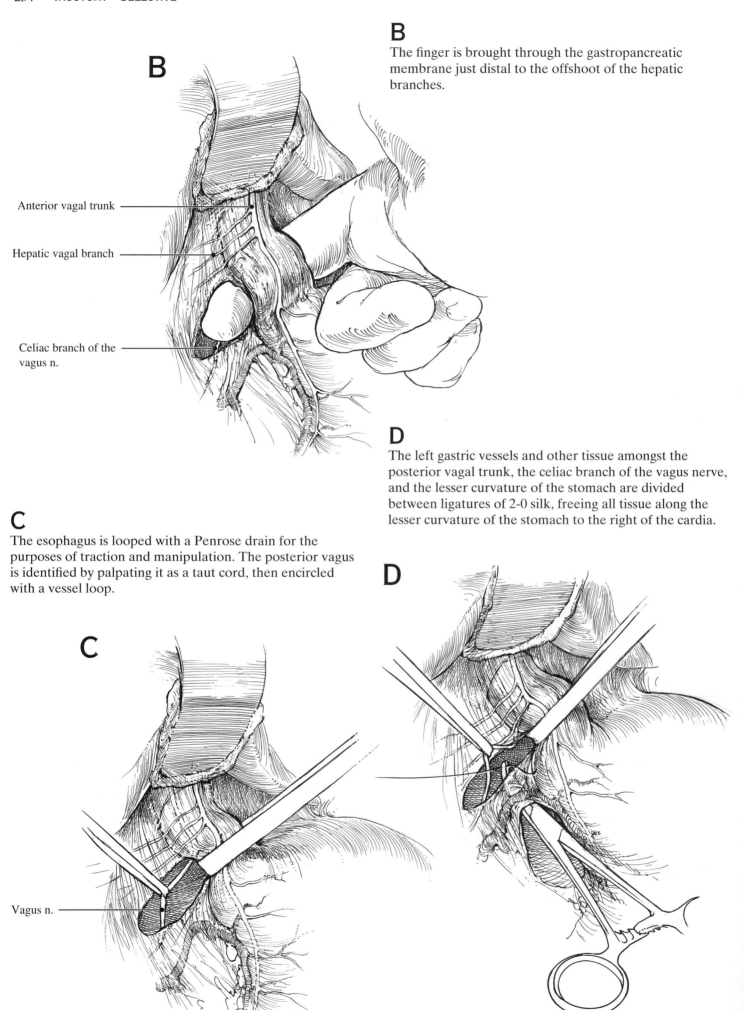

B

The finger is brought through the gastropancreatic membrane just distal to the offshoot of the hepatic branches.

Anterior vagal trunk

Hepatic vagal branch

Celiac branch of the vagus n.

D

The left gastric vessels and other tissue amongst the posterior vagal trunk, the celiac branch of the vagus nerve, and the lesser curvature of the stomach are divided between ligatures of 2-0 silk, freeing all tissue along the lesser curvature of the stomach to the right of the cardia.

C

The esophagus is looped with a Penrose drain for the purposes of traction and manipulation. The posterior vagus is identified by palpating it as a taut cord, then encircled with a vessel loop.

Vagus n.

E, F

The anterior vagal trunk is pulled upward with a nerve hook, clips are applied to the nerve at least 3 cm apart, and the portion of the intervening nerves are resected for microscopic confirmation.

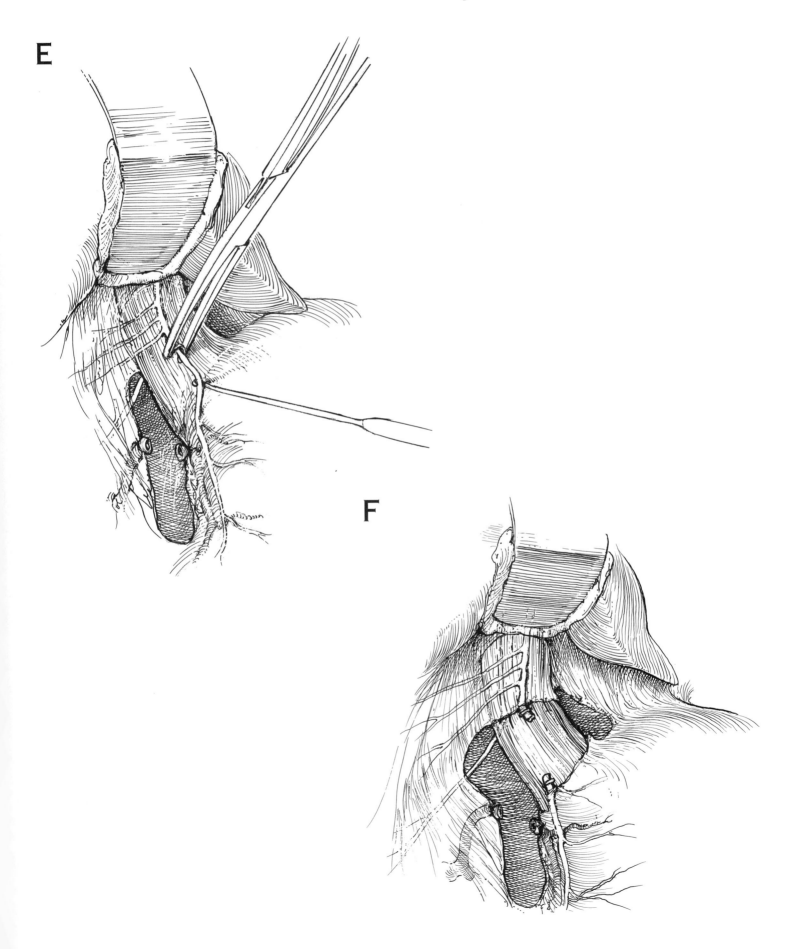

E

F

HIGHLY SELECTIVE

The purpose of highly selective vagotomy is to denervate only the acid-bearing parietal cell mass; in addition, the surgeon should do so without a stomach drainage procedure.

A

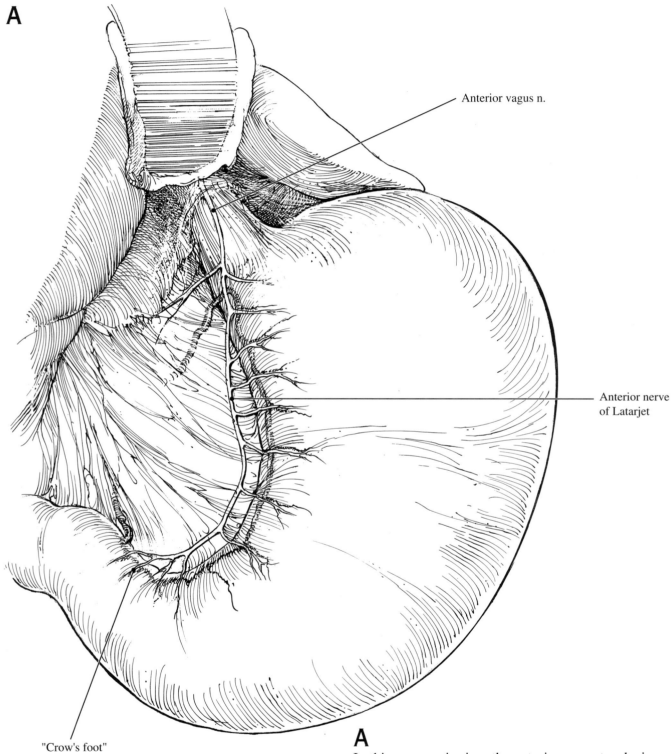

Anterior vagus n.

Anterior nerve
of Latarjet

"Crow's foot"

A

In this panoramic view, the anterior vagus trunk gives off the hepatic branch and continues caudally anteriorly on the lesser curvature of the stomach as the anterior nerve of Latarjet. Dorsal to this, in the posterior leaf of the lesser omentum, the right vagus gives off a celiac branch and continues as the posterior nerve of Latarjet. Both these nerves terminate in the antral-parietal area of the lesser curvature; because of their trifurcate configuration at this point, they are often referred to as the "crow's foot."

B

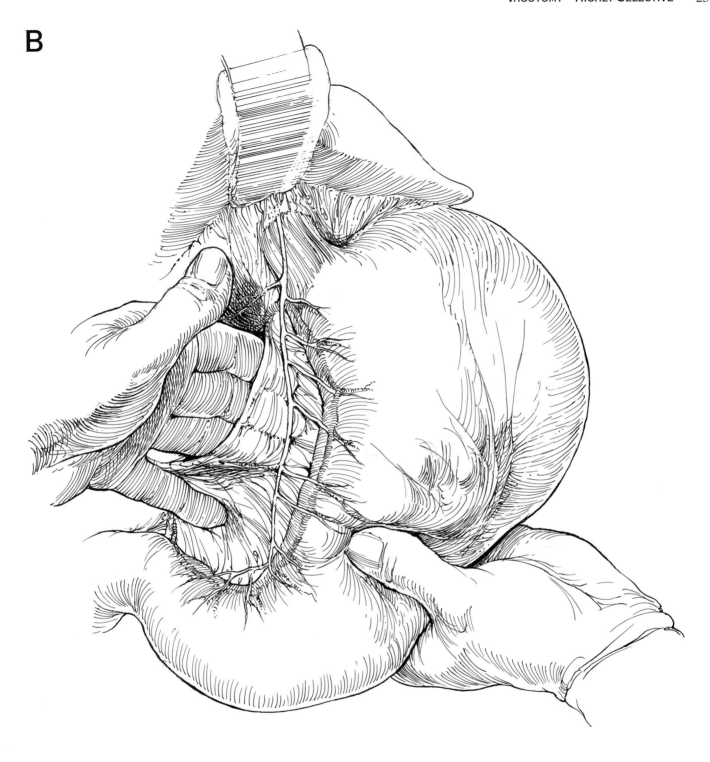

B

The lesser sac is entered, and a hand is placed under the superficial layer of the lesser omentum. With one hand grasping and retracting the body of the stomach to the patient's left, the nerve trunk and its gastric branches are fully exposed.

C

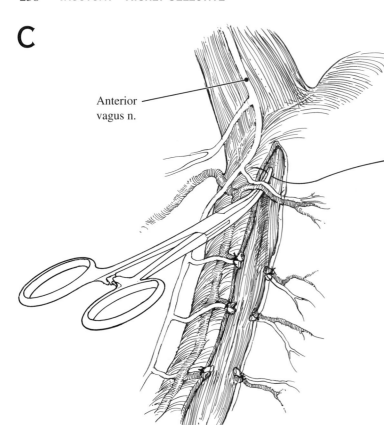

Anterior
vagus n.

C, D

A fine forceps, preferably an Adson, which is long handled
and has a fine, curved tip—both features favorable for
working with such tissue and especially in deep-chested
patients—is used to isolate each branch about 1 cm from
the main trunk. The branches are then ligated with 3-0 silk
and divided. This is done in serial fashion as far caudally as
the crow's foot and then repeated with the branches of the
posterior vagus nerve.

D

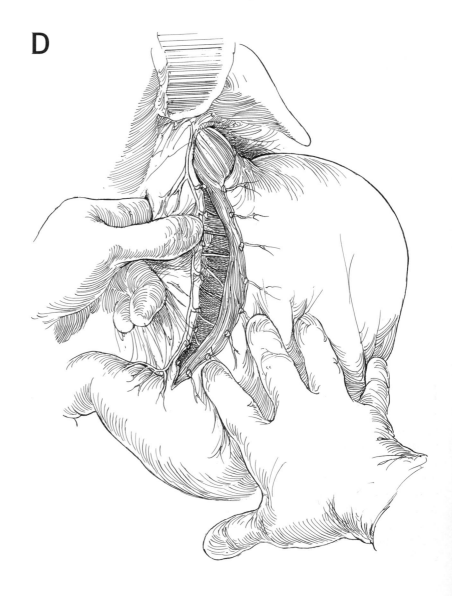

E

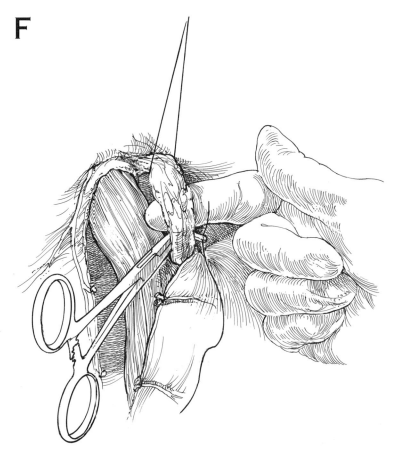

Attention is focused on dividing nerve branches and blood vessels that enter high on the lesser curvature. A Penrose drain is used to retract the esophagus firmly to the patient's left, exposing the branches of the left gastric artery as they enter the cardia and lower esophagus. An acutely curved forceps is used to encircle all this tissue and to ligate it doubly with 2-0 silk before division. This effectively creates a window that makes the next step easier.

F

F

A nasogastric tube positioned at the beginning of the operation is particularly helpful while working near the esophagus; in this instance it helps define the tissue around it, because the aim is to clear the esophagus of all nerve fibers for a length of 5 cm. Division of the major branches of the vagus at the upper lesser curvature allows the trunk of the vagus to be moved upward and to the patient's right. The tissue to the left of the esophagus that remains to be divided includes fat, vessels, and nerves. This tissue is doubly ligated on each side with 2-0 silk and divided.

G

The next task is to clear all of the intra-abdominal and 4 to 5 cm of the thoracic esophagus of all nerve filaments. This is done with fine instruments in a methodical fashion. The finger and thumb handling the esophagus can be used to "roll" it somewhat to gain a clear inspection of the dorsal surface. Bleeding points can be controlled with electrocoagulation or clips.

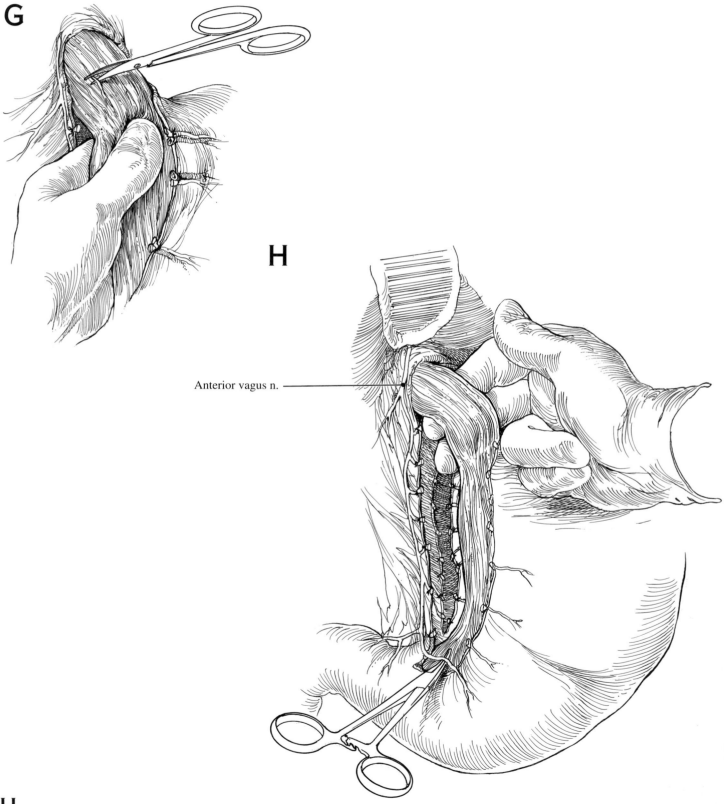

Anterior vagus n.

H

The dissection is completed with the hemostat demonstrating the uppermost branch of the crow's foot.

I

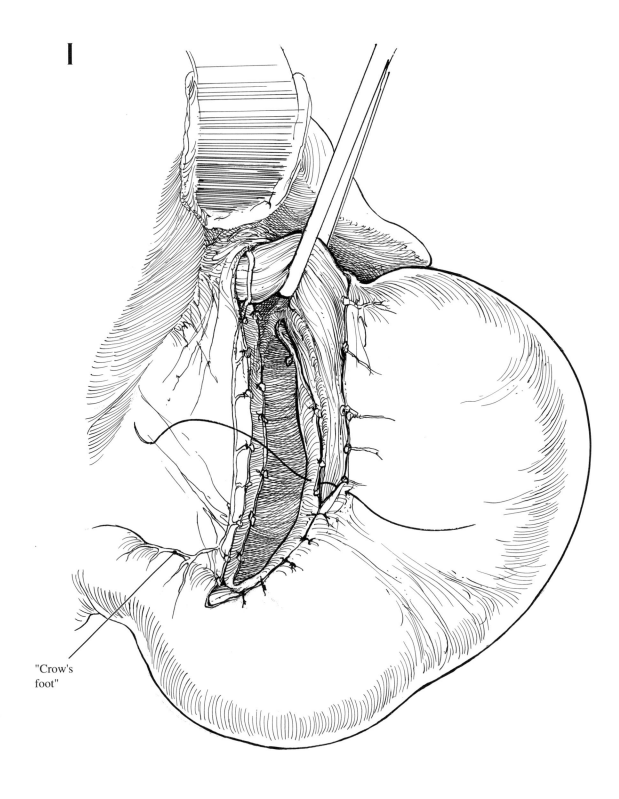

"Crow's
foot"

I

Reapproximation of the serosa covering the denuded
stomach is done with 4-0 silk, taking small superficial bites
with the needle. Implicit in this operation is the absence of
a drainage procedure. The abdomen is closed in a routine
manner.

LAPAROSCOPIC (HIGHLY SELECTIVE)

Relatively few of the very large number of patients with peptic ulcer disease require an operation, but of those that do, the majority have an acid-reducing operation. Laparoscopic vagotomy is an evolving operation for this problem, and the technique of highly selective vagotomy is an attempt to eliminate the need for an emptying procedure and the problems of dumping and diarrhea that are seen with the more easily performed truncal vagotomy.

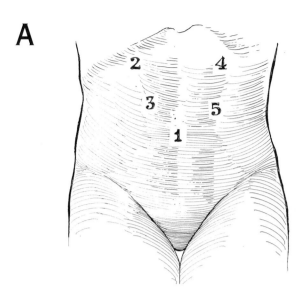

A

The patient is anesthetized and positioned horizontally, and the entire abdomen and lower thorax are prepared and draped. The port placement is as follows: no. 1 at the umbilicus for the laparoscope; no. 2 at the costal margin for the liver retractor; no. 3 midway between no. 1 and no. 2 for the main operating port; and no. 4 for gastric esophageal retraction. No. 5 is an example of an additional port if further exposure is needed.

B

The dissection is begun by incising the peritoneum over the esophagogastric junction and opening the gastrohepatic omentum. A Babcock forceps applied to the gastric fundus and retracting it to the patient's left helps with the dissection that is to follow. A previously inserted Maloney dilator helps identify the lower esophagus.

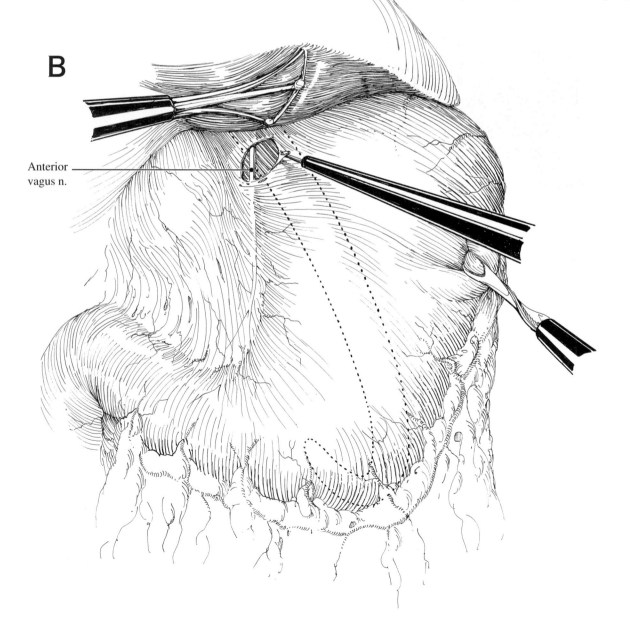

Anterior vagus n.

C

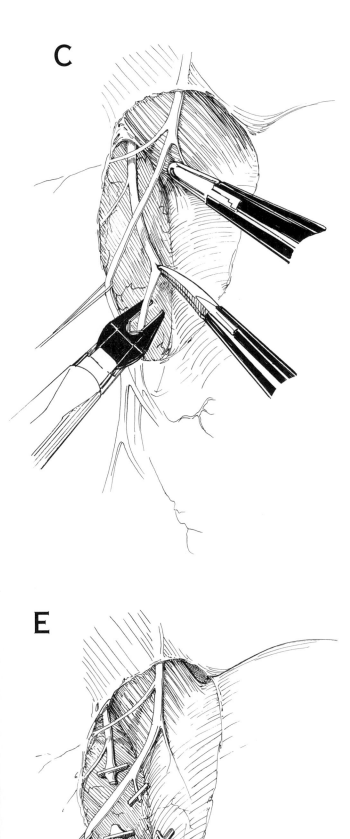

C, D

The posterior vagus is dissected for 4 to 5 cm before dividing the nerve between clips and sending a short segment of it to the pathologist for histologic confirmation.

D

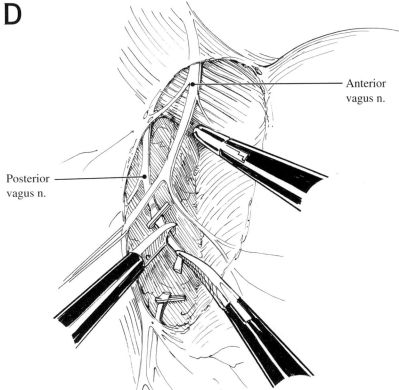

Anterior vagus n.

Posterior vagus n.

E

E

With continued traction on the gastric fundus, the anterior vagus nerve is made taut in preparation for the highly selective vagotomy. The hepatic branch of the anterior vagus nerve is spared whenever possible.

F, G

Once the "crow's foot" has been identified, the branches of the anterior vagus nerve are serially secured between clips and divided up to the esophagogastric junction.

No emptying procedure is necessary. Bleeding points are looked for and coagulated as necessary. The trocar sites are closed in an appropriate manner.

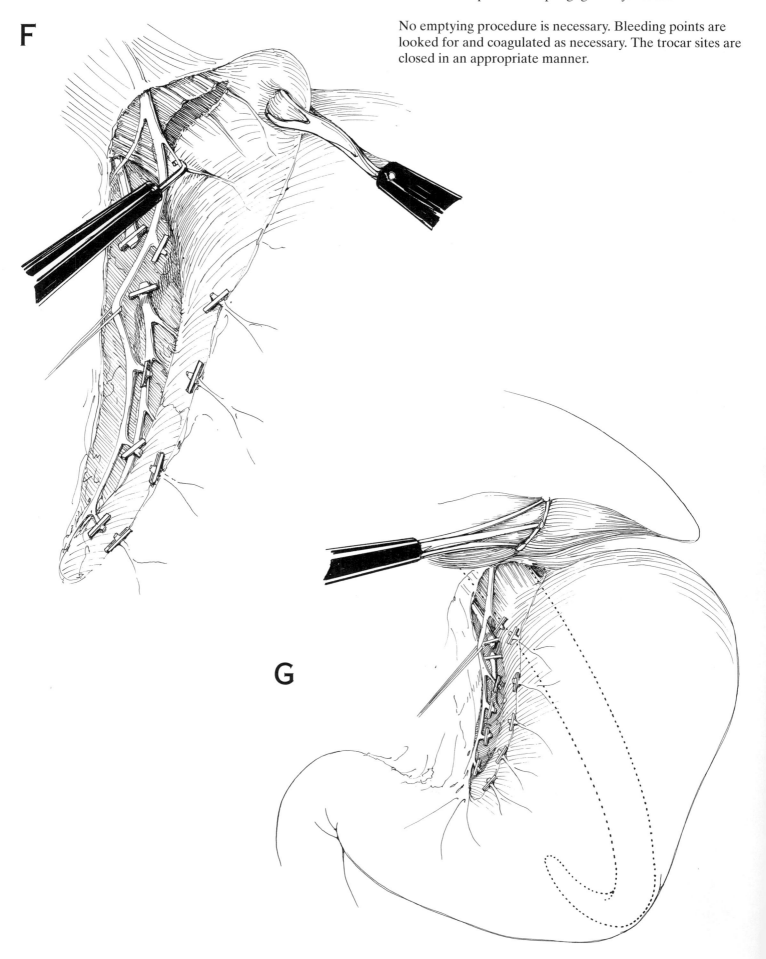

F GASTROSTOMY

STAMM

Gastrostomy is used widely to prevent distention of the stomach or to feed the patient. The increasing application of endoscopic or percutaneous techniques for accomplishing this notwithstanding, the techniques described herein are essential components of the general surgeon's armamentarium, and knowledge about them and skill in performing them should become second nature.

A

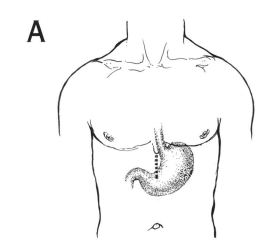

B

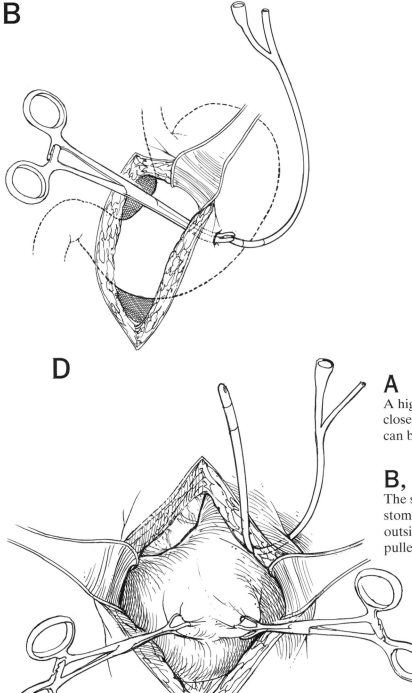

C

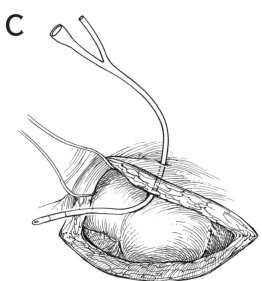

D

A

A high midline incision is best because it can be made and closed swiftly and easily, it provides adequate access, and it can be enlarged if necessary.

B, C

The skin incision is made overlying the body of the stomach, and a hemostat is forced from within to the outside to grasp the tip of the Foley catheter, which is pulled into the abdominal cavity.

D

The gastric entry site is selected and grasped on either side with Babcock forceps.

E, F, G, H, I

A purse-string suture of 2-0 silk is applied and the intended puncture site electrocoagulated (*E*). A hemostat is passed through the electrocoagulated site down to the mucosa, at which point the hemostat is spread and advanced to grasp the mucosa; this too is electrocoagulated (*F, G, H*). Taking these steps obliterates any potential bleeding points. With the Babcock forceps to hold the stomach up and suction at the ready, the mucosa is then perforated with the hemostat (*I*).

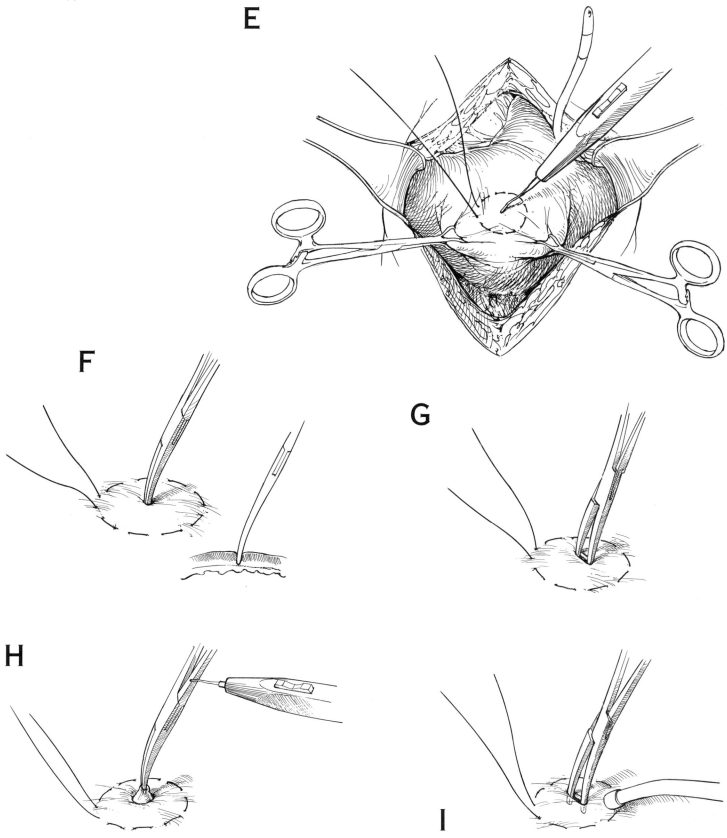

J, K, L, M

The Foley catheter is inserted and the purse-string suture drawn and tied (*J, K*). Anchoring stitches are placed between the stomach and the parietal peritoneum at the cephalad and caudal side of the gastrostomy (*L*). The Foley balloon is now inflated. The anchoring stitches are drawn and tied as the Foley is pulled; this snugs the stomach to the parietal peritoneum. A stitch is used to anchor the Foley catheter to the skin (*M*).

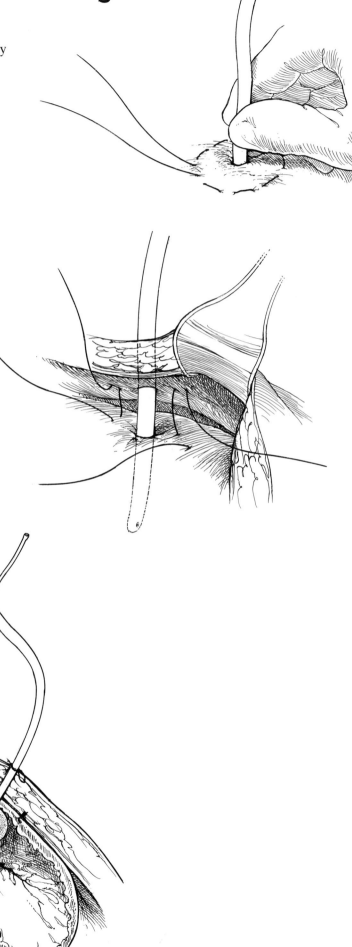

JANEWAY

A Janeway gastrostomy is preferred over a Stamm gastrostomy when more permanent access to the stomach is needed.

A, B

With the abdomen opened and in preparation for creation of the gastrostomy, two Babcock forceps are used to grasp the stomach in a transverse fashion; they will delineate the direction and length of the tube. The GIA instrument is applied with the tip of it at 3 cm from the greater curvature. The instrument is closed and the staples fired.

A

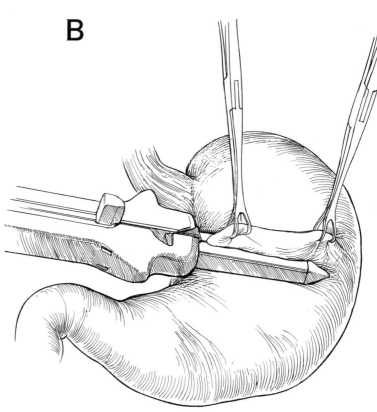

B

C

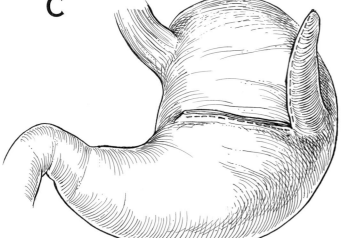

C

The tip of the tube is included in the staple line; this seals it and lessens the degree of contamination.

D

The tube is oversewn with a continuous stitch of catgut. A counterincision is made in the skin, and the tube is brought to the surface.

D

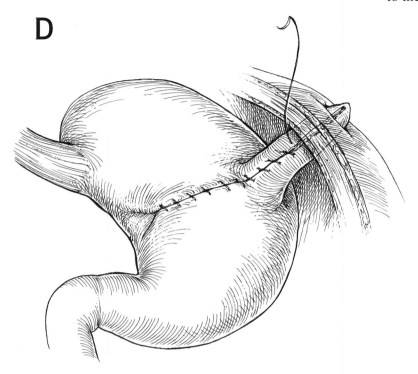

E

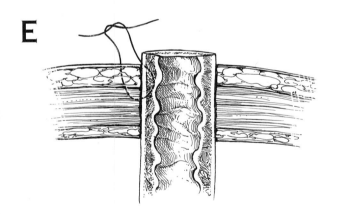

F

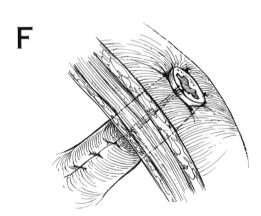

E, F

When the tube is brought to the surface, the pointed tip is cut off, creating an opening, which then is sewn as shown both to anchor the tube and to tent it open for easy cannulation. The abdominal cavity is closed in a preferred manner.

Chapter

11

SMALL INTESTINE

$\overline{A}$ MECKEL'S DIVERTICULECTOMY

A Meckel's diverticulum is the congenital remnant of the omphalomesenteric duct and usually is located about 25 cm proximal to the ileocecal valve. The majority are asymptomatic but can be affected in a variety of clinical scenarios requiring emergency surgery. If found incidental to a celiotomy, removal is advised unless they are short and wide based, or when resection might interfere with addressing the primary intra-abdominal pathologic condition. The incision usually is that employed in the celiotomy for an unrelated problem; otherwise, a low midline incision is preferred.

A

The diverticulum with the associated small intestine is delivered into the wound. Here, the mesodiverticulum and its associated vessel are being secured with a suture ligature. The base of the diverticulum should be amputated in a manner that will least compromise the ileum.

B

In this instance, the Meckel's diverticulum is amputated with a stapler in a direction perpendicular to the long axis of the intestine.

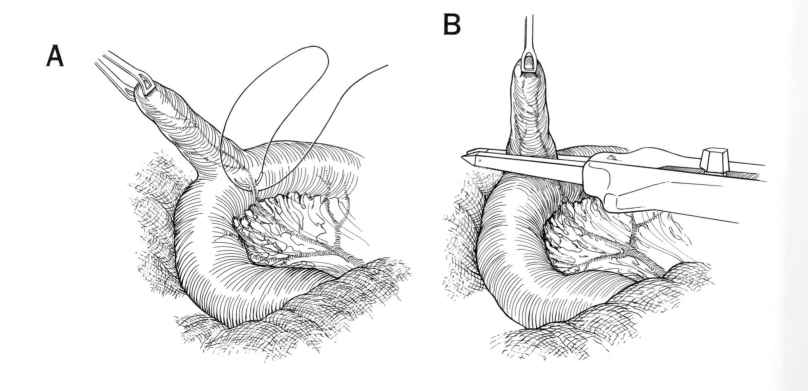

A

B

C, D

The stapled line is oversewn with a continuous, simple stitch of 4-0 chromic catgut.

E

Sometimes, the dimensions and configuration of the diverticulum indicate the need for resection with primary anastomosis. The mesenteric vessels are ligated and divided, after which the intestine is divided between intestinal clamps proximal and distal to the diverticulum.

C

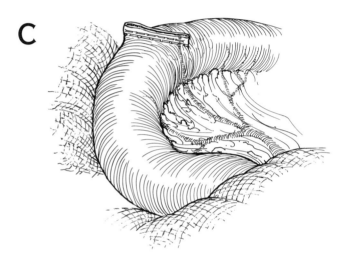

D

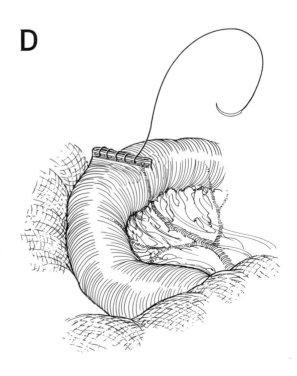

E

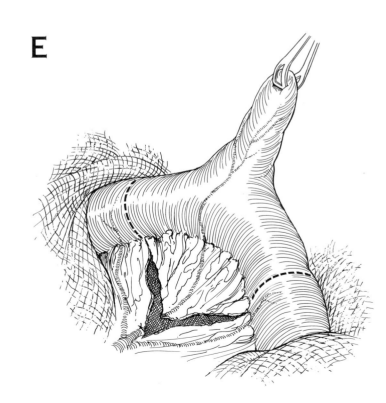

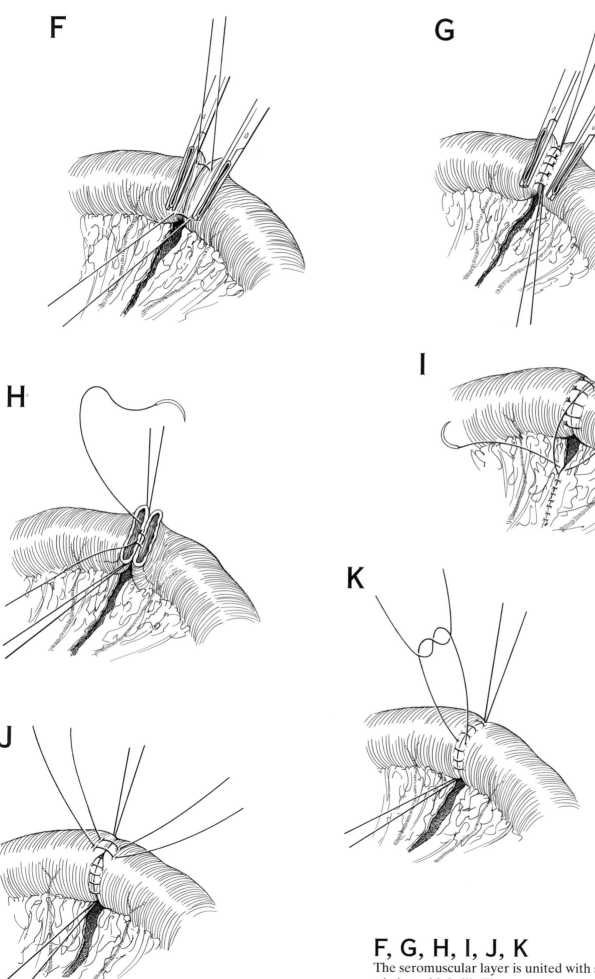

F, G, H, I, J, K

The seromuscular layer is united with simple, interrupted stitches of 3-0 silk. The mucosa is approximated with continuous or interrupted 3-0 chromic catgut.

B INTUSSUSCEPTION—REDUCTION

B

A

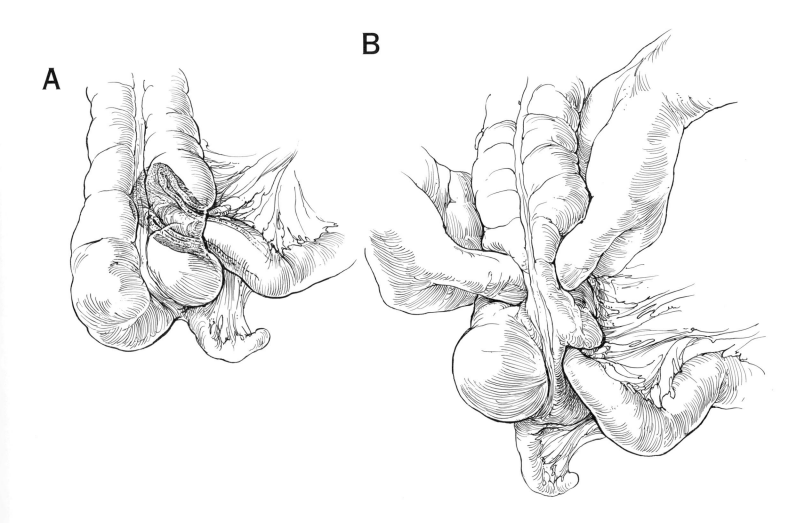

C

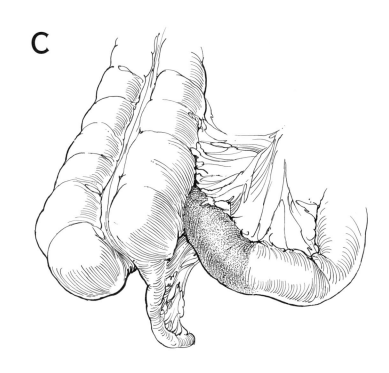

A

Intussusception, usually the invagination of the ileum into the colon—sometimes all the way to the transverse colon, and even farther—most commonly occurs in infants. If operative reduction becomes necessary, the intussuscepted mass is delivered through an incision in the right lower quadrant.

B

The intussusception is reduced by "milking" it out of the colon; never by pulling on the ileum. Intussusception that is not reducible, or when reduced, raises concern about the viability of the intestine, calls for resection of the affected intestine.

C

Often, a reduced ileum has an erythematous surface. It can simply be observed for a few minutes to be assured of its viability. An appendectomy is advisable in most instances. The abdomen is closed in a routine manner.

12

APPENDIX

A APPENDECTOMY

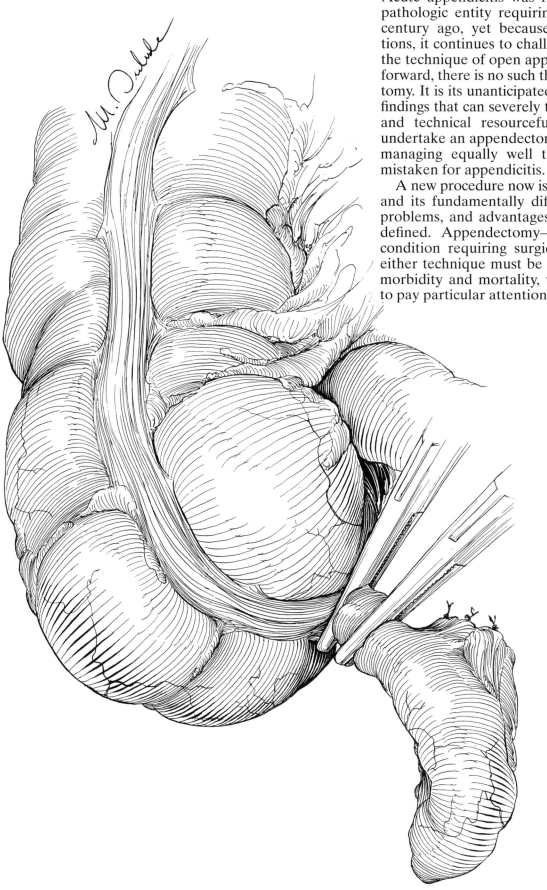

Acute appendicitis was recognized as a clinical and pathologic entity requiring surgical therapy about a century ago, yet because of its protean manifestations, it continues to challenge the surgeon. Although the technique of open appendectomy is quite straightforward, there is no such thing as a "simple" appendectomy. It is its unanticipated location or the unexpected findings that can severely test the surgeon's knowledge and technical resourcefulness. No surgeon should undertake an appendectomy without being capable of managing equally well the conditions that can be mistaken for appendicitis.

A new procedure now is laparoscopic appendectomy and its fundamentally different technical guidelines, problems, and advantages, all still not unequivocally defined. Appendectomy—the most common acute condition requiring surgical therapy—performed by either technique must be accompanied by a very low morbidity and mortality, which is what prompted us to pay particular attention in presenting this chapter.

A

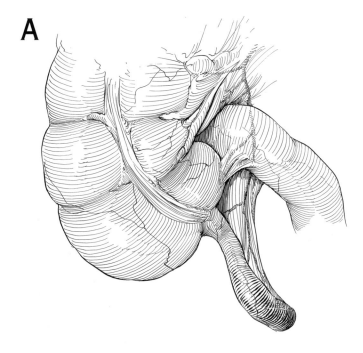

OPEN

A

The base of the appendix comes off the tip of the cecum, the anterior tinea serving as a reliable guide to it if the cecum appears first in the operative incision. This can be helpful in that the tip of the appendix can be found at a number of positions but is most commonly pelvic, next retroileal but still intraperitoneal, and then retrocecal or retroperitoneal. The appendicular artery, a branch of the superior mesenteric artery, courses behind the terminal ileum to run along the free edge of the mesoappendix as it gives off its branches to the appendix itself. This makes it possible to ligate the appendiceal artery and the appendices epiploica with a single stout absorbable ligature. Otherwise, the mesoappendix and its contained branches to the appendix need to be ligated in several steps.

B

The most commonly used incisions for an appendectomy are the McBurney and the lower-positioned Rocky Davis. Modest variations of the McBurney are equally satisfactory for the surgeon in the habit of using it. If the diagnosis is uncertain, a midline incision provides the surgeon with the greatest latitude. It is reasonable to expect, however, that with the advent of minimal access (laparoscopic) techniques, cases of uncertain diagnosis will be better defined so that the incision for an open operation can be positioned accordingly or the appendectomy simply will be performed laparoscopically.

C

The incision is carried down and parallel to the fibers of the aponeurosis of the external oblique muscle; the incision of the aponeurosis is performed in the same plane. Notice the rectus abdominus muscle (with its sheath intact) at the medial aspect of the incision.

B

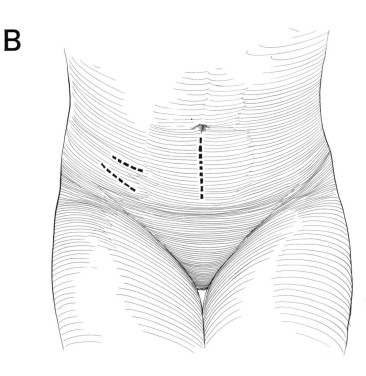

C

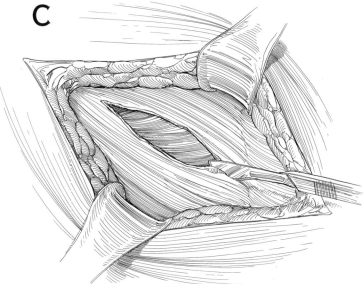

D

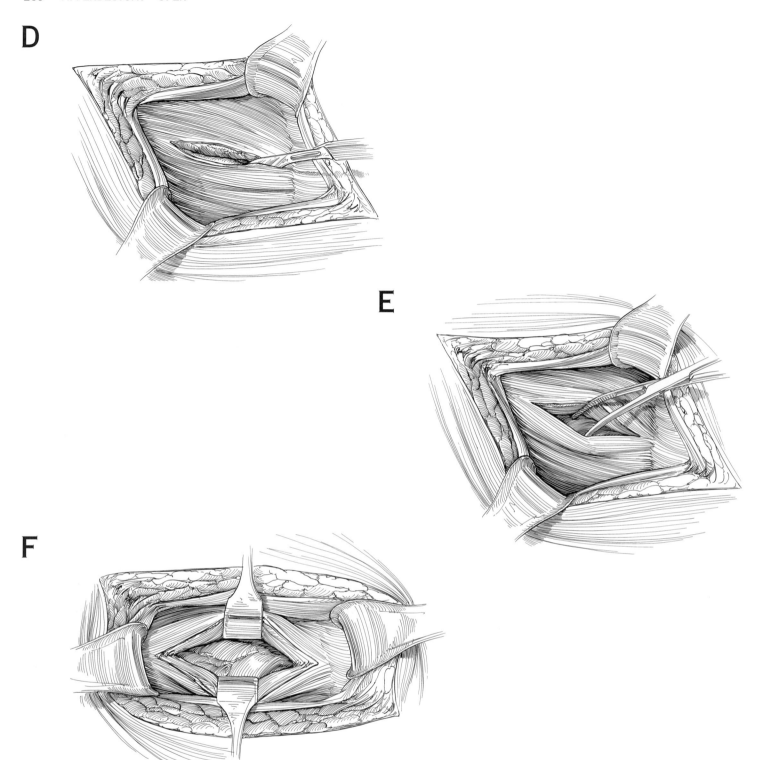

E

F

D, E, F

Techniques are described in which the external and internal oblique muscles and the transversalis fascia are split as separate layers. This seems to be excessive dissection with benefits that likely are more apparent than real. We prefer to start the dissection by incising the aponeurosis of the external oblique fibers and then using a hemostat to begin separating them as one. It is premature to insert two fingers (there is not enough room) and to begin separating the muscle at this point. Instead, the separation should continue with the hemostat (often two) until the transversalis fascia is reached and separated first for one finger, then for two. The index finger of each hand or small Richardson retractors are maneuvered into position, and all the layers are separated as one by a steady, firm pull.

G

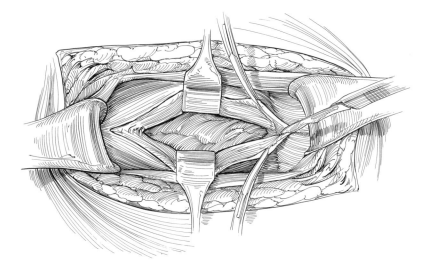

G

If it is felt that the opening should be longer, it can be accomplished by dividing the rectus abdominis muscle sheath for approximately 2 cm (but leaving the muscle intact).

H

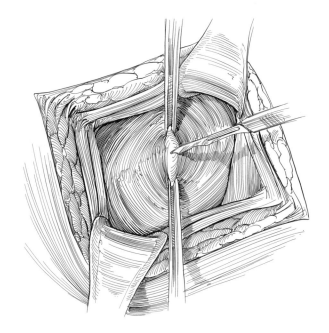

H

After the muscles have been separated maximally, larger Richardson retractors are inserted. The surgeon and assistant grasp the peritoneum, making certain this grasp does not include underlying viscera. The peritoneal incision is made cautiously, and any free fluid encountered is swabbed for bacterial examination.

I

The peritoneum is opened further, and the retractors are positioned to now retract all layers of the abdominal wall. Usually the cecum comes into view. The surgeon should slide the index finger along the tinea in the direction of the appendix. Doing so not only confirms the location of the appendix but also alerts the surgeon to an abscess that might be opened and spill more freely if the cecum is retracted forthwith.

I

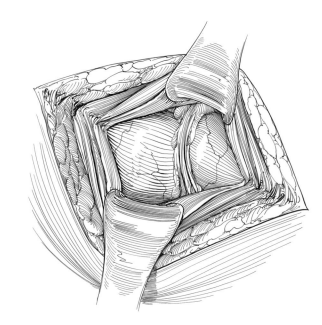

J

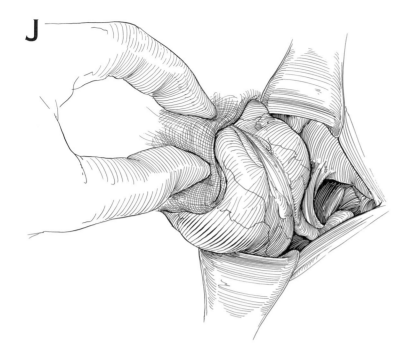

K

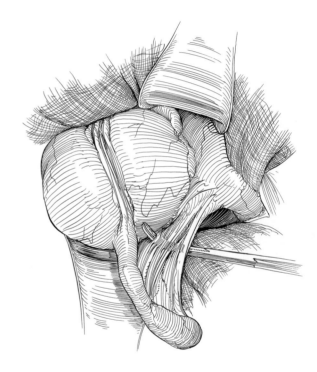

J

The cecum is grasped with a moistened sponge between it and the fingers; otherwise it slips away during the course of the operation. The cecum is delivered into the wound, bringing the appendix into view or into the wound. Sometimes, minimal fibrinous adhesions need to be cleared by a sweep of the finger to permit the appendix to follow the cecum into the wound.

K, L

The appendiceal artery is close to the free edge of the mesoappendix; a very small branch often courses very close to the appendix. A Mixter or curved hemostat is passed through the mesoappendix as close to the appendix as possible, thus encompassing all of the blood supply to the appendix. The mesoappendiceal tissue with the incorporated appendiceal vessels is ligated with 3-0 chromic catgut, and the tissue is divided, leaving a 1-cm stub.

L

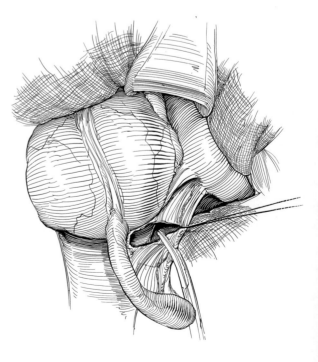

M

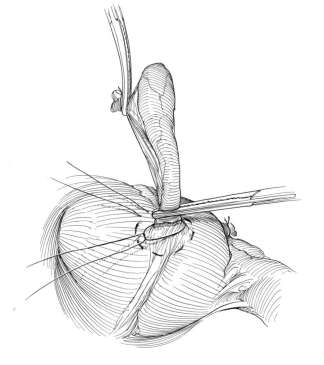

M

A purse-string suture of 3-0 silk is stitched through the seromuscular tissue that should be of sufficient circumference to accommodate the inverted appendiceal stump.

N, O, P

The base of the appendix is crushed with a hemostat and tied with 4-0 catgut. The appendix is clamped distal to this and divided with a scalpel, leaving a 5-mm stump. The purse-string suture is tightened as the appendiceal stump is inverted.

N

O

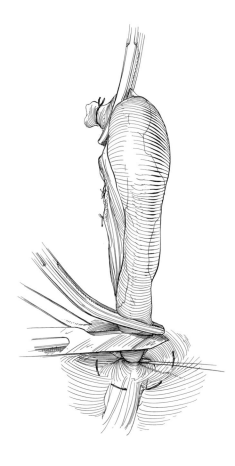

P

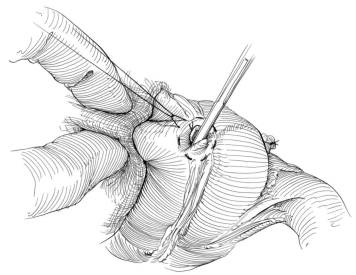

Q, R

Occasionally, the inflamed appendix is *paracecal* and adherent to the surrounding tissue. Accordingly, it is removed in a retrograde manner by encircling the appendix, crushing its base, tying it, and using this tie for manipulating the appendix as it is dissected off the cecum. The mesoappendix and appendiceal artery are tied and divided as encountered. A purse-string suture is applied, and the appendix is amputated and inverted as before.

Q

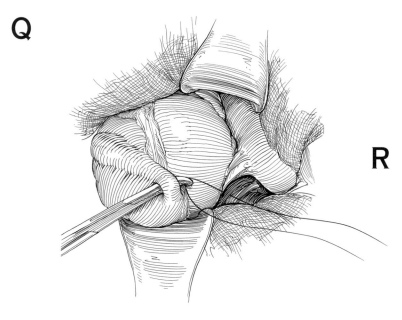

R

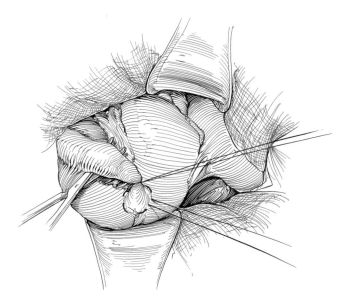

S

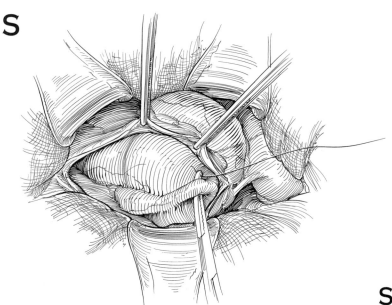

S

Occasionally, the appendix is *retrocecal,* making it necessary to incise the peritoneum—usually quite edematous by virtue of the confined infection—lateral to the cecum to reach it. The base of the appendix is isolated, crushed, and ligated. The appendix is dissected free, and the mesoappendix and appendiceal artery are ligated as encountered. The appendix is amputated and inverted with a purse-string suture of 3-0 silk. The lateral peritoneum is not closed.

T

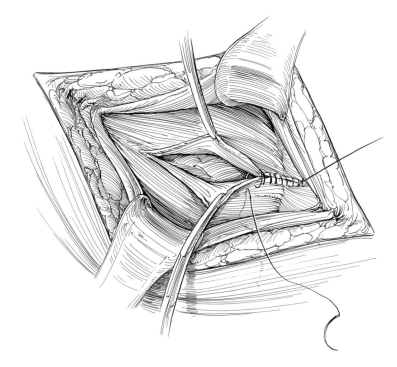

U

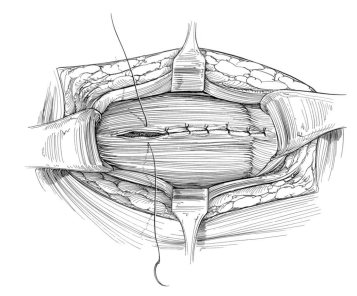

V

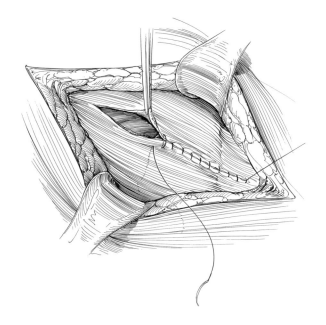

T, U, V

The peritoneum, often incorporating some of the transversalis fascia, is closed with a continuous simple stitch of 3-0 chromic catgut. The muscles are reapproximated with simple interrupted stitches using similar suture material and tied gently so as not to cut through the muscle fibers. The external oblique muscle is reapproximated with a continuous stitch of catgut only through the aponeurosis; the underlying muscles invariably come together and stay so postoperatively with contraction of the abdominal muscles. Drains are rarely used. The skin is closed in a preferred manner. We rarely practice delayed closure.

A

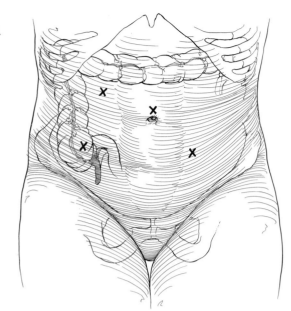

LAPAROSCOPIC

A

Laparoscopic appendectomy is steadily gaining acceptance for a variety of reasons: (1) Exploration of the abdominal cavity can be more inclusive than is possible through a McBurney incision; (2) a "negative" appendix can be removed with minimal morbidity; (3) perhaps there is less inhibition to having an "early look"; (4) patients with a certain body habitus—obesity, for example—experience less operative trauma than with an open exploration; and (5) there is minimal abdominal scarring.

One customary pattern of trocar placement is shown.

B

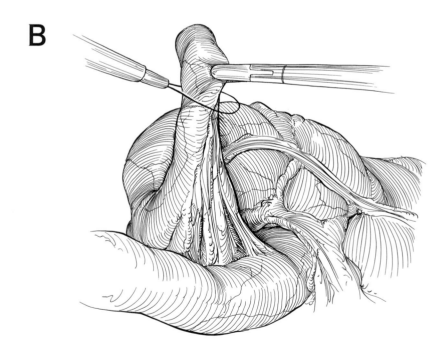

B

The appendix is snared with an endoloop and displaced toward the midline. This loop also is used to manipulate the appendix during the procedure, thus avoiding fragmentation of the appendix and possible fecal spillage.

C, D, E

Although the mesoappendix can be ligated by various means, here a rent in an avascular area of the mesoappendix adjacent to the base of the appendix is created by a blunt dissector (*C*), and the endo-GIA stapler with a vascular clip is insinuated and fired. This secures the vessels and divides the mesoappendix.

C

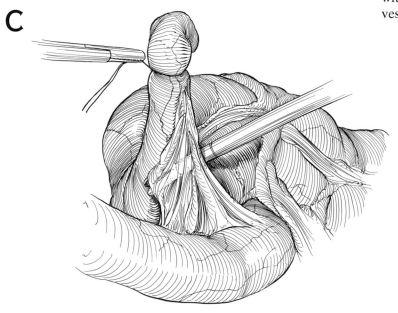

D

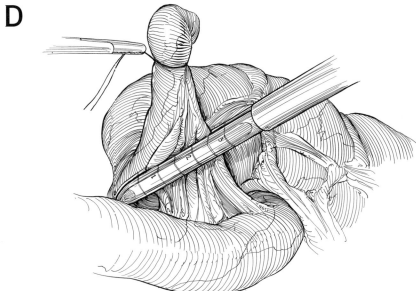

E

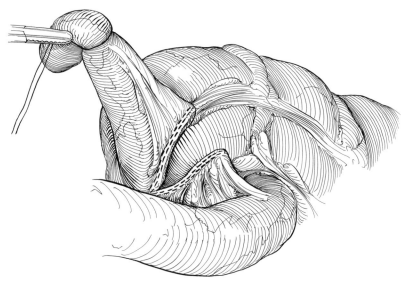

F

The endo-GIA stapler is placed across the base of the appendix and fired. Alternatively, this step can be performed before transection of the mesoappendix.

G

The stapled mesoappendiceal vessels and stump of the amputated appendix are shown. The staple line is carefully examined for hemostasis.

F

G

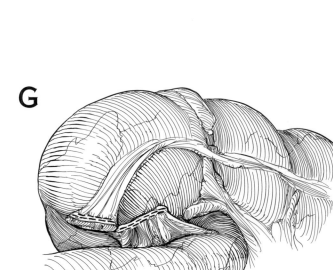

H

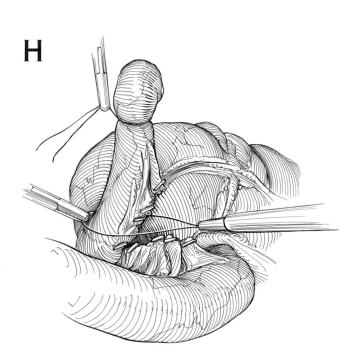

H

An alternative method of handling the mesoappendix is to secure the appendiceal artery and lesser vessels with clips until the base of the appendix is reached. The appendix then is ligated twice with an endoloop and amputated between ligatures.

I

The specimen is herniated into the 12-mm trocar, and both are withdrawn.

J

For bulky or particularly phlegmonous specimens that are too large to herniate into the trocar or that might fragment and contaminate the tract excessively, the specimen can be placed into a specimen retrieval bag and withdrawn from the abdominal cavity through the largest trocar site.

I

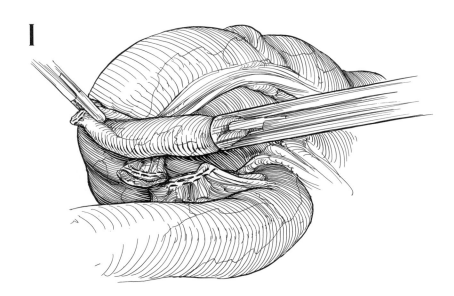

J

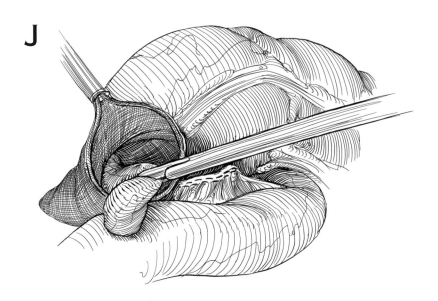

13

COLON

Ā RIGHT COLECTOMY

OPEN

A

The purpose of this operation, usually performed for cancer, is to remove the right colon and all its lymph node–bearing area. The blood supply is predominantly from the ileocolic and right and middle colic arteries. The resection includes the right colon just short of the middle colic artery and the attached mesentery.

Some surgeons place ties around the upper right colon and on the very terminal ileum to isolate any cancer cells that may shed into the bowel lumen during the course of the operation and implant themselves in the anastomotic line. The "no touch" technique, in which draining vessels are also tied and the tumor-bearing area of the colon is not handled, has lost favor.

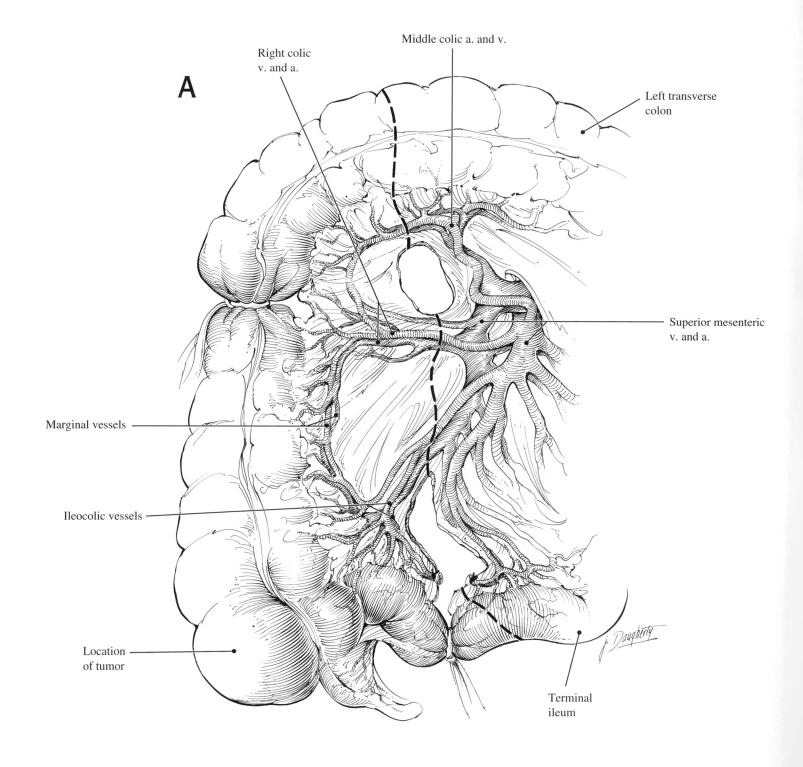

Right colic
v. and a.

Middle colic a. and v.

Left transverse
colon

A

Superior mesenteric
v. and a.

Marginal vessels

Ileocolic vessels

Location
of tumor

Terminal
ileum

B

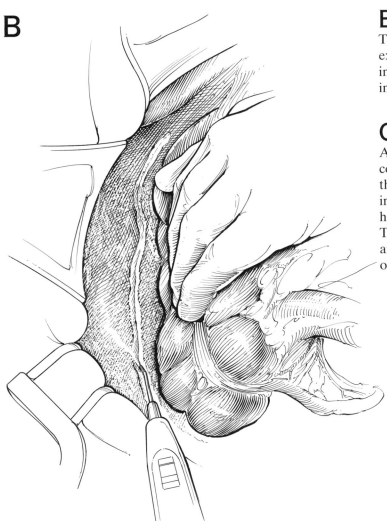

The resection is begun by retracting the colon medially to expose the rather avascular peritoneal reflection, which is incised by electrocautery applied with a fine-tipped instrument.

C

At the hepatic flexure, the hepatocolic ligament often contains sizable vessels, making it advisable to ligate or clip this tissue. The dashed line indicates the full extent of the intended mobilization. The duodenum lies deep to the hepatic flexure and can be injured by inattentive dissection. The ureter lies deep to the mesentery and can be injured at any point along its course but especially at the pelvic brim or close to primary or metastatic tumor.

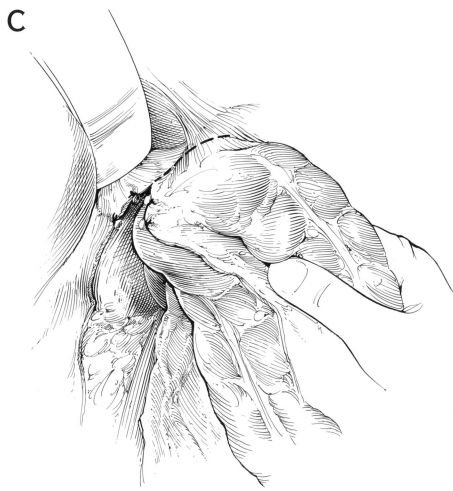

D

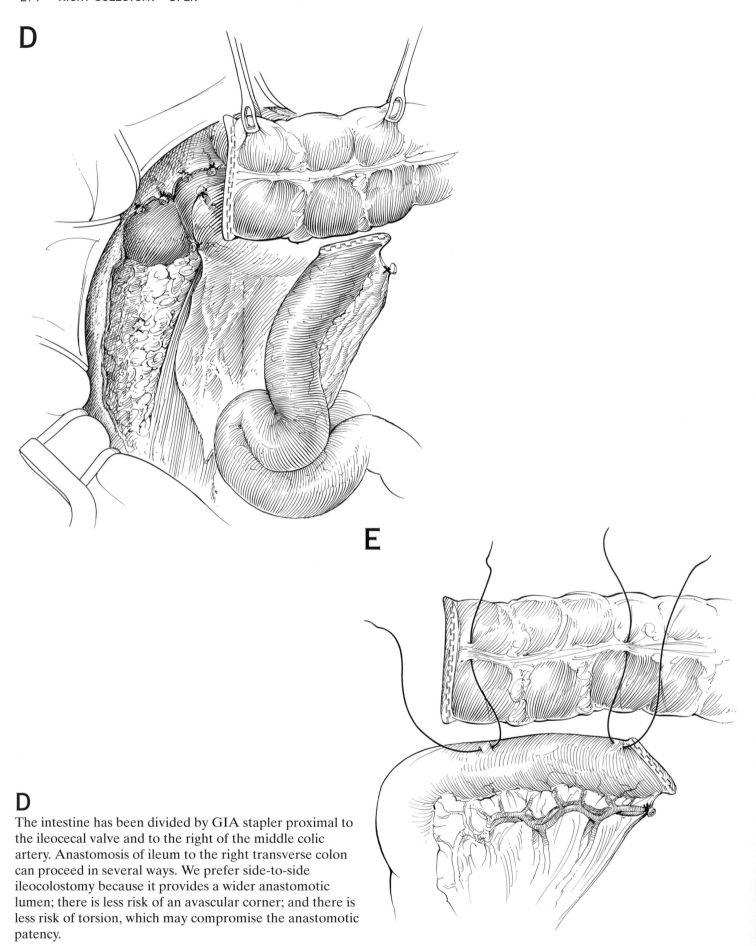

D

The intestine has been divided by GIA stapler proximal to the ileocecal valve and to the right of the middle colic artery. Anastomosis of ileum to the right transverse colon can proceed in several ways. We prefer side-to-side ileocolostomy because it provides a wider anastomotic lumen; there is less risk of an avascular corner; and there is less risk of torsion, which may compromise the anastomotic patency.

E

Two anchoring stitches of 3-0 silk are applied to the ileum and transverse colon; the distance between them is determined by the size of the desired anastomosis.

F

The entry site for the instrument is on the distal side of the intended anastomosis, because any swelling at the anastomotic site will not pose as serious a risk of obstructing the ileum.

G

The stapler is fired and withdrawn; a Babcock clamp is used to lift one side of the opening, from which the staple line is inspected for any bleeding.

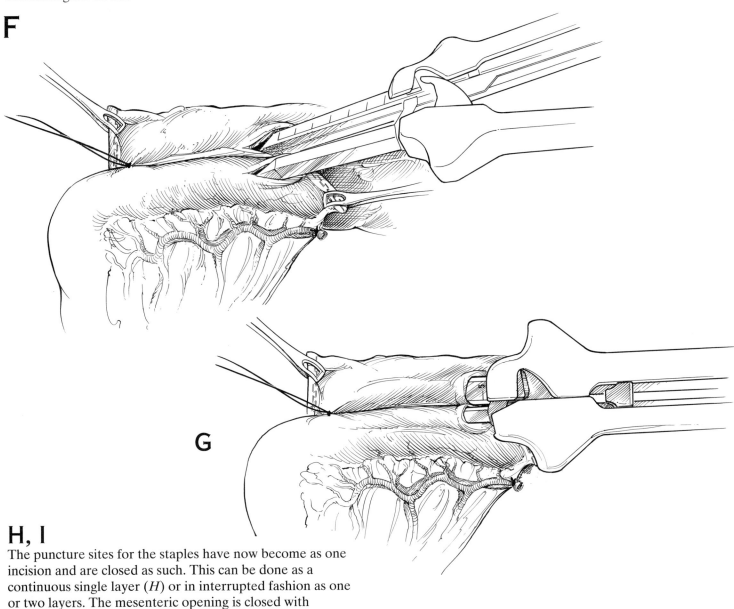

F

G

H, I

The puncture sites for the staples have now become as one incision and are closed as such. This can be done as a continuous single layer (*H*) or in interrupted fashion as one or two layers. The mesenteric opening is closed with continuous 3-0 chromic catgut.

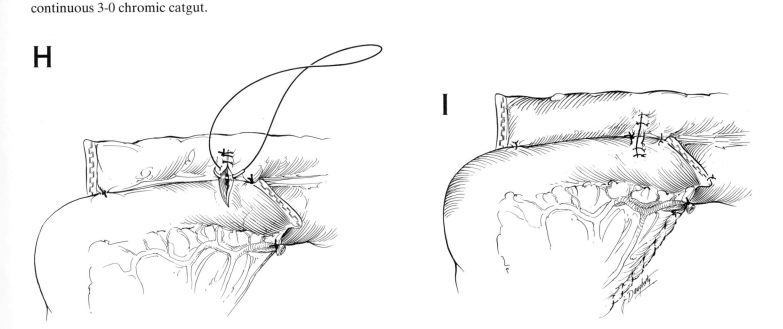

H

I

LAPAROSCOPIC-ASSISTED

Laparoscopic-assisted right colectomy for benign and early malignant disease is gaining favor, even as the procedure is undergoing modification in technological and operative techniques.

A

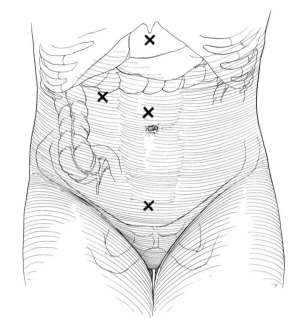

A

Preparations are as for a customary colon resection. The patient is anesthetized, and the table is placed in a 20- to 30-degree Trendelenburg position during work on the lower abdomen. The pattern of trocar placement is substantially influenced by the surgeon's preference. One such pattern is illustrated.

The initial trocar should be placed with special care if an open technique is not used so that the underlying intestine is not pierced. To have sufficient thrust to penetrate the abdominal wall yet sufficient restraint to avoid the trocar's uncontrollable piercing of the peritoneal cavity, the following procedure is used. The trocar is held with the handle in the cup of the surgeon's hand, the index finger firmly along its shaft just short of the tip. The trocar is placed at the desired spot, and firm, twisting pressure is applied mainly by the ball of the hand. Thus, should the trocar begin to advance unexpectedly swiftly, the index finger along its shaft prevents an unimpeded plunge.

B

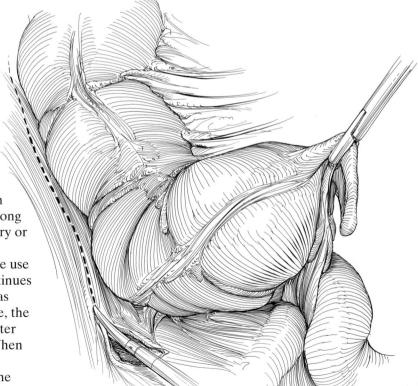

B

The appendix is grasped and used to retract the colon toward the patient's left as the parietal peritoneum along the entire length of the right colon is incised by cautery or scissors. At the hepatic flexure, the vascular supply is plentiful and the peritoneum sufficiently thick that the use of clips and cautery is prudent. The mobilization continues to a point to the right of the middle colic artery. Just as when performing this operation by an open technique, the surgeon should visualize the duodenum and right ureter during the dissection and protect them from harm. When the hepatic flexure can reach down to the left lower quadrant and the cecum to the left upper quadrant, the surgeon can feel confident that there is enough mobilization to proceed with exteriorization.

C

An approximately 6-cm transverse incision is made at the location of the right subcostal trocar, and the intestines from the terminal ileum to the midtransverse colon are brought to the outside. The mesenteric vessels are ligated in continuity (doubly on their proximal side) with 2-0 silk before being divided. The exteriorized intestine is first divided at the terminal ileum by a GIA stapler.

C

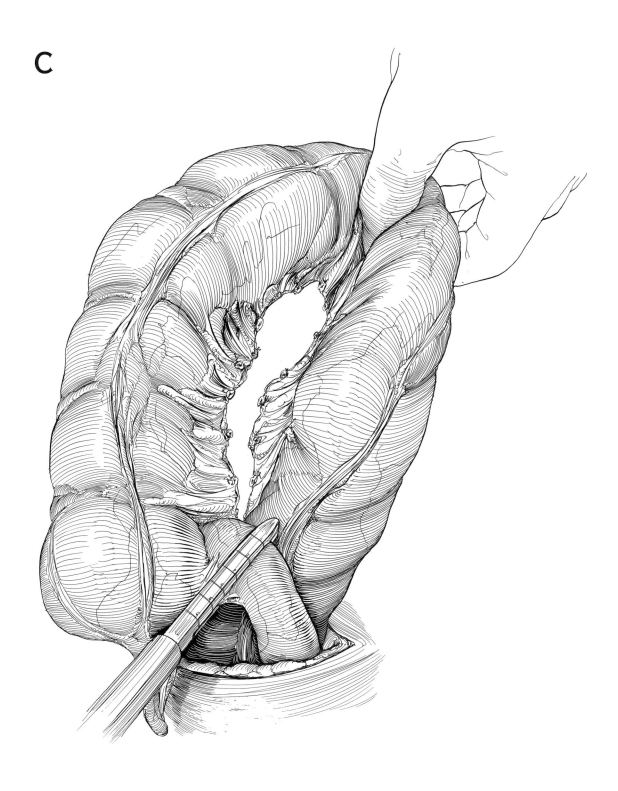

D

The exteriorized colon is divided just to the right of the
midcolic artery.

D

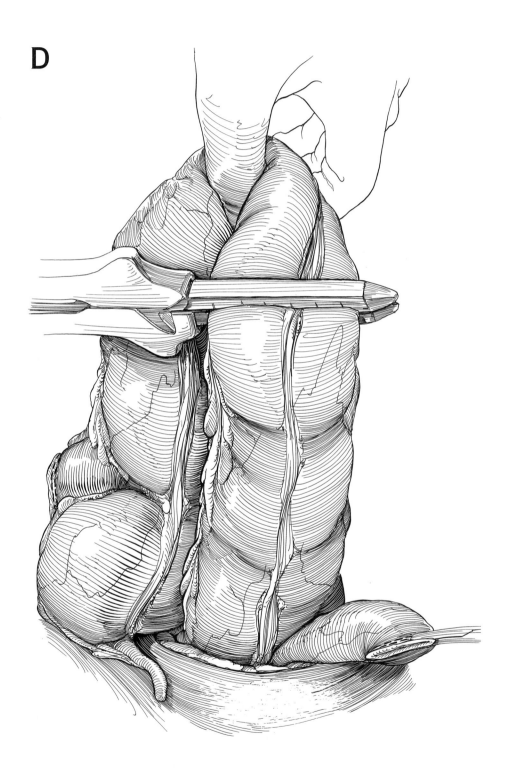

E

The resected colon is removed from the operative field. The open ileum and transverse colon are held straight up with Babcock forceps, their respective antemesenteric borders abutting. Each jaw of the stapler is inserted into each intestinal lumen and fired, thus connecting the lumina. The staple lines are inspected for bleeding. An alternative technique leaves the intestinal segments stapled until just before the anastomosis, at which time a corner of each intestinal segment is snipped off to permit entry of the jaws of the GIA stapler. This technique does not allow for inspection of the staple line for bleeding. Both the side-to-side and end-to-end anastomoses can also be performed by hand.

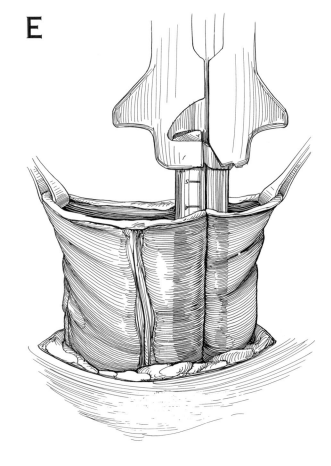

E

F, G

With the two intestines still held up, both openings are closed with a TA stapler, thus completing the anastomosis. The excess tissue is trimmed with a scalpel swept across the still-closed stapler. The mesenteric defect is closed with continuous 3-0 chromic catgut. The intestines are returned to the peritoneal cavity and the operation terminated in the usual manner.

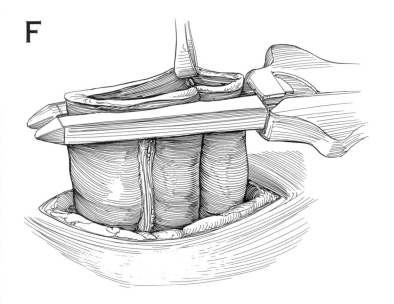

F

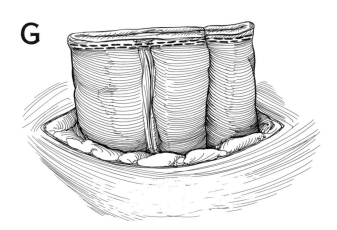

G

B LOW ANTERIOR RESECTION

Low anterior resection is done primarily for lesions of the rectum. The special circumstances of having to adequately resect a cancer and to effect a primary anastomosis deep inside the pelvis have resulted in the development of several techniques by which this can be done.

A

The proposed incision of the pelvic peritoneum (indicated by the dashed line) is defined with an Adson hemostat placed just under it and divided by electrocautery.

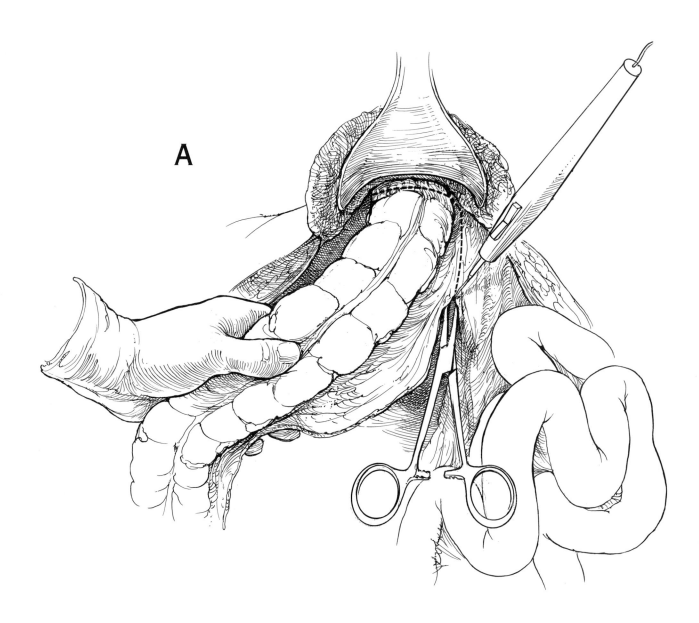

A

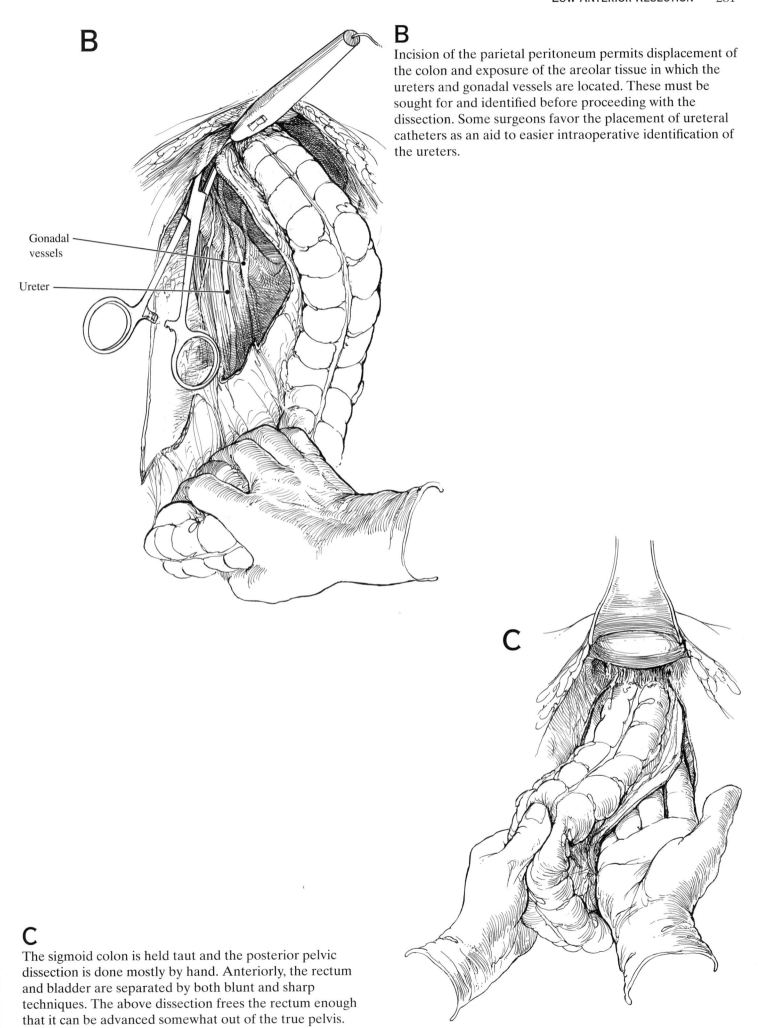

B

B

Incision of the parietal peritoneum permits displacement of the colon and exposure of the areolar tissue in which the ureters and gonadal vessels are located. These must be sought for and identified before proceeding with the dissection. Some surgeons favor the placement of ureteral catheters as an aid to easier intraoperative identification of the ureters.

Gonadal vessels

Ureter

C

C

The sigmoid colon is held taut and the posterior pelvic dissection is done mostly by hand. Anteriorly, the rectum and bladder are separated by both blunt and sharp techniques. The above dissection frees the rectum enough that it can be advanced somewhat out of the true pelvis.

D, E

The sigmoid colon is divided between two Kocher clamps. Moving down into the pelvis, a right angle clamp is applied across the rectum appropriately distal to the tumor, and the rectum is divided immediately distal to the clamp. The clamp is removed; the crushed portion provides adequate hemostasis. Traction stitches are applied laterally on the rectum.

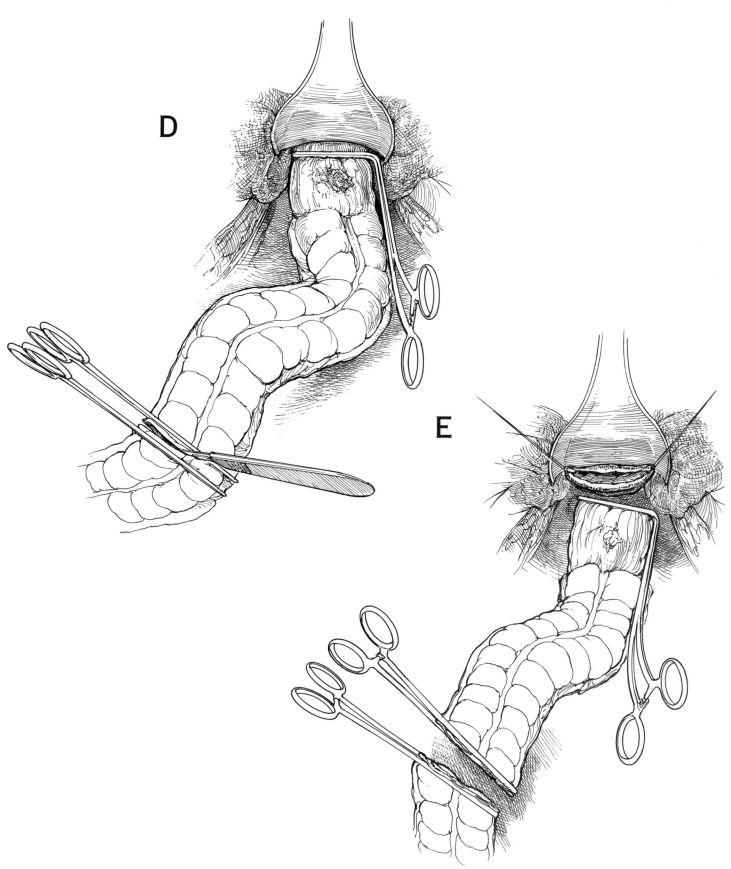

D

E

F

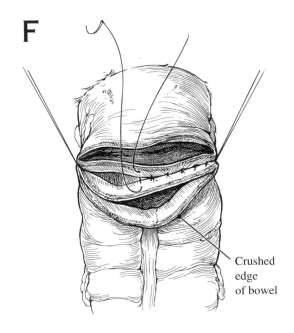

Crushed
edge
of bowel

END-TO-END ANASTOMOSIS (HAND SEWN)

The colon must be scrupulously cleansed of liquid or solid stool because the open end of the lumen distal to the occluding intestinal clamp drips into the depth of the dissected pelvis.

F

The ends of the bowel with the crushed edges intact are apposed and stitched together at the right and left extremes with interrupted 3-0 silk. A row of simple interrupted stitches of 3-0 silk is applied, catching the tissue several millimeters behind the crushed edge.

G

Following completion of this layer, the mucosal layer is approximated with a continuous stitch of 3-0 absorbable suture, incorporating both the crushed tissue and the noncrushed tissue immediately adjacent to it.

H, I

The continuous anterior mucosal stitch is continued; somewhere along its course, the direction of the needle and stitch is reversed so that the two stitches meet naturally as they approach and then are tied to each other. The anastomosis is completed with an anterior row of interrupted seromuscular stitches using 3-0 silk.

G

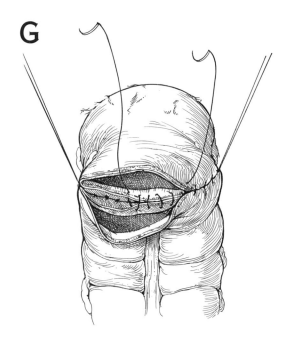

H

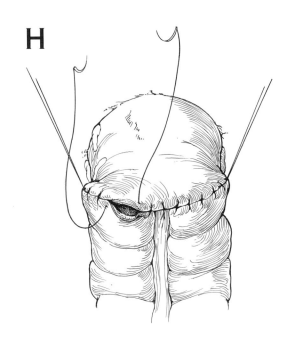

I

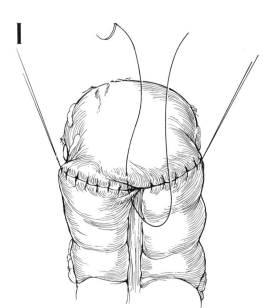

SIDE-TO-END ANASTOMOSIS (HAND SEWN)

J

Side-to-end anastomosis can be useful in several clinical settings: when the disparity between the two bowel lumina is excessive (the colon usually is smaller than the rectum) and when the colon mesentery and its vasculature are short, making it difficult to straighten out the colon from its "fish-hook" configuration.

The stapled bowel is laid across the opened rectum (notice that the crushed rim of tissue remains with the specimen). Stitches of 3-0 silk are applied at the lateral extremes of the colon, the distance between the two determined by the width of the rectum.

K, L

The interrupted simple seromusclar stitches are applied in the rectum just behind the crushed portion of tissue. The dashed line indicates where the colon will be incised.

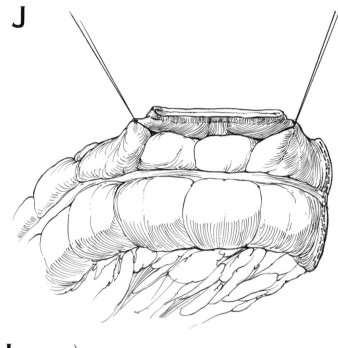

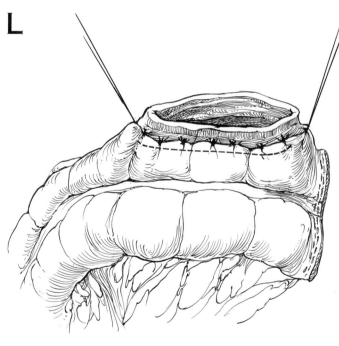

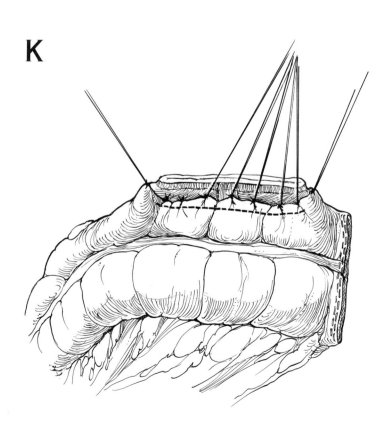

M

The mucosal approximating stitch is applied in continuous or interrupted fashion.

N

The anterior mucosal stitch can be continuous or interrupted; here it is the latter with the knots of the tied stitches facing the lumen.

O

The anastomosis is completed with seromuscular simple interrupted stitches of 3-0 silk.

M

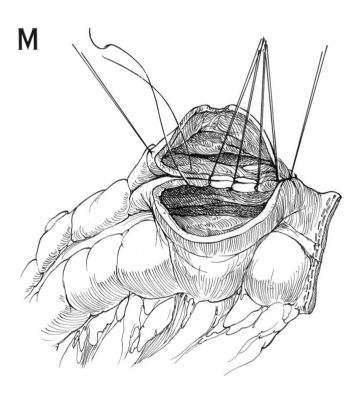

N

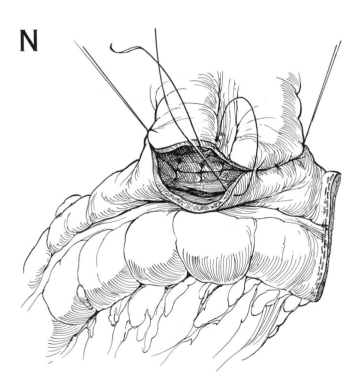

O

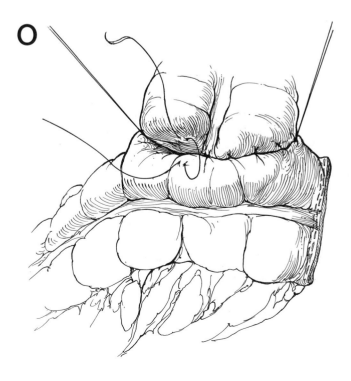

End-to-End Anastomosis (Stapled; Transanal)

P, Q

A purse-string of stout vascular suture is loosely stitched around the entire circumference of the opened bowel.

P

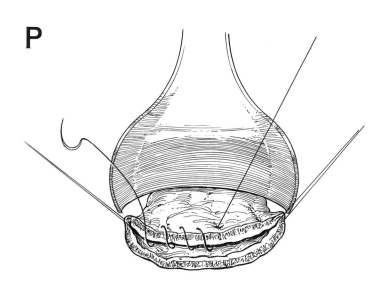

Q

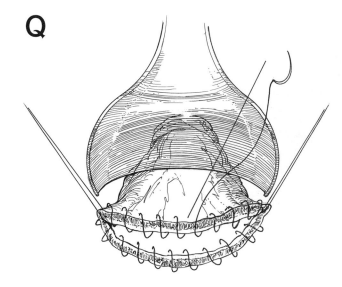

R

The tumor-bearing segment of large bowel is removed from the immediate operative field. The curved CEEA stapler is introduced transanally and advanced to the level of the purse-string.

R

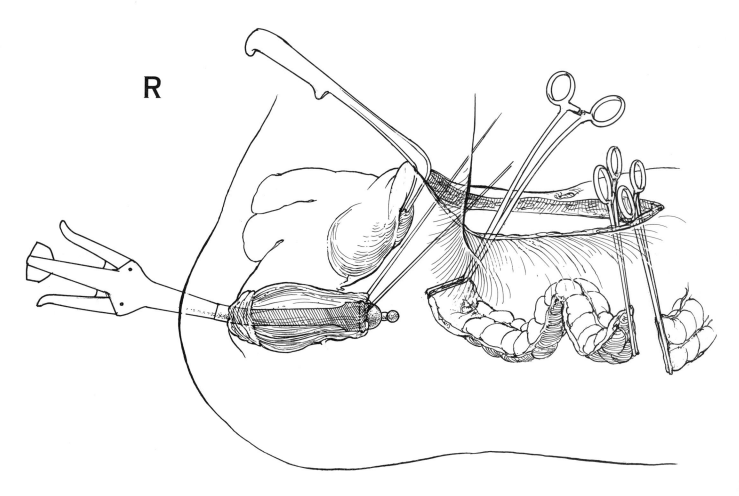

S, T

The anvil is opened to provide room for the purse-string to
be tied.

S

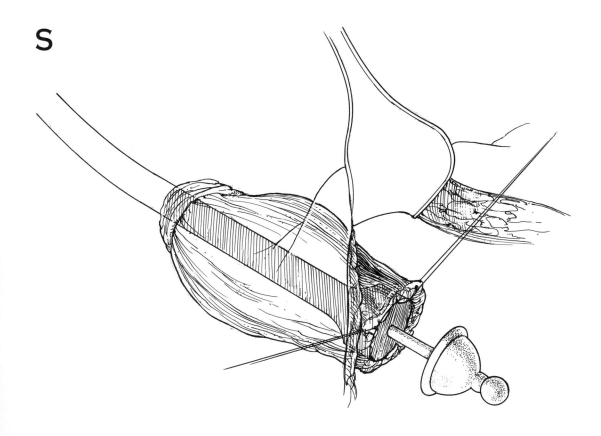

T

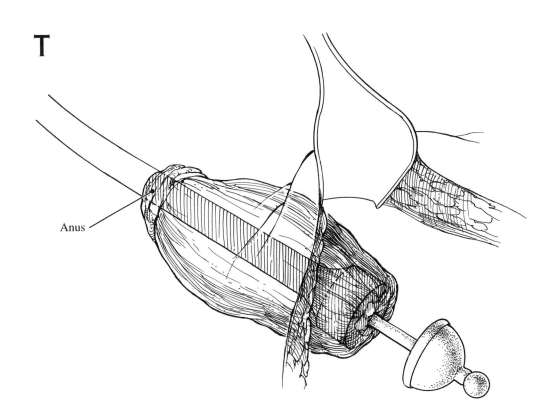

Anus

U, V

Any excess tissue outside the Kocher clamps is trimmed and a similar purse-string suture of monofilament material applied to the proximal colon. With the help of two Babcock forceps to keep the colon open and aligned properly, the anvil is maneuvered into the colon. The purse-string is tightened and tied in readiness for bringing the two ends of the bowel into apposition.

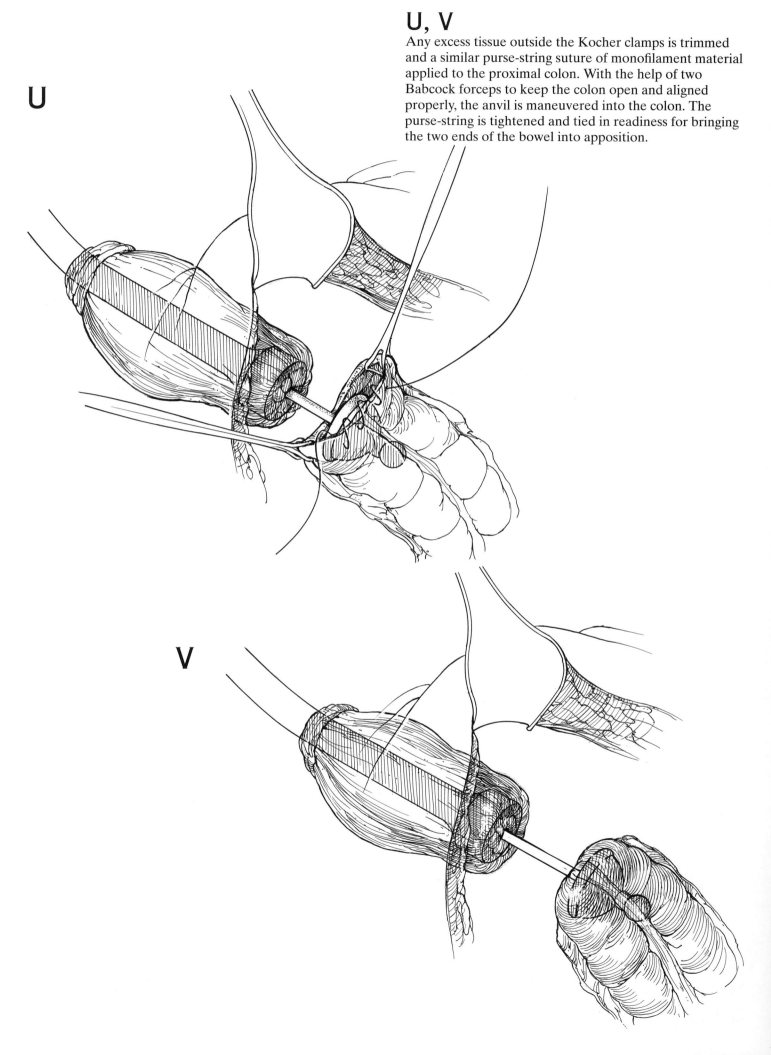

U

V

W

Sometimes physical constraints in maneuvering the entire stapling instrument are such that alternative techniques must be used: Anvil and anvil shaft are inserted into the colon, and the purse-string suture is tied. The stapler without the anvil is introduced transanally and is advanced through the open rectum; the purse-string is then secured. Or the rectum is divided by linear stapler. The curved stapler with a recessed trocar tip is introduced transanally. The trocar is advanced and poked through the middle of the staple line on the rectum, and the trocar is removed. The anvil and shaft are then engaged in the instrument shaft.

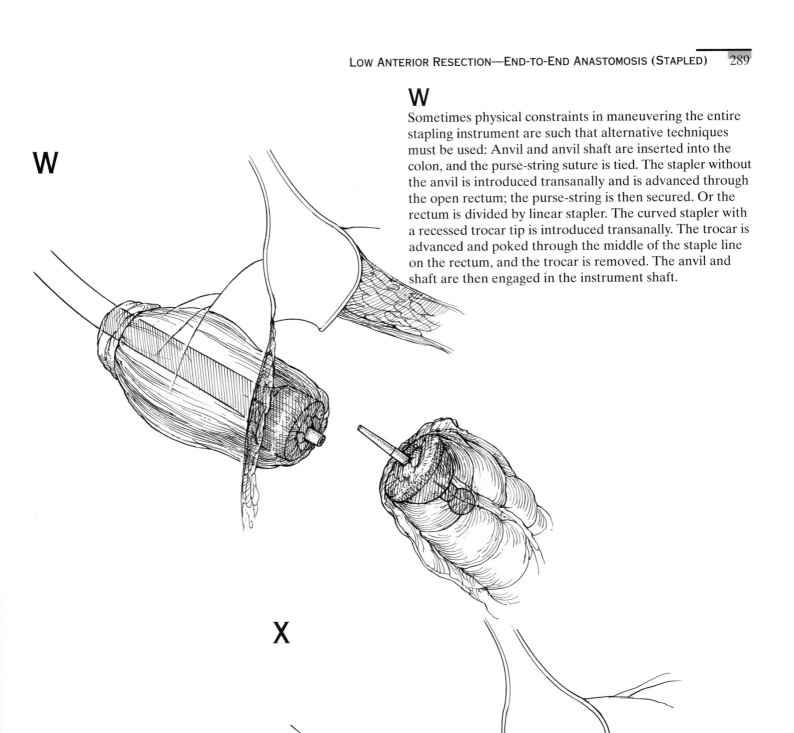

W

X

X

The area is inspected to be certain that all layers of the two apposing bowel segments are incorporated within the stapler; the instrument is closed and fired.

Y

The stapler is opened slightly and withdrawn over the staple line with a rotary motion. The tissue within the cartridge is inspected for purse-string continuity and the presence of all tissue layers.

Z

A proctoscope is used to inspect the suture line for adequate hemostasis and absence of a leak.

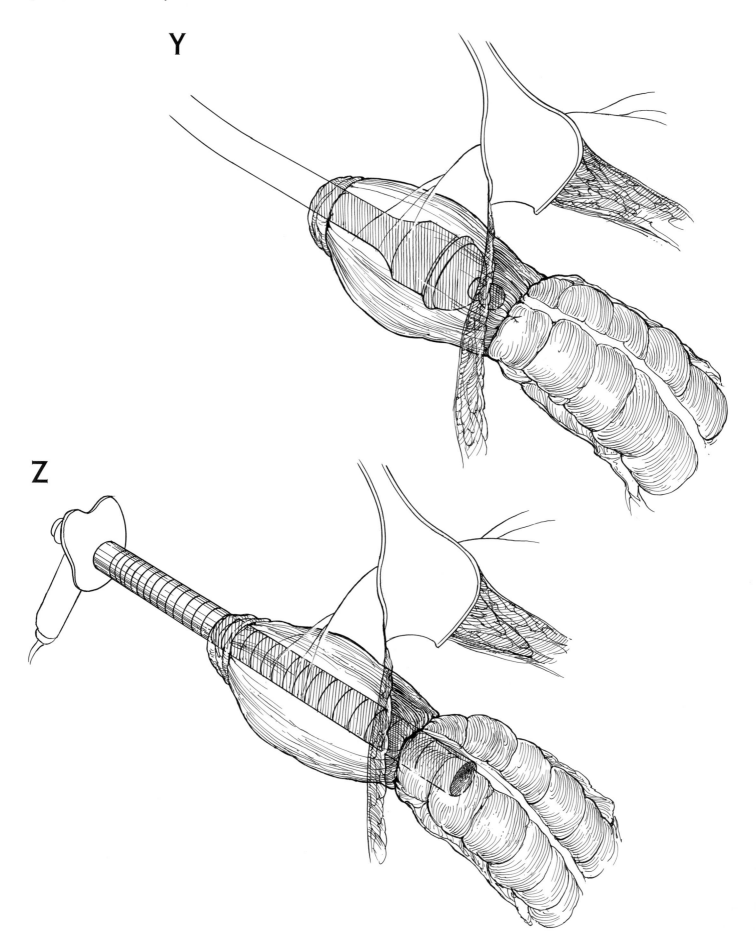

Y

Z

C TOTAL COLECTOMY—WITHOUT PROCTECTOMY; BROOKE ILEOSTOMY

The most common indication for total abdominal colectomy is fulminant ulcerative colitis and its complications of toxic megacolon, hemorrhage, and perforation. Less common, relative indications for total colectomy include massive colonic bleeding whose exact origin is not known, polyposis, and synchronous multiple cancers. Most patients with the latter indications have intestinal continuity retained or restored by ileorectal anastomosis.

A

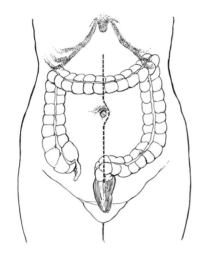

The abdominal cavity is opened for its full length through a midline incision and is explored for unanticipated abnormalities and extent of the known disease.

B

The right colon is being displaced medially as the lateral peritoneal reflection is incised with a fine-tipped electrocautery.

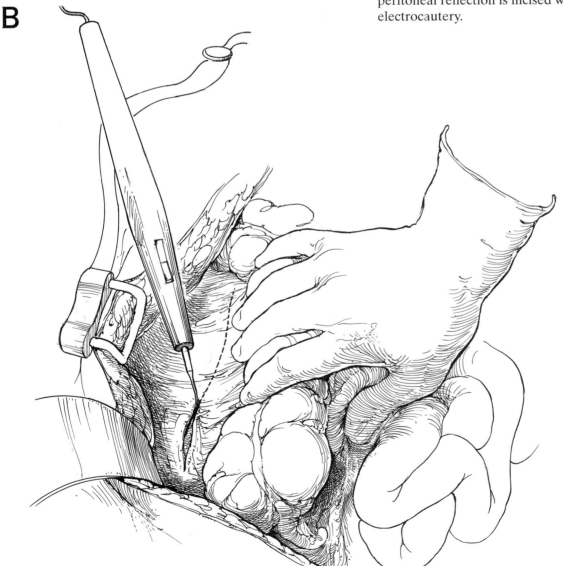

C

Some of the parietal peritoneum of the terminal ileum also must be divided so that the ileum can be addressed properly.

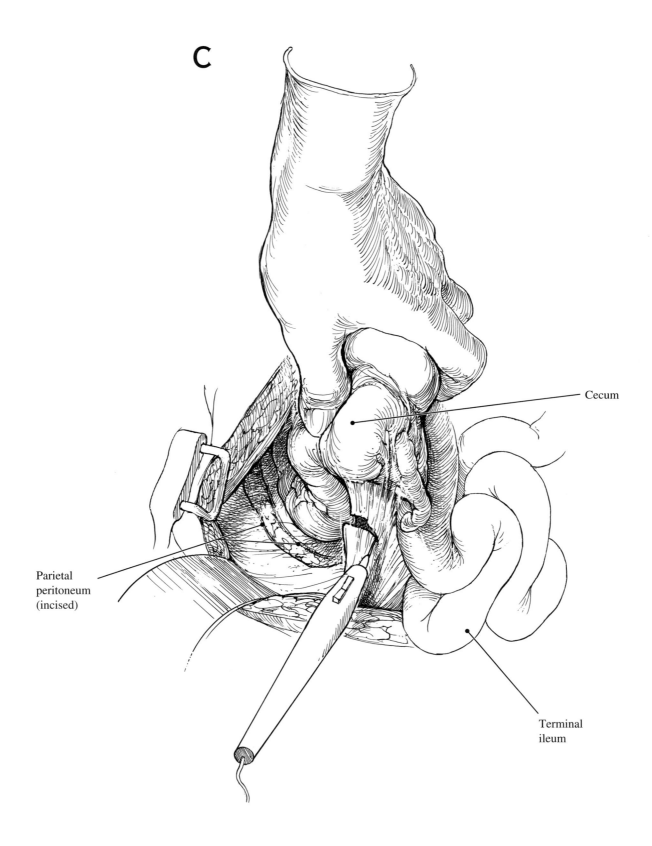

C

Cecum

Parietal
peritoneum
(incised)

Terminal
ileum

D

The phrenocolic and hepatocolic ligaments are tied or
clipped before being divided because the vessels within
them can bleed persistently if not secured.

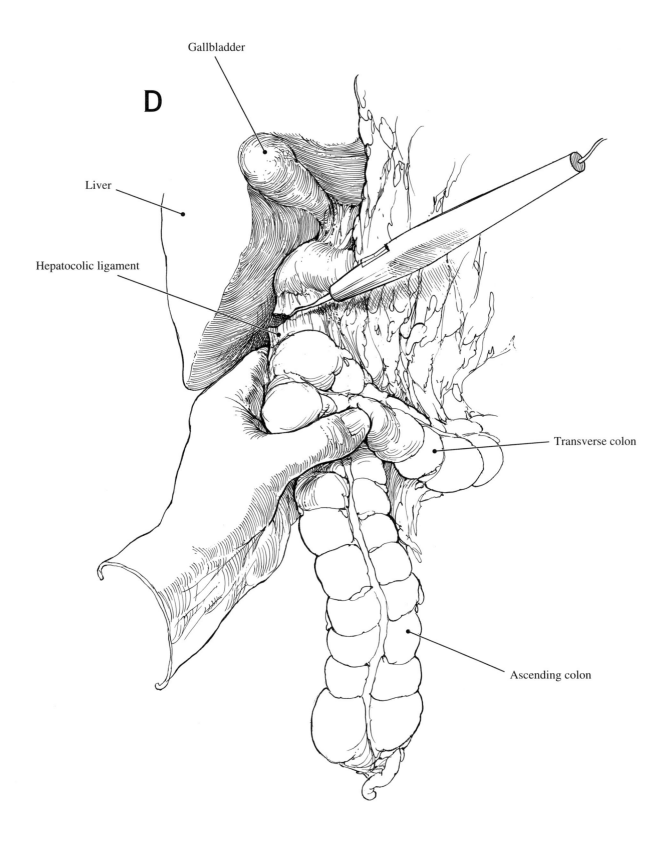

Gallbladder

D

Liver

Hepatocolic ligament

Transverse colon

Ascending colon

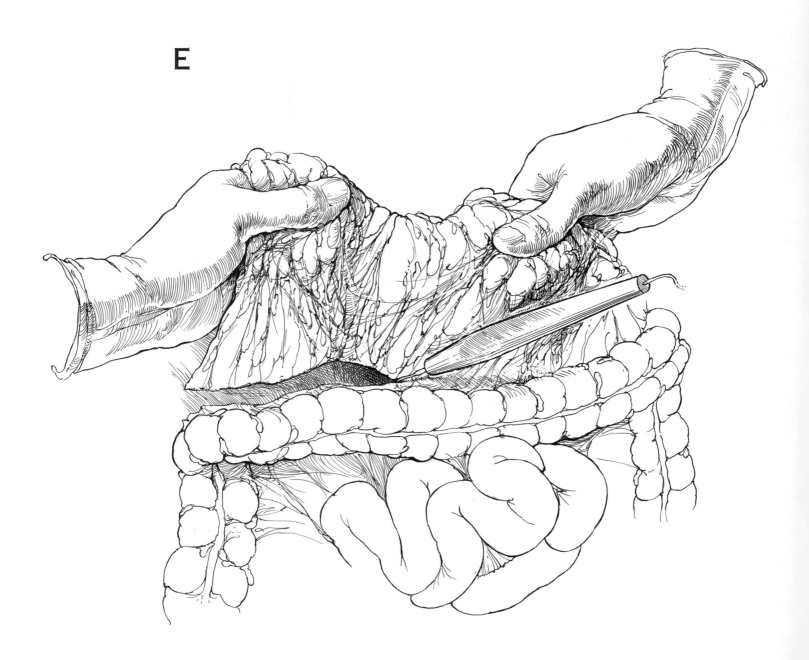

E

The entire right colon has been mobilized. If the operation is being performed for chronic inflammatory disease, the pericolic inflammation will not permit easy separation of the colon from the surrounding tissue, so the right ureter and retroperitoneal portion of the duodenum may be injured. Also, the omentum cannot safely be freed from the colon. Otherwise, as in this case, the omentum is disengaged from the colon and left behind.

F

As the splenic flexure is approached, the omentum becomes thicker and its attachment to the colon broader. Electrocautery, judiciously applied, can be used here, but if any vessels are seen therein, the tissue should be serially tied or clipped before it is divided.

F

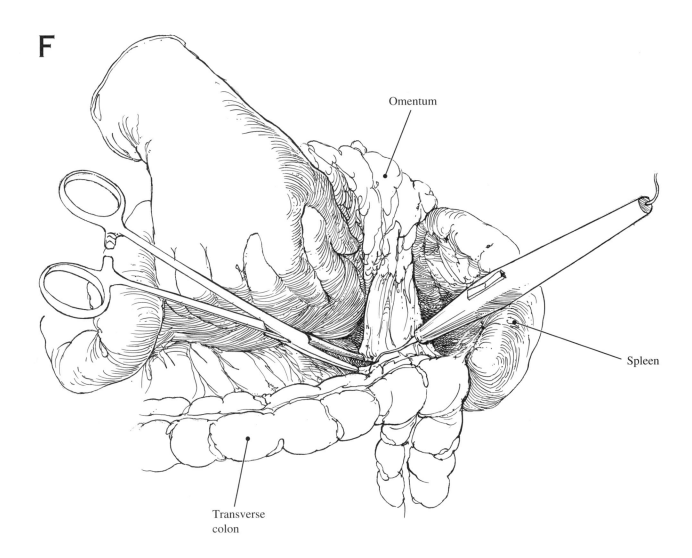

Omentum

Spleen

Transverse
colon

G

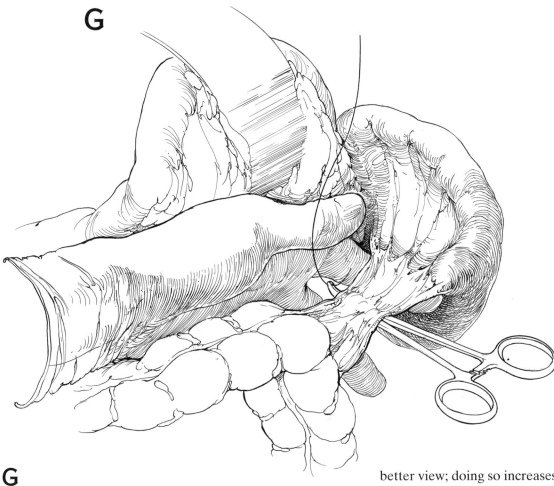

G

The operation shifts to the descending colon, which is retracted medially as the peritoneal reflection is incised up to the splenic flexure. For this reason, the hand is placed near the splenic flexure as shown, and the index finger is insinuated under the splenocolic ligament, which is clamped, cut, and ligated with 2-0 silk. If the splenic flexure is unusually high, the surgeon may be tempted to pull too hard on the colon to bring the splenocolic ligament into better view; doing so increases the risk of tearing the splenic capsule in this area.

H

The left colon is detached from its lateral fixation and displaced medially as its mesentery is separated from the underlying psoas muscle, Gerota's fascia, spermatic or ovarian vessels, and ureter.

H

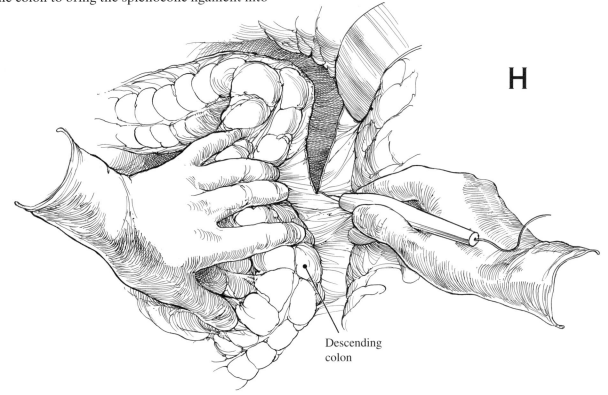

Descending colon

I

The colon is returned to its natural position so that its vasculature, here of the right colon, can more easily be visualized and divided. If the surgeon remains proximal to the vascular arcades, relatively few vessels need to be divided. This is done doubly with 2-0 silk.

I

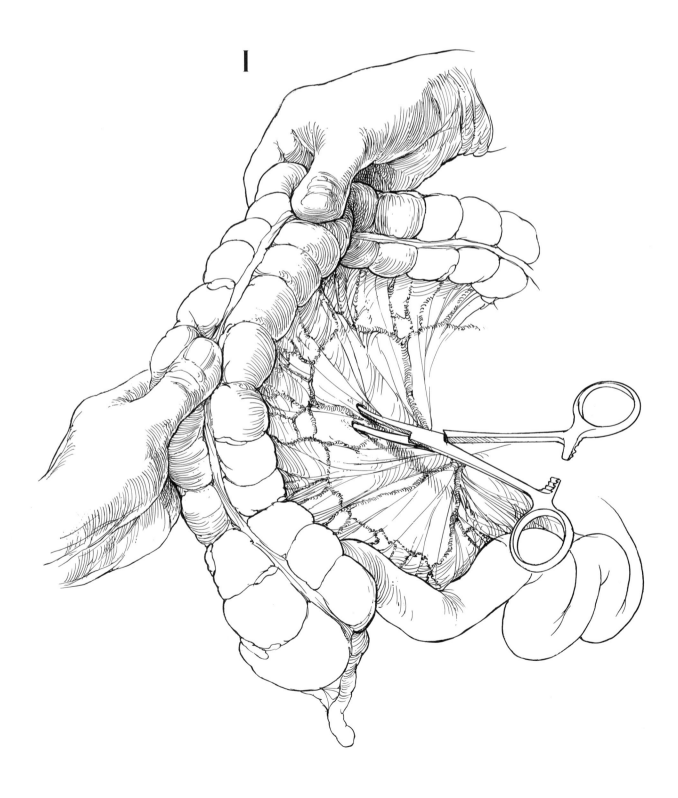

J

The vessels of the transverse mesocolon are serially ligated with 2-0 silk and divided as mobilization of the colon proceeds toward the splenic flexure.

K

The left colon has been repositioned so as to lie naturally and its vasculature ligated. The left ureter can be injured easily during ligation of the sigmoidal or superior rectal artery; therefore, caution should be exercised during this maneuver.

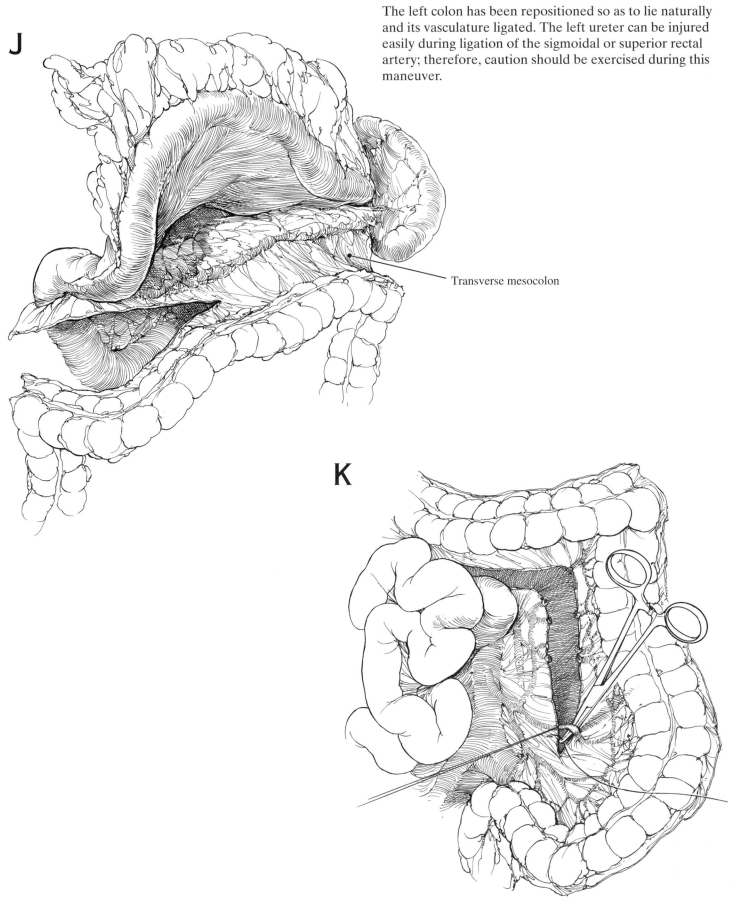

J

Transverse mesocolon

K

L

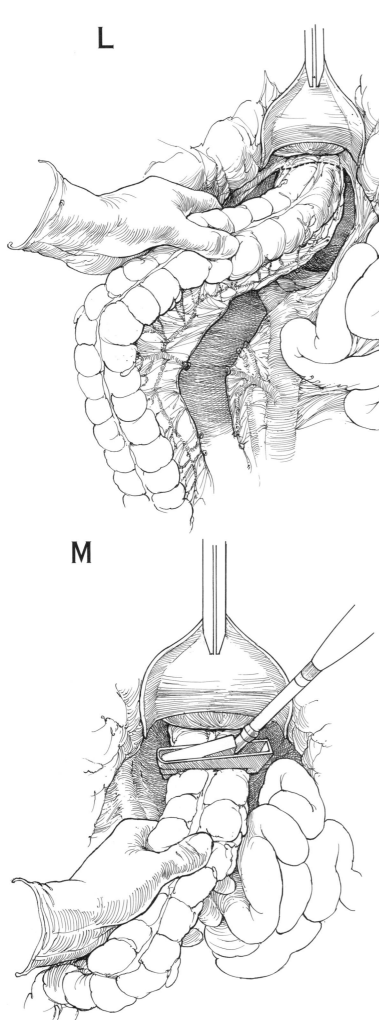

M

L, M

The colon is divided at the peritoneal reflection and oversewn or stapled. If the surgeon is certain that the rectum will be removed at a later date, it is desirable to carry out the dissection below the peritoneal reflection. Division of the rectum at this low level makes it easier to perform a delayed transperineal proctectomy.

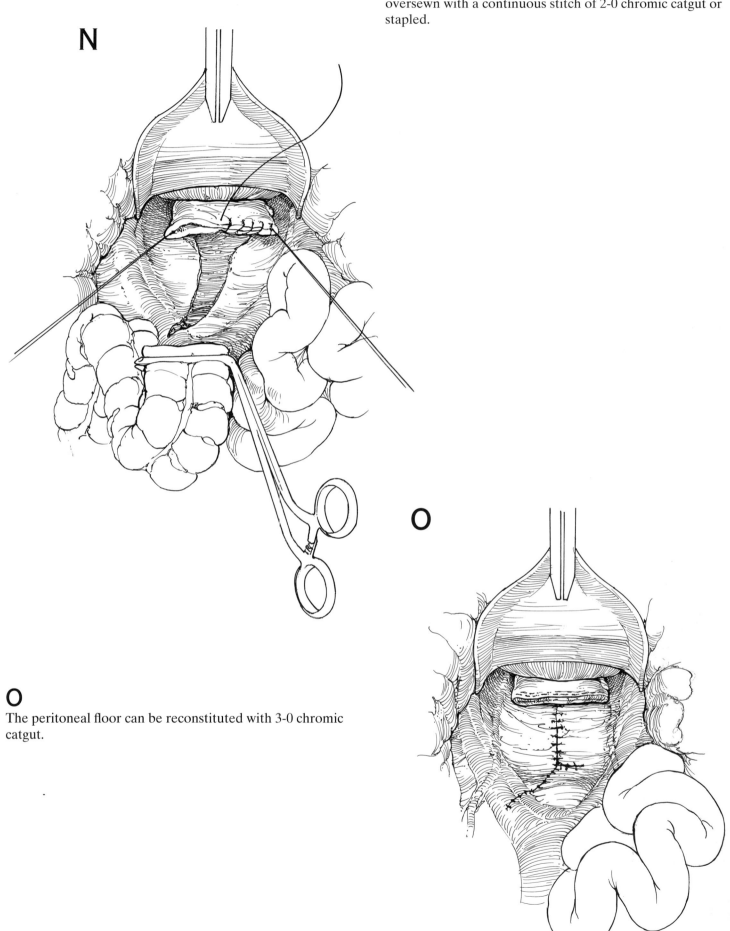

N

The sigmoid colon or rectum, as the case may be, is oversewn with a continuous stitch of 2-0 chromic catgut or stapled.

O

The peritoneal floor can be reconstituted with 3-0 chromic catgut.

P

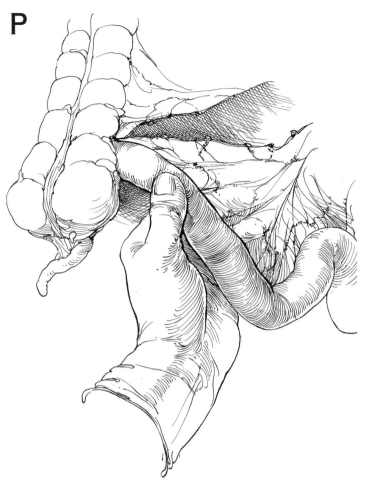

P, Q

Division of the ileum is left until last because it coincides with the subsequent construction of the ileostomy. Every vessel in its mesentery should be handled gently. In addition, the mesentery should be tailored in a fashion that will enable the vessels within it to carry blood to the very edge of the transected ileum. The stapling should be on a slight bias as shown; this configuration obliges the vessels to travel the shortest distance to the cut edge.

Q

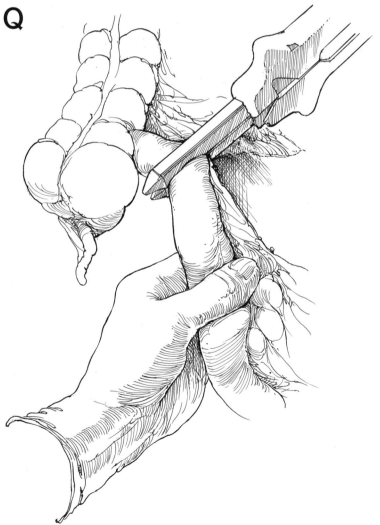

R

The ileostomy is best placed midpoint between the umbilicus and the anterior iliac spine within the rectus sheath on a smooth surface without scars or natural skin creases. The patient should be examined for the latter preoperatively while lying down as well as while standing and leaning over.

S, T, U

A circular piece of skin, fascia and peritoneum equal in diameter to that of the ileum, is cut out at the selected spot on the abdomen.

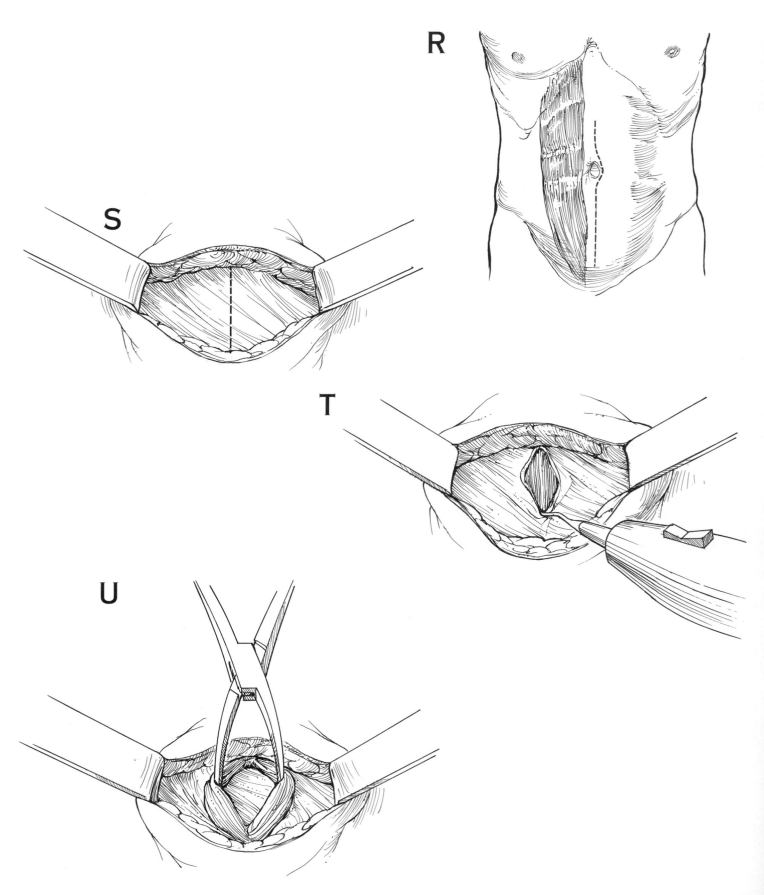

V

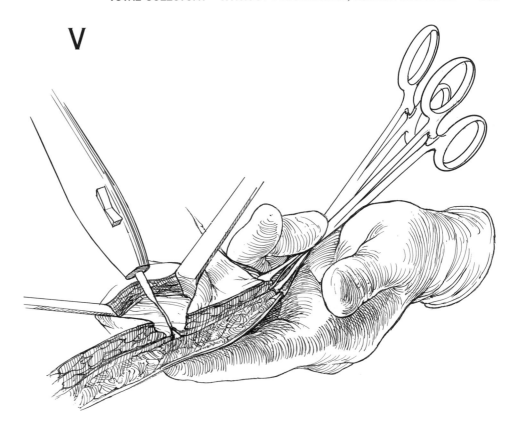

V, W, X

The skin, anterior rectus sheath, and peritoneum are grasped and held in proper line while this cut is being made so that the cut through the various layers will remain in line later. Dissociation between tissue planes can result in a shearing effect and possible obstruction of the terminal ileum.

W

X

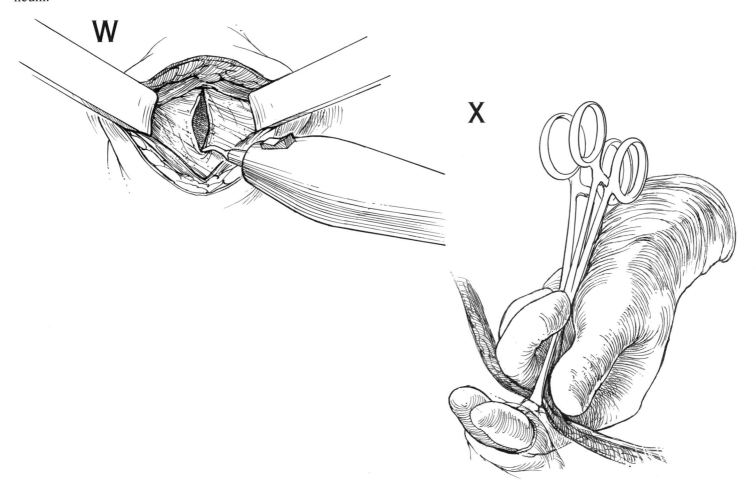

Y

A Babcock clamp is inserted through the abdominal opening to grasp the ileum and pull it to the outside for a length of 5 cm.

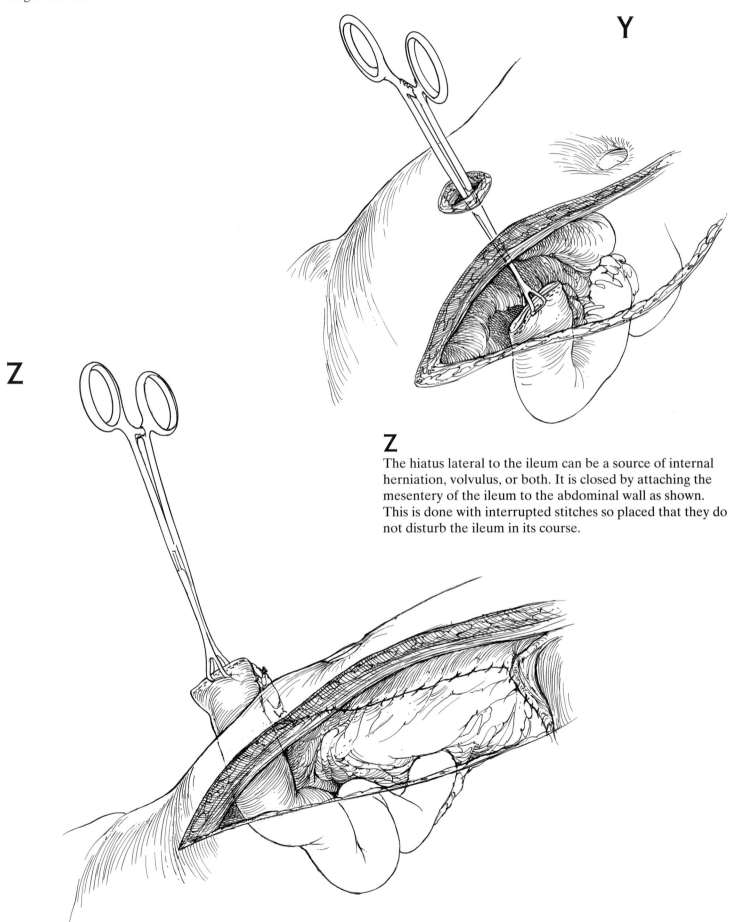

Y

Z

The hiatus lateral to the ileum can be a source of internal herniation, volvulus, or both. It is closed by attaching the mesentery of the ileum to the abdominal wall as shown. This is done with interrupted stitches so placed that they do not disturb the ileum in its course.

AA, BB

At this point the very end of the ileum containing the staples is excised. Simple exteriorization of the ileum often is attended by inflammation with proximal progression and subsequent dysfunction of the ileostomy. These are avoided by eversion of the ileum so that no serosa remains exposed. Stitches are placed so that they both anchor the ileum and keep the mucosa everted, with no suture remaining buried. The needle should traverse the full thickness of the mucosa, then the seromuscularis of the underlying ileum at the skin level, and then the skin itself. The ileostomy bag is placed in position in the operating room.

The abdomen is closed in a preferred manner.

AA

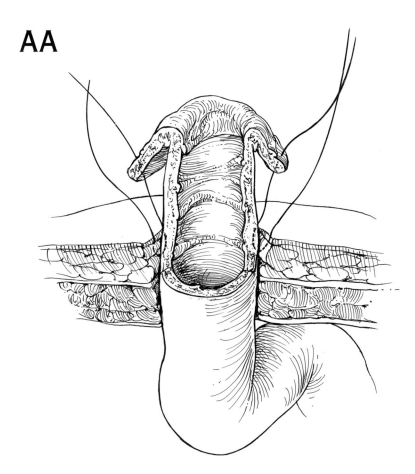

BB

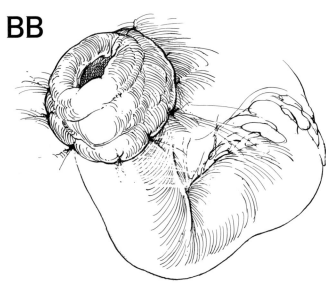

D COLOSTOMY

CREATION

Colostomy is performed primarily to defunctionalize or decompress bowel or as a permanent means of stool evacuation. This operation is carried out under emergency, elective, or adjunctive circumstances and functions as either a temporary measure or a permanent one. Corrective surgery for bowel obstruction can be performed in one stage (resection of obstructing tumor with primary anastomosis), in two stages (resection of obstruction and use of this or a more proximal site for a colostomy to be closed later), or in three stages (decompressing colostomy, later followed by resection of the obstructing pathology without disturbing the colostomy, and closure of the colostomy in a third operation). With recent advances, fewer stages are the rule. The more common types of colostomy are featured in this chapter.

Loop

For obstruction distal to the transverse colon, the upper midabdomen is the favored colostomy site, as it interferes least with interim work on the lower abdomen. The descending sigmoid colon is best for permanent or long-term use.

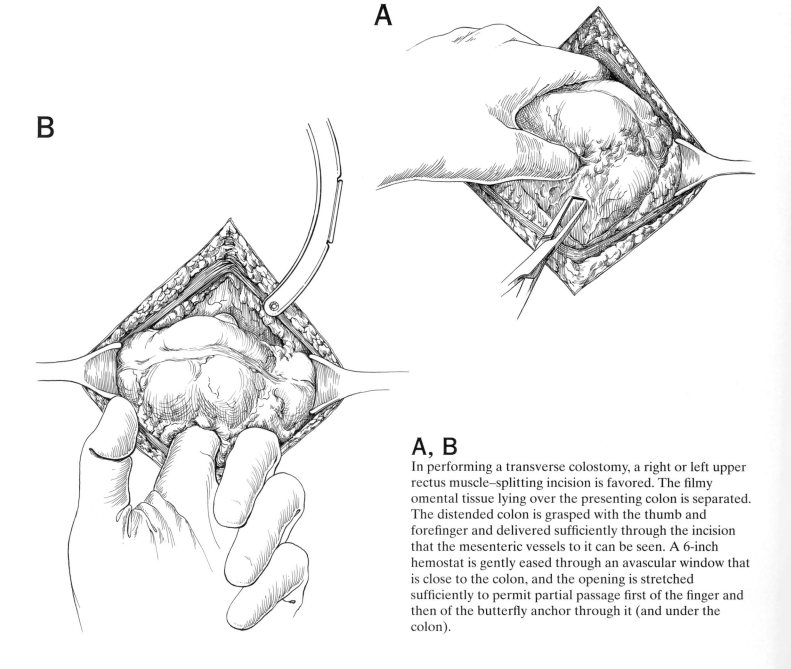

A

B

A, B

In performing a transverse colostomy, a right or left upper rectus muscle–splitting incision is favored. The filmy omental tissue lying over the presenting colon is separated. The distended colon is grasped with the thumb and forefinger and delivered sufficiently through the incision that the mesenteric vessels to it can be seen. A 6-inch hemostat is gently eased through an avascular window that is close to the colon, and the opening is stretched sufficiently to permit partial passage first of the finger and then of the butterfly anchor through it (and under the colon).

C

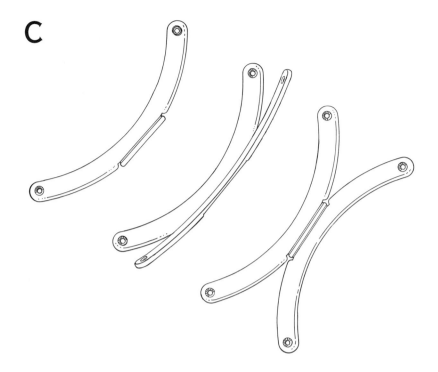

C, D, E

The butterfly anchor is passed through the created opening and spread and anchored by the four available needle ports.

D

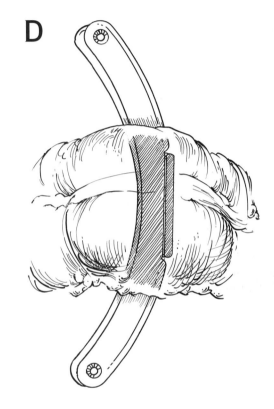

E

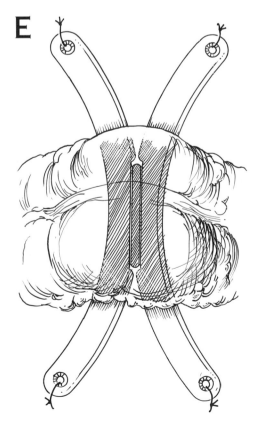

F

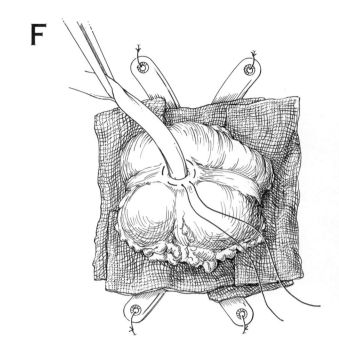

The decision as to when to open the colostomy depends on how urgently the colon must be vented. If it needs to be opened promptly, the area around the base is generously surrounded with protective gauze pressed closely against the colon and a purse-string suture of 3-0 silk is applied in the area of the tinea. An opening is made along the tinea, a multifenestrated catheter is inserted into the proximal limb, and the purse-string suture is tightened. Air and some liquid feces in the immediate area are evacuated; this tends to decompress the colon locally, making it easier to deliver more of it to the outside. Invariably, however, the tube becomes clogged, limiting the long-term usefulness of this maneuver.

G, H, I

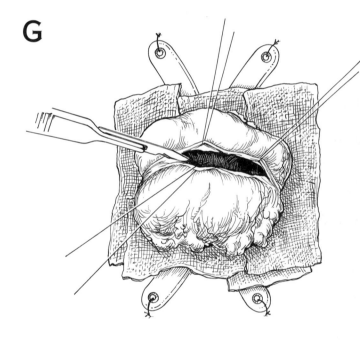

The colon is opened longitudinally along the course of the tinea. The circular muscle fibers of the colon cause the cut edges to evert. The protective gauze is now removed, and the edges of the incised skin and open colon are stitched to each other with interrupted 3-0 chromic catgut. A temporary colostomy bag is applied in the operating room.

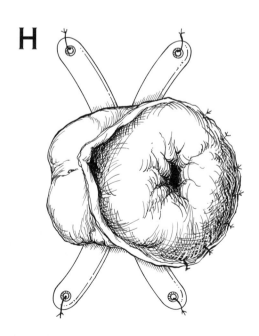

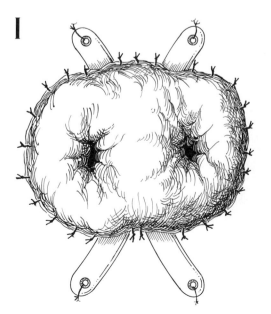

Double-Barrel

J

The double-barrel colostomy is performed as two end colostomies separated by some distance and "matured" at the operating table, with a colostomy bag inserted over the proximal stoma at that time. In a few weeks, the orifice of the distal colostomy shrinks remarkably. At the time of reanastomosis, a formal celiotomy is necessary to dismantle both colostomies and perform an end-to-end anastomosis.

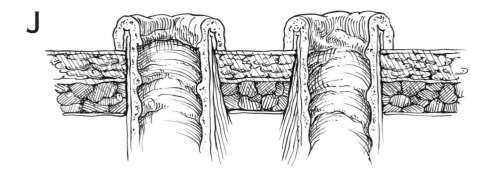

End

K

An end colostomy is easy to construct, fit with a bag, and keep clean. If, however, the patient is scheduled to have the colon reconnected, the operation to retrieve the distal bowel can be more difficult if it has been simply placed back into the abdominal cavity. For patients requiring a short-term end colostomy, therefore, we favor dividing the colon and placing a small-caliber Foley catheter in the distal segment. The Foley catheter is exteriorized at a conveniently separate spot from the proximal limb, so that a colostomy bag can be fitted to the protruding colon. Parenthetically, the Foley catheter can, on occasion, be used for prograde radiologic studies.

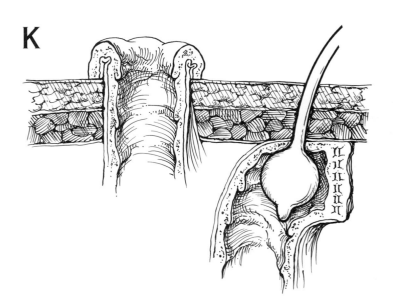

TAKEDOWN

Reestablishment of continuity following a loop colostomy can be performed in two principal ways: (1) the dismantling of both stomas with a formal end-to-end anastomosis; (2) the bringing together of the separate anterior portions of them as is shown here.

A

A "matured" colostomy, or one in place for 6 weeks or longer, contains more mature fibrous tissue, making it easier to handle. The skin is incised within 5 mm of the mucosa; sacrificing more is simply unnecessary.

B

The mucosa can be torn easily, so the tissue is maneuvered by the forceps applied to the rim of skin around the stoma. The fat is dissected to the colon serosa, following this plane down to just inside the peritoneum.

A

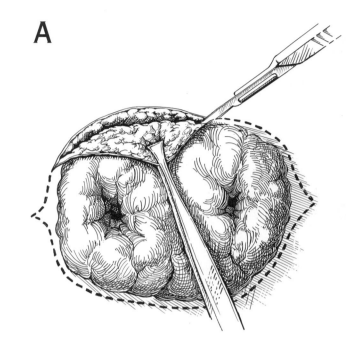

B

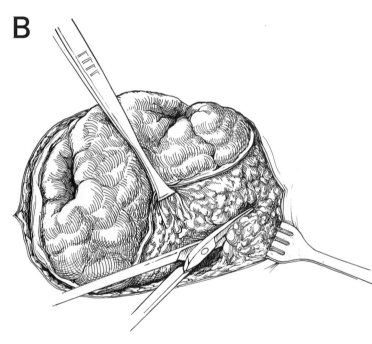

C

As a colostomy matures, the serosa curls up to become adherent to the adjoining serosa, thus forming the "rosebud" of the stoma. This now is undone by grasping the attached skin with an Allis forceps and, with a no. 15 scalpel blade or fine scissors, separating one adherent serosal surface from the other.

C

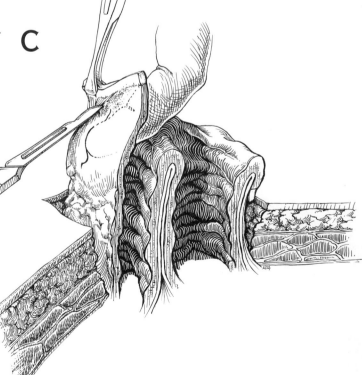

D

With the seroso-serosal adherence now lysed circumferentially, the skin attached to the colon is removed with a fine scissors or scalpel in readiness for closure.

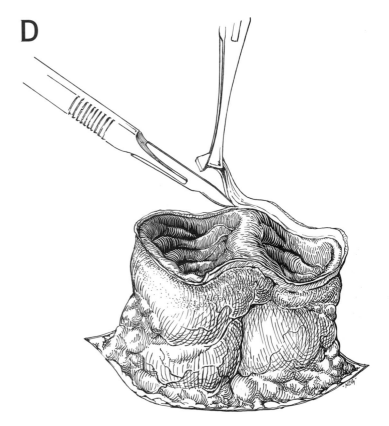

E, F

The mucosal edges are now approximated with a continuous stitch of 3-0 chromic catgut, followed by an inversion of the serosa with simple interrupted stitches of 3-0 silk.

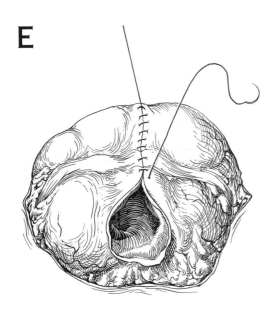

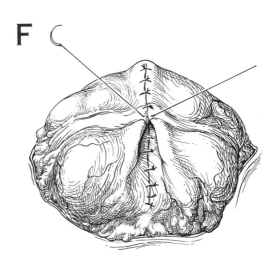

G

The rectus fascia is closed with stout absorbable suture material. The skin is closed loosely with nylon.

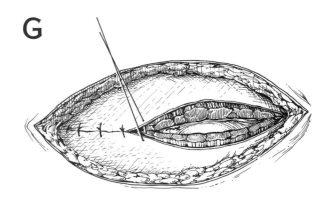

14

RECTUM

A ABDOMINOPERINEAL RESECTION

The abdominoperineal operation includes removal of the sigmoid colon and its mesentery, the rectum and mesorectum, some of the pelvic musculature, ischiorectal fat, and an ellipse of perianal skin. It is becoming a less commonly performed operation because of the availability of stapling devices to effect low anastomoses and because of a greater willingness on the part of surgeons to use rectal ultrasound to select certain tumors to excise locally. Nevertheless, it is an important and necessary operation for bulky tumors in the distal rectum that invade the sphincter. The site of the colostomy should be marked preoperatively on a spot midway between the umbilicus and the anterior iliac spine, over the rectus sheath, and on skin without scars or natural creases. The anus is occluded with a purse-string suture of 0 silk.

A

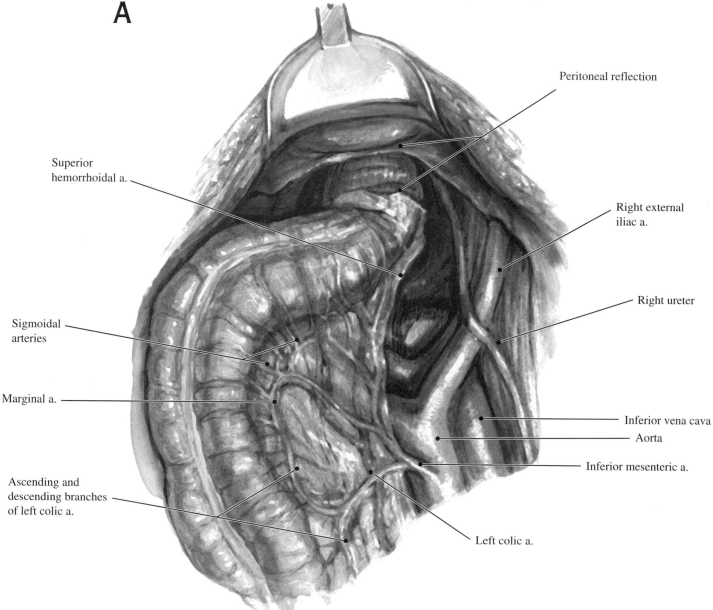

Superior hemorrhoidal a.

Sigmoidal arteries

Marginal a.

Ascending and descending branches of left colic a.

Peritoneal reflection

Right external iliac a.

Right ureter

Inferior vena cava

Aorta

Inferior mesenteric a.

Left colic a.

A

The pertinent anatomic structures to be encountered in the abdominal portion of the operation are shown. The pubic symphysis is at the top of the illustration. The right ureter is rarely in jeopardy, but the left can be damaged easily during mobilization of the sigmoid colon. A cystoscopy is advisable for rectal lesions that are located anteriorly. Also, we often catheterize the ureters for easier identification and lessened risk of injury to them. An intravenous urogram will have shown the number of ureters. The inferior mesenteric artery is shown as it typically arises approximately 4 cm proximal to the aortic bifurcation. The left colic artery is given off approximately 5 cm from the origin of the inferior mesenteric artery. The left colic artery then divides into an ascending and descending branch. Preservation of this bifurcation when ligating the descending branch at its origin from the left colic artery helps to ensure blood supply to the distal sigmoid via the marginal artery. The vascular anatomy of this area varies considerably, which must be taken into account to ensure a viable colostomy. When the mesentery is fat, the major vessels can be better palpated than seen.

B

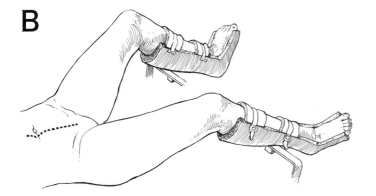

B

The patient is anesthetized and placed in the horizontal position. Or, if a two-team approach is used, the patient is placed in a semilithotomy position as shown. The abdomen is opened through a midline incision in the lower two thirds of the abdomen. On entry, there should be an exploration for metastases to other organs. The presence of several metastatic nodules in the liver need not preclude an abdominoperineal resection because, among other considerations, the metastases can be treated for cure by resection or cryodestruction. In addition, palliation of troublesome symptoms such as tenesmus and spasm must be considered.

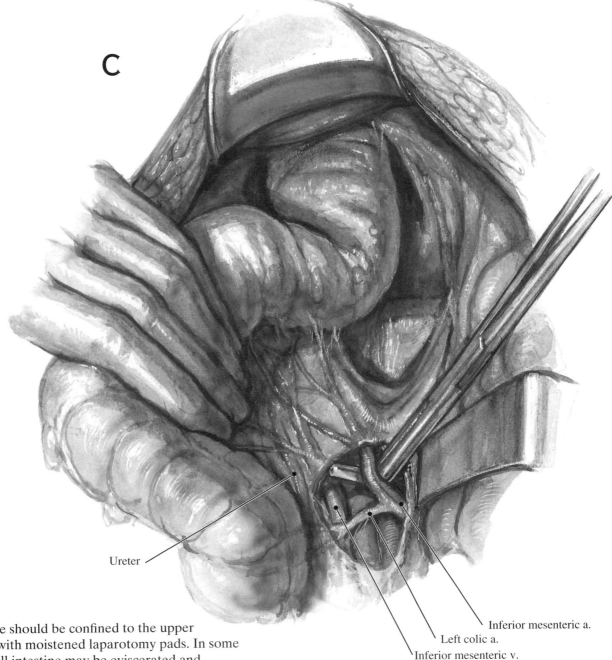

Ureter

Inferior mesenteric a.
Left colic a.
Inferior mesenteric v.

C

The small intestine should be confined to the upper peritoneal cavity with moistened laparotomy pads. In some instances, the small intestine may be eviscerated and covered with moist pads, but if this is done it should be watched for torsion or excess tension. Through a short incision in the peritoneum of the mesentery, the inferior mesenteric artery is isolated just distal to the origin of the left colic artery and ligated with 2-0 silk. The inferior mesenteric vein just lateral, but not parallel, to it is handled likewise. Alertness is necessary during the performance of these steps so that the adjacent ureter is not injured.

D

The sigmoid is mobilized by reflecting it medially and incising the mesentery at the lateral peritoneal reflection. Incision of the peritoneum over the mesosigmoid is continued downward to and across the rectovesical or rectouterine sulcus. Traction on the sigmoid makes the mesosigmoid taut and easier to cut. The left ureter and iliac vessels are now exposed and should be protected. This dissection allows the surgeon to free the mesocolon to the midline.

D

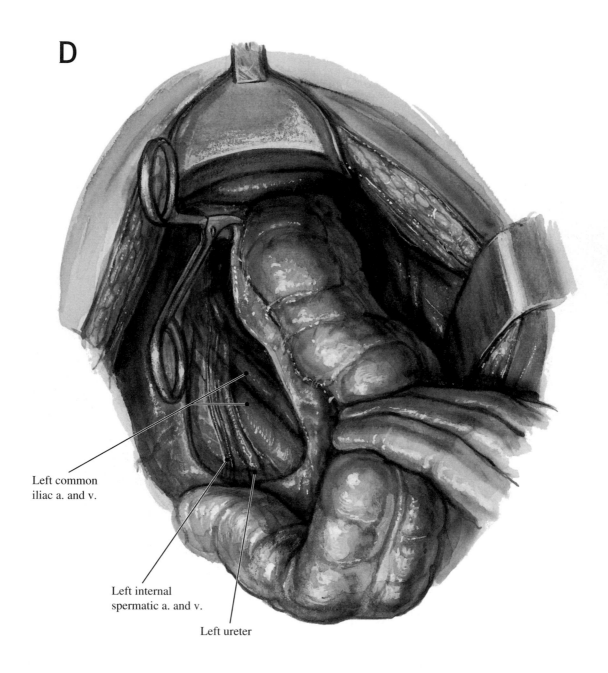

Left common
iliac a. and v.

Left internal
spermatic a. and v.

Left ureter

E

The sigmoid is reflected to the left, and again the peritoneum over the mesosigmoid is carried to its counterpart from the left. The ureter and iliac vessels must likewise be searched for and safeguarded.

F

With traction on the sigmoid and rectum, the lateral rectal stalks containing the middle hemorrhoidal vessels are exposed, clamped, cut, and ligated with 2-0 silk as laterally as possible.

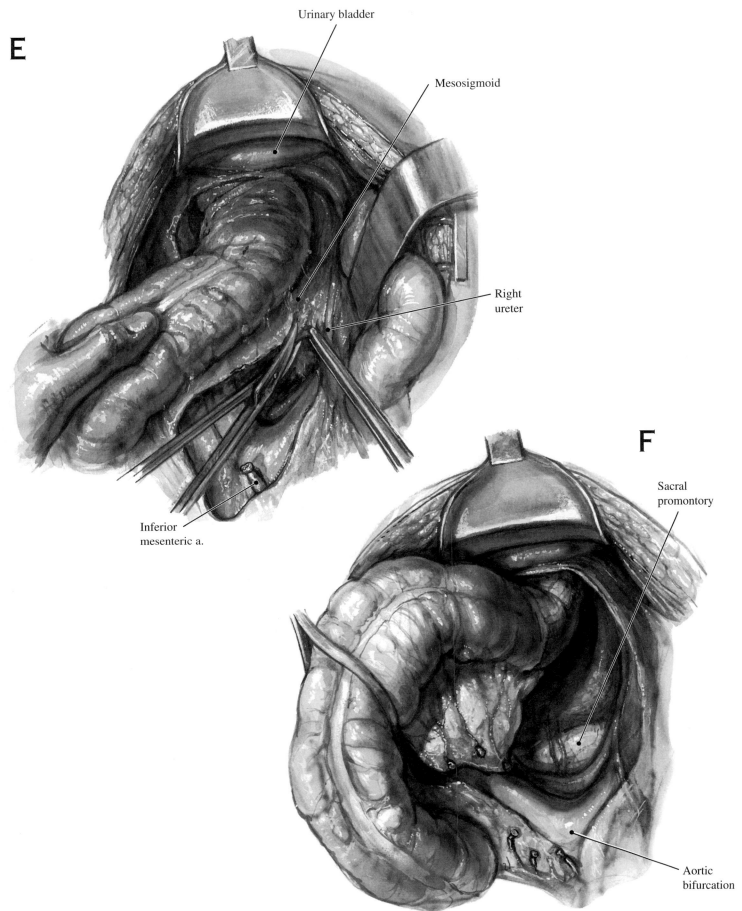

E

Urinary bladder

Mesosigmoid

Right ureter

Inferior mesenteric a.

F

Sacral promontory

Aortic bifurcation

G

The mesosigmoid is divided by clamping, dividing, and ligating all tissue to just below the sacral promontory but avoiding the midsacral vessels. The dissection in the hollow of the sacrum can then be carried out by careful but firm blunt dissection. When in the right plane, the ease and feel of the dissection is unmistakable, and the surgeon will save time and avoid trouble if care is taken to establish this plane. One must be alert not to dissect deep to the presacral fascia or tear the sacral veins in this area, as the hemorrhage can be considerable and difficult to control. Anteriorly, the importance of the suprapubic retractor having a deep blade with a lip on it cannot be overemphasized.

G

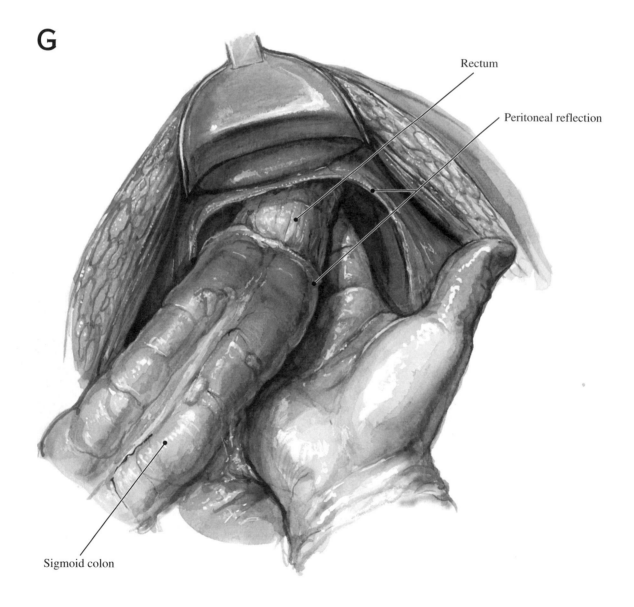

Rectum

Peritoneal reflection

Sigmoid colon

K

The most accessible peritoneum for a reperitonealization of the pelvis is over the bladder anteriorly. Lateral mobilization also helps to release available peritoneum. In females in whom no alternative is feasible, the uterus may be tipped backward to help to close this defect.

L

The pelvic peritoneum is approximated with a continuous stitch of 2-0 chromic catgut. The ureters are close by and should be avoided. A colostomy is created in the customary manner, as is the closure of the abdomen.

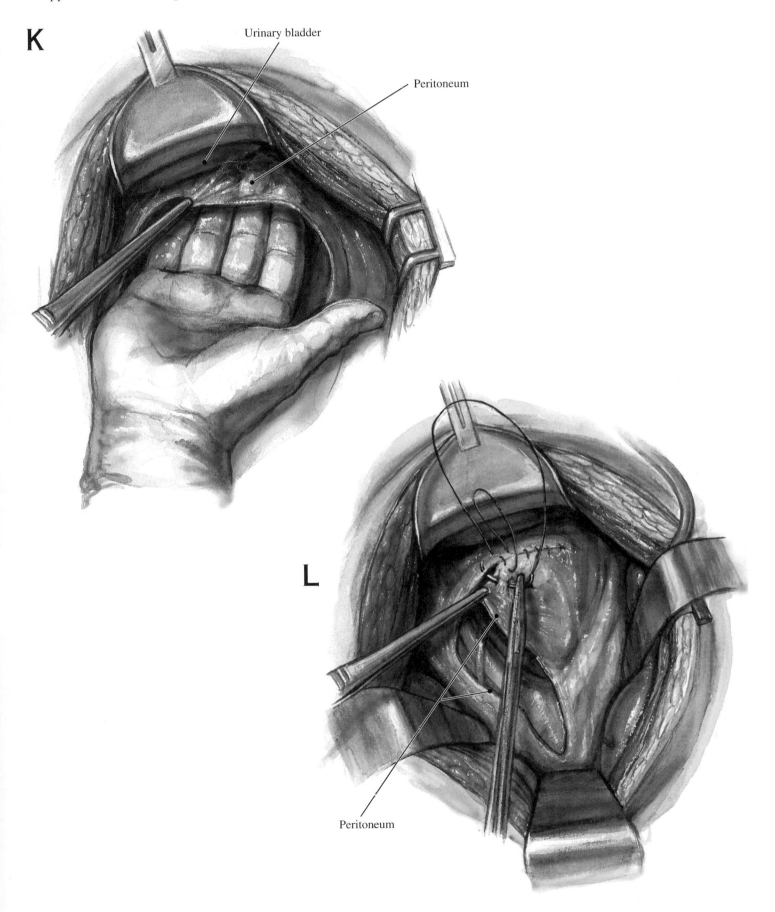

K

Urinary bladder

Peritoneum

L

Peritoneum

M

The position of the patient for the perineal dissection is as
depicted in *B*, for a synchronous two-team approach.
Otherwise a formal lithotomy position should be used.
Some of the pertinent anatomy is shown. After the patient
is positioned, a purse-string suture is used to seal the anus,
after which the area is cleansed and draped. A urinary
catheter will have been placed in position.

M

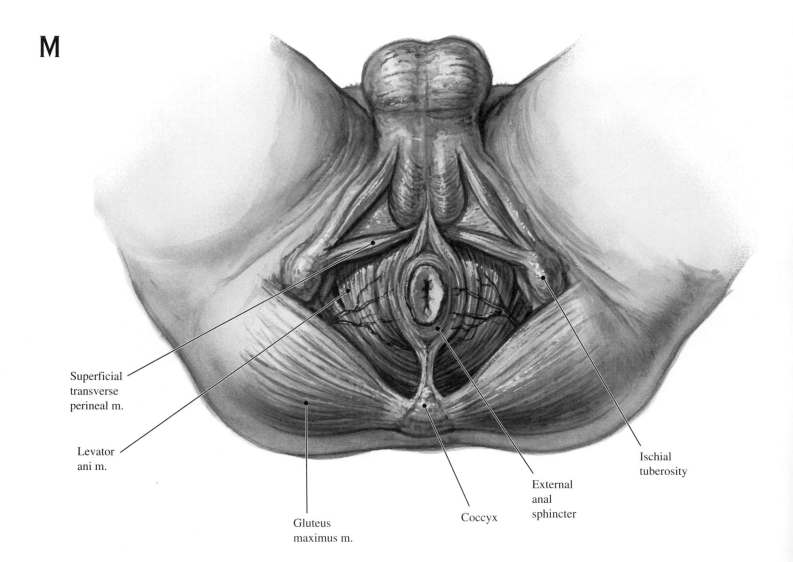

Superficial
transverse
perineal m.

Levator
ani m.

Gluteus
maximus m.

Coccyx

External
anal
sphincter

Ischial
tuberosity

N

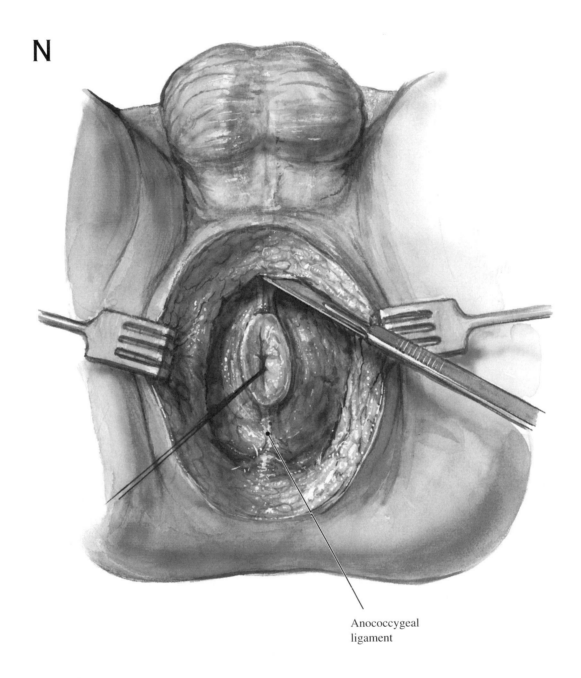

Anococcygeal
ligament

N

The elliptic perineal incision extends from the ischial
tuberosities laterally to the coccyx posteriorly and to the
perineal region anteriorly. The anococcygeal ligament is an
important ligament that should be looked for. Sharp
dissection can be used with electrocoagulation to secure
bleeding points, or electrocautery can be used throughout.
The latter is swifter, and there seems to be little difference
in the final healing.

O, P

The inferior hemorrhoidal arteries and branches from the internal pudendal vessels are clamped, cut, and ligated with 2-0 chromic catgut (*O*). This exposes the inferior surface of the levator ani muscles which are divided by electrocautery or sharp technique (*P*).

O

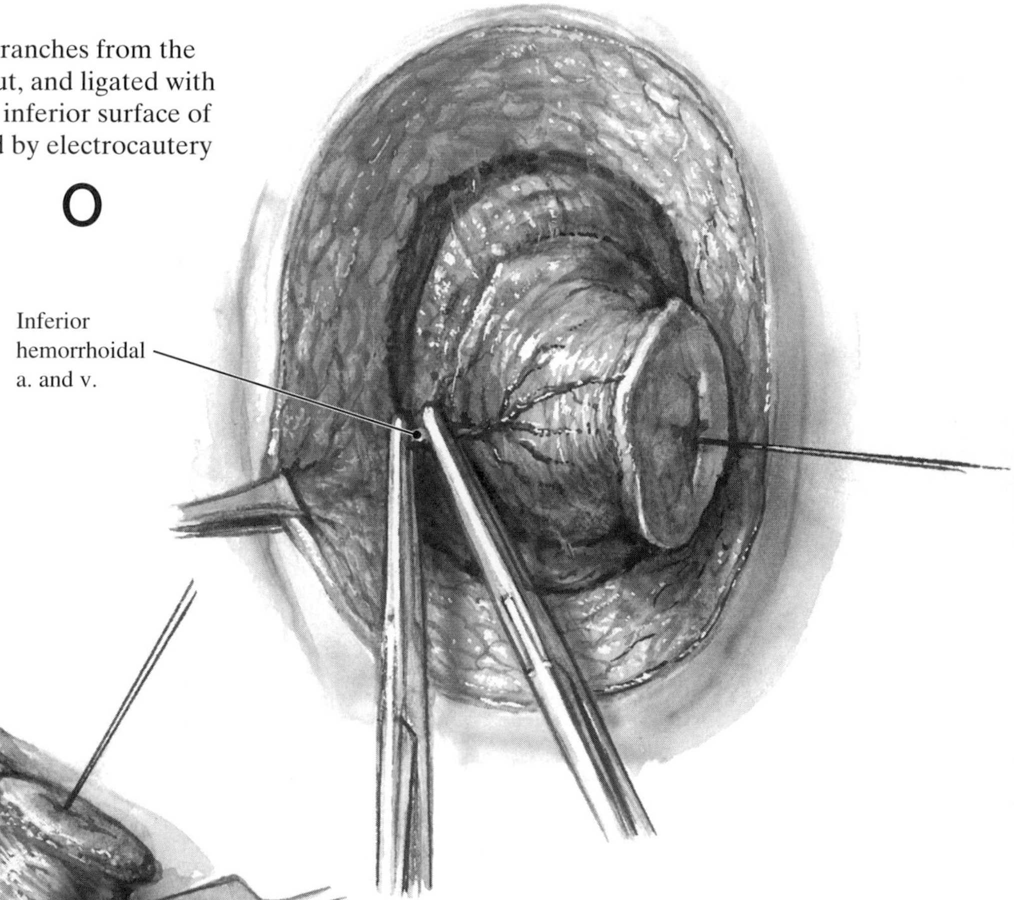

Inferior hemorrhoidal a. and v.

P

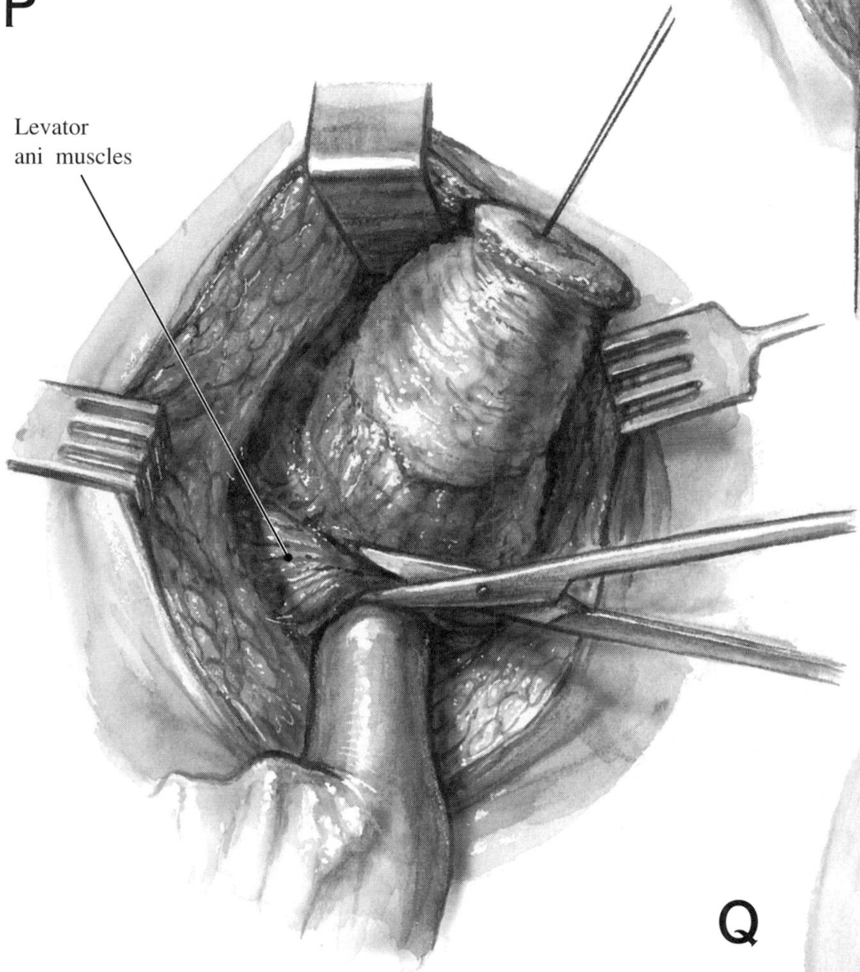

Levator ani muscles

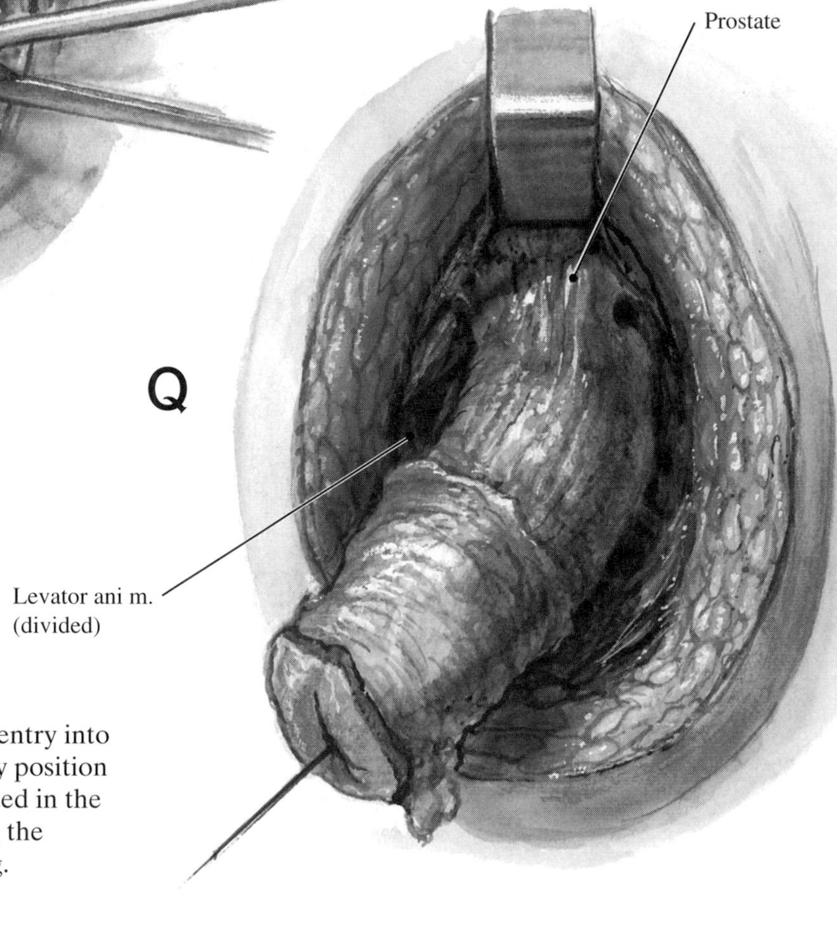

Prostate

Q

Levator ani m. (divided)

Q

The anococcygeal ligament is incised, permitting entry into the pelvic cavity. With the patient in the lithotomy position during the abdominal phase, the blood accumulated in the hollow of the pelvis pours out, sometimes leading the unwary to think that there is brisk active bleeding.

R

The hand is inserted in the hollow of the sacrum and the lower sacral dissection completed. The levator ani muscles are divided as far anteriorly as the superficial transverse perineal muscles, where the latter are divided, resulting in the anterior levators holding the specimen in place.

R

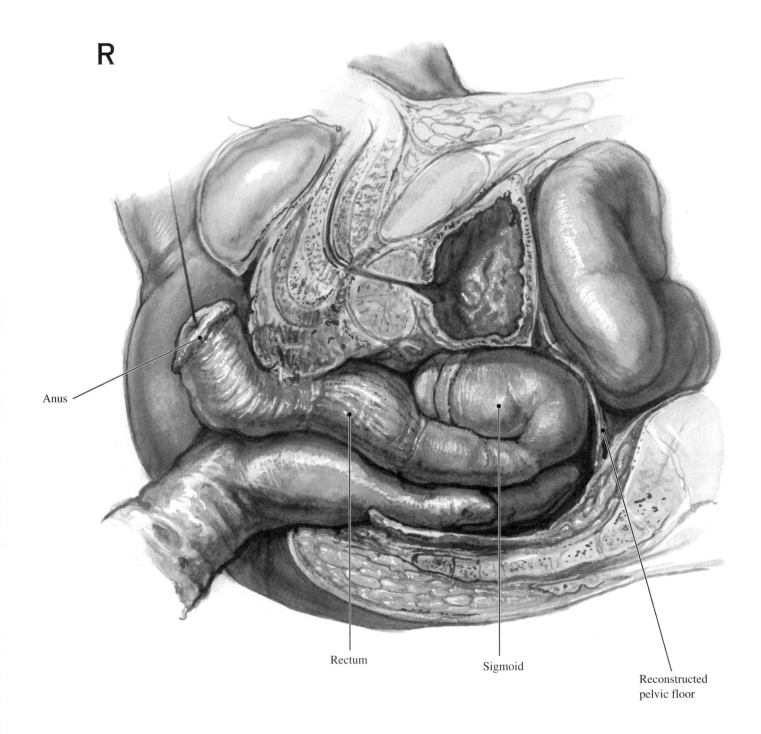

Anus

Rectum

Sigmoid

Reconstructed
pelvic floor

S

The largely freed rectum has been exteriorized. The specimen remains attached by the retroprostatic tissue. As a consequence, the urethra can be pulled perilously close to the plane of dissection, especially when resecting an anteriorly placed rectal lesion.

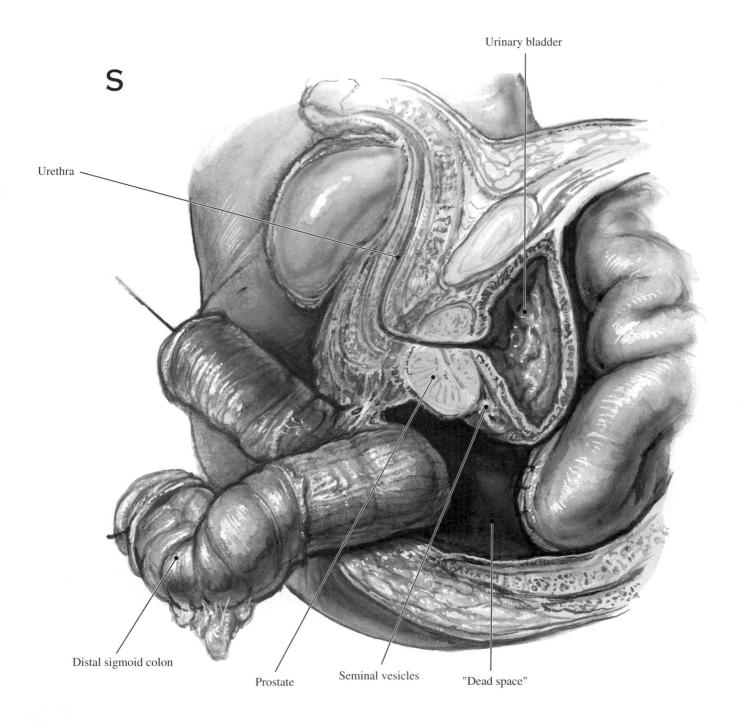

S

Urinary bladder

Urethra

Distal sigmoid colon

Prostate

Seminal vesicles

"Dead space"

T

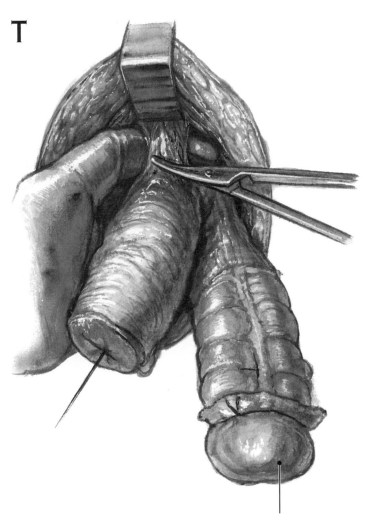

Transected sigmoid
(covered with rubber dam)

T

With a finger behind the anterior portion of the levator ani muscles, a more accurate dissection can be carried out with less risk of urethral trauma in the male. In the female, vaginal tissue is taken if indicated by virtue of proximity of the tumor.

U

U

The pelvic hollow is examined minutely for bleeding points. A large Penrose drain is exteriorized from the sacral hollow and the perineal wound closed with interrupted stitches of 3-0 nylon. If the hemostasis in the pelvis seems suboptimal or if the wound was somehow grossly contaminated, it should be left open. A rubber dam backed by rolls of fluffed gauze is used to fill the pelvic space and to apply mild pressure for hemostasis. Removal of such a pack is begun in several days.

B REPAIR OF RECTAL PROLAPSE

ABDOMINAL

Because of their advanced age, most patients with rectal prolapse usually have one or more associated diseases, some of which are more serious than the prolapse. All patients presenting for treatment of their rectal prolapse should have a thorough evaluation of their cardiothoracic and gastrointestinal systems and, not the least, their emotional state.

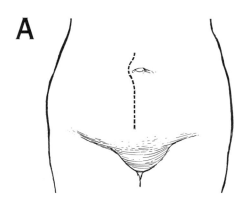

A

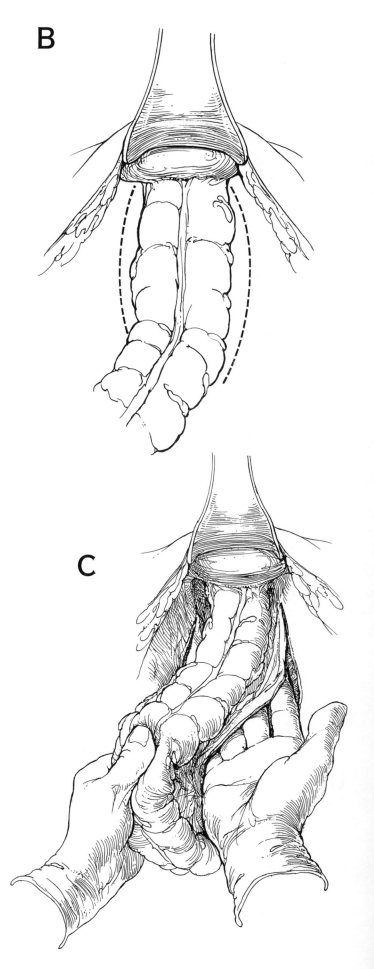

B

C

A, B

The intent of the operation is to retract the prolapsed rectum, as high as possible in this instance, and to anchor it securely to the sacrum with Teflon. The expectation is that the ingrowth of fibrous tissue from the rectum into the Teflon will ensure permanent fixation.

A low midline incision is best. Having the patient in a modest Trendelenburg position helps keep the small intestine out of the pelvis during the operation. The dashed line indicates the intended position of the posterior parietal peritoneum that precedes mobilization of the rectum.

C

Most of the dissection is by hand through rather loose areolar tissue. One hand applies a steadying pull of the rectum; the other hand, palm side up, is inserted into the hollow of the sacrum and is used to bluntly dissect the rectum free down to the pelvic floor. There is some minimal oozing that can be controlled by temporary packing with laparotomy pads.

D

The presacral fascia is dissected clean with special diligence in the area just below the promontory, as this is where the Teflon will be anchored. A strip of Teflon 3 to 4 cm wide and 15 or so cm long is slipped under the bowel and positioned on the sacrum.

E

The Teflon is anchored to each side of the vertebra with three stitches of 2-0 black silk, making certain that each passage of the needle engages the presacral fascia. Orthopedic staples can also be used to anchor the Teflon.

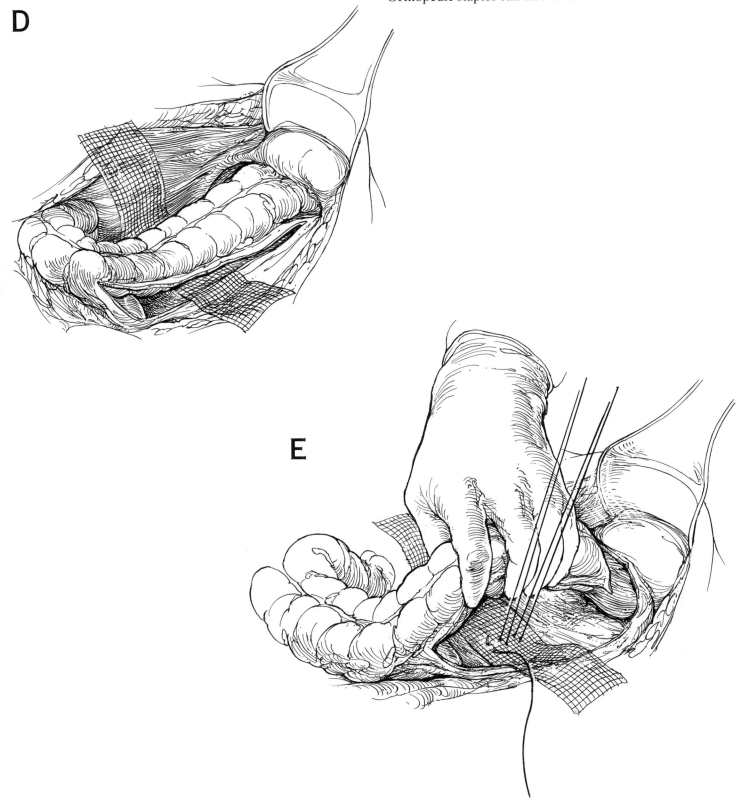

F

The bowel is repositioned, and cephalad traction is applied on the sigmoid. This brings the rectum up substantially, so much so that it likely will reach the level of the sacral promontory. The Teflon is folded over the bowel and trimmed so that the ends are 1 to 2 cm apart, and then the ends are stitched to the rectum with simple stitches of 3-0 black silk. The hiatus between the ends of the trimmed Teflon permits some distention of the rectum, obviating an iatrogenic obstipation.

F

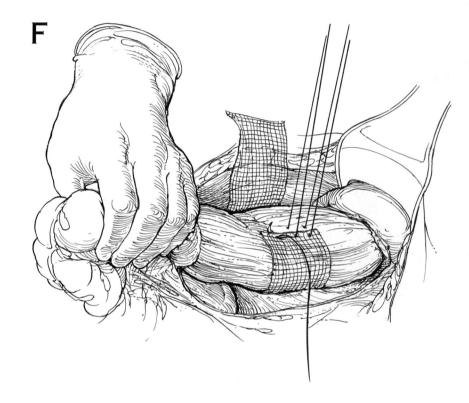

G

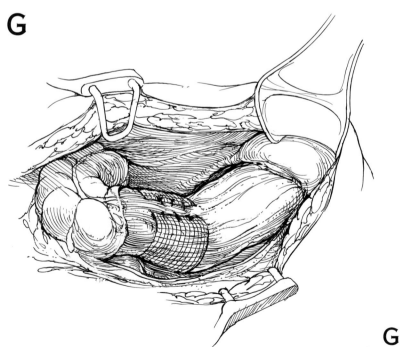

G

With the anchoring completed, the sigmoid is returned to a normal position. The small intestine is returned to its normal position in the pelvis, and the abdomen is closed in the preferred fashion.

PERINEAL
Hand Sewn

A

This diagram shows prolapse without a hernia in the pouch of Douglas and is the type whose repair is described here.

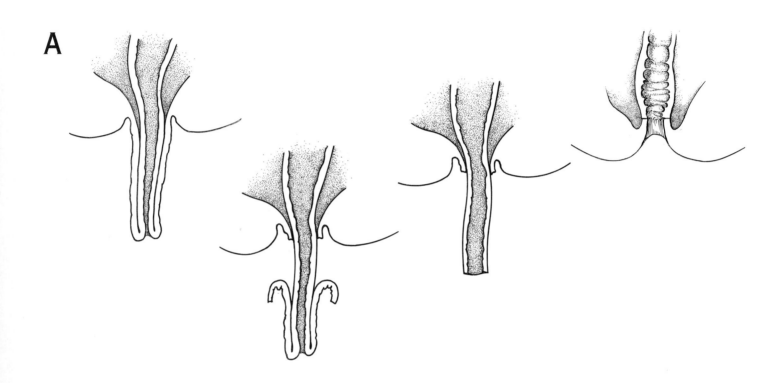

B

When the patient is in the lithotomy position, the prolapse protrudes and identifies itself. A Babcock clamp is attached to the lowermost end of the prolapse and gently pulled down to its fullest extent. The incision, which is through the full thickness of the telescoped segment, is circumferential and made about 3 cm proximal to the dentate line; this length of rectum suffices postoperatively to allow normal defecation. The incision is followed by generous bleeding from this vascular area. Hemostasis here can be obtained by electrocoagulation with a fine-tipped instrument. Beyond this point, all tissue is clamped, cut, and ligated because the prolapsed segment carries with it its thick mesentery and associated vessels. This mesentery retracts when divided, so if the hemostasis with electrocautery is incomplete it can easily lead to the formation of a hematoma with the accompanying risk of an anastomotic infection or disruption.

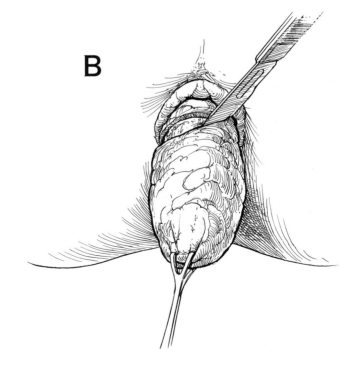

C

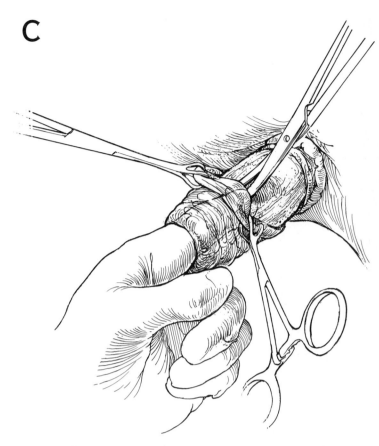

The index finger is inserted into the rectal lumen and Babcock forceps applied to the mucosa and muscle at the distal incision. With gentle traction on the Babcock forceps, fine Metzenbaum scissors are used to separate the two segments of bowel.

D, E

The bowel is now fully unfolded and left to hang. The levator ani muscles are dissected sufficiently to identify their course, and their diastatic condition is corrected by approximating them with interrupted simple stitches of 2-0 black silk.

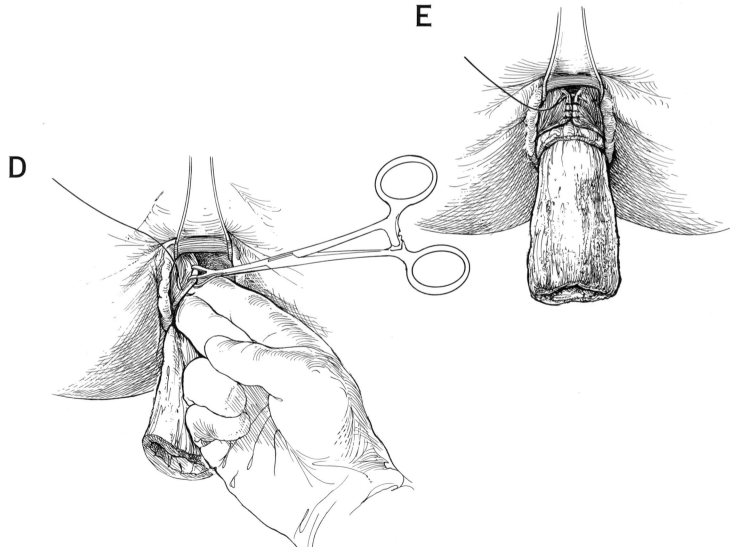

F

The excess rectum is divided with electrocautery in the direct posterior and anterior positions up to the level of the original circumferential cut.

G

At the apices of the longitudinal cuts, simple stitches of 3-0 long-lasting absorbable suture, made taking generous bites of tissue, are used to approximate the intestine.

F

G

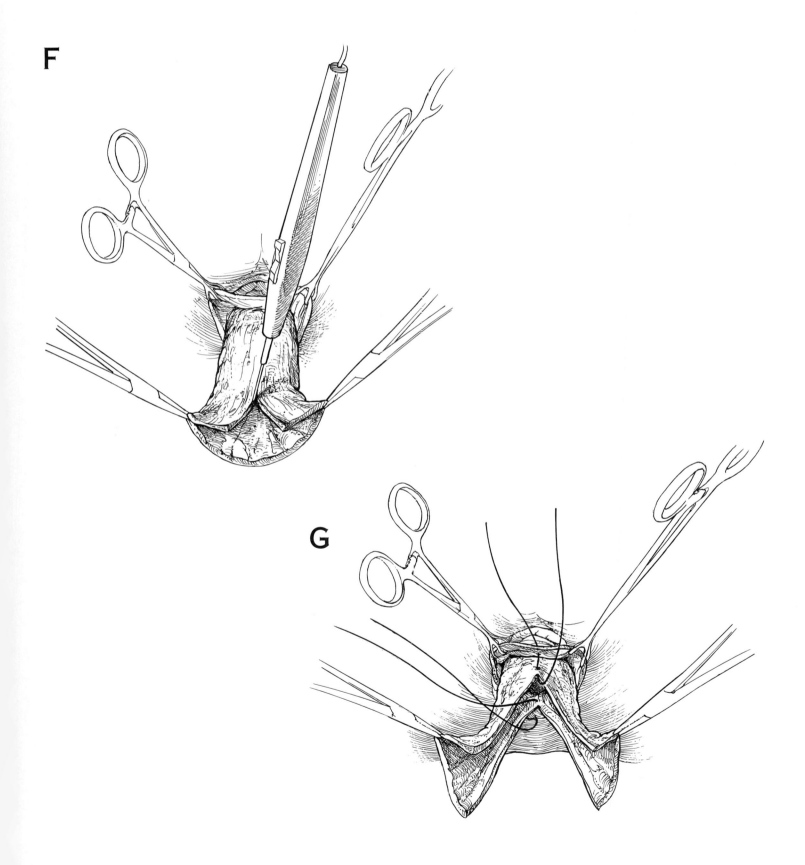

H

At the apex of the cut, the trimming is done circumferentially. At short intervals, the two sectioned segments of bowel are sutured to each other with interrupted 3-0 long-lasting absorbable suture. Doing this in a "stitch as you go" method easily holds the tissue in clear view, ensuring accurate placement of the stitches.

H

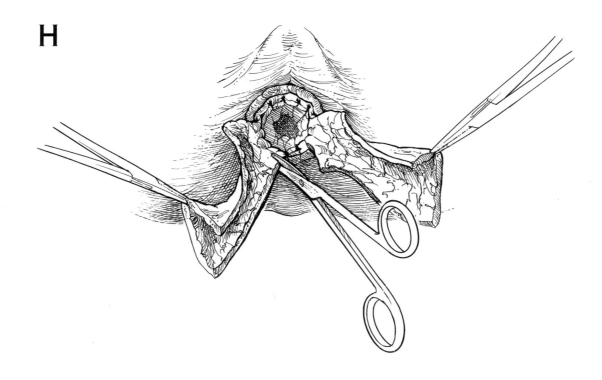

I

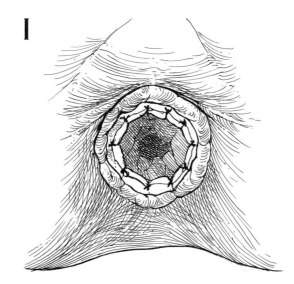

I

The repair is complete. The anus is patulous from chronic dilation preoperatively, and the tissues are edematous both from its extended dependency and from the operation. This swollen tissue is replaced inside the anus.

Stapled

A

With the patient in the lithotomy position, the prolapse is brought down to its fullest extent and a circumferential cut through the muscularis mucosa is made about 3 cm from the pectinate line. Generous oozing is controlled by electrocoagulation.

B

The prolapsed rectum has been dissected free from itself. A longitudinal cut is made for easier insertion of the stapling device. A purse-string suture of stout monofilament material is applied just caudal to the initial circumferential cut.

C

The purse-string suture is tied snugly just below the anvil. Next, a circumferential purse-string suture of similar material is applied to the divided distal rectum, making certain it incorporates all layers of the rectum.

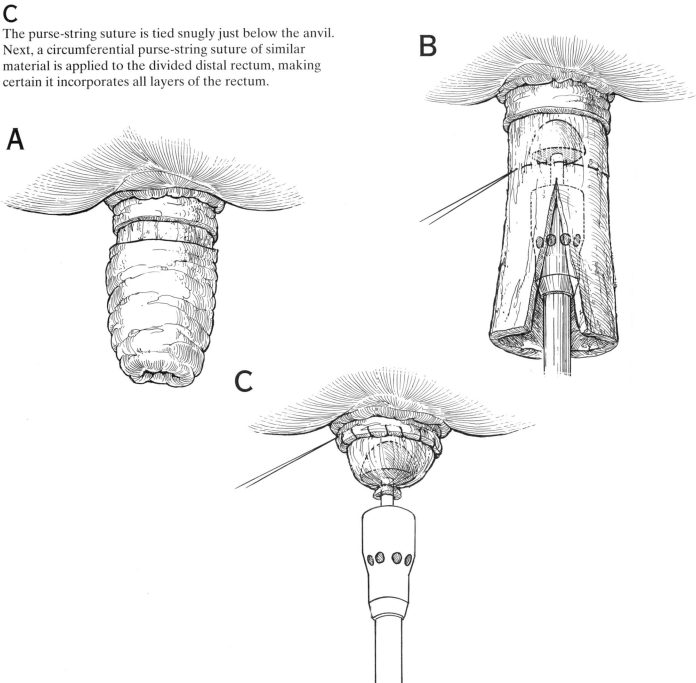

D

The center rod is extended so that the anvil lies at the level of the anal sphincter or even higher. This maneuver invaginates the divided rectum that was purse-string sutured to it.

E

The purse-string on the distal segment of rectum is tied firmly around the center rod.

F

Both segments of bowel with purse-string sutures securing them are now abutting each other.

The anvil and the stapling instrument are brought together snugly, and the gun is fired. The stapling instrument is gently eased out, and the tissue within the cartridge is examined for integrity of the ring of tissue.

G

The anastomosis is completed with the stapled suture line lying within the rectum.

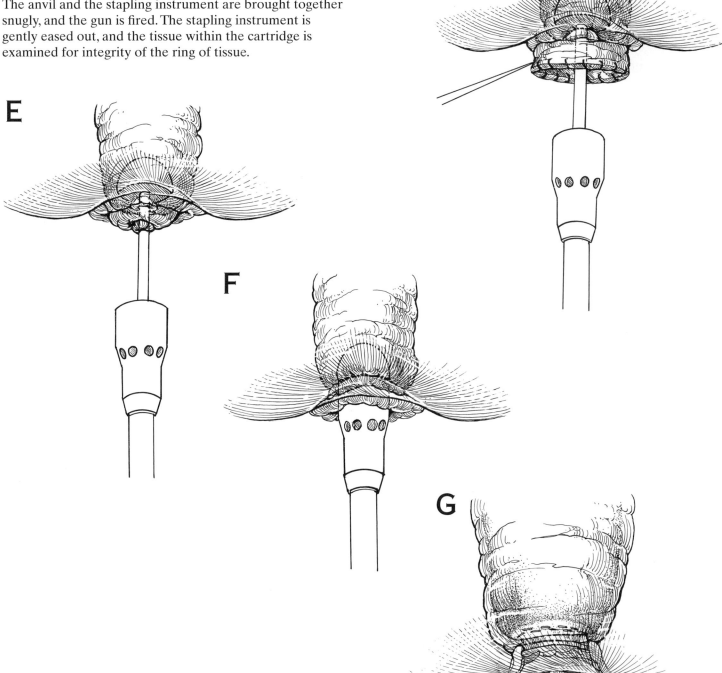

Chapter 15

ANAL AND PERIANAL PROCEDURES

A HEMORRHOIDECTOMY

Many anorectal conditions that are common can produce great distress and disability if not diagnosed or treated correctly. The general surgeon is obliged, therefore, to be thoroughly conversant with the anatomy of the anus and rectum and of the pathophysiologic processes at play. The operations selected for inclusion here confront the general surgeon in a number of clinical settings yet are straightforward and can be approached in logical manner.

A

This three fourths synoptic view of the anal, perianal, and rectal areas provides an anatomic backdrop for a better understanding of the operations to be described.

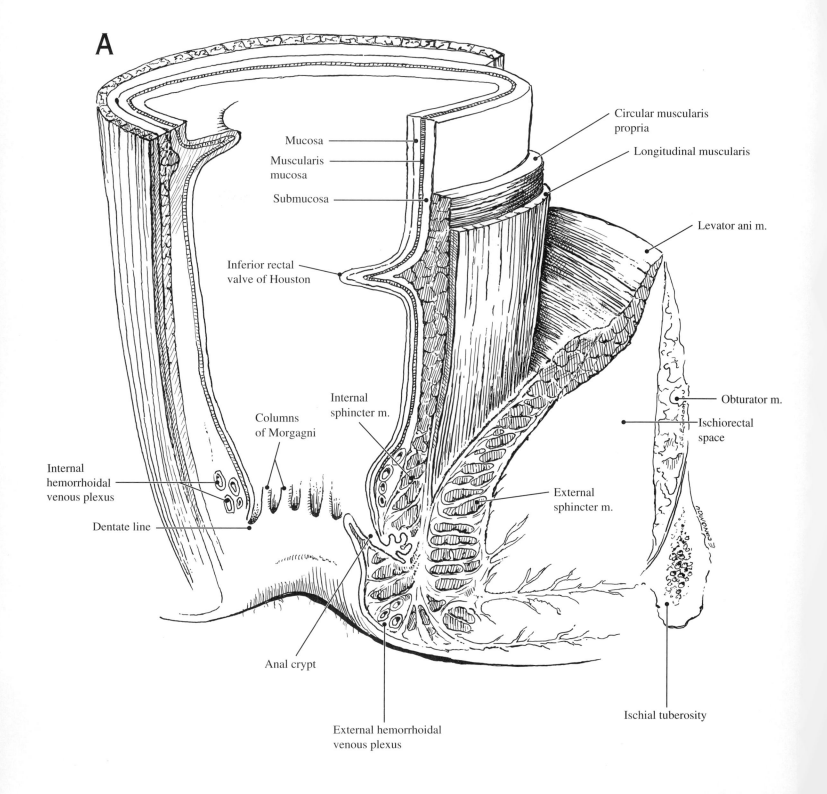

A

- Circular muscularis propria
- Longitudinal muscularis
- Mucosa
- Muscularis mucosa
- Submucosa
- Levator ani m.
- Inferior rectal valve of Houston
- Internal sphincter m.
- Columns of Morgagni
- Obturator m.
- Ischiorectal space
- Internal hemorrhoidal venous plexus
- External sphincter m.
- Dentate line
- Anal crypt
- External hemorrhoidal venous plexus
- Ischial tuberosity

B

Most operations on the anus and rectum can be performed with the patient in the lithotomy position; the lateral or prone position may be used as well, depending on the surgeon's preference.

The anus is gently dilated with one and then two fingers before the anoscope (single or double blade) is inserted. Forceful dilation risks tearing the anal mucosa and internal sphincter, potentially adding to the postoperative pain.

The hemorrhoidal clusters usually occur at the left lateral, right anterior, and right posterior positions. Here, a single one in the direct dorsal location is exposed for treatment.

B

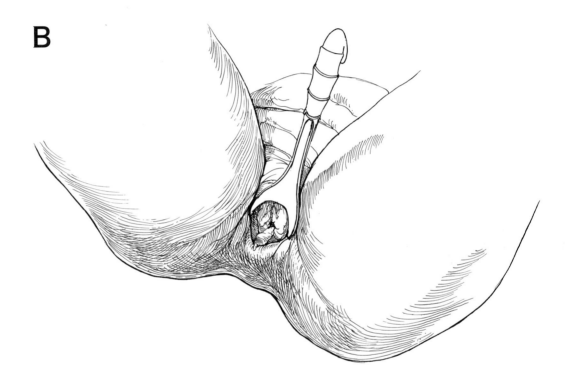

C

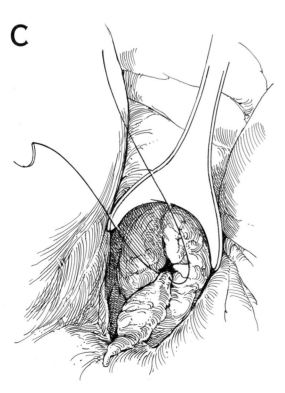

C

A stitch of 3-0 chromic catgut is placed through the apex of the hemorrhoidal complex; it should traverse deeply enough to incorporate the submucosal hemorrhoidal vessels.

D

The hemorrhoidal complex is grasped fully with a Babcock forceps and encompassed with an elliptic incision begun at the lowermost apex. The amount of skin to be excised should be such that when the tissue is reapproximated, the result is a smooth surface, without tension on the suture line.

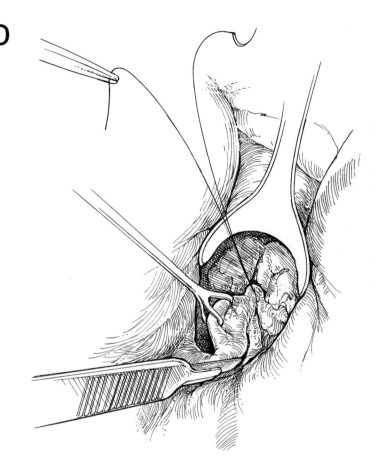

D

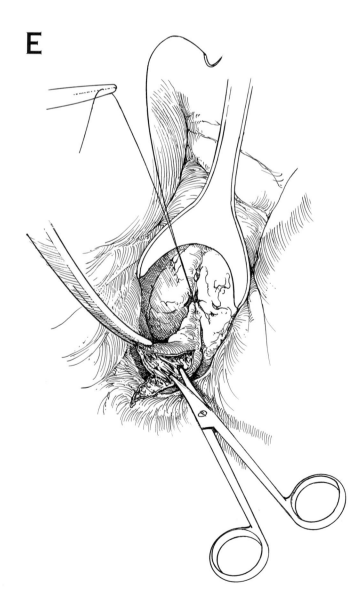

E

The lowermost apex of the skin incision is grasped with a hemostat and used to elevate the hemorrhoidal and submucosal tissues as they are dissected off the sphincter muscles.

F

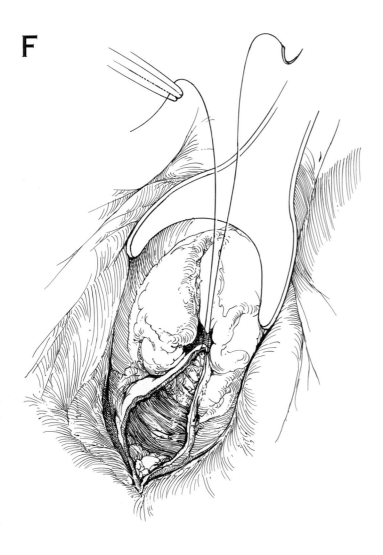

F

When the dissection is completed, the base of the dissected area is examined for bleeding vessels. Usually bleeding is controlled with delicately applied electrocoagulation. Minimal oozing from the cut edges of the mucosa is controlled by the continuous mucosal stitch that is to follow.

G

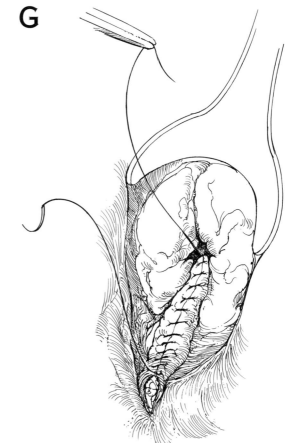

G

One arm of the 3-0 chromic catgut that has been applied to the proximal apex of the dissected area is used to place a continuous over-and-over stitch down to the dentate line. Leaving the external aspect of the incision open may allow escape of a submucosal fluid collection. A variety of drains, stents, or hemostatic agents have been left in the anal canal. The purpose and value of anything placed in the anal canal whose mucosa has been reapproximated is not clear and may only serve to worsen postoperative pain.

B FISSURE—LATERAL SUBCUTANEOUS SPHINCTEROTOMY

For reasons not entirely clear, chronic midline anal fissures are much more likely to heal following a lateral subcutaneous sphincterotomy.

A

The anesthetized patient is placed in the lithotomy position. The anus is gently dilated, and the retractor is inserted to expose the fissure, which is most commonly found in the dorsal midline. Ventral midline fissures are seen, although less frequently.

B

An incision is made in the posterolateral aspect of the anal canal mucosa and is extended up to the dentate line.

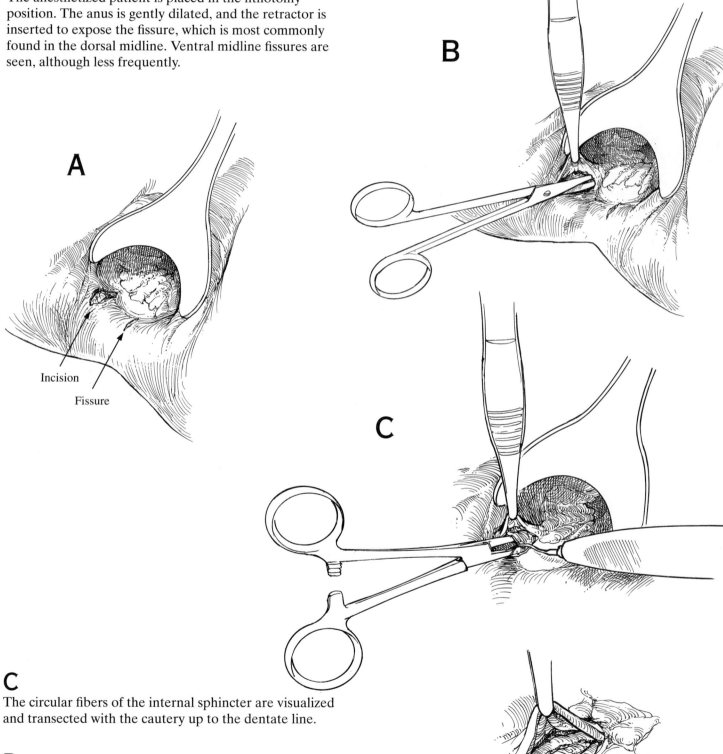

C

The circular fibers of the internal sphincter are visualized and transected with the cautery up to the dentate line.

D

Hemostasis should be obtained diligently. The wound may be left open or closed primarily.

C FISTULA-IN-ANO

SAUCERIZATION

A, B

The anal canal is gently dilated and a speculum placed to expose the affected area. A malleable probe is introduced into the internal opening and manipulated gently until it appears internally, usually at an inflamed or deep crypt. With the probe in position, the fistula is saucerized with electrocautery. If granulation tissue in the fistula is minimal, it can be curretted. With chronic intermittent inflammation with associated dense scarring, the fistulous tract can be excised, with the probe therein acting as a guide.

A

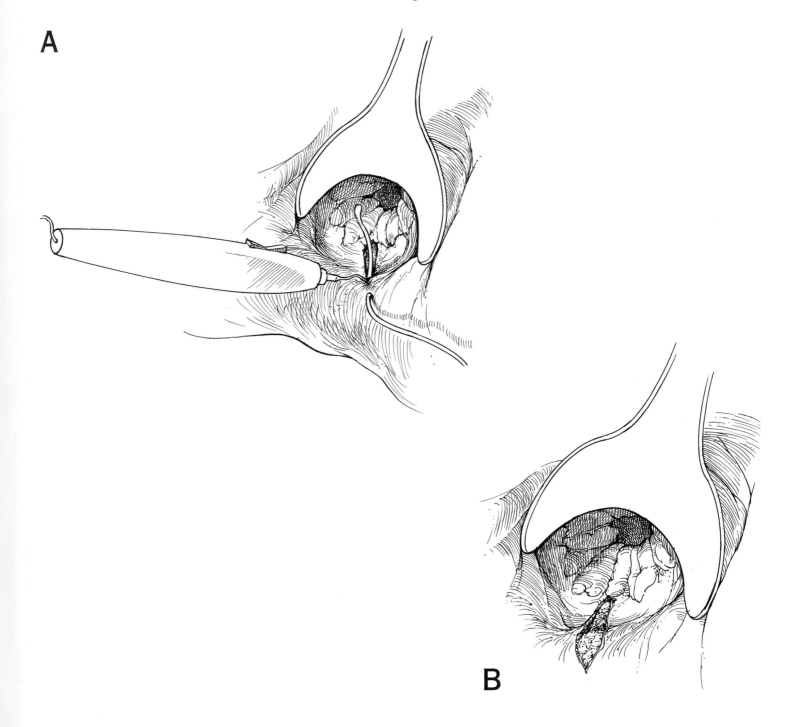

B

SETON SUTURE

A, B, C

A fistula whose extent is superficial to the deep portion of the external sphincter can be treated by a simple fistulotomy. However, one whose extent is deeper to the levators cannot be performed in one stage; the Seton suture technique addresses this problem well.

The malleable probe with its bulbous tip is passed through the fistula, at which time a small Penrose drain is tied to it. It then is withdrawn through the external opening of the fistula.

D

With firm traction on both ends of the drain, the ends are tied together firmly with stout silk. The tight Penrose drain gradually cuts through the sphincters it is encircling. As the Penrose cuts through tissue and is thus less constricted, the process of tightening it can be repeated until the process of division is complete.

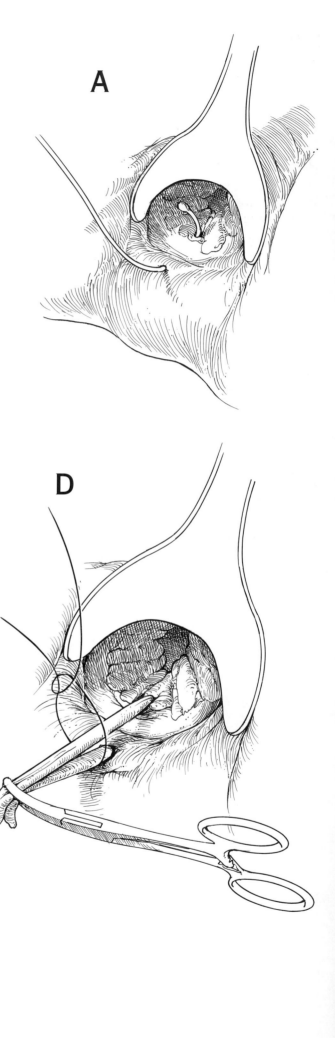

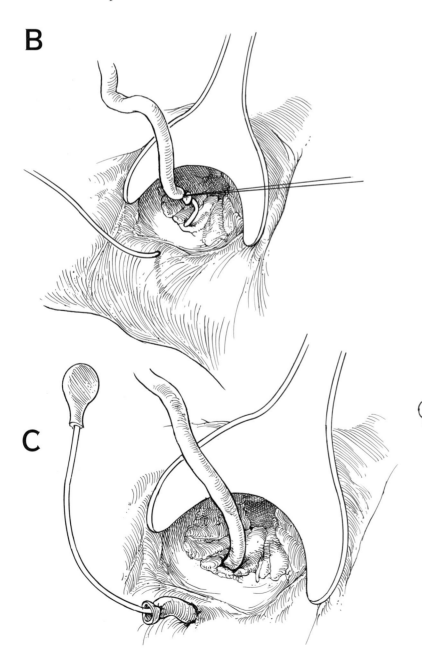

D ABSCESS

Surrounding the anal canal are several glands, which are located either within the internal sphincter or in the intermuscular space between the internal and external sphincters. Their ducts enter the anal canal at the base of the crypts within the dentate line. Infection within the anal glands may progress into surrounding tissues, producing four categories of abscess that have different presentations and treatment.

Perianal Abscess. This is the most common variety of abscess. The infectious process remains within the intersphincteric space and points caudally, producing a tender, erythematous, fluctuant mass. Externally, the abscess is easily identifiable and is treated by incision and drainage. One should make the incision as close to the anal verge as possible; in the event an underlying fistula is present, the subsequent fistulotomy wound will be smaller and will heal more rapidly.

Intersphincteric Abscess. Infection progressing cephalad in the intersphincteric space produces an abscess that may lack external evidence of an inflammatory process. In such instances, patients may complain of constant deep rectal pain that usually is unrelated to defecation. This entity must be considered in any patient who presents with these symptoms and a tender, boggy area that is noted on digital rectal examination. Treatment consists of transanal internal sphincterotomy over the entire length of the abscess, thereby providing internal drainage.

Ischiorectal Abscess. An abscess that traverses both the internal and the external sphincter into the ischiorectal fossa produces a tender, fluctuant mass that is easily identifiable on examination. Treatment is with incision close to the anal verge, débridement, and external drainage.

Supralevator Abscess. Abscesses within the supralevator, subperitoneal space may follow infectious intra-abdominal processes (e.g., diverticulitis, inflammatory bowel disease, pelvic inflammatory disease) or infections in the anal glands. In the latter circumstance, intersphincteric or ischiorectal abscesses may progress cephalad through the levator ani muscle, producing deep rectal or pelvic pain. If the abscess is due to an extension of an intersphincteric abscess, transanal extended internal sphincterotomy provides adequate internal drainage. The ischiorectal space should not be violated in these instances because doing so would create a suprasphincteric fistula. If a supralevator abscess is due to a cephalad extension of an ischiorectal abscess, incision and drainage through the ischiorectal fossa and perhaps packing or catheter drainage of the cavity is the preferred treatment.

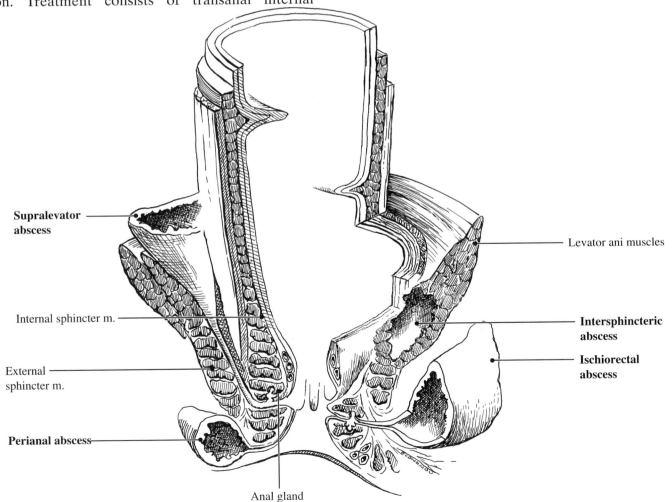

Supralevator abscess

Levator ani muscles

Internal sphincter m.

Intersphincteric abscess

Ischiorectal abscess

External sphincter m.

Perianal abscess

Anal gland

PILONIDAL CYST

A PILONIDAL CYSTECTOMY

A pilonidal cyst or sinus can manifest as an acute abscess, a recurrent inflammation, a simple sinus, a complicated sinus, and, of course, as a recurrent problem following previous therapy.

A

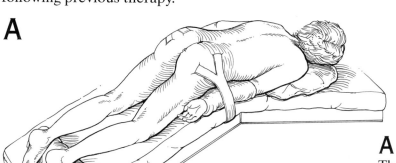

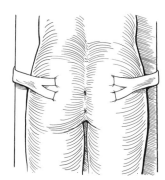

A

The patient is placed in the prone position with the table broken at the hip and slightly at the knees. A rolled blanket under the ankles protects the great toes from bearing the full weight of the legs. The buttocks are spread with tape as shown so that they do not interfere with exposure. A local anesthetic is administered.

B

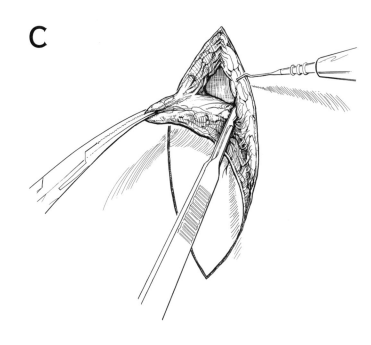

C

D

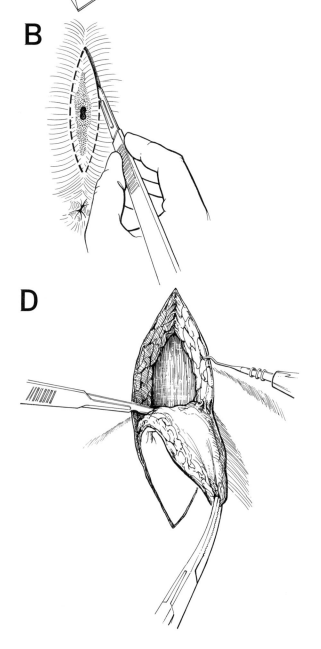

B

The purpose of excisional therapy is to remove all the diseased tissues yet not to remove too much tissue without a valid reason, for doing so makes primary closure difficult. Generally, excising a breadth of tissue 1 cm on either side of the affected tissue is adequate. Often the extent of involvement is not apparent. If so, a probe can be inserted into the sinus track, which then is opened; the excision can then proceed the necessary distance wide of the affected area.

E

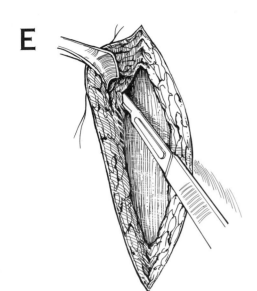

C, D

The tissue is cut sharply and straight down; trying to conserve skin by cutting obliquely in lateral fashion preserves the skin but creates an overhang that increases the amount of dead space following skin closure. The skin usually heals, but the deeper tissue is more likely to separate, setting the stage for a recurrence and sinus formation. The incision is carried down to the fascia; the fascia itself is not penetrated. A fine-tipped cautery is ideal for obtaining pinpoint hemostasis.

E, F

If the surgeon intends to close the wound primarily, the tissue at the level of the fascia is undercut laterally to a sufficient extent that the deep tissue can be approximated with minimal tension.

F

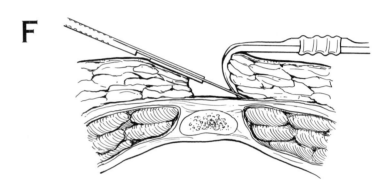

G

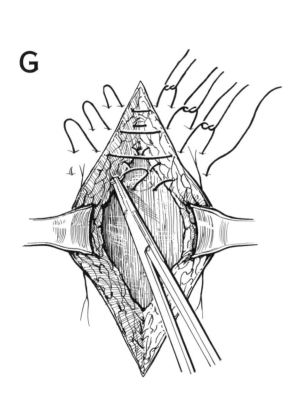

G, H

The wound is approximated with vertical mattress stitches using stout, nonabsorbable suture material and spacing the stitches approximately 1 cm apart.

H

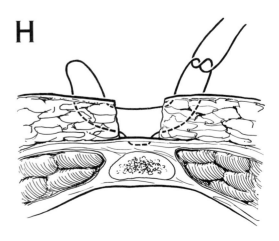

I, J, K, L

If the inflamed tissue is more extensive than anticipated, or if the sinus has a serpiginous course, it is best marsupialized. The sinus is excised as necessary and the skin and fascia approximated with 3-0 chromic catgut. The stitches through the fascia should be placed directly perpendicular to the skin; attempting to narrow the wound by positioning the stitches more medially is ill advised. An overhang of the skin is created with dead space underneath it.

I

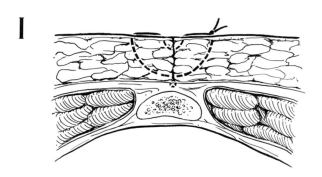

J

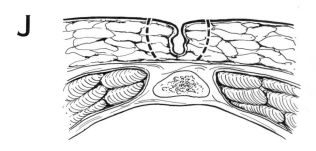

L

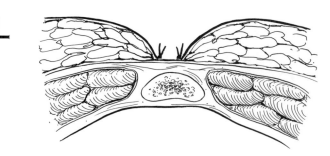

K

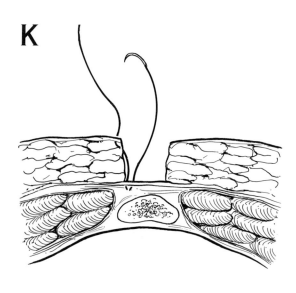

M

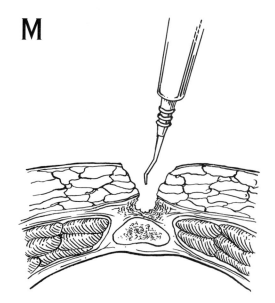

M

The choice may be to simply marsupialize the sinus without excising the inflamed tissue. This can be performed under local anesthesia and on an outpatient basis. With a probe in the sinus, the fine-tipped electrocautery is used to divide the tissue down to the probe; at the same time it provides hemostasis. The granulation tissue in the sinus is firmly wiped off with gauze, and a simple dressing is applied.

Chapter

17

HERNIA

A HERNIORRHAPHY—INGUINAL

INDIRECT; OPEN—NO MESH

A

This illustration demonstrates some of the surface anatomy encountered during an inguinal herniorrhaphy. The ilioinguinal nerve exits with the spermatic cord; the iliohypogastric nerve is located more cephalad to this. Injury to either can cause annoying symptoms in the areas they innervate. The patient is placed in the supine position and the skin prepared and draped from the costal margin to the upper thighs.

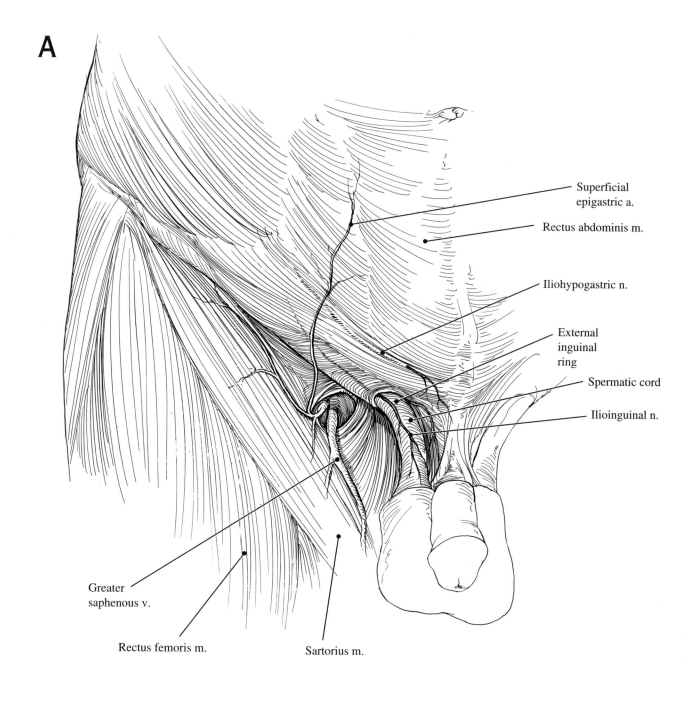

A

Superficial epigastric a.

Rectus abdominis m.

Iliohypogastric n.

External inguinal ring

Spermatic cord

Ilioinguinal n.

Greater saphenous v.

Rectus femoris m.

Sartorius m.

B

The incision is made 2 cm above and parallel to Poupart's ligament, extending from the anterior superior iliac spine to the pubic tubercle. The superficial epigastric and the external pudendal veins are encountered and require clamping and ligation with 4-0 chromic catgut. All other vessels are small and can be electrocoagulated. The aponeurosis of the external oblique muscle is cleansed of attached fatty tissue.

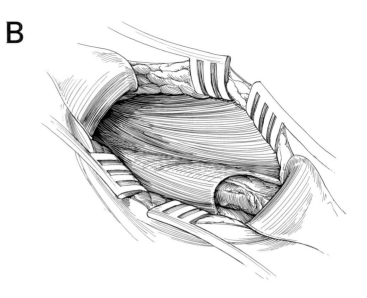

C, D

The ilioinguinal nerve is tight against the external ring and may be injured if the incision of the external oblique muscle is begun here. Instead, an index finger is placed in the ring and lifted while the external oblique muscle is incised several centimeters more proximally. The cut edges are grasped with hemostats, and the incision to the external ring begins at this point.

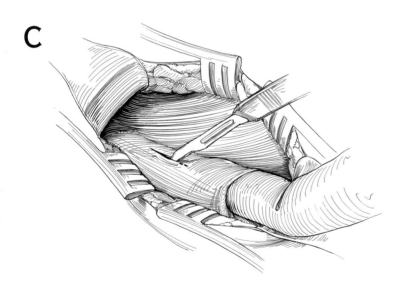

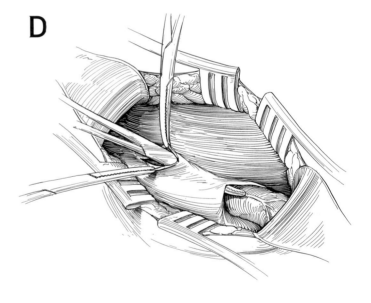

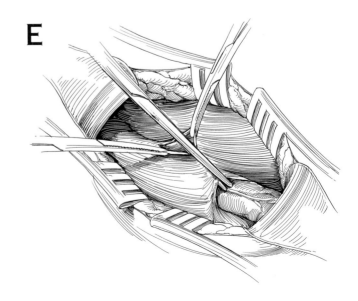

E

The ilioinguinal nerve lies on the cord and should not be grasped directly with thumb forceps. Neither should it be dissected clean—the perineural fat should be left attached, as much as possible.

F, G

The nerve is encircled with Babcock clamp to allow manipulation as the loose dissection is performed; the nerve is shifted laterally and kept out of harm in this position. The external oblique muscle can be freed from the underlying cord with a sweep of the finger.

H, I, J

A tightly rolled pledget of gauze on a 6-inch forceps (locally referred to as a "peanut") is used to free the cord sufficiently that the index finger and then a small Penrose drain can be passed deep to it. The Penrose drain is used to lift the cord as it is mobilized from the pubic tubercle to the internal ring.

F

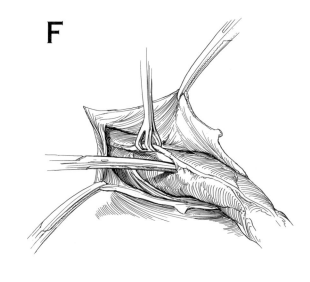

G

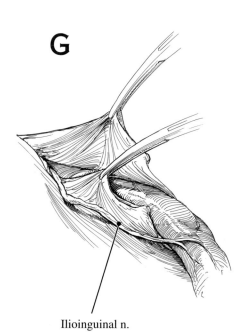

Ilioinguinal n.

H

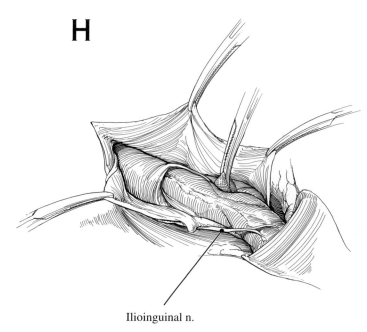

Ilioinguinal n.

I

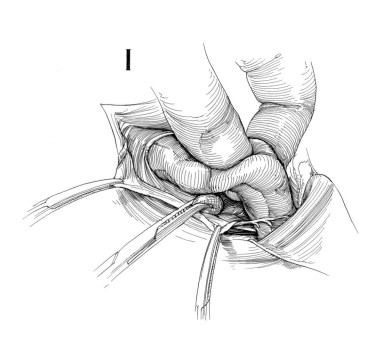

J

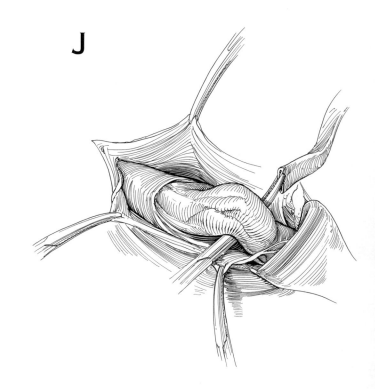

K

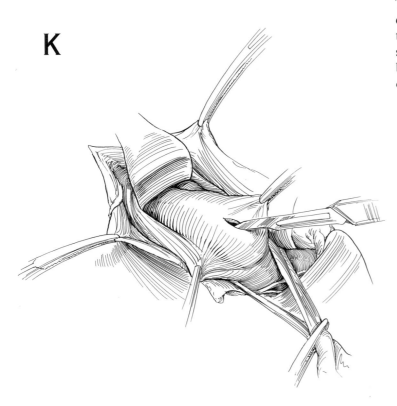

The cremasteric fibers are held up with forceps as they are divided with cautery parallel to their course and down to the hernia sac, which usually is found on the anteromedial side of the cord. The sac is opened cautiously with a no. 15 blade so as not to also open intestine that may be at the tip of the sac.

L

The left index finger is inserted into the sac and the other fingers used to hold hemostats placed along the rim of the opened sac to pull it up taut. The assistant provides counterresistance as the surgeon's other hand uses the peanut to separate the sac from the surrounding tissue. If the dissection is in the right plane—immediately superficial to the sac—the dissection is blunt and bloodless. The exception is the area in which the vas deferens and some of the cord are adherent to the sac; these are best freed by sharp dissection.

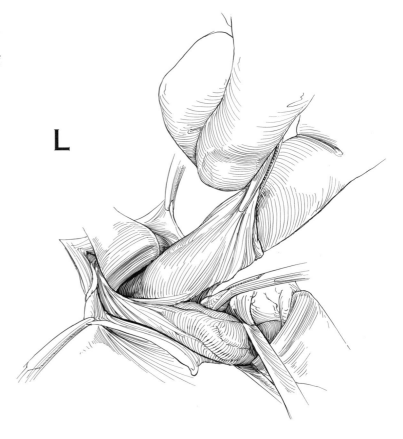

M, N, O, P, Q, R

For larger hernial openings, a purse-string closure seems best and more secure. Careful attention is directed to not including intestine in the constricting purse-string. Once the purse-string is in position, the index finger is inserted in the sac, keeping the intestines in front of it. As the purse-string is pulled taut, closing the hernial sac, the finger is gradually withdrawn, thus effectively preventing entrapment of the intestine.

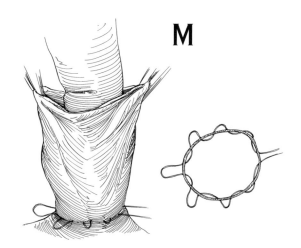

M

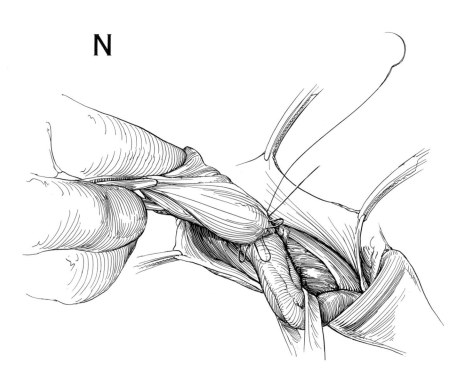

N

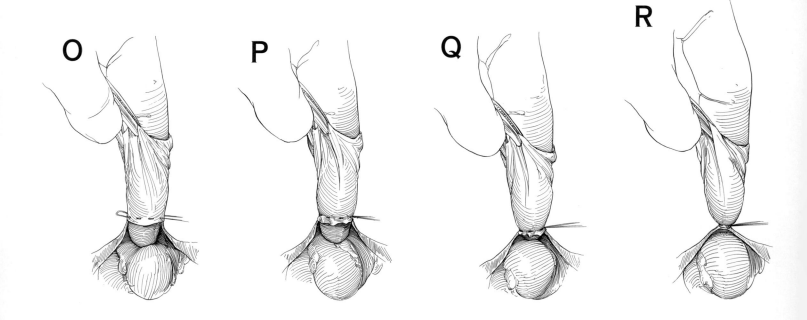

O   P   Q   R

S

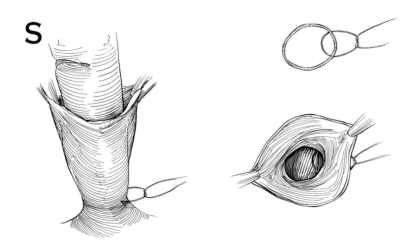

T

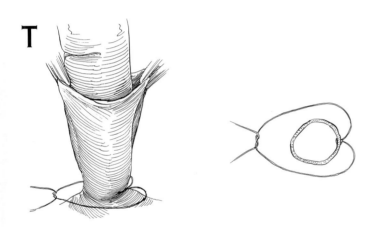

U

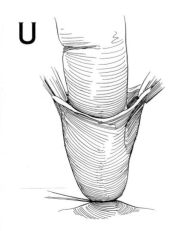

S, T, U

For smaller hernial openings, a transfixion ligature is used.

V

The neck of the sac is ligated as high as possible. Excess tissue is trimmed, leaving a 10-mm stub.

W, X, Y

The conjoined tendon and adjacent fibers of the internal oblique muscle are sutured to Poupart's ligament with simple interrupted stitches of 0 Neurolon and tied once all are in place. Several additional stitches can be placed cephalad to the internal ring if they seem to be necessary.

V

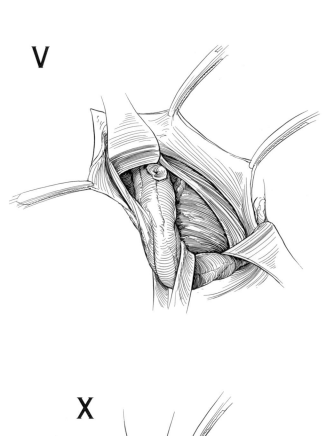

W

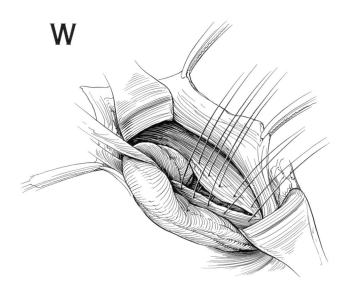

X

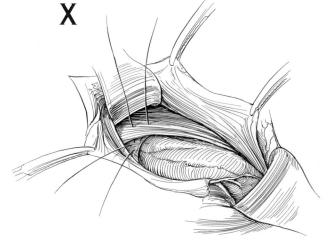

Y

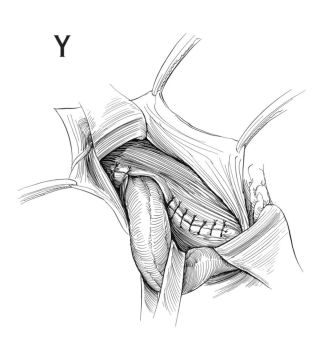

Z

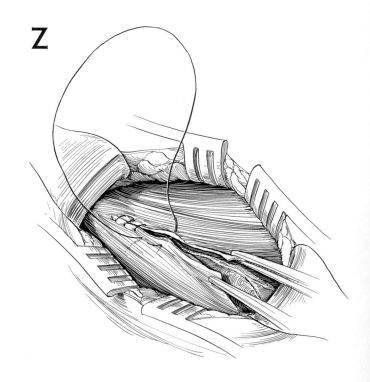

Z

The external oblique muscle is closed with a continuous stitch of 3-0 Maxon. Each bite of the needle should be observed to make certain that it does not snare the underlying ilioinguinal nerve.

AA, BB

Scarpa's fascia is reapproximated with a continuous stitch of 4-0 Maxon.

CC, DD

The skin can be closed with interrupted vertical mattress stitches of 5-0 nylon or with a fine nonabsorbable subcuticular stitch. The faint crosshatching applied at the beginning of the operation is a useful guide to an exact reapproximation.

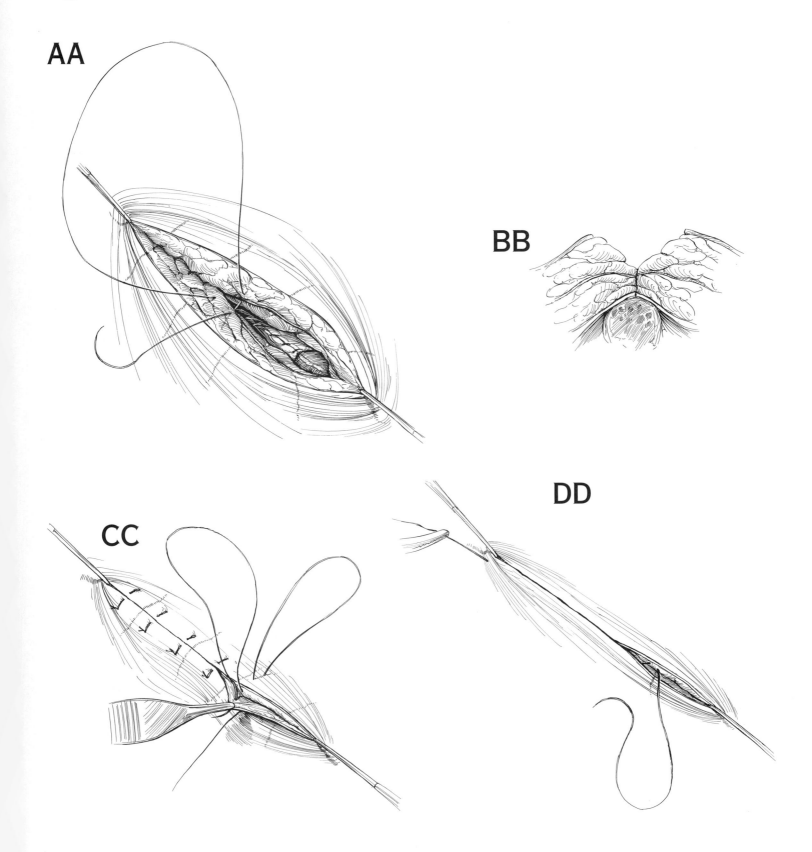

DIRECT; OPEN—NO MESH

A

The patient is placed in the supine position and anesthetized, and then the operative field is prepared and draped in a preferred manner. The incision is 2 cm above and parallel to Poupart's ligament, exposing the bulging aponeurosis of the external oblique muscle.

B

The external oblique muscle is opened proximal to the ring, the nerve is identified, and the incision is continued with the ilioinguinal nerve in view and safeguarded.

C, D

The spermatic cord is looped with a small drain that is used to manipulate the cord as it is dissected its full length. Care is taken to avoid injury to the external spermatic vessels and genital branch of the genitofemoral nerve that lie posterior to the cord. They are preserved with the cord structures.

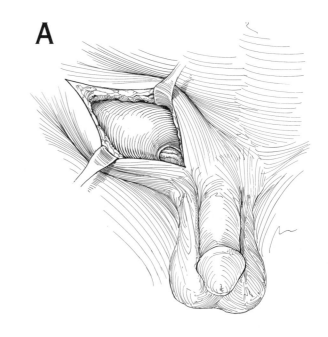

A

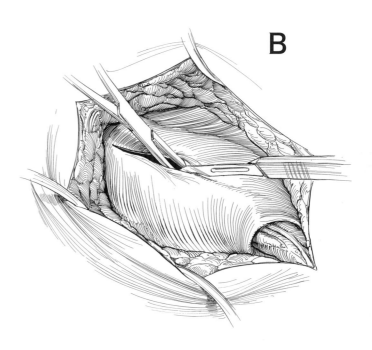

B

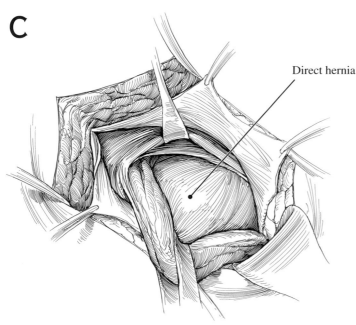

C

Direct hernia

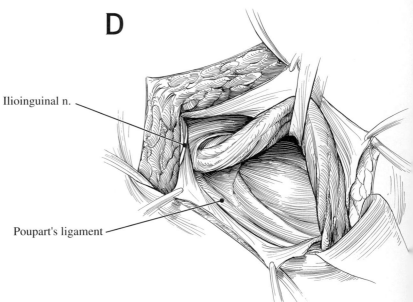

D

Ilioinguinal n.

Poupart's ligament

E, F

The posterior wall of the inguinal canal is incised completely. Cooper's ligament is dissected clean of any fatty areolar tissue. The cord can be lifted to expose the proximal reaches of Cooper's ligament.

E

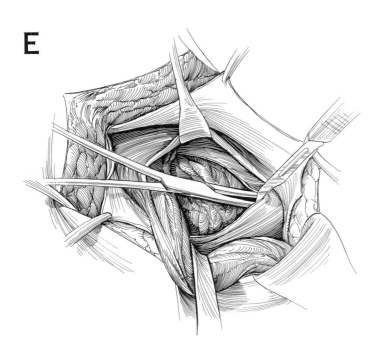

F

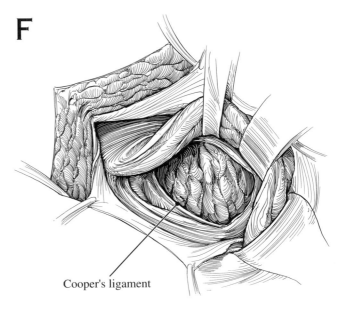

Cooper's ligament

G

The cremasteric fibers are divided circumferentially at the internal ring, further reducing extraneous bulk that may interfere with a snug repair.

H

A relaxing incision is made just at the line of fusion of the aponeurosis of the external oblique muscle and the rectus muscle sheath and carried down just short of the pubic tubercle.

G

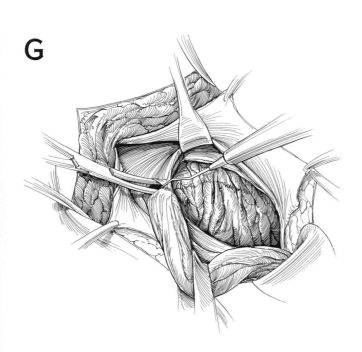

H

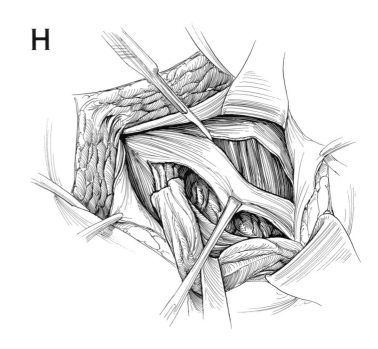

I

The repair is begun at the pubic tubercle, where interrupted simple stitches of 0 Neurolon are placed between the transversus abdominis muscle of the abdomen and Cooper's ligament.

J, K

The repair continues to the medial edge of the femoral vein.

L

The sutures are tied after all are in position. The internal ring should admit the tip a 6-inch hemostat.

The cord is repositioned, and the external oblique muscle is closed with a continuous stitch of 3-0 chromic catgut; the skin is closed with 4-0 nylon.

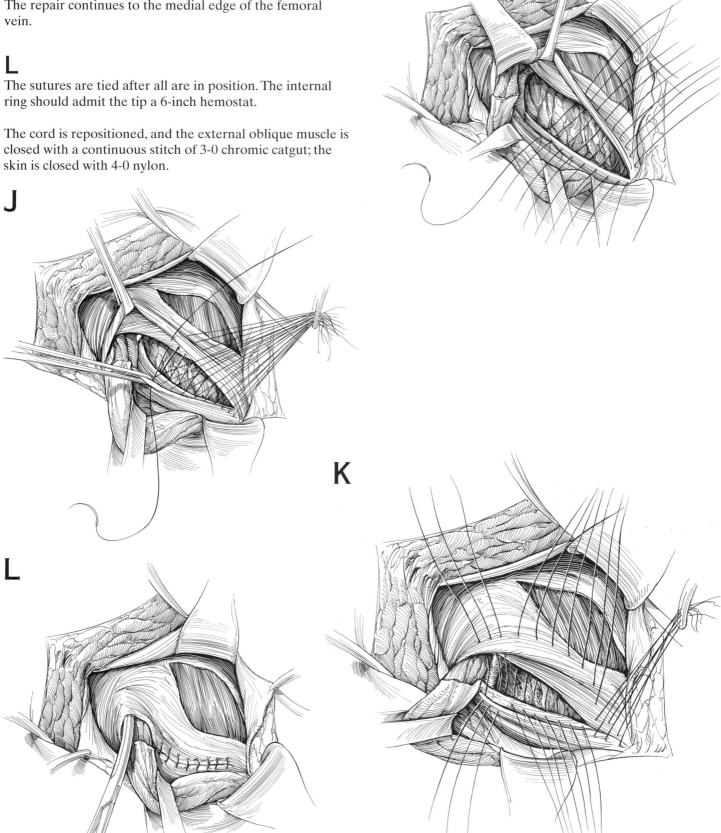

I

J

K

L

DIRECT; OPEN—MESH

In this type of repair, Marlex mesh or Gore-Tex is used to cover the entire inguinal floor rather than to bring the tissue together, thus making it a tension-free repair.

A

The exposure is as for a traditional repair, and the dissection proceeds to the inguinal floor. An oval patch of mesh is anchored to the iliopubic track with a continuous stitch of 2-0 Prolene, beginning just above the pubic tubercle and continued proximally along this route.

B

When the internal ring is reached and the surgeon can see how the mesh will lie in this area, a circular piece of mesh is cut out to accommodate the cord.

C

The mesh is maneuvered around the cord, and suturing of the mesh is continued peripherally.

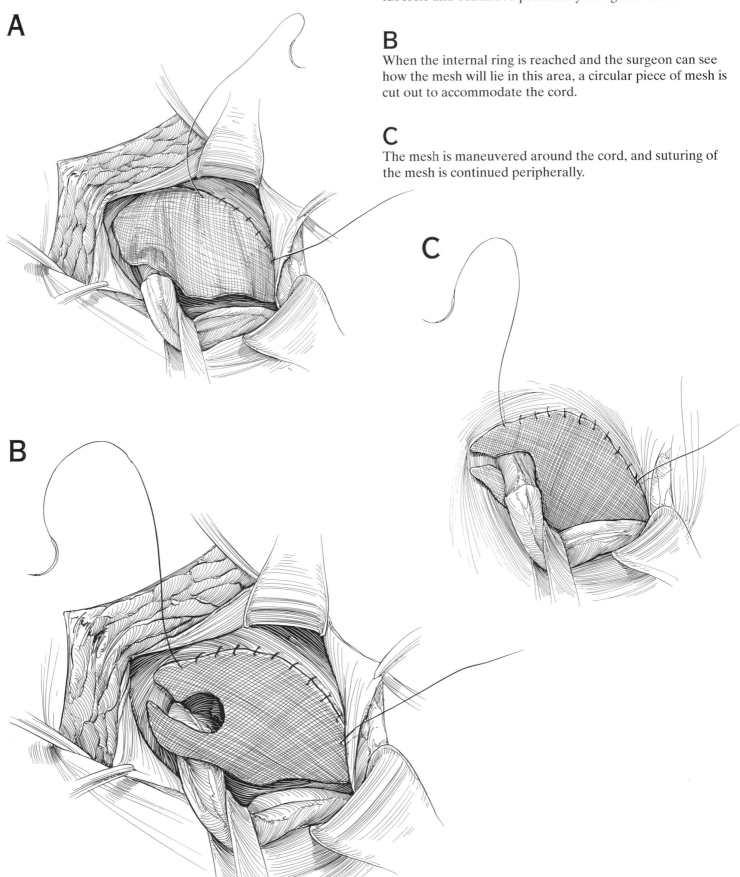

D

With the cord in position, the slit in the mesh is reapproximated with interrupted simple stitches of 2-0 Prolene.

E

The circumferential stitching of the patch is completed as the Prolene suture is tied to the end left free at the beginning of stitching.

F

The external oblique muscle is closed with a continuous stitch of 3-0 Maxon, and the remainder of the wound is closed in the customary manner.

D

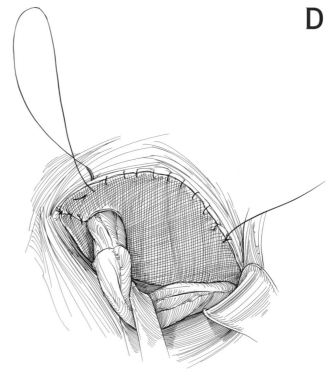

E

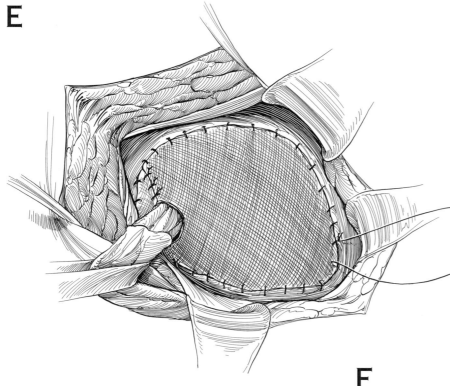

F

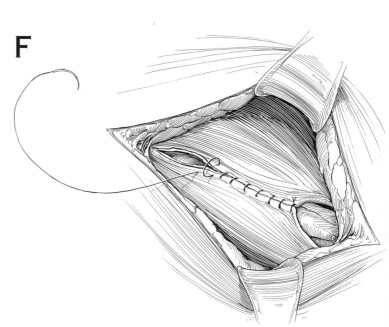

LAPAROSCOPIC

A

The pelvic anatomic features pertinent to this operation are depicted with the peritoneum removed for easier identification of anatomic landmarks. A number of structures shown are essential to the stability of the herniorrhaphy, or must not be injured while performing the dissection, or must be avoided when placing the staples. They include the following: Cooper's ligament, transversus abdominis aponeurosis, iliopubic tract, epigastric vessels, external femoral artery and vein, vas deferens, cord vessels, and lateral femoral cutaneous nerve.

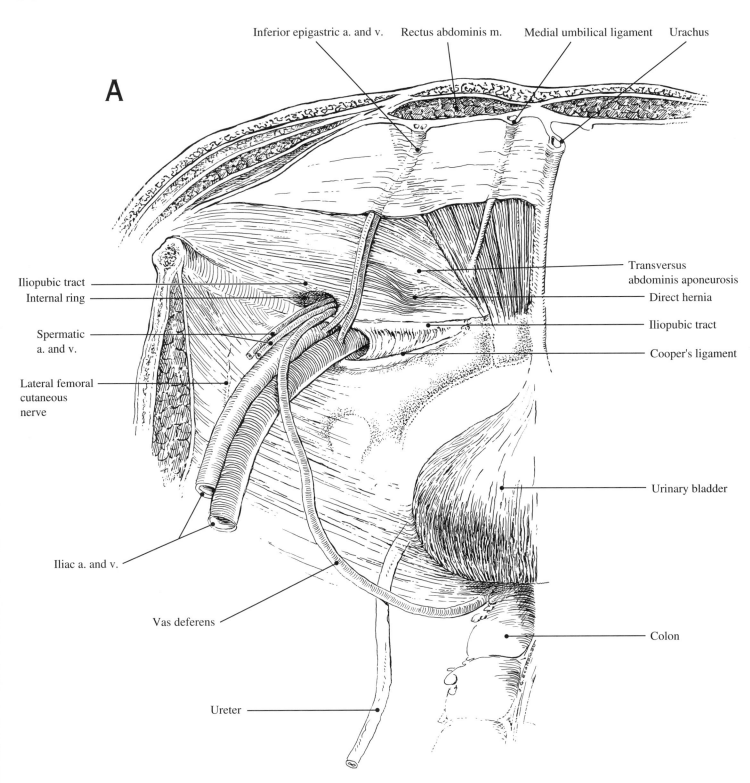

Inferior epigastric a. and v.   Rectus abdominis m.   Medial umbilical ligament   Urachus

A

Transversus abdominis aponeurosis

Direct hernia

Iliopubic tract

Cooper's ligament

Iliopubic tract

Internal ring

Spermatic a. and v.

Lateral femoral cutaneous nerve

Iliac a. and v.

Urinary bladder

Vas deferens

Colon

Ureter

B

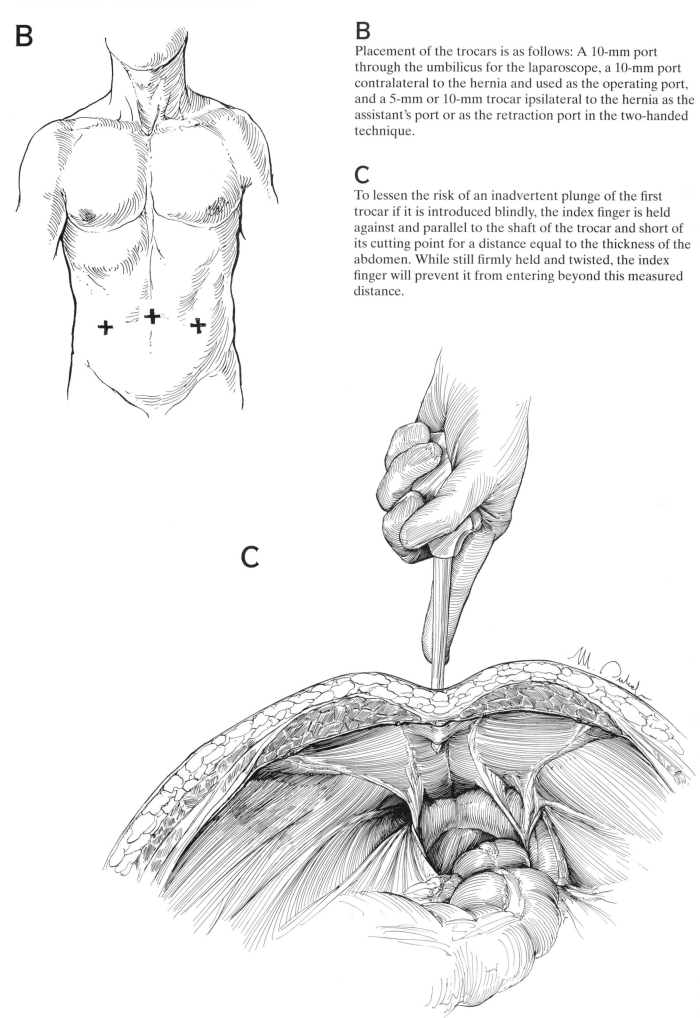

B

Placement of the trocars is as follows: A 10-mm port through the umbilicus for the laparoscope, a 10-mm port contralateral to the hernia and used as the operating port, and a 5-mm or 10-mm trocar ipsilateral to the hernia as the assistant's port or as the retraction port in the two-handed technique.

C

To lessen the risk of an inadvertent plunge of the first trocar if it is introduced blindly, the index finger is held against and parallel to the shaft of the trocar and short of its cutting point for a distance equal to the thickness of the abdomen. While still firmly held and twisted, the index finger will prevent it from entering beyond this measured distance.

C

D

This is the appearance of the field with the peritoneum intact as first viewed by the surgeon. The somewhat opaque anatomic outline of the anatomy demonstrates convincingly the need to be spatially well acquainted with the structures in this area.

D

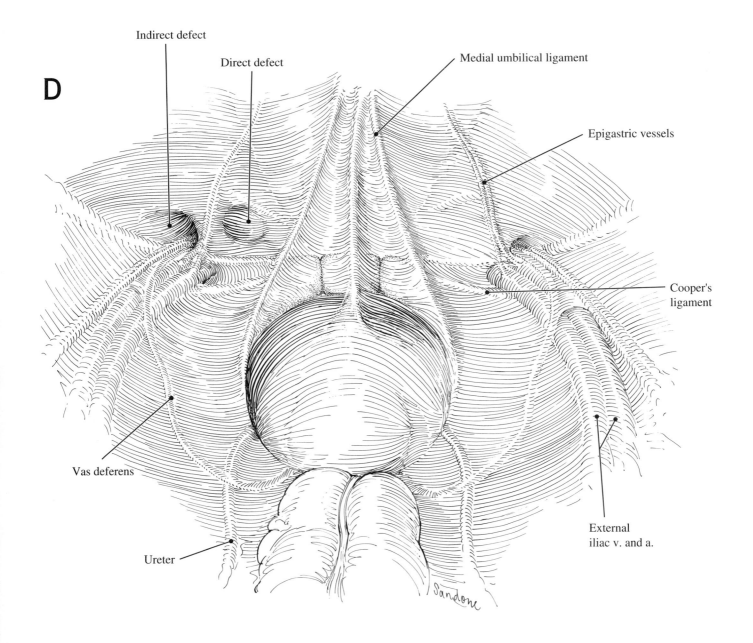

Indirect defect

Direct defect

Medial umbilical ligament

Epigastric vessels

Cooper's ligament

Vas deferens

External iliac v. and a.

Ureter

Sandone

E, F

For a sizable *indirect* hernia, the peritoneum at the neck of the sac is opened transversely and the hernia sac dissected away from the cord structures. The transverse peritoneal flap is then developed medially along the dashed line to expose Hesselbach's triangle. In contrast, for a *direct* hernia the transverse peritoneal incision is made 3 to 4 cm above the hernia, and the posterior flap is developed dorsally, exposing the defect without excising the sac.

E

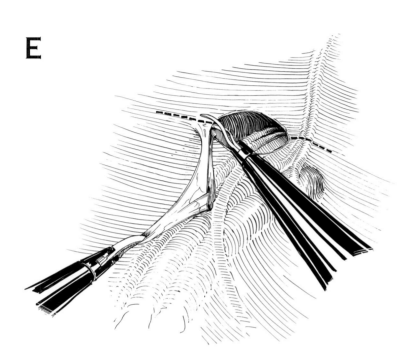

F

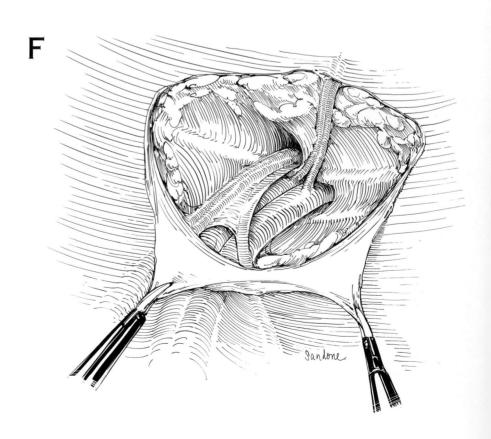

G

The cord vessels approaching laterally and the vas deferens medially form a triangle called the "triangle of doom;" one should not dissect or place staples in this area because of risk of injury to the structures within.

This diagram shows the pertinent anatomic structures and the customary number and location of staples.

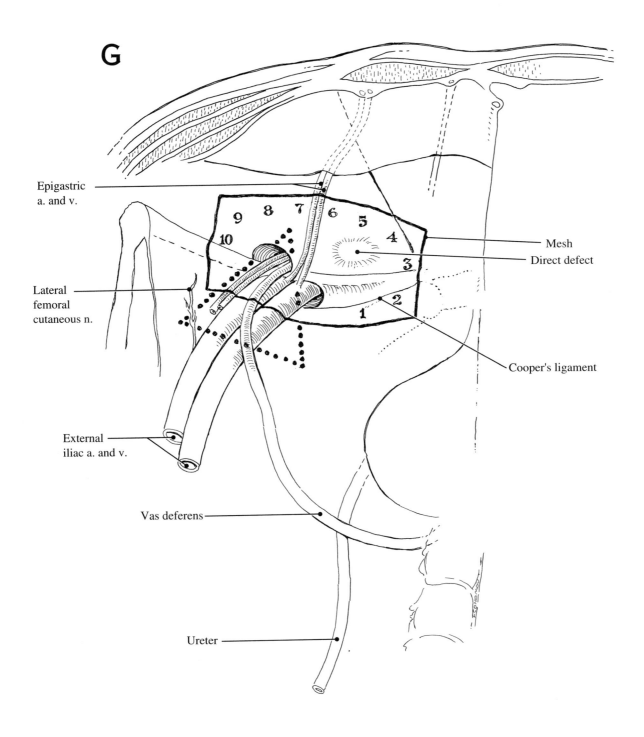

G

Epigastric a. and v.

9 8 7 6 5

10 4

Mesh
Direct defect

3

Lateral femoral cutaneous n.

2

1

Cooper's ligament

External iliac a. and v.

Vas deferens

Ureter

H

A sheet of Marlex mesh is placed under the developed peritoneal flaps and over the hernia defect. It is important that the mesh overlap the hernial defect by at least 2 cm before stapling is begun. The mesh usually is not slit but simply positioned over the cord structures.

H

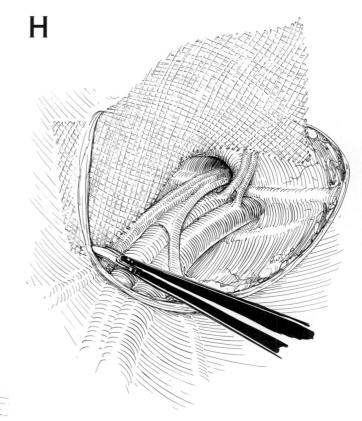

I

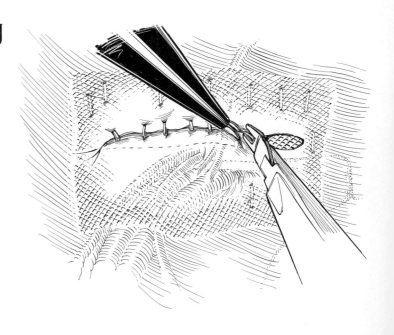

I

The staples are placed in Cooper's ligament, the transversus abdominis aponeurosis, and the abdominal wall musculature lateral to the epigastric vessels and above the iliopubic tract. Ten or so staples are usually required. No staples are placed within the previously described "triangle of doom."

J

J

The peritoneal flaps over the mesh are reapproximated with staples, clips, or sutures, thus preventing contact between the mesh and the intestines and the formation of potentially troublesome adhesions between the two.

The peritoneum should be overlapped 1 cm or more before applying the staples. This almost eliminates the gaping seen between staples if the peritoneum is reapproximated edge to edge.

B HERNIORRHAPHY—FEMORAL

A femoral hernia becomes incarcerated or strangulated with sufficient frequency that it should always be repaired unless there is a medical contraindication to an operation. Several methods of repair are possible, depending on clinical circumstances and the surgeon's preference. The operation is performed using general anesthesia, local anesthesia with sedation, or regional anesthesia. The preparation and draping include the abdomen, groin, and upper thigh. The incision is made 2 cm above the inguinal crease.

A, B

These plates illustrate some parts of the anatomy pertinent to this operation with which the surgeon should be thoroughly familiar.

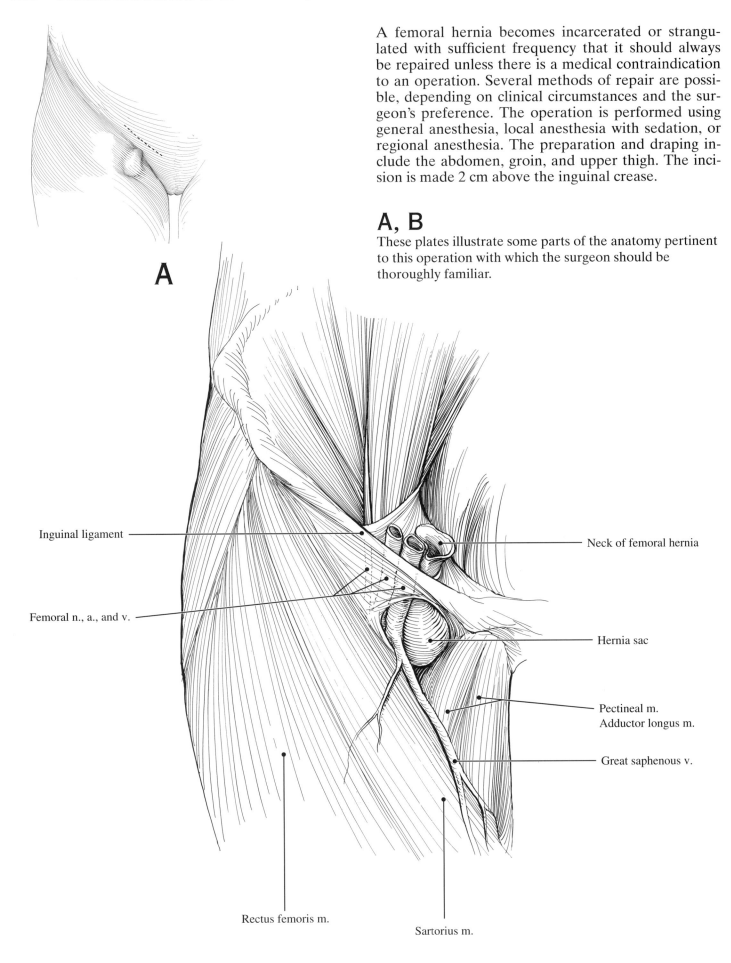

A

Inguinal ligament

Neck of femoral hernia

Femoral n., a., and v.

Hernia sac

Pectineal m.
Adductor longus m.

Great saphenous v.

Rectus femoris m.

Sartorius m.

B

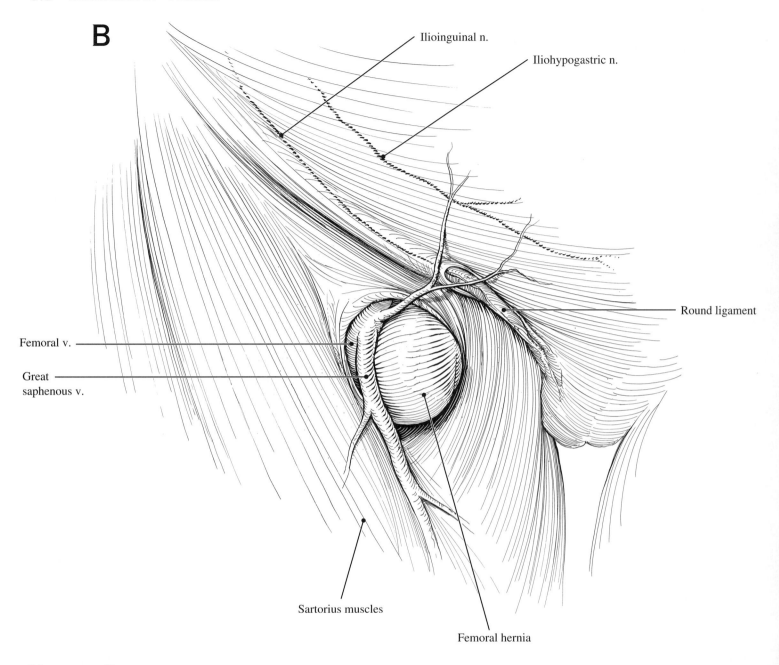

Ilioinguinal n.

Iliohypogastric n.

Round ligament

Femoral v.

Great
saphenous v.

Sartorius muscles

Femoral hernia

METHOD ONE

C

The neck of the hernia is suprainguinal, which is the reason
the incision should be made above the inguinal crease, very
much as in an inguinal herniorrhaphy. The inguinal incision
is developed by carrying it through the inguinal floor to the
transversalis fascia, under which the hernia is located.

C

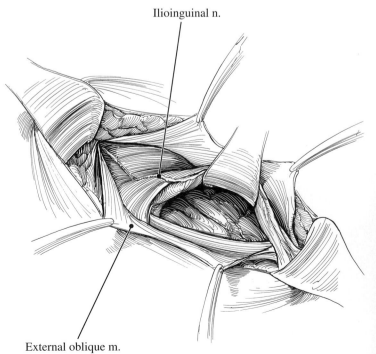

Ilioinguinal n.

External oblique m.

D, E

Pressure on the infrainguinal area produces a bulge, which is the hernia. The bulge is grasped with a forceps, delivered fully into the wound, and dissected with a fine Metzenbaum scissors down to its neck.

F, G, H, I

If the neck is broad, it is best to cut and sew the sac while closing it with a continuous running stitch of 2-0 silk. The femoral canal is closed as in a Cooper's repair.

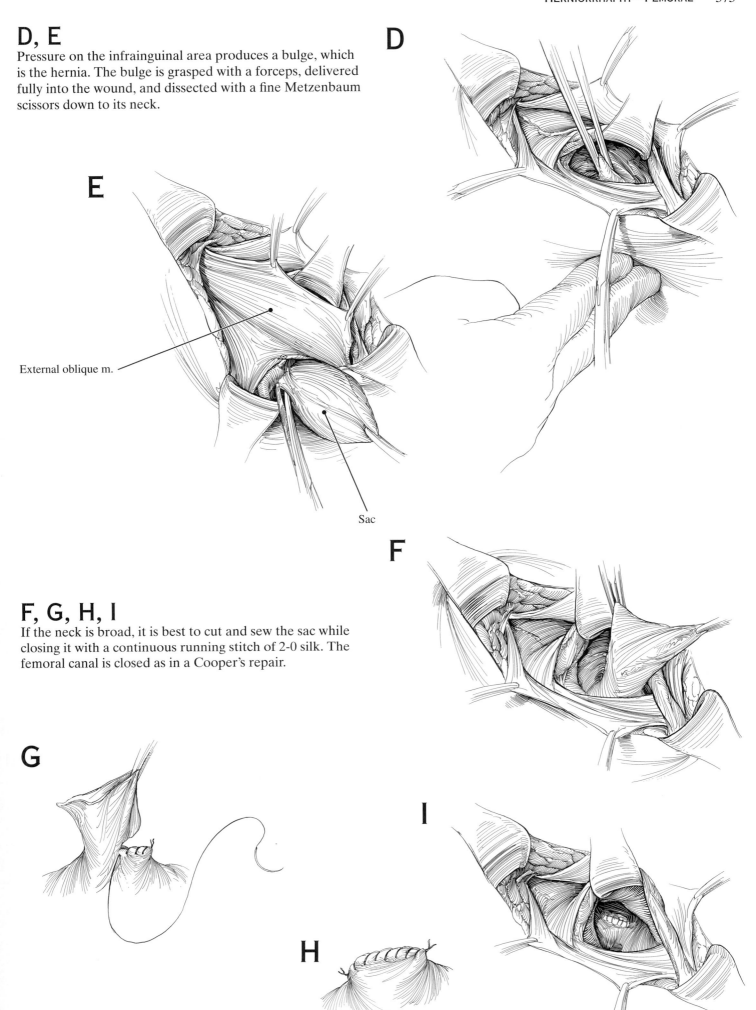

D

E

External oblique m.

Sac

F

G

I

H

J, K

For a hernia with a narrow neck, a transfixion ligature buttressed by a more superficial simple ligature is adequate.

J

K

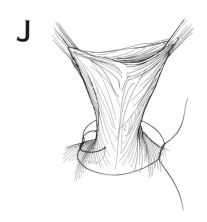

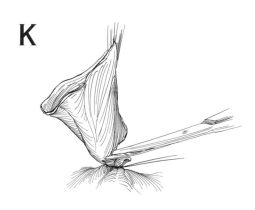

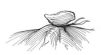

METHOD TWO

L, M

The hernia appears incarcerated, so it is exposed both above and below Poupart's ligament. It needs to be delivered above the inguinal ligament. Once the suprainguinal component is opened, Poupart's ligament is lifted and firmly pulled cephalad. Now the sac can be opened and the intestine assessed as to its viability before replacing it into the abdominal cavity.

L

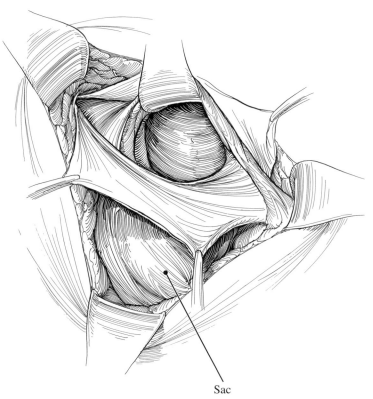

Sac

M

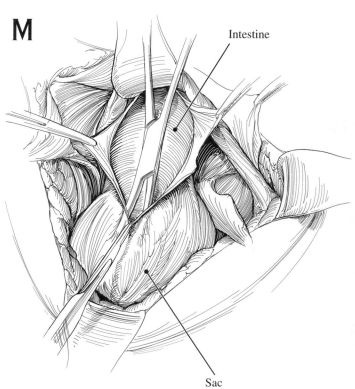

Intestine

Sac

N

The sac is dissected and closed as necessary. The herniorrhaphy is completed in a preferred manner.

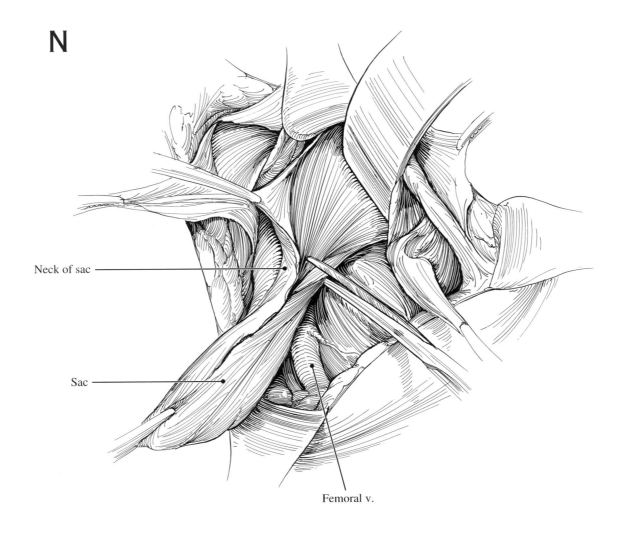

N

Neck of sac

Sac

Femoral v.

METHOD THREE

O, P

As in the previous case, the intestine is incarcerated but now is also seen to be nonviable. The task here is to excise this bowel without spillage or otherwise grossly contaminating the operative field.

A GIA stapler is placed across both limbs to incorporate this segment of bowel and fired.

Q

The nonviable bowel is still in the sac but has now been isolated.

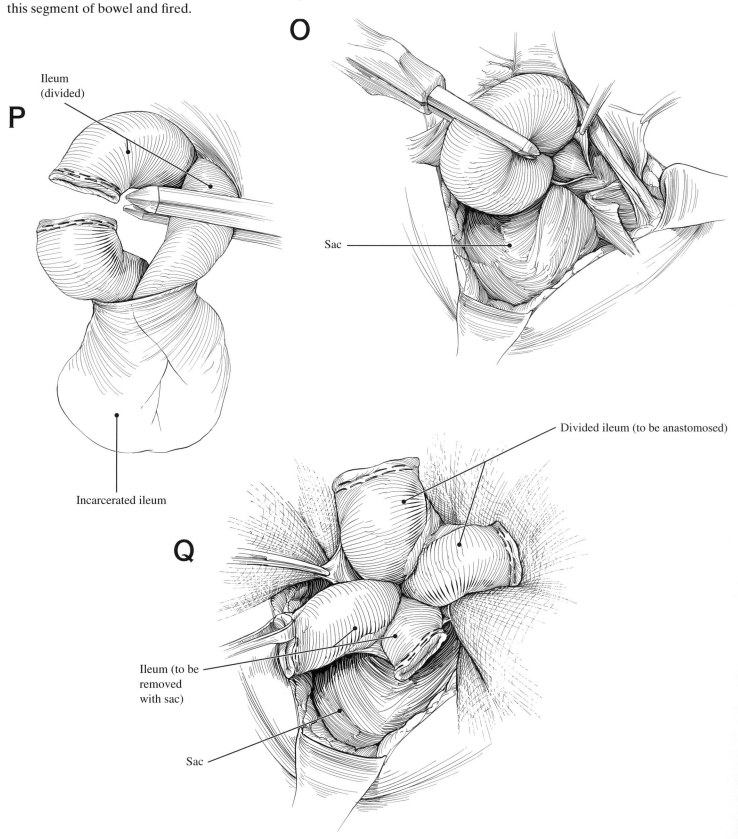

O

Sac

P

Ileum (divided)

Incarcerated ileum

Q

Divided ileum (to be anastomosed)

Ileum (to be removed with sac)

Sac

R

The sac is pulled downward to expose its posterior aspect, which is cut, thus fashioning the posterior rim of the hernial opening.

R

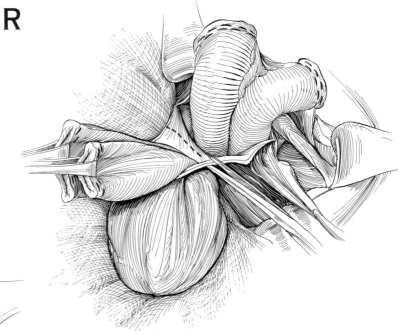

S

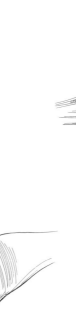
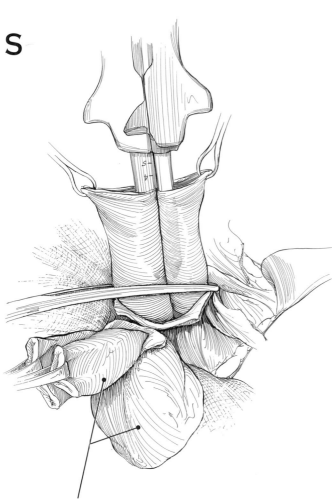

Ileum in sac

S

The stapled tissue is removed from both limbs of the intestine, and the limbs are held up as a side-to-side anastomosis is performed.

T, U

Both limbs are united with a TA-55 stapler, and the reunited intestine is replaced into the abdominal cavity. The nonviable segment of intestine and the sac are dissected free and discarded. The remainder of the operation is as in a Cooper's repair.

T

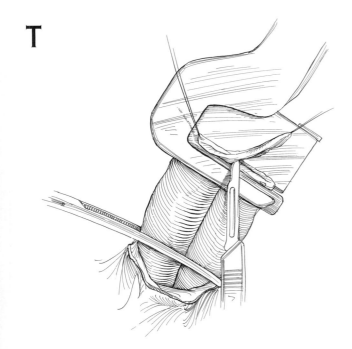

U

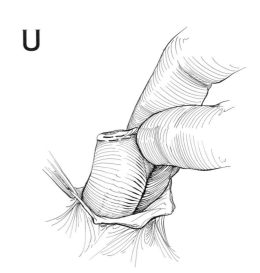

METHOD FOUR

V

The occasional patient has a sizable, reducible hernia with a small neck, yet also has associated medical problems that preclude any but the simplest operation. This operation can be done under sedation and local anesthesia.

W, X

The hernia is located and dissected clean in the usual manner. The sac is opened, and the intestine is replaced into the peritoneal cavity, the neck ligated, and the excess tissue discarded.

Y, Z, AA

A piece of Marlex mesh 1 inch wide is tightly rolled to form a plug the size of the femoral canal. It is squeezed into the femoral canal and held in place with a few stitches of 2-0 Prolene. The wound is closed in the customary manner.

V

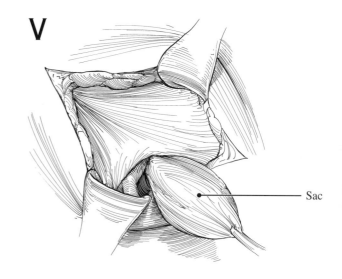

Sac

X

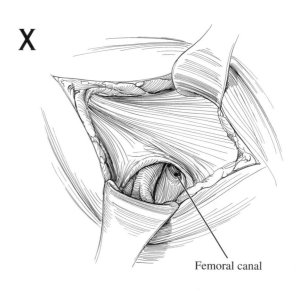

Femoral canal

W

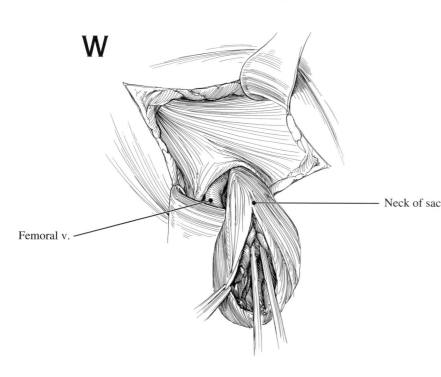

Neck of sac

Femoral v.

Z

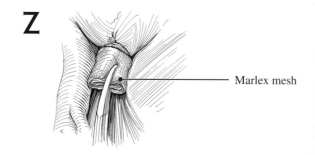

Marlex mesh

Y

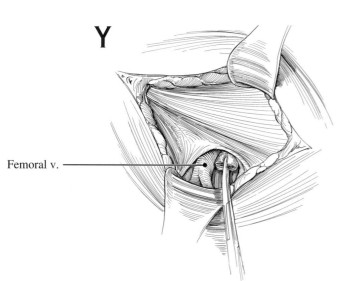

Femoral v.

AA

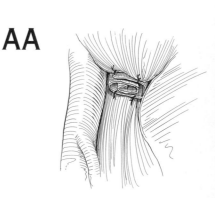

C HERNIORRHAPHY—UMBILICAL

Umbilical hernia occurs at all ages but poses a greater risk of strangulation in adults. Thus, it necessitates repair when diagnosed, other conditions permitting.

A

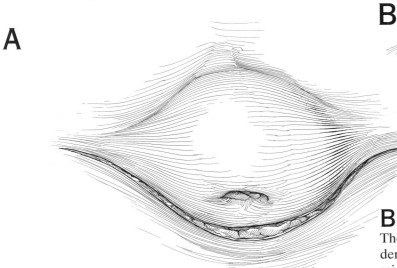

B

B, C

The incision is extended down to the hernia sac. As is demonstrated in this sagittal view (*C*), the dissection is with scissors and directly on the sac.

C

A

Except for patients with very large hernias in whom overlying skin will have to be sacrificed, an attempt should be made to retain the umbilicus. An infraumbilical transverse incision whose length should be several centimeters lateral to the medial borders of the rectus muscles is preferred. Such a breadth of excision is valuable later when the fascial flaps are developed.

D

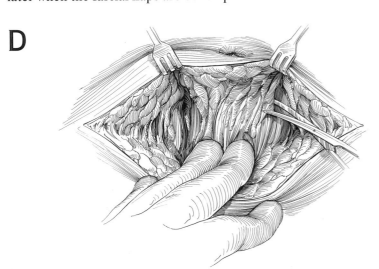

D

The process is facilitated by using small rakes to retract the flaps upward as the surgeon provides countertraction during the resection.

E

The fascia is exposed as broadly as shown to facilitate the repair.

F

F

The sac is lifted and opened with care, keeping in mind that omentum—even intestine—may be incarcerated within it. Any such adhesions that may be present are carefully lysed down to the neck of the sac.

G

G

The rectus fascia is incised several centimeters lateral to the medial border of the rectus muscles.

H

The surgeon opens the sac to its base, still inspecting its inside in the event omentum or intestine is present at the point the sac will be amputated.

H

I

I

With the neck free of any attachments, a stitch of 2-0 Maxon is started at one of the lateral extremes. In a cut-and-sew manner, the sac is amputated and oversewn.

J

The rectus fascia should be closed by imbricating the top flap over the lower one by the time-honored "pants-over-vest" technique. Here the fascia is being dissected off the rectus muscle in preparation for the lower flap to be brought as high as possible under the upper flap. An attempt can be made to lessen the diastasis of the rectus muscles by reapproximating them. However, because the diastasis extends a considerable distance cephalad and caudad, the opportunity for a meaningful reapproximation is limited.

K, L

Stitches of 2-0 Prolene are passed through the margins of the lower flap and brought out as high as possible on the upper flap. With traction applied to the upper flap, the stitches are serially brought down snugly and tied.

M, N, O

The free edges of the upper flap are sutured to the lower flap (M). Several stitches of fine catgut are used to tack the undersurface of the umbilical skin to the adjacent fascia (N). The subcutaneous closure is done with interrupted 2-0 Maxon and the skin with interrupted vertical mattress stitches of 4-0 nylon (O).

J

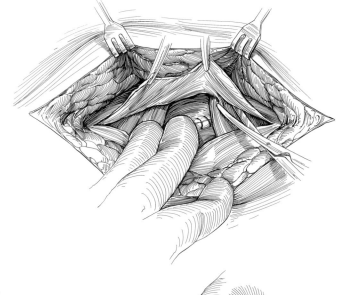

L

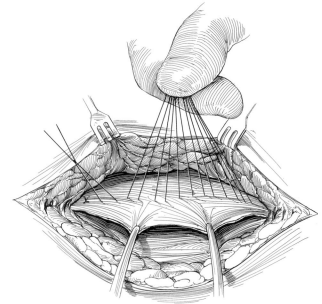

K

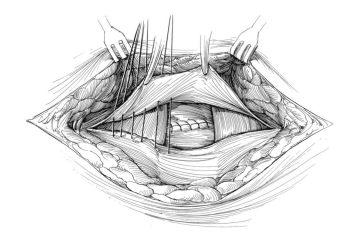

N

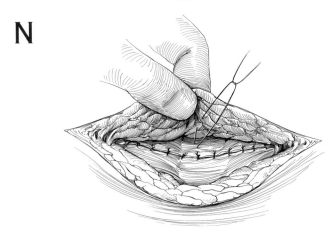

M

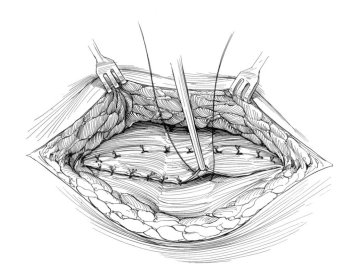

O

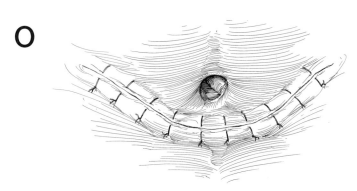

D HERNIORRHAPHY—VENTRAL

NO MESH

A, B

Ventral herniation most commonly is a postoperative
sequela. Despite outward appearances, the surgeon must
be prepared for the unexpected in the way of size of the
herniation, associated smaller defects, or more than the
expected weakness of the tissues surrounding the frank
herniation. All these should be factors in deciding whether
mesh should be used in the repair.

The peritoneum and intestine lie directly under the skin
that often is devoid of fat. This is important to remember
when making the incision.

A

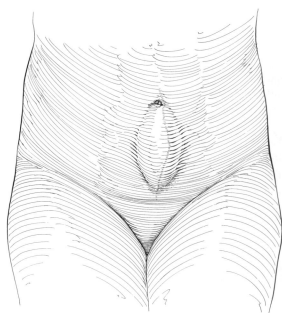

B

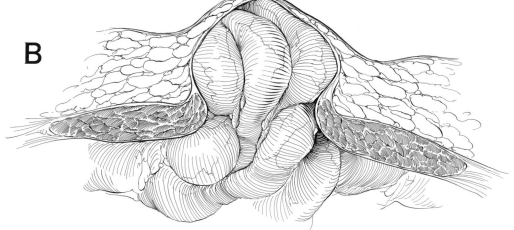

C

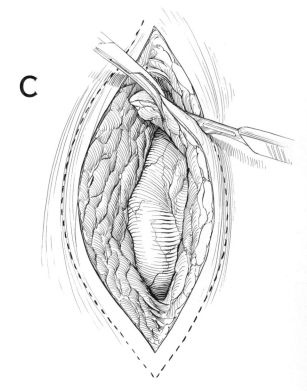

C

The scar is excised. Doing so makes thicker skin available
during closure. It also makes it natural not to have to enter
the peritoneum at the most prominent aspect of the hernia.

D

On opening the peritoneal cavity, the findings may range from glistening clean intestine with the only abnormality being the hernia to numerous adhesions that dominate the operative field. The extent to which adhesions other than those to the hernia are addressed in the course of proceeding with the repair is a surgical judgment.

The illustrated technique is one that can be used while dissecting the fascia peripherally to a point at which it is thick enough to be incorporated into the repair. The fascial edges are grasped securely with Kocher toothed forceps and placed under uniform tension while several fingers of the surgeon's left hand (not shown here) are positioned intraperitoneally opposite the scissors and serve as a palpatory guide while the cutting proceeds along the fascial plane. Such an interplay of scissors, traction, and palpating fingers facilitates a brisk dissection with little risk of damaging the fascia as well as the advantage of being able to determine when adequately strong fascial tissue has been reached.

D

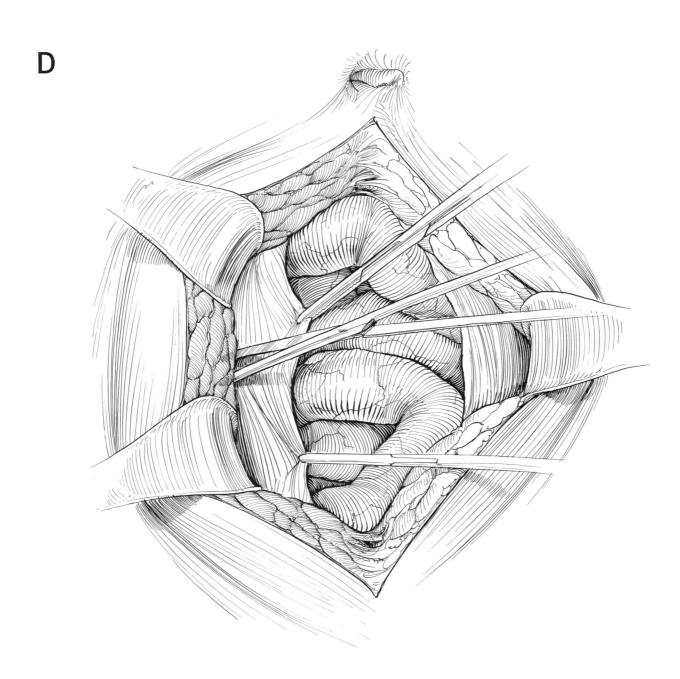

E

E

With the fascial flaps developed, interrupted 2-0 silk is used to anchor one leaf as far as possible under the opposite leaf.

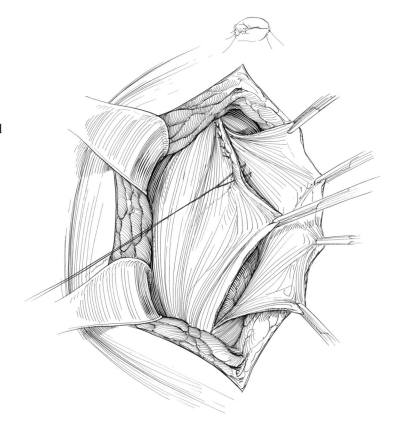

F, G

With the above step completed, the loose flap is next laid flat and anchored to the opposite flap with interrupted stitches of 3-0 silk. These must be placed in a shallow manner with great care that there is no injury to any underlying intestine.

G

F

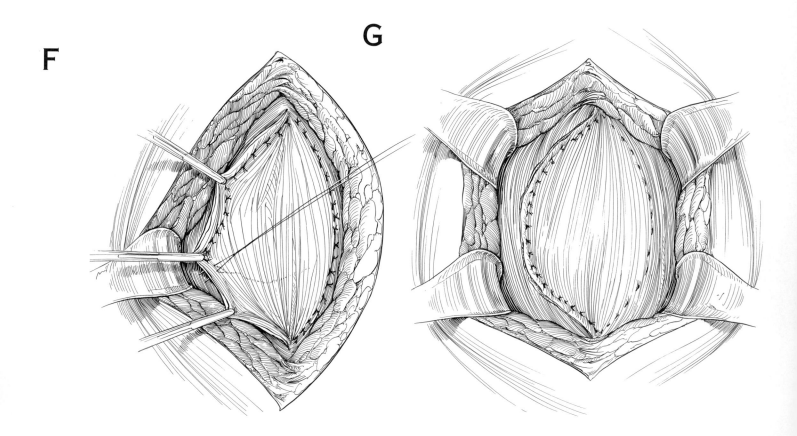

H

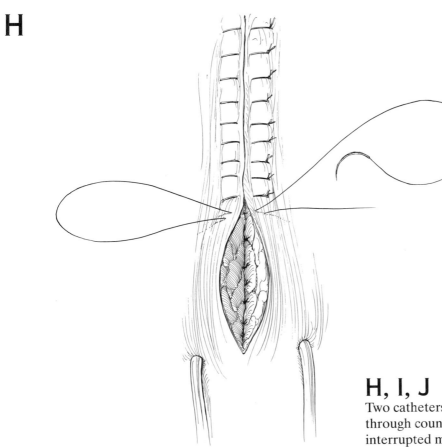

H, I, J

Two catheters are placed over the repair and exteriorized through counterincisions. The wound can be closed with interrupted monofilament stitches, a continuous subcutaneous stitch, or skin clips. The catheters are placed on suction.

I

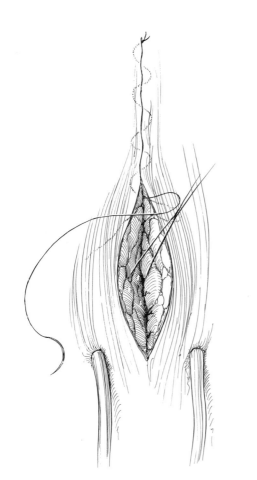

J

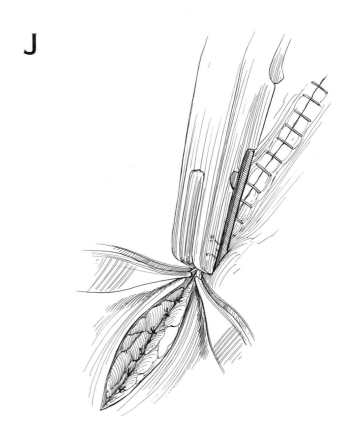

MESH

A

There are several reasons for using mesh in the repair of ventral hernia: (1) The area of weakened tissue is too broad to make reapproximation possible and reliable; (2) the tissue can be dissected sufficiently to undergo reapproximation, but the increased duration of the operation and the commonly occurring prolonged postoperative discomfort make this choice undesirable; and (3) the surgeon may want to stay out of the peritoneal cavity, for a number of reasons. It is wise for the surgeon to decide whether mesh will be used before beginning the operation. What is to be avoided is dissecting for several hours before deciding that mesh is needed after all.

B

The dissection is carried laterally and cephalocaudad to strong fascia. The extent of the dissection is determined by the findings at operation. A desirable feature of this approach is that there need not be any inhibition about the breadth of the necessary dissection. The relaxed tissue does not need to be excised. This and strong fascia that is peripheral to it will be covered with mesh. A sheet of mesh that is trimmed so that one side has a curvilinear shape is placed over the area to be repaired. Stout, monofilament suture material is used as a continuous stitch to anchor the mesh to the underlying fascia.

A

B

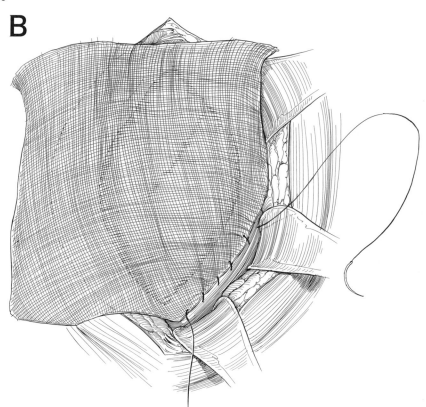

C

When one side is stitched in place, the assistant applies traction to the mesh as the surgeon serially trims and sews the remainder of it in place.

D

The use of a continuous stitch using monofilament suture facilitates equilibration of tension along the entire suture line. Despite the seemingly ample porosity of the mesh, serum coagulates on its surface, impeding escape of fluid directly into the peritoneal cavity. For this reason, two catheters are placed on the mesh and brought to the outside through counterincisions.

E

The subcutaneous tissue is approximated with a continuous stitch of 3-0 chromic catgut. The skin can be closed in any of several ways.

C

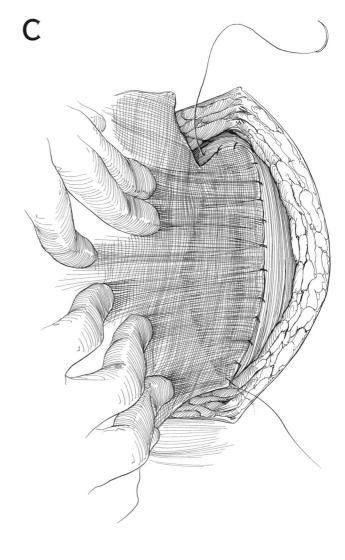

D

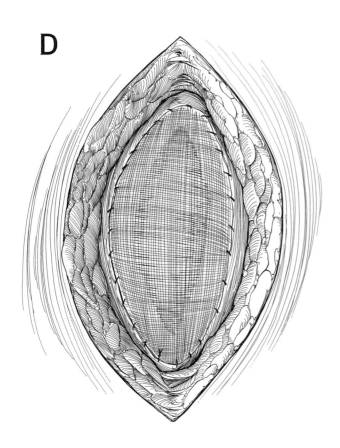

E

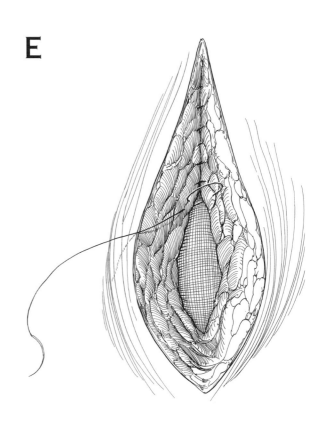

E HERNIORRHAPHY—SLIDING

A hernia is termed sliding when some portion of the retroperitoneal viscus slides downward to form part of the wall of the sac. Featured here will be a right-sided repair in which the cecum or right colon may be the sliding component.

A

The preparation and draping of the patient is as for other inguinal hernias. The incision is carried down to the transversalis fascia. The sac is identified and opened, demonstrating its characteristic appearance.

A

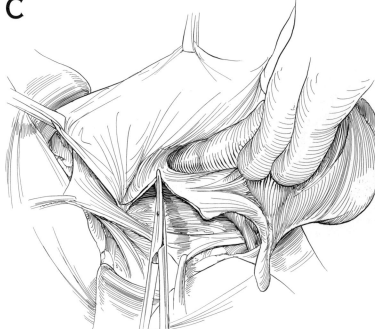

B

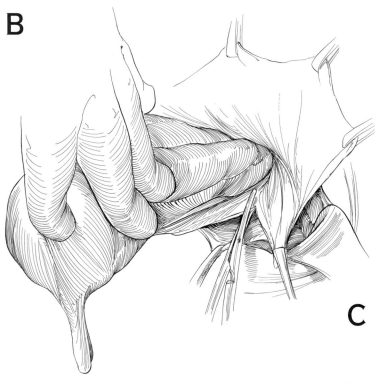

C

B, C

The sac is trimmed several centimeters or so from the colon, and bleeding points are electrocoagulated.

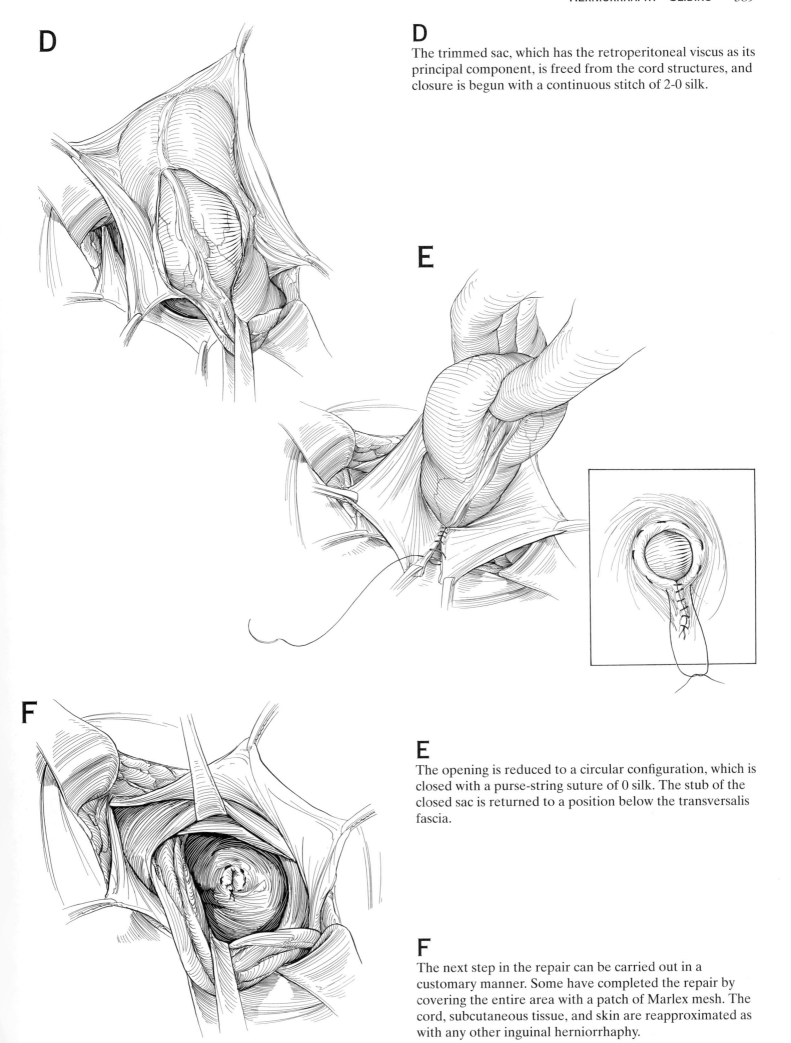

D

D

The trimmed sac, which has the retroperitoneal viscus as its principal component, is freed from the cord structures, and closure is begun with a continuous stitch of 2-0 silk.

E

E

The opening is reduced to a circular configuration, which is closed with a purse-string suture of 0 silk. The stub of the closed sac is returned to a position below the transversalis fascia.

F

F

The next step in the repair can be carried out in a customary manner. Some have completed the repair by covering the entire area with a patch of Marlex mesh. The cord, subcutaneous tissue, and skin are reapproximated as with any other inguinal herniorrhaphy.

A̅ HEPATIC RESECTION—RIGHT LOBECTOMY

A

The liver has a dual blood supply: the hepatic artery and the portal vein. The middle hepatic vein courses through segments 5 and 6 of the right lobe. Although the middle hepatic vein must be divided in the performance of a trisegmentectomy, this vein should be left intact in the course of a right lobectomy; its loss would require the extension of the resection along a plane parallel to the ligamentum teres.

A

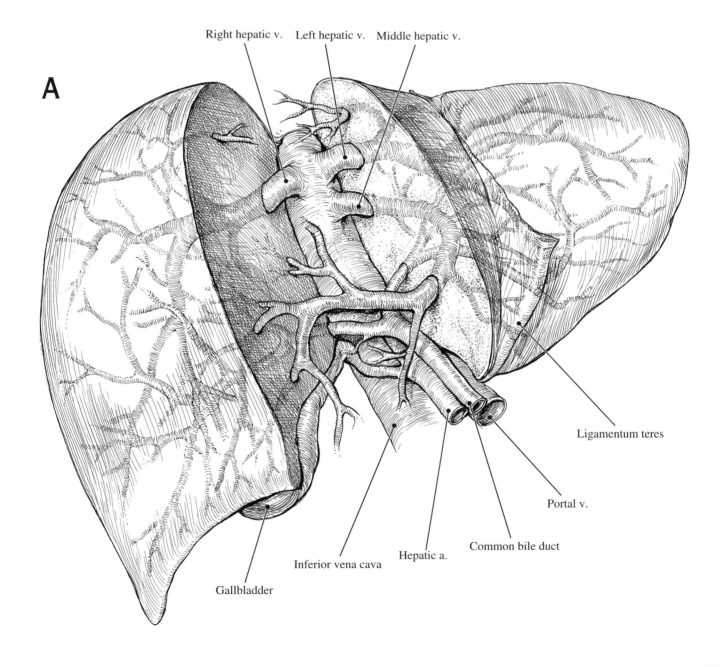

Right hepatic v.   Left hepatic v.   Middle hepatic v.

Ligamentum teres

Portal v.

Common bile duct

Hepatic a.

Inferior vena cava

Gallbladder

B

This illustration shows the retroperitoneum with the liver absent. The accessory hepatic veins empty into the vena cava in a fairly ordered, paired fashion. When retracting the liver toward the left and dissecting in this area, the right accessory (short) hepatic veins are first encountered, and their appearance is the signal that the row of left veins is nearby.

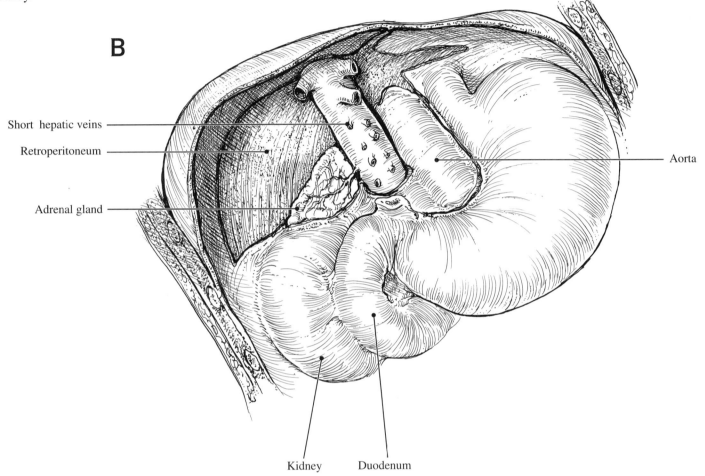

B

Short hepatic veins

Retroperitoneum

Adrenal gland

Aorta

Kidney   Duodenum

C

Segments 5 and 8 of the right lobe—the usual extent of resection for a right hepatic lobectomy—are in line with the gallbladder. In a trisegmentectomy (in which the middle and the right hepatic veins are sacrificed), the line of demarcation is slightly to the right of the course of the ligamentum teres.

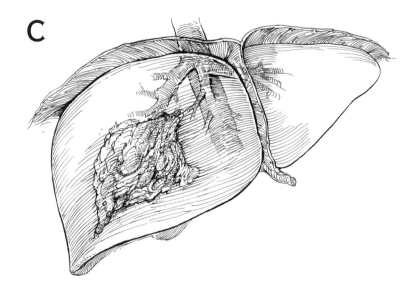

C

D

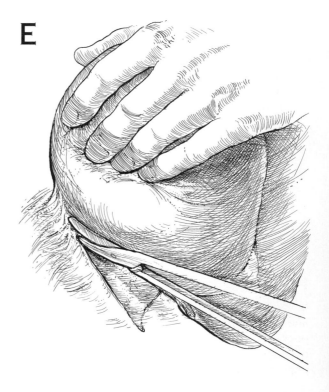

D

The patient is in the supine position with the right side elevated slightly by a rolled blanket under the right scapula and right hip. This permits the full development of the right side of a subcostal incision if it is necessary. Often there is a midline T extension of the subcostal incision to the xyphoid process. An "upper arm" retractor that is fixed to the table allows the extra lift and cephalad retraction of the incision.

On peritoneal entry, the extrahepatic sites should be examined for metastases, which, if present, foreclose the possibility of a curative lobectomy. Sometimes the diaphragm seems to be invaded by contiguous cancer when, in fact, there simply is adherence between it and the tumor; in such cases, that portion of the diaphragm is excised en bloc with the liver.

E

The right lobe is mobilized toward the left by dividing the triangular ligament with scissors on electrocautery. The retrohepatic area itself is relatively avascular. The adrenal gland is not disturbed. The right side of the vena cava and the right accessory hepatic veins are exposed.

At the upper aspect of the dissection, the right hepatic vein will come into view. It is dissected circumferentially using a Mixter hemostat. This provides ready access to it should the need arise for swiftly securing it in the course of the operation. Dividing it before interrupting the arterial and portal vessels is not advisable; such a measure leads to a congested liver with a bloodier subsequent dissection.

E

F

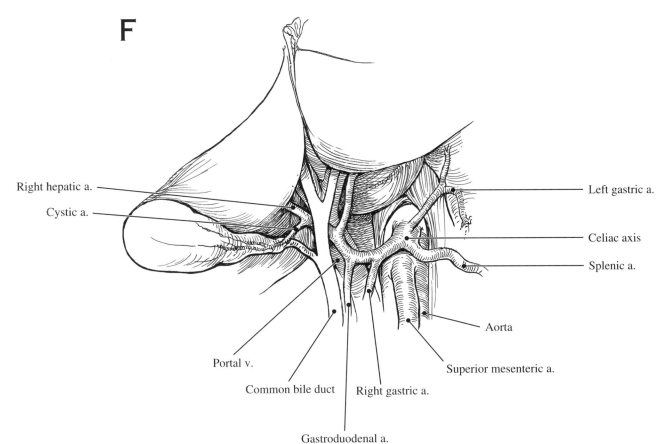

Right hepatic a.

Cystic a.

Left gastric a.

Celiac axis

Splenic a.

Aorta

Portal v.

Superior mesenteric a.

Common bile duct   Right gastric a.

Gastroduodenal a.

G

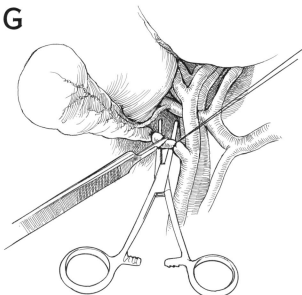

F

With no further dissection in the area of the hepatic vein, the liver is returned to its natural position so that the blood supply to the right lobe can be secured in the area of the porta hepatis. This illustration demonstrates the anatomy of the hepatic hilum that is pertinent to this operation.

G

The cystic duct and cystic artery are dissected free, ligated in continuity with 3-0 silk, and divided.

H

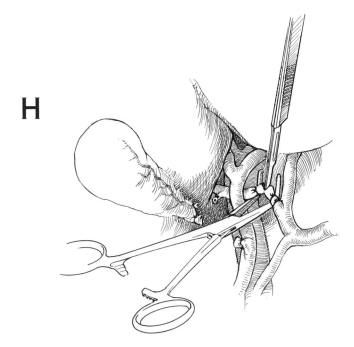

H

Division of the cystic duct and artery facilitates exposure and dissection of the right hepatic artery. Confirming its point of bifurcation from the common hepatic artery by dissecting distally to verify its entry into the liver must precede its ligation and division.

I

The previous step brings the right hepatic bile duct into better view. The surgeon should identify its origin and course, as well as that of the hepatic artery, before ligating the duct in continuity and dividing it.

I

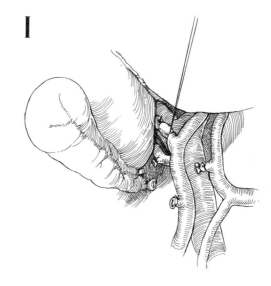

J

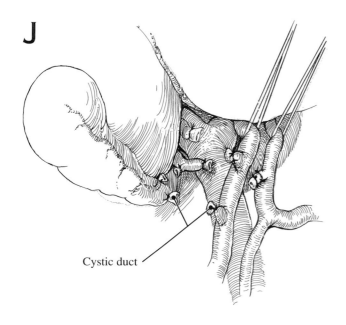

Cystic duct

J

The right hepatic artery and duct are separately encircled with vessel loops and retracted medially to expose the right and left branches of the portal vein.

Right branch of portal v.

K

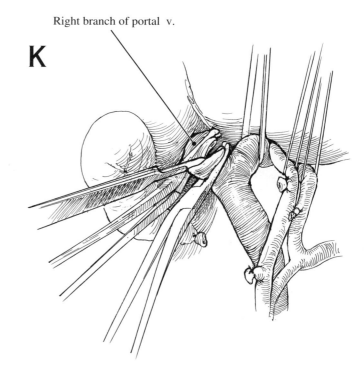

K

A Mixter hemostat is insinuated around the right branch of the portal vein so that it can be manipulated at its origin from the common portal vein and its entry into the liver can be confirmed.

L

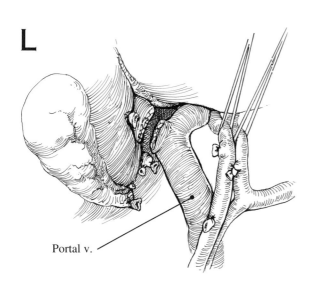

Portal v.

L

Regardless of the available length of the right portal vein, we prefer to oversew its proximal portions with a vascular suture. The distal segment can be ligated or oversewn.

M

Steps H through L effectively interrupt the blood supply to the right lobe. This becomes evident quite soon, as the right side of the liver becomes dusky to the right of a line running cephalocaudad in a plane with the gallbladder.

M

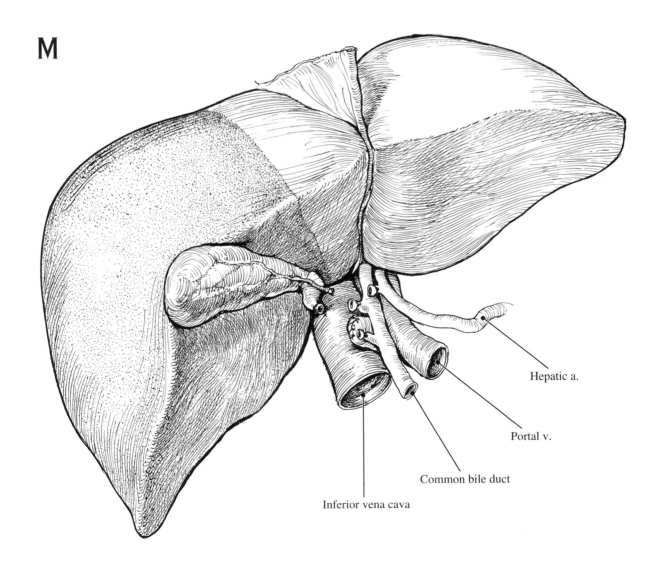

Hepatic a.

Portal v.

Common bile duct

Inferior vena cava

N, O, P, Q, R

The right lobe is returned to its normal position once again. The line of dissection is delineated by scoring the liver capsule with electrocautery. The parenchyma is divided at the leading liver edge and progressing cephalad and dorsal to the more deeply situated vessels. Division of the liver parenchyma is carried out by a variety of techniques, all of which depend on the experience of the surgeon and the area being dissected. Some of these methods are as follows: Finger fracture (N); use of a blunt instrument, such as a scalpel handle or a suction tip; electrocautery using a low current for parenchymal division and securing the vessels as they are encountered; using maximum current and charring most things in sight except the larger vessel; and ultrasonic dissection, which is slower but more precise. As illustrated here, individual vessels whose lumina are larger than 1 mm or so (O) are secured by ligation (P), suture ligation (Q), or vessel clips (R). Some surgeons use a cell saver during this part of the dissection, if the operation is for a noncancerous mass. A Pringle maneuver with a vascular clamp during the parenchymal dissection decreases blood loss. One can maintain this maneuver for 15 to 20 minutes before risk of liver ischemia occurs.

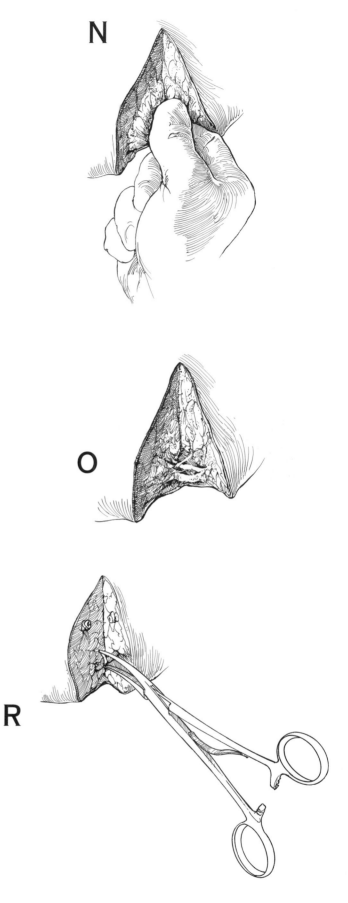

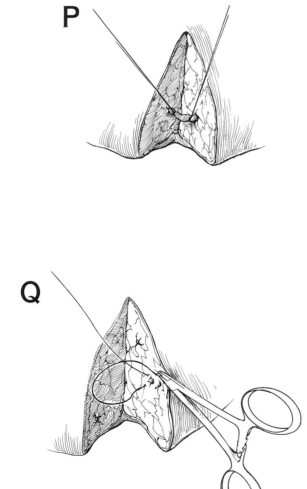

Although the various dissecting techniques can be used with equivalent success, securing the vessels as the dissection progresses is much better than proceeding pellmell with the resection and expecting to secure the vessels later. Such an approach is untidy and more risky because bleeding obscures the field and results in greater blood loss.

S

Despite ligation of the right hepatic artery and vein, there may still be collateral vessels from the left lobe. Therefore, the right hepatic vein is ligated after the parenchyma is divided; otherwise the collateral vessels would continue to fill the right lobe, causing it to become congested and bleed more during the transection. At this point, an angled vascular clamp is placed across the right hepatic vein; this vein is transected, and the specimen is removed from the field. The vein is oversewn with 3-0 monofilament suture material.

S

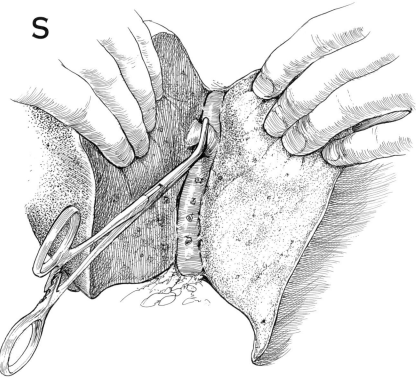

T

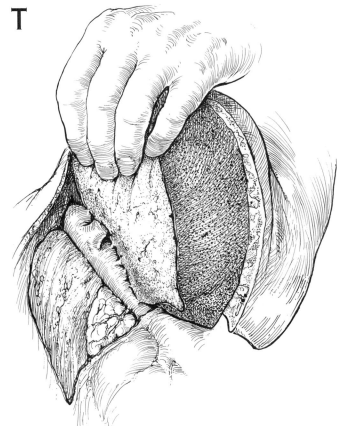

T

In the event it is difficult to gain access to the junction of the right hepatic vein and the vena cava at the depth of the hepatic division, the liver is rotated toward its left.

U

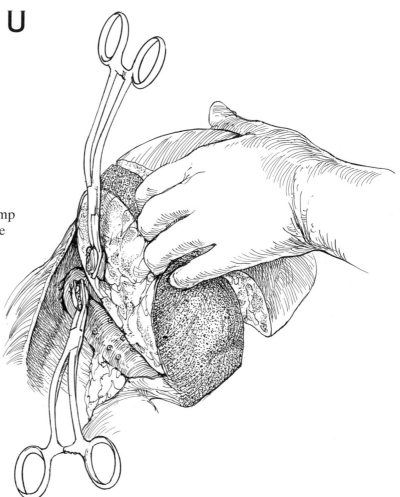

The vein is circumferentially dissected with a Mixter clamp whose long, blunt tip is more likely to glide over the edge of a vein rather than to puncture it. The vein is secured with vascular clamps and divided. The caval stump is oversewn with 3-0 monofilament vascular suture.

V

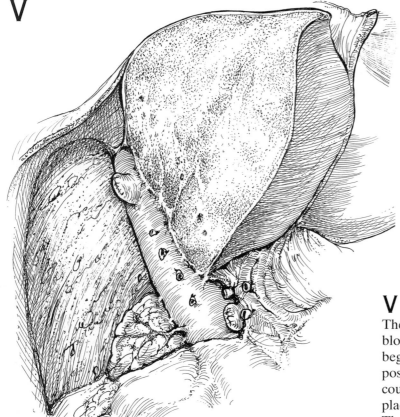

The transected liver surface should be examined for any blood or bile ooze and this condition corrected before beginning the closure. Two Jackson-Pratt drains are positioned across the dissected liver and exited through counterincisions. Available omentum is mobilized and placed over the drain and onto the transected liver surface. The abdominal incision is closed in a preferred manner.

B HEPATIC RESECTION—TRISEGMENTECTOMY

A trisegmentectomy—an extended right lobectomy—is much like a right hepatic lobectomy, but because the neoplasm extends farther toward the left, the operation includes the medial aspect of the left lobe.

The anesthetized patient is tilted slightly toward the left and is supported in this position with a rolled blanket under the right shoulder and the pelvis. A right subcostal incision is favored, and the patient is draped so that a simple T extension toward the sternum can be made if additional exposure is necessary. An upper arm adjustable retractor that is fixed to the operating table is used to retract the central portion of the wound cephalad for even further exposure. At exploration, a search should be made for extrahepatic involvement, which, if present, makes it inappropriate to proceed with liver resection.

A

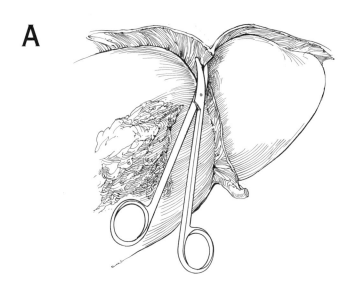

A, B

The liver is mobilized by dividing the ligamentum teres and looking for retrohepatic involvement. The use of intraoperative ultrasound has been of great value in detecting deep lesions that otherwise are nonpalpable and often not detectable preoperatively by other means.

B

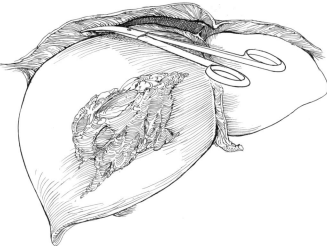

C

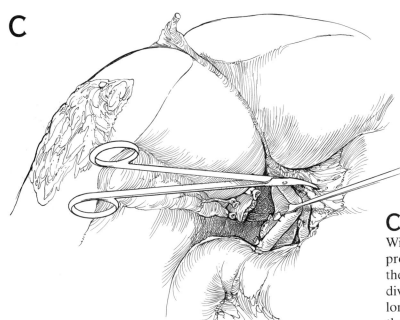

C

With the liver in its natural position, the hilar dissection proceeds as with a right lobectomy except that the artery to the medial segment of the left lobe is sought, ligated, and divided. With the blood supply interrupted, the longitudinal demarcation line will be seen in a plane with the ligamentum teres.

D

D, E

The division is begun on the demarcation line in a caudocephalad direction and from ventral to dorsal. This can be done with either electrocautery or ultrasonic dissector. Small blood vessels and bile ducts can be further secured with clip or stitch ties.

E

F

Right
hepatic v.
Middle
hepatic v.
Left
hepatic v.

F

Near the apex of the dissection, the right, middle, and left hepatic veins are encountered. The right hepatic vein drains directly into the vena cava, and division can be carried out at this point. The middle hepatic vein empties directly into the vena cava, or it may empty into the left hepatic vein. In any event, both the right and middle hepatic veins must be sacrificed. The middle hepatic vein requires special attention if it is to be dissected from the all-important left hepatic vein and should not be injured, as it is the only drainage access from the left lobe.

G

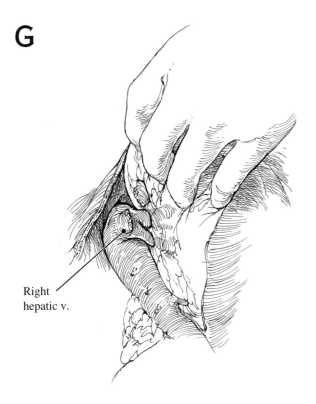

Right
hepatic v.

G

If it is not possible to ligate the hepatic veins from the anterior approach, the liver is rotated toward the patient's left and the short hepatic vein ligated in continuity and divided. The right hepatic vein comes into view and can be clamped and divided; the severed ends can be oversewn with vascular material, at least on the caval side.

H

The triangular ligament is resewn to lessen the risk of the left lobe twisting on itself. The cut liver surface is examined carefully for bleeding or bile leakage points, which, if found, are secured.

Two Jackson-Pratt or similar drains are placed across the surface of the liver and are exited through counterincisions. The abdomen is closed in a routine manner.

H

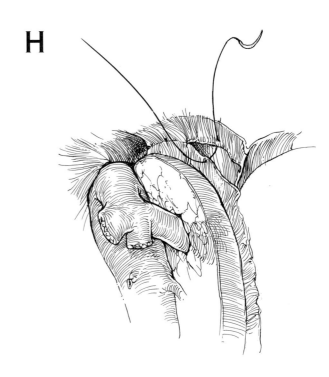

C HEPATIC RESECTION—LIMITED

On occasion, resectable lesions on the surface of the liver are of a size or are so situated that a formal anatomic resection is not necessary. Instead, saucerization or wedge resection is sufficient.

A, B, C, D

The lesion is excised with at least a 1-cm margin. Ligature, suture ligature, clip, or cautery is used to stop any bleeding or leakage of bile.

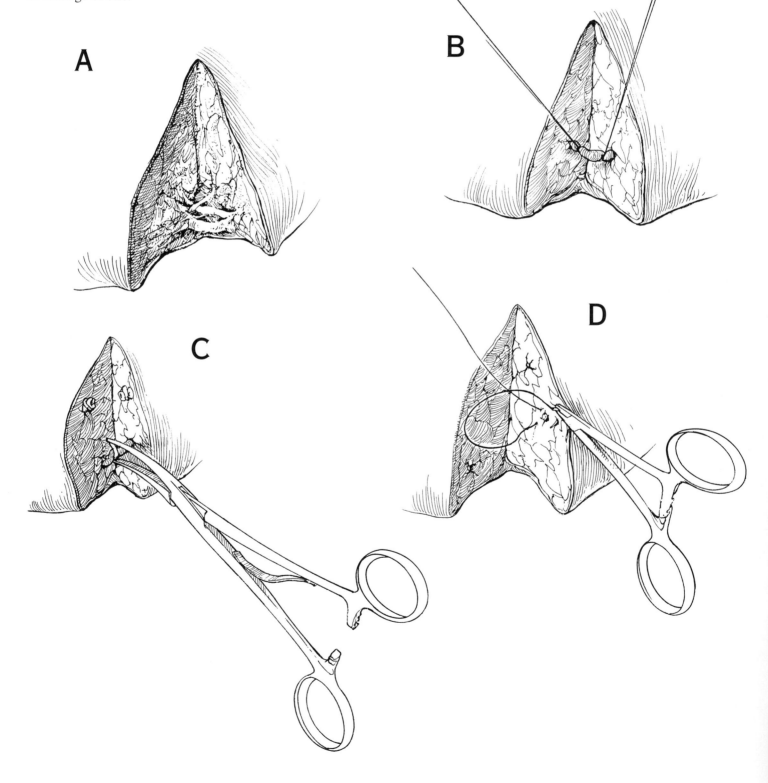

E, F, G, H

If coaptation of the cut liver surface is not possible, compression of the cut surface is utilized. Horizontal mattress stitches of monofilament suture material that are buttressed by Teflon bolsters are positioned and tied just tightly enough to achieve a dry field as the specimen is removed; no attempt is made to approximate the liver capsule (E, F, G). Or the lesion is simply excised by saucerization (H).

E

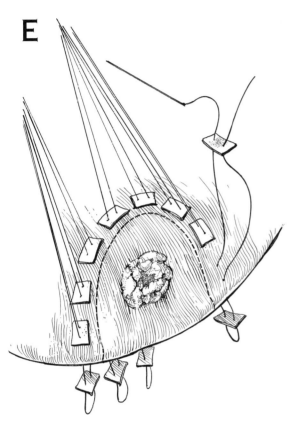

F

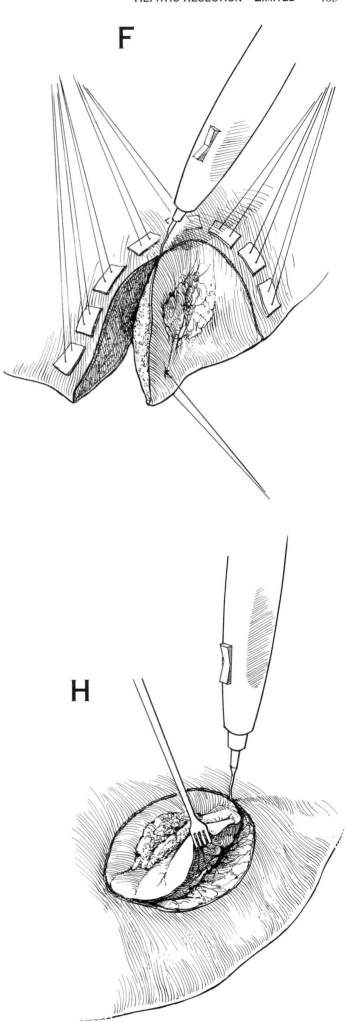

G

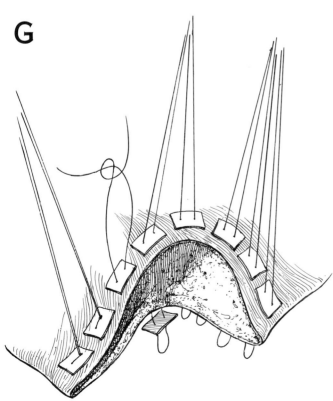

H

BILIARY SYSTEM

A CHOLECYSTECTOMY

OPEN
Retrograde
Cholangiography

A

Cholecystectomy is a common operation performed in several ways, each suited to the clinical needs and the surgeon's capabilities and preferences. Until very recently, open cholecystectomy was the principal method of removing a diseased gallbladder, but it is being replaced swiftly by methods utilizing endoscopic techniques. Such variations are proper as long as the patient's welfare remains paramount and the results are equivalent or superior to those using traditional methods.

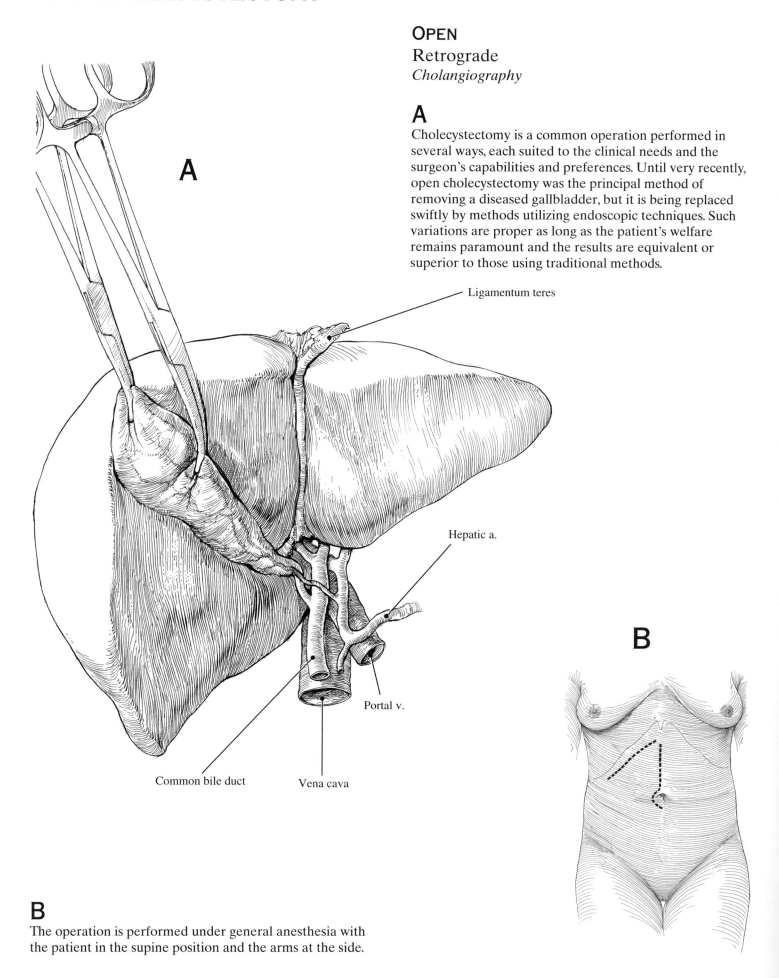

A

Ligamentum teres

Hepatic a.

Portal v.

Common bile duct

Vena cava

B

B

The operation is performed under general anesthesia with the patient in the supine position and the arms at the side.

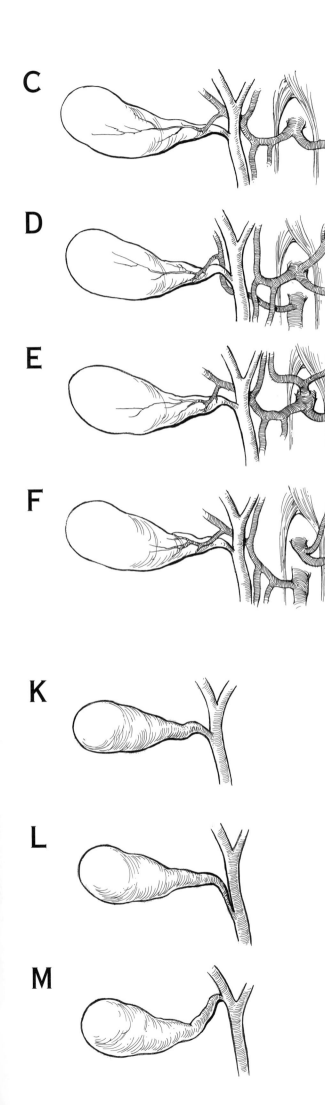

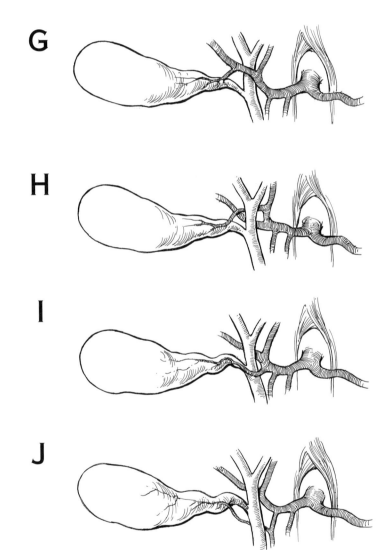

C, D, E, F

The surgeon should be prepared for a considerable variation in the origin of the hepatic arteries, as indicated here.

G, H, I, J

Of even greater immediate importance for the surgeon, the same variation can be found in the relationship of the cystic artery to the hepatic duct. It is in this location that most mishaps in tying the wrong vessel occur.

K, L, M

Three variations in the shape and termination of the cystic duct are shown; others include a low posterior insertion of the cystic duct or a cystic duct from a separate and low-lying segmental right hepatic duct. A surgeon can best avoid a mishap by not dividing the cystic duct before visualizing the afferent and efferent limbs of what it is draining into.

N

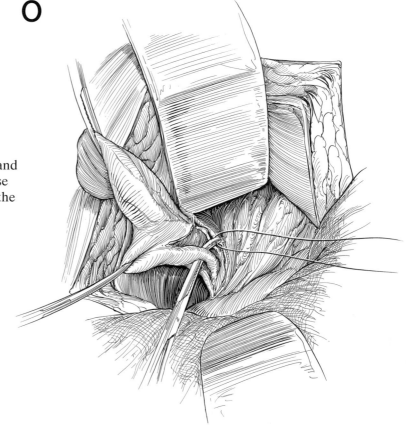

N

On opening the abdomen, a general exploration is conducted before the focus is fixed to the right upper quadrant. The ligamentum teres is clamped with a 6-inch curved hemostat and gentle traction is applied to it, bringing the liver down to a more accessible position in the operative field. The undersurface of the liver is kept exposed with a Deaver retractor.

The gallbladder is clamped with a 6-inch curved hemostat, and traction is applied on Hartmann's pouch in a caudal direction, thus putting the peritoneum over the junction of the cystic and common ducts on a stretch. The peritoneum in this area is incised with long-handled fine Metzenbaum scissors.

O

O

The dissection continues until the junction of the cystic and common duct is identified, and the cystic duct is tied close to the gallbladder with 2-0 silk to prevent leakage from the gallbladder during the subsequent manipulations.

P

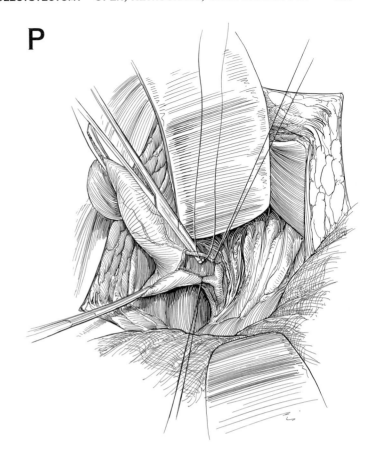

P, Q

The cystic artery is then tied with 2-0 silk and divided.

Q

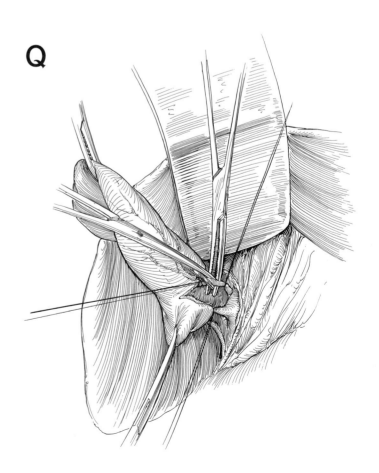

R, S, T

This series of illustrations shows the sequence of catheter placement for the cholangiography. The cystic cholangiogram is begun by making an incision halfway across the cystic duct (*R*). The semiflexible cholangiogram catheter is attached to the syringe, which is filled with dye, as is the catheter, so that air bubbles are not introduced into the common duct during the procedure that would create a false reading of stones on the cholangiogram. The catheter is inserted into the cystic duct and is advanced into the common duct (*S*). A ligature is looped doubly around both the cystic duct and the catheter within it and is pulled taut; this is used to prevent leakage and to secure the catheter in preparation for the cholangiography (*T*).

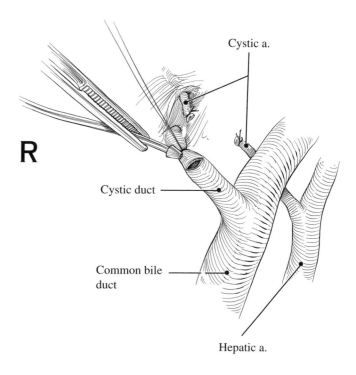

R

Cystic a.

Cystic duct

Common bile duct

Hepatic a.

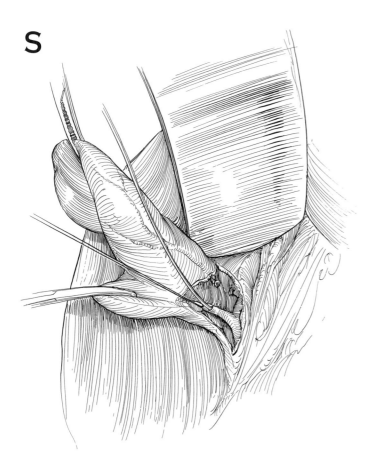

S

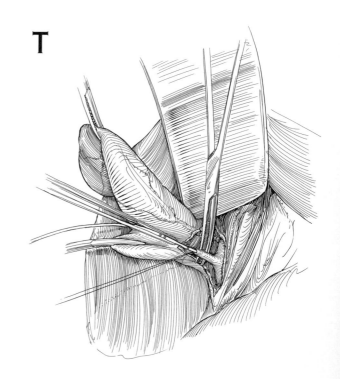

T

U, V, W, X, Y

The semiflexible catheter with a conical arrow tip is introduced into the cystic and common duct, and a double loop of 2-0 silk is placed around both the cystic duct and catheter (U). Tension is maintained on the looped silk to prevent leakage around the catheter as the cholangiogram is performed (V). After a satisfactory cholangiogram is obtained, the double-looped silk is removed and the catheter withdrawn (W). The cystic duct is ligated with 2-0 silk (X), leaving a 5-mm stub. The cystic duct is transected (Y) and the cholecystectomy continued.

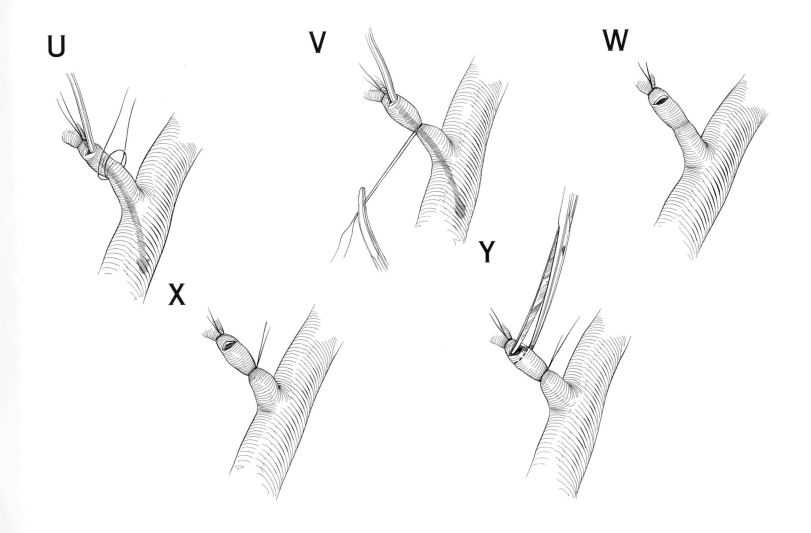

Z, AA, BB

With the cystic duct and arteries ligated and divided, the retrograde cholecystectomy is begun. It is less bloody when cut with cautery and safer if a fine instrument, such as an Adson hemostat, is placed under the issue as it is divided. The gallbladder is gradually mobilized, each step preceded by dividing the serosa of the gallbladder. A fine-tipped electrocoagulation unit is used for cutting or coagulation, or both. The gallbladder bed is examined for bleeding venules or small accessory bile ducts. These are coagulated or secured with secure ligatures.

The gallbladder bed is left open. A drain is not used routinely.

Z

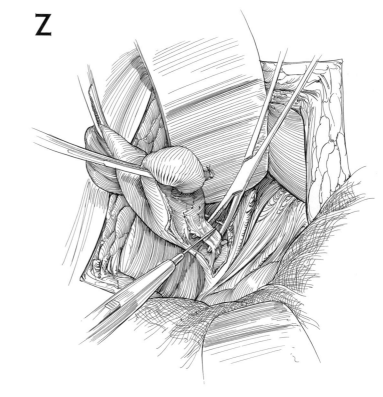

AA

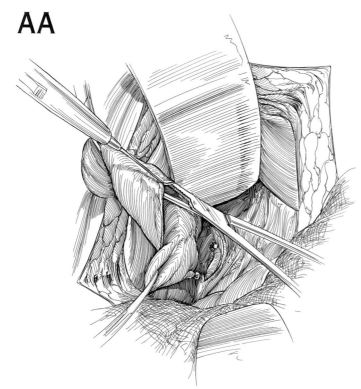

BB

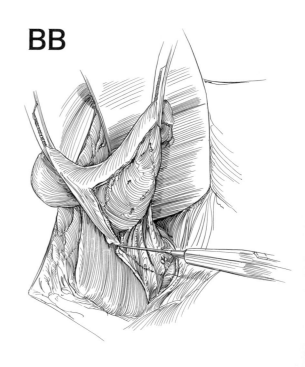

Common Duct Exploration
In addition to the need for radiologic visualization, some clinical circumstances call for the manual exploration of the inside of the bile duct.

A

The peritoneum lateral to the duodenum is incised, and the duodenum is mobilized medially so that the terminal common duct is exposed. The duct, especially the distal segment, is palpated bidigitally for any abnormal masses.

B, C

A 1-cm longitudinal incision is made on the common duct distal to the entrance of the cystic duct. A stitch of 4-0 chromic catgut is applied on each side of the opening, and mosquito hemostats are attached; their weight serves to keep the incision gaping.

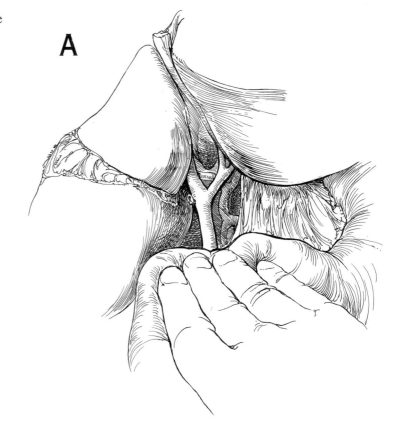

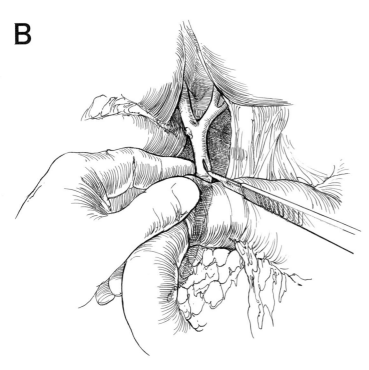

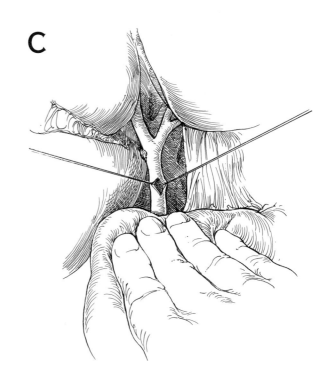

D

A very small sized rubber catheter attached to a 20-ml syringe filled with saline is introduced distally into the common duct. The plunger of the syringe is pushed while slowly withdrawing the catheter. As long as the tip is in the duodenum, there is no return of saline; return occurs the instant the catheter is on the proximal side of the sphincter of Oddi. At this point, it is hoped that the flow of saline will flush any distal stones retrogradely.

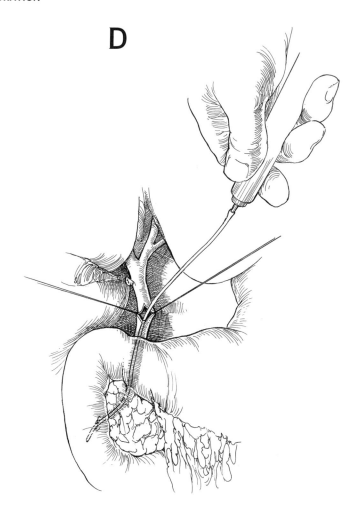

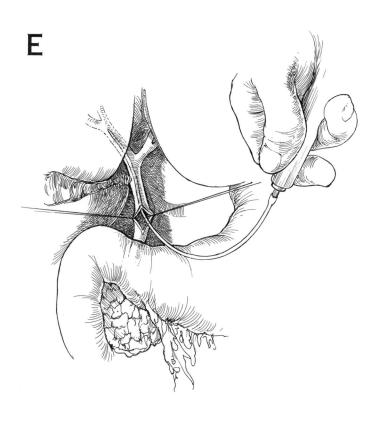

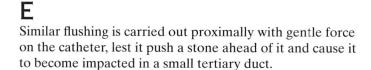

E

Similar flushing is carried out proximally with gentle force on the catheter, lest it push a stone ahead of it and cause it to become impacted in a small tertiary duct.

F

Next, a very small sized Foley catheter is inserted proximally, its balloon is gently inflated, and the catheter is withdrawn, with the intention of bringing out ahead of the balloon any stones in this area.

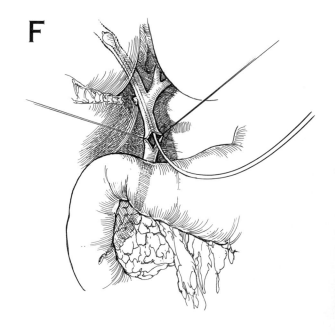

G, H, I, J, K

This step is subdivided as follows: With the balloon deflated, the Fogarty is inserted distally into the duodenum (*G*); the balloon is inflated, and the catheter is withdrawn gently until it meets resistance at the sphincter (*H*); the balloon is deflated sufficiently (*I*) and only enough to withdraw it immediately inside the sphincter (*J*), at which point it is instantly reinflated (*K*); and withdrawal is continued. Ideally, any stones in the terminal duct will be withdrawn ahead of the balloon.

H

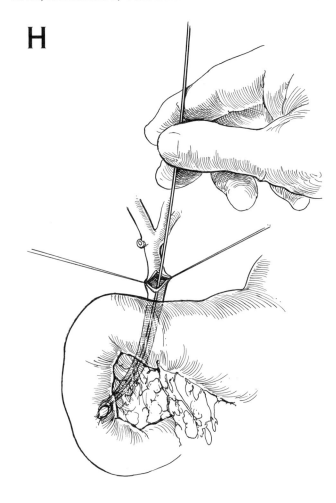

G

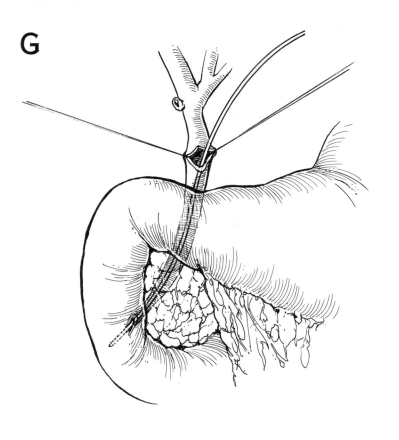

J

I

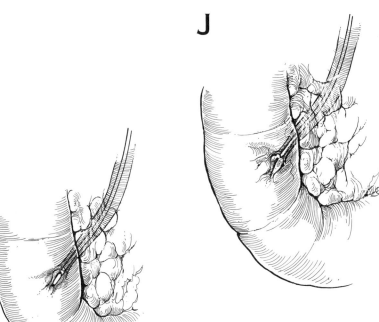

K

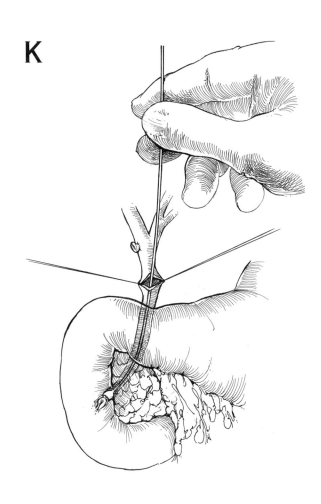

L

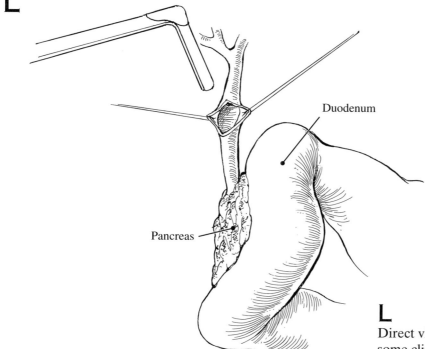

Duodenum

Pancreas

L

Direct visualization of the common duct can be decisive in some clinical settings, and the surgeon should be skilled in the use of the choledochoscope and the accessory attachments designed for removal of stones or biopsy of suspicious lesions. The irrigating channel of the choledochoscope is attached to a 1-liter plastic bag containing normal saline solution, which then is placed in a pneumatic pressure bag apparatus and set at 150 mm Hg. The choledochoscope is introduced into the already opened duct with care that the duct is not damaged by the rigid arm of the instrument. Nor should the instrument be forced into a common duct unless it can be accommodated easily.

M

Saline flow is instituted; the overflow of saline is aspirated. The distal end of the duct usually is examined first. Any observed stones should be removed directly using the balloon, forceps, or Dormia basket attachments. Biopsies can be performed on suspicious lesions.

M

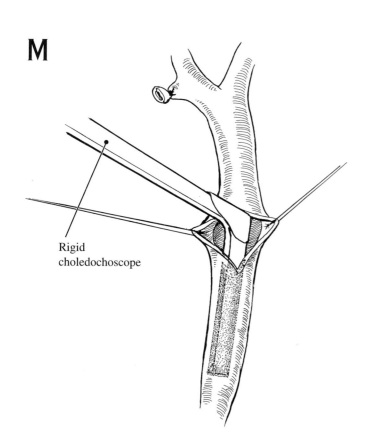

Rigid
choledochoscope

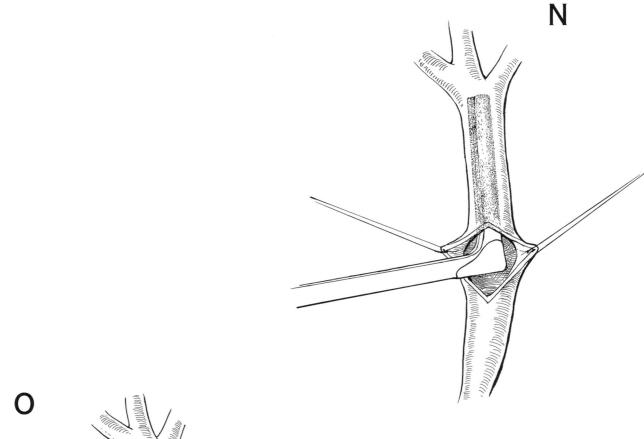

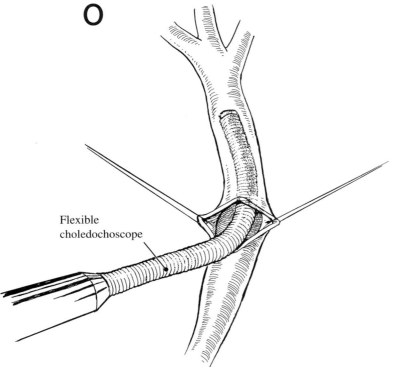

Flexible
choledochoscope

N

The choledochoscope is removed and reinserted to view the proximal ducts. The surgeon should be viewing as the instrument is being advanced lest a stone that is present in the duct be pushed proximally into an hepatic radicle.

O

The flexible choledochoscope is more difficult to use, but more of the ductal system can be visualized when it is employed. Also, it is of particular value in circumstances in which the common duct may have a curvilinear course and does not yield to the rigid arm of a standard choledochoscope.

P

Depending on the clinical circumstances, the patency of the common duct and the possible presence of stones can be further tested by passing a soft lead probe distally. It is easy and misleading to merely feel the sphincter pushed ahead of an obstructed duct and thus believe that the probe has passed through it. More reliable is faintly seeing and actually feeling the tip of the probe as it is pushed against the duodenal wall opposite the duct opening.

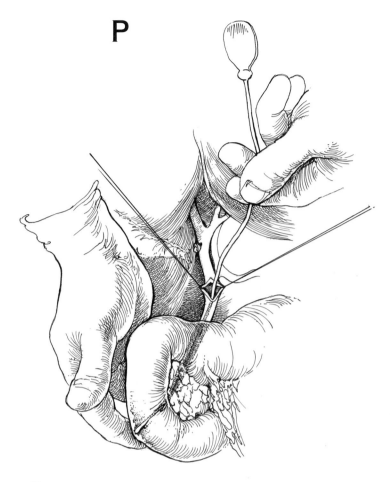

Q

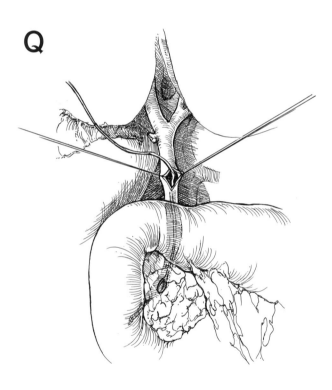

A soft lead spoon can be used to feel for a stone but especially to remove known stones and sometimes to scrape clean the duct wall that may be encrusted with calcific deposits.

R

A stone forceps can also be used to remove stones or gross debris. Ultrasonography also can play an important role in evaluating the status of the common duct. Finally, it is possible that any or none of this array of instruments and techniques will be successful. It is incumbent on the surgeon, however, to be familiar with their purposes and uses.

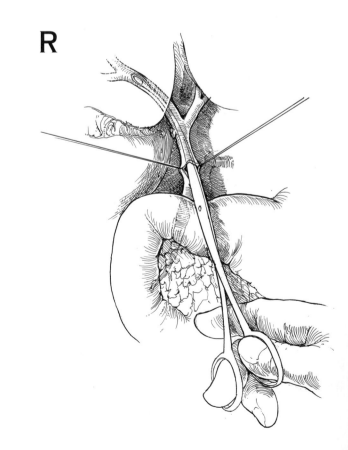

S, T

A T-tube is prepared for insertion into the common duct. Trimming as shown enables it to be used properly and also offers a streamlined, nontearing configuration at the time of its withdrawal.

U, V, W

The T-tube is grasped with a Mixter clamp at the junction of the vertical and horizontal parts of the T-tube (*U*), and one arm is inserted proximally as far as possible (*V*). The distal arm can then be inserted with minimal difficulty.

X

The T- tube is slid back and forth and is flushed with saline to be certain there is no occlusion or twisting.

Y

The closure is with 3-0 chromic catgut, with the first stitch applied next to the vertical arm of the tube. All sutures are positioned before being tied.

Z

Following closure, saline is injected into the T-tube to reveal any gross leaking, and a completion T-tube cholangiogram is obtained to evaluate any residual filling defects and assess free flow into the duodenum. A suction drain is placed in this area and is exteriorized through a counterincision. The abdomen is closed in a customary manner.

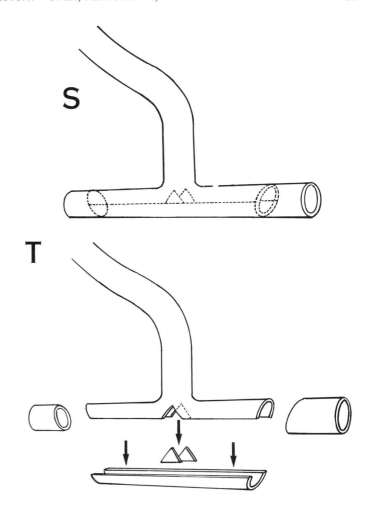

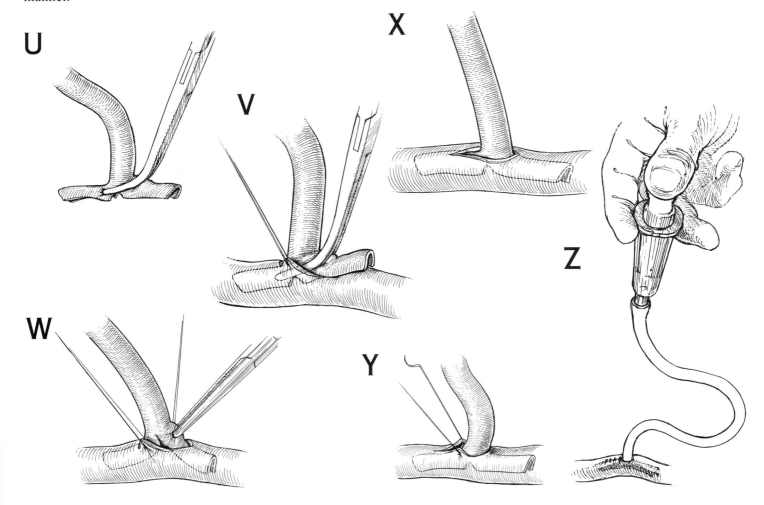

Antegrade

A

The abdomen is opened through a subcostal incision, and a general exploration is conducted. A 6-inch curved hemostat is placed across the falciform ligament, and with the assistance of one hand over the dome of the liver, traction is applied, thus lowering the liver and bringing it into better working position.

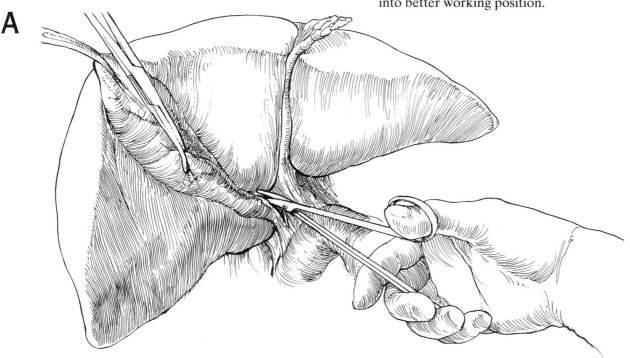

B

The loose peritoneum over the junction of the cystic and common ducts is incised and gently spread, exposing the cystic duct. An Adson hemostat is used to pass a strand of 2-0 silk around the duct that is then double looped and placed under some tension. This serves to occlude the duct so that no stones will be squeezed into the common duct during subsequent manipulations. This silk also can be used to move the cystic duct and the surrounding anatomy about as the gallbladder is being freed. It is not tied until the dissection has progressed to this point and the identity of tissues being ligated is certain.

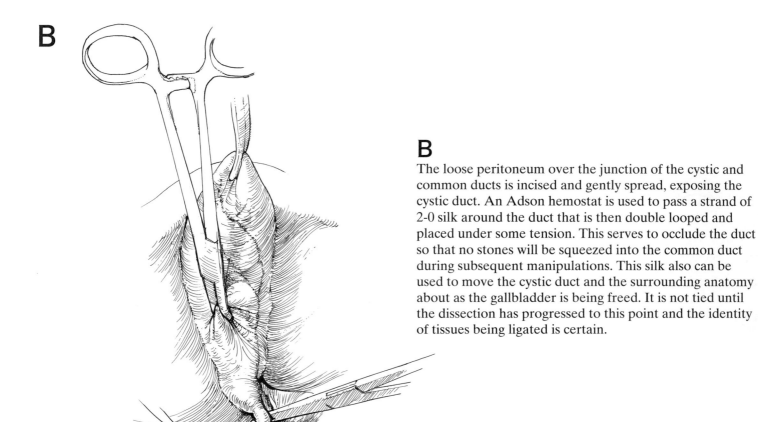

C

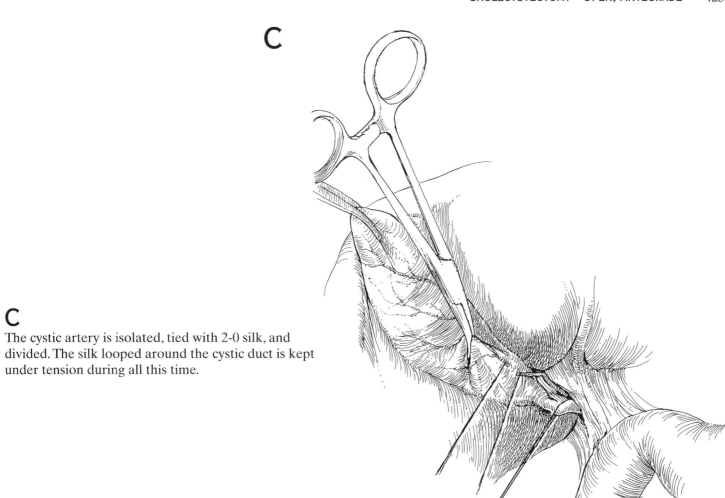

C

The cystic artery is isolated, tied with 2-0 silk, and divided. The silk looped around the cystic duct is kept under tension during all this time.

D

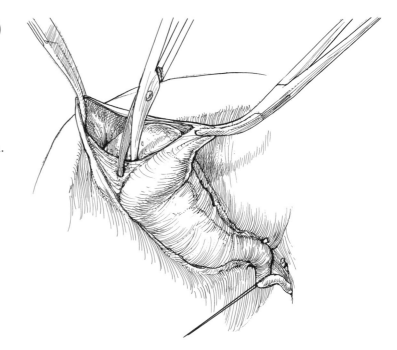

D

The gallbladder is dissected off its bed with a Metzenbaum.

E

E

Bleeding points are electrocoagulated. Larger vessels are clipped or stitch tied. If a bile duct is encountered, the surgeon must reassess and verify the anatomy to avoid injuring a segmental right hepatic duct. Occasional tiny bile ducts are clipped or suture ligated.

F

F

When the gallbladder is completely free from the liver, the cystic duct is tied with 2-0 silk and the cholecystectomy completed. The gallbladder bed is not closed, and no drain is used on a routine basis.

The abdomen is closed in a preferred manner.

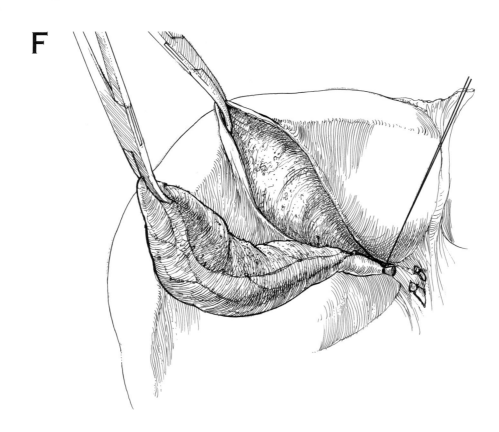

LAPAROSCOPIC

A

Laparoscopic cholecystectomy has become the preferred surgical treatment for most patients with symptomatic cholelithiasis. The advantages of a laparoscopic approach in terms of minimizing patient discomfort and hastening recuperation have been readily apparent. Initially, the procedure was limited to the elective management of chronic cholecystitis. As experience has accumulated, the technique has been extended successfully to include the treatment of acute cholecystitis and associated choledocholithiasis (with or without retrograde endoscopic stone removal). However, the potential for certain complications related to the laparoscopic technique has raised concern. In particular, bile duct injuries have been more frequent than traditionally anticipated during open cholecystectomy. Safe performance of laparoscopic cholecystectomy requires adequate training, appropriate patient selection, proper technical execution, and an operative strategy that provides exposure and allows clear definition of the anatomy. The surgeon must exercise good judgment and maintain a low threshold for converting to an open procedure whenever circumstances are not optimal.

A

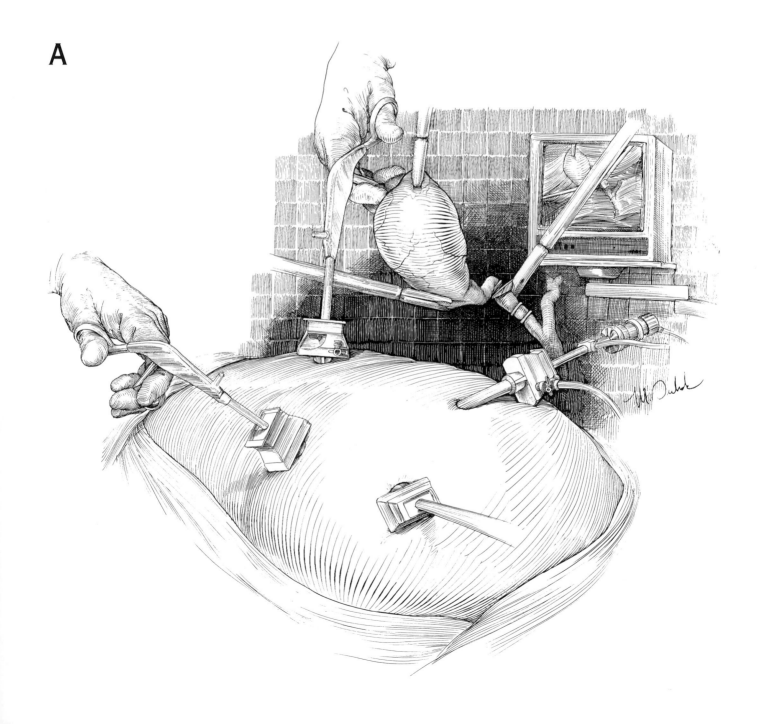

B

Standard cannula positions for laparoscopic cholecystectomy include a 10-mm umbilical port for the laparoscope, a 10-mm epigastric port for the operating surgeons, and two lateral 5-mm ports. The lateral ports are placed at the midclavicular line just below the costal margin and at the anterior axillary line at or above the level of the umbilicus.

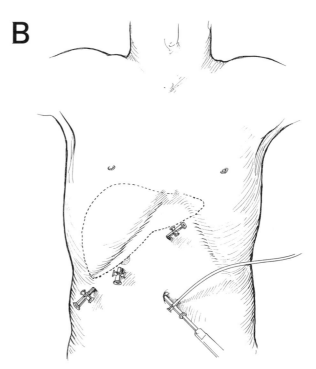

B

C

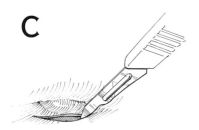

D

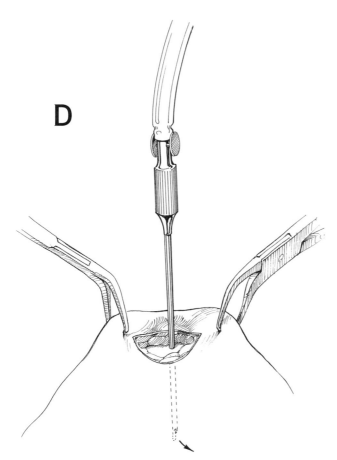

C, D

A short subumbilical skin incision is made, and the Veress needle is introduced. Alternatively, a vertical incision directly through the umbilicus may be made. Following confirmation of free intraperitoneal entry, gas is insufflated to establish an adequate pneumoperitoneum. Firm support of the abdominal wall fascia facilitates safe needle placement.

E

An open technique for gaining access to the peritoneal cavity avoids blind placement of the insufflation needle. The incision is continued under direct vision through the fascia and peritoneum. A blunt Hasson-type trocar and cannula is placed through the opening. Fascial stay sutures secure the cannula, and the tapered collar prevents escape of intraperitoneal gas.

F

The pneumoperitoneum is established by gas insufflation to 15 mm Hg intraperitoneal pressure. If an insufflation needle has been used, a 10-mm trocar and cannula is then introduced at the umbilicus.

E

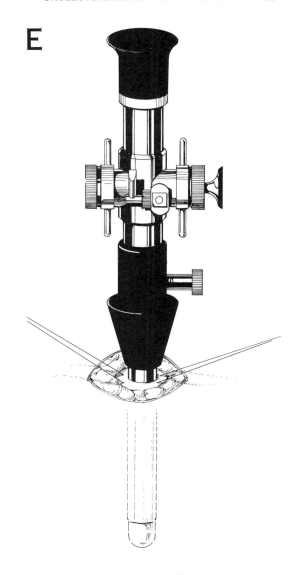

F

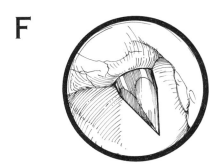

G

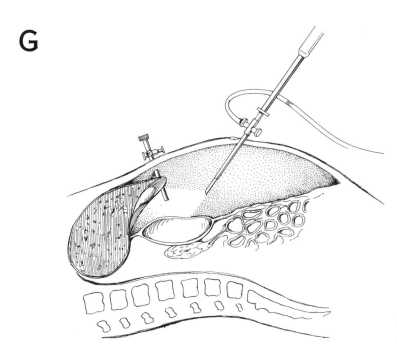

G

The videolaparoscope is introduced through the umbilical cannula, and exploration is begun. Additional trocars are placed under direct videolaparoscopic vision (*G*).

H

The gallbladder fundus is grasped through the lowest lateral port and retracted cephalad above the edge of the liver. The infundibulum is retracted *laterally* through the midclavicular port. Lateral retraction is critical to provide exposure to Calot's triangle. Dissection is begun high on the gallbladder.

I

The junction of the cystic duct and the gallbladder is circumferentially dissected. The cystic duct should be clearly seen enlarging into the neck of the gallbladder.

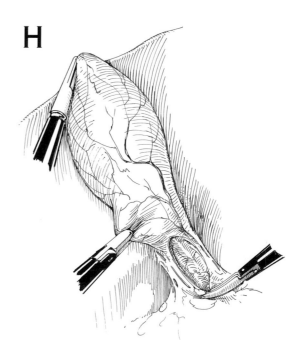

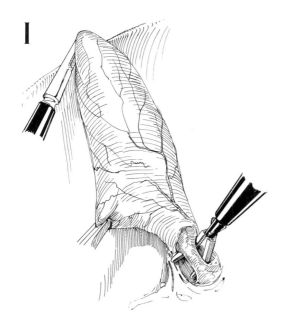

J, K

If cholangiography is not to be performed, the cystic duct is clipped—doubly on the common duct side—the cystic duct is divided, and gallbladder removal is begun. The space between the presumed cystic duct and the liver must be dissected first to verify the anatomy.

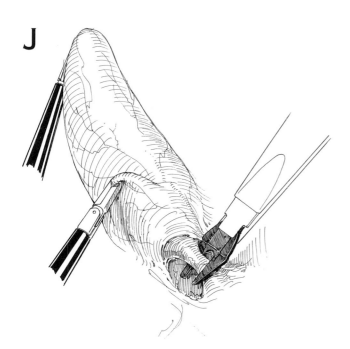

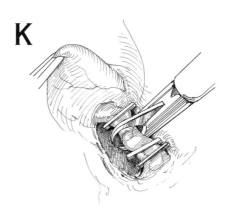

L

If a cholangiogram is to be done, it is performed at this time. A clip is placed on the cystic duct near the gallbladder.

M

The cystic duct is opened well away from the common bile duct in preparation for cholangiography.

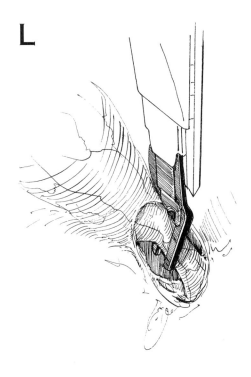

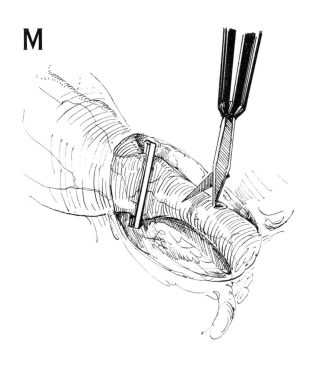

N, O

A no. 5 or no. 4 French urethral catheter is advanced over a guide wire and secured with a cholangiogram catheter clamp. The catheter is flushed before placement and is aspirated after the wire is removed to eliminate air. Alternative methods of securing the catheter include the use of a clip or a balloon catheter.

When cholangiography has been completed, the catheter is removed and the cystic duct is handled in the same manner as when a cholangiogram is not done (J, K). Two clips are placed on the cystic duct, taking care not to impinge on the common duct or to incorporate other tissue; the cystic duct is divided proximal to these.

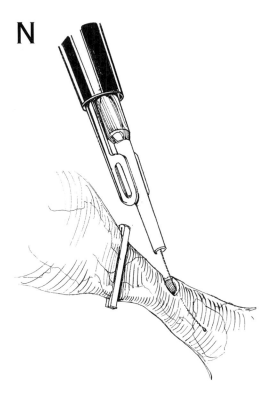

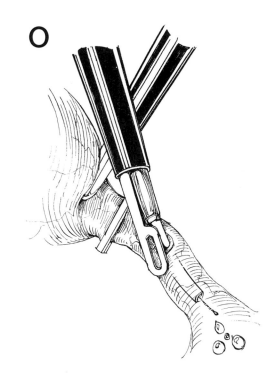

P, Q

The cystic artery is identified, clipped, and divided near the gallbladder. Not uncommonly, the posterior branch of the cystic artery must be separately dissected and ligated.

P

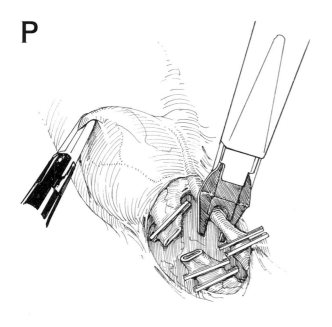

Q

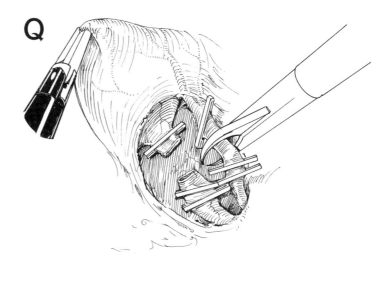

R

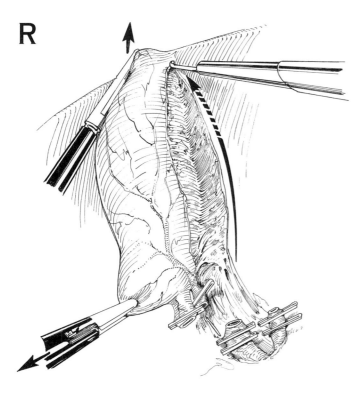

R, S

The anterior and posterior peritoneal reflections between the gallbladder and the liver are divided with monopolar electrocautery. Alternating lateral and medial retraction of the proximal gallbladder provides exposure and necessary tension.

S

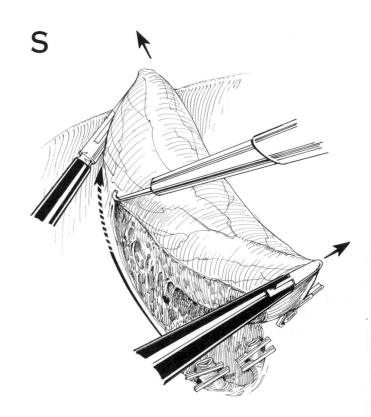

T, U

The gallbladder is dissected from the liver bed while cephalad retraction of the fundus is maintained and retraction on the proximal gallbladder is adjusted as necessary. Before completely detaching the gallbladder, the liver bed and stumps of the cystic artery and cystic duct are inspected for any sign of bleeding or bile leak.

T

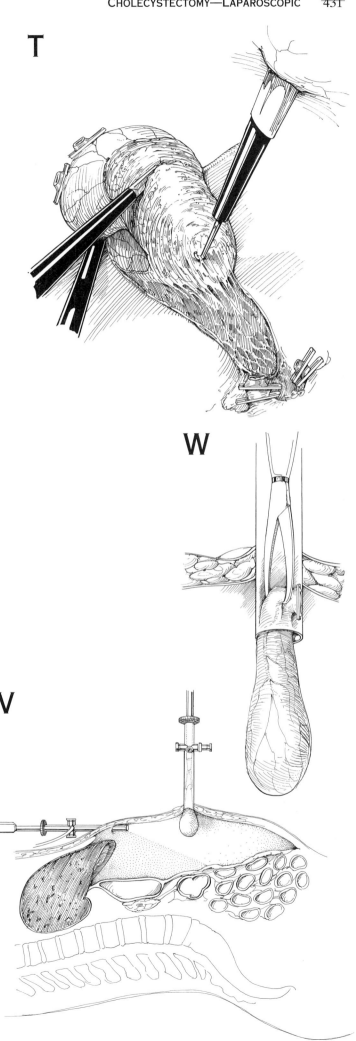

U

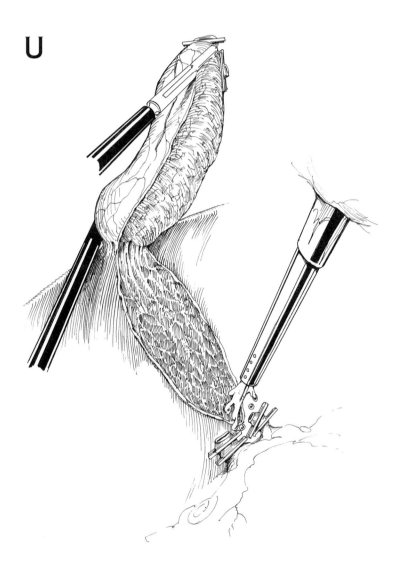

W

V

V, W

The laparoscope is moved to the epigastric port, and the detached gallbladder is delivered to the umbilical port from which it is extracted. External gallbladder decompression, stone extraction, or extension of the fascial incision may be required to remove the gallbladder. Once the gallbladder has been removed, the pneumoperitoneum is reestablished and the surgical field reinspected. A drain may be placed at the discretion of the surgeon. Accessory cannulas are removed under direct videolaparoscopic vision to ensure that there is no bleeding at any of these sites. The pneumoperitoneum is released. The umbilical fascia and the small skin incisions are closed.

B SPHINCTEROPLASTY

Sphincteroplasty is used principally for the extraction of common duct stones, for easy egress of gravel and even recurring stones following transphincteric stone removal, and for fibrosis of the sphincter of Oddi.

A

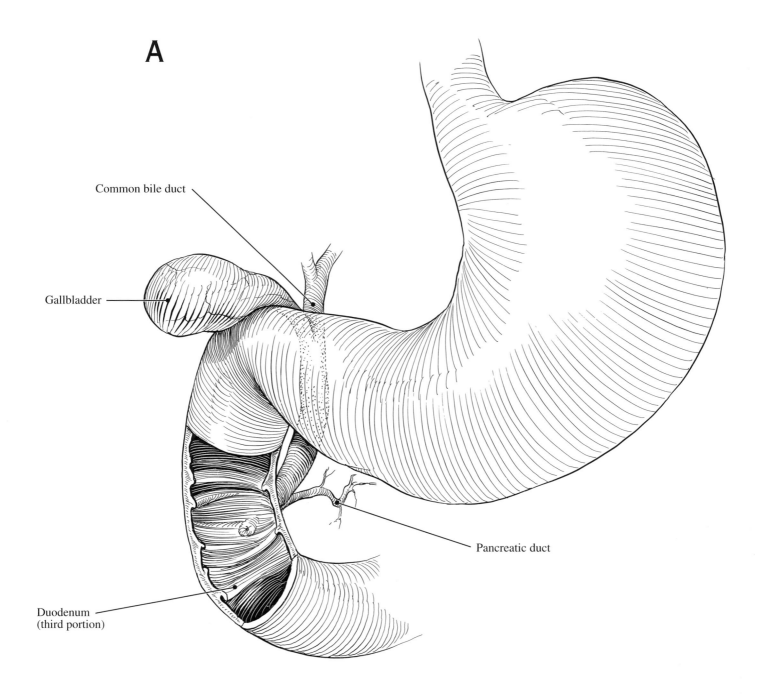

Common bile duct

Gallbladder

Pancreatic duct

Duodenum
(third portion)

A

The sphincter of Oddi surrounds the terminal 1 to 2 cm of the common duct as it enters the duodenum at the junction of its second and third portions. The easiest and most reliable way to identify the sphincter of Oddi is to advance a tube already in the common duct through the sphincter and into the duodenum. The duodenum is opened opposite to the exit of the tube.

B

In the absence of such a preexisting tube, a grooved director is inserted into the terminal duct, and two stitches of 3-0 chromic catgut are applied, with the groove serving both as a guide and as a protector of tissue in the opposite wall.

B

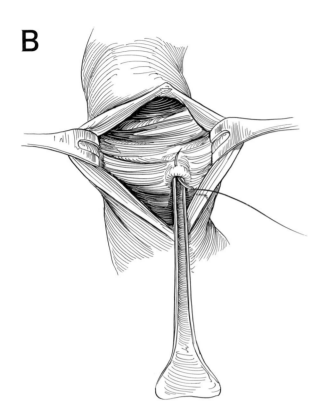

C

The sphincter is divided with a no. 15 blade.

C

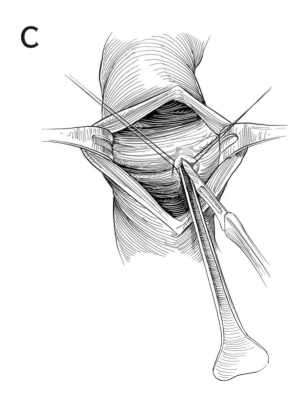

D, E, F

A Fogarty or other catheter can be passed retrogradely if not already placed antegradely. With the catheter as a guide, the division of the sphincter and wall is continued for a distance of 1 to 2 cm as determined by the length of the intramural segment of common bile duct. The duct is serially stitched to the duodenal mucosa with interrupted simple stitches of fine, absorbable sutures, as is shown in these magnified illustrations (E, F).

D

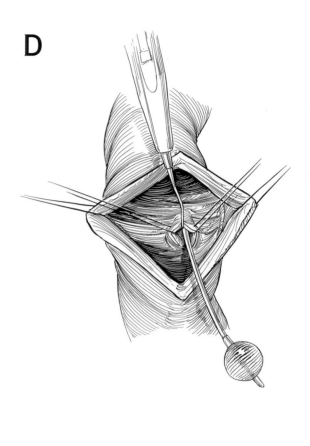

E

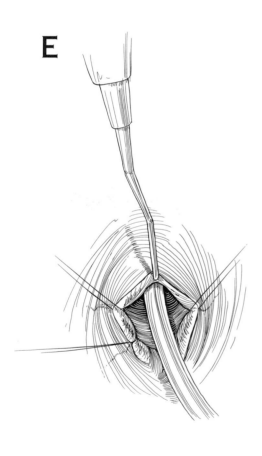

F

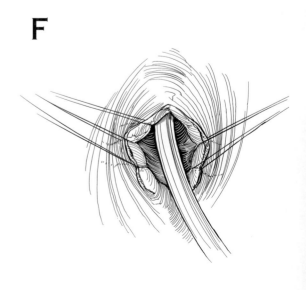

G

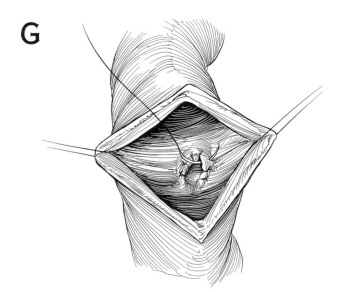

G

The sphincteroplasty is now completed; the tangential plane at which this takes place results in the opening of the duct to a bit larger than normal.

H, I, J

The duodenum is closed in a transverse manner, using continuous 3-0 chromic catgut for the mucosa (*H, I*) and interrupted inverting stitches of 3-0 silk for the seromuscularis.

H

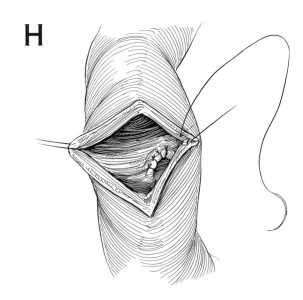

I

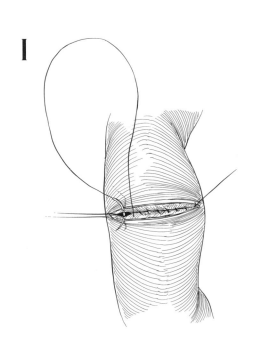

J

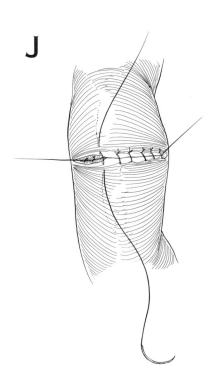

C CHOLEDOCHOJEJUNOSTOMY—ROUX-EN-Y

Roux-en-Y choledochojejunostomy is one way to reestablish extrahepatic biliary continuity following its irreparable damage, usually sustained intraoperatively and most often of its proximal portion. It is also used for reconstruction after resection or for bypass of unresectable cancers.

A

Preferably the abdomen is entered through a subcostal incision. If, however, there is a longitudinal incision from a previous operation, the use of a subcostal incision might place the surgeon in difficulty if it became necessary to mobilize the small bowel in the abdomen to bring it up as a roux-en-Y.

B

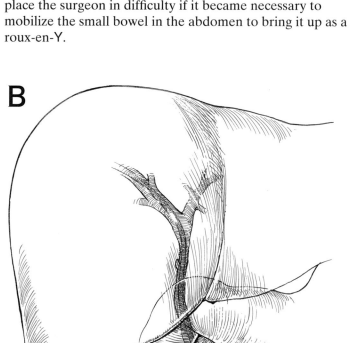

C

When approaching the subhepatic area, the surgeon should be prepared for dense, seemingly impenetrable adhesions that nonetheless need to be lysed with persistent yet restrained aggressiveness.

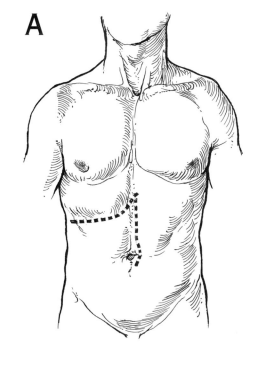

A

B

Often a decompressing catheter has been positioned in the common duct percutaneously and transhepatically. This can be of considerable assistance as the surgeon searches for the proximal common duct.

C

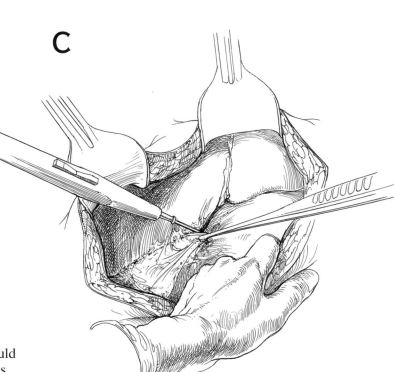

D

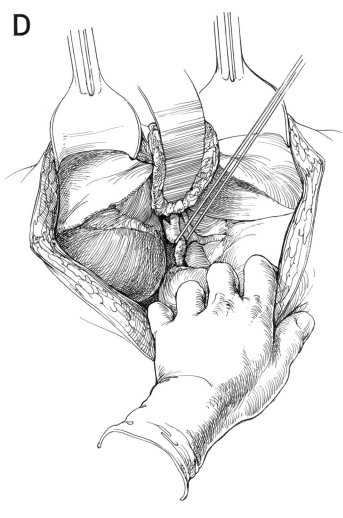

D

The common and hepatic ducts are located and dissected circumferentially. Sometimes the duct is barely recognizable as such; often it does not look as "clean" as it does in this illustration. Care should be taken to avoid excessive skeletonization and devascularization of the proximal duct.

E

The anterior duct wall is divided and the tube within it brought to the outside. A vessel loop around the duct helps position it as necessary for these steps.

E

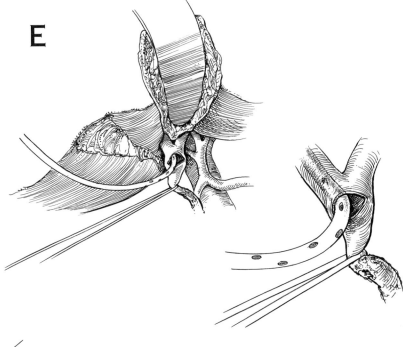

F

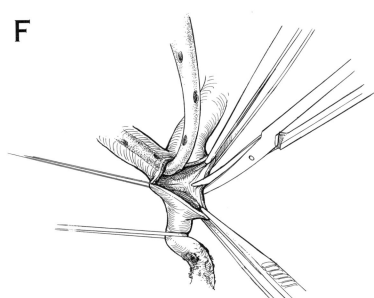

F

The duct is completely transected sharply.

G

The damaged duct is amputated and the distal opening closed with a running stitch of 3-0 chromic catgut.

H

The operative field is now dissected sufficiently that the reconstruction can begin.

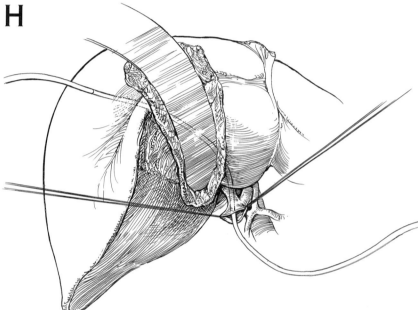

G

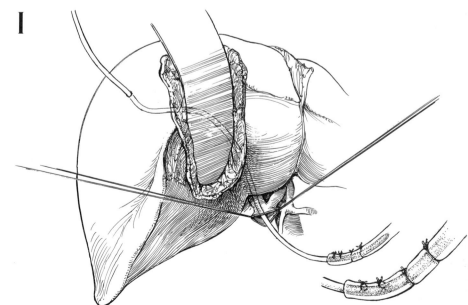

I

If a stent is desired, a larger caliber Silastic catheter can be securely attached to the original decompressing choledochostomy and pulled out through the skin retrogradely.

I

J, K

If no decompressing tube has been placed in position, this can be done now by advancing a semirigid probe retrogradely and out through the skin. A Silastic tube is placed over the bulbous tip of the probe to prevent it from slipping off and is tied several times tightly with 2-0 silk. The Silastic tube now can be pulled through the liver parenchyma and the duct into the operative field.

J

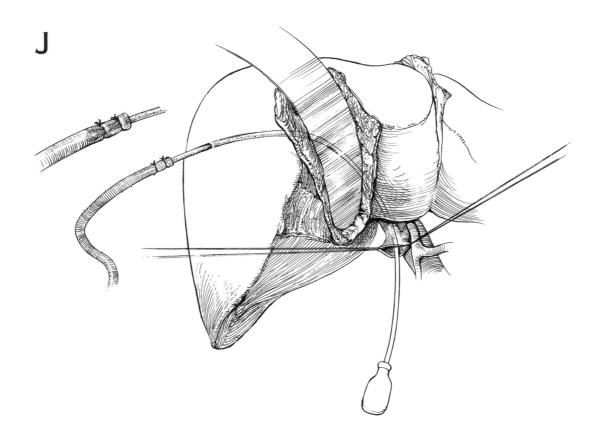

K

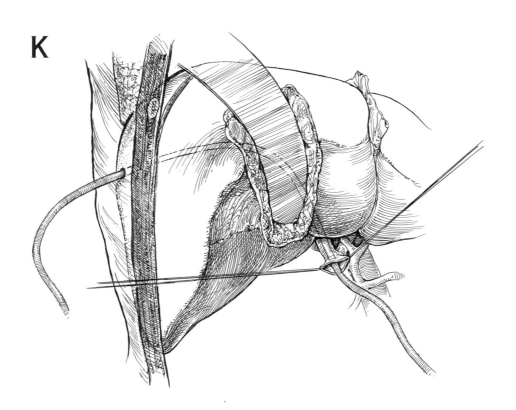

L

The Roux-en-Y limb is now fashioned by first preparing the mesentery and then transecting the jejunum with a linear stapler approximately 20 cm from the ligament of Treitz.

L

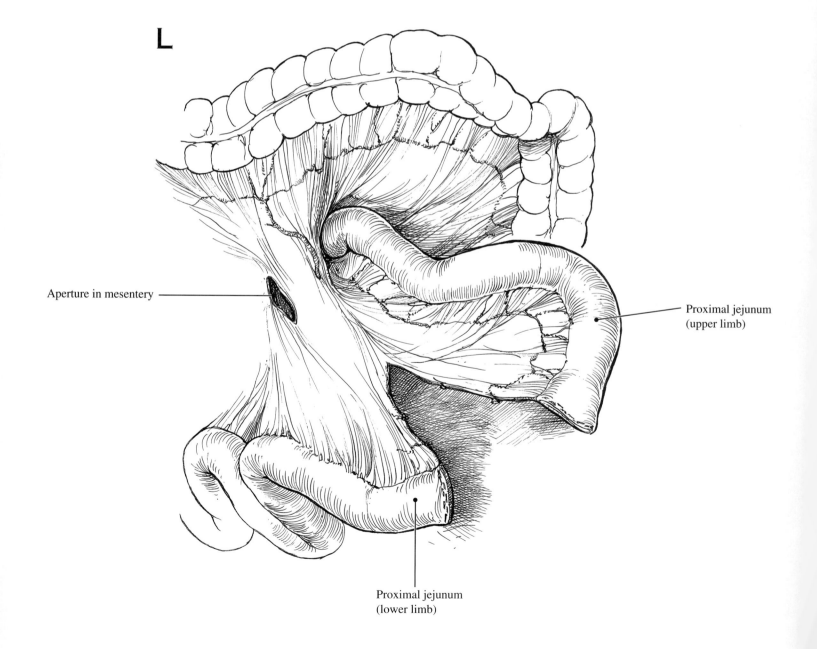

Aperture in mesentery

Proximal jejunum
(upper limb)

Proximal jejunum
(lower limb)

M

A Babcock clamp is passed through a previously fashioned window in the mesocolon, and the distal limb of the divided jejunum is pulled up to the hilum of the liver.

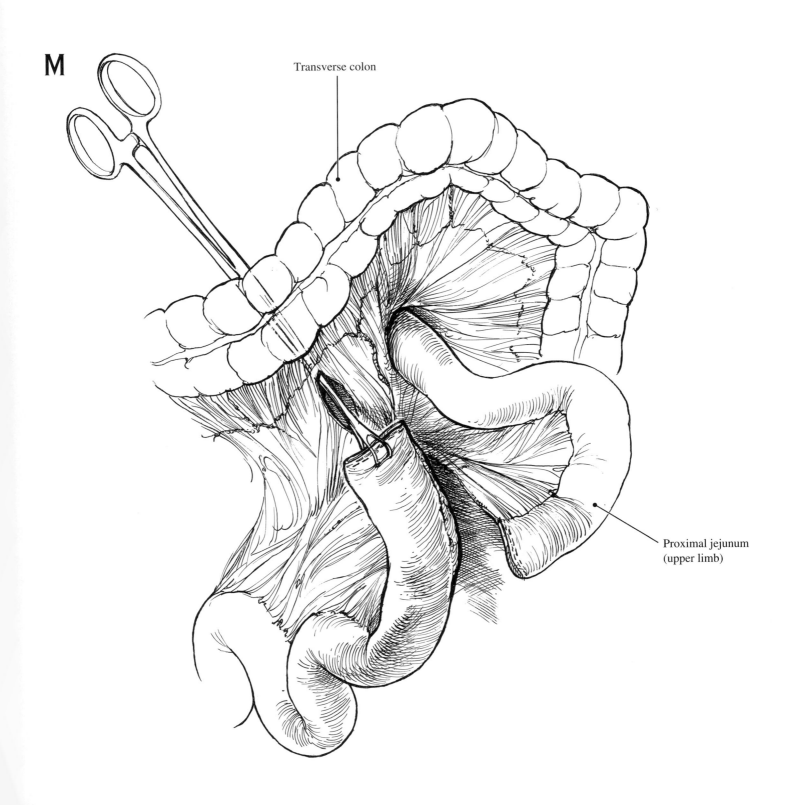

M

Transverse colon

Proximal jejunum
(upper limb)

N

The limb of the jejunum has been brought through the
aperture in the transverse mesocolon in readiness for the
anastomosis. The side of the jejunum is brought in
juxtaposition to the prepared proximal common duct.

N

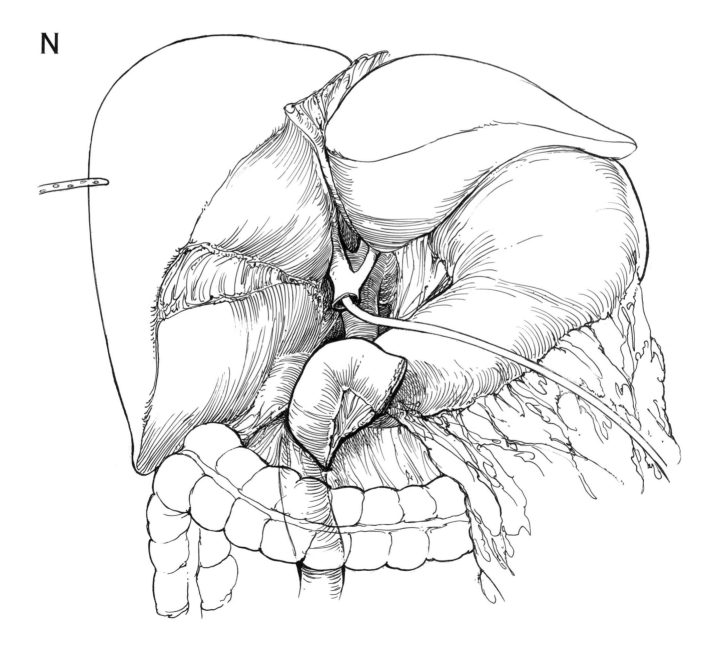

O, P

The anastomosis is in one layer and is begun with two separate sutures of fine nonabsorbable vascular material. Stitching is begun on the far side first and is done so that the knots end outside the lumen. It continues until the posterior portion is completed.

Q, R, S

The stenting Silastic tube is introduced into the distal limb of the Roux-en-Y, and the anterior closure is continued to completion.

O

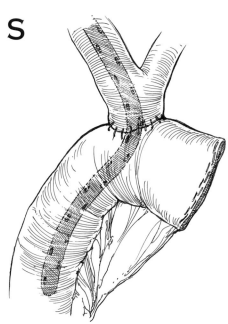

P

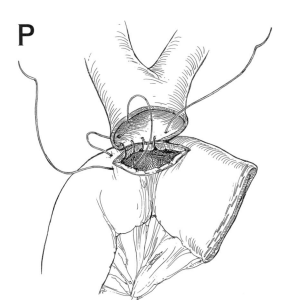

Q

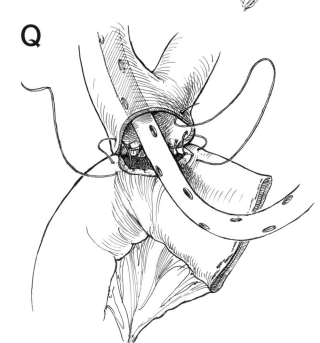

R

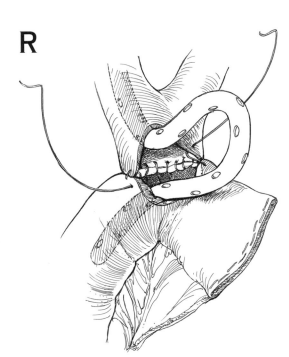

S

T

Sometimes it is desirable or the surgeon's preference to perform the anastomosis with interrupted stitches of 4-0 Maxon. Anchoring stitches incorporating duct and intestine are placed at each side of the proposed anastomosis.

U, V

The stitches are tied only after they are all in position. A fine-tipped electrocautery is used to make an opening in the intestine somewhat smaller in dimension than that of the opened common duct, as the opening invariably stretches.

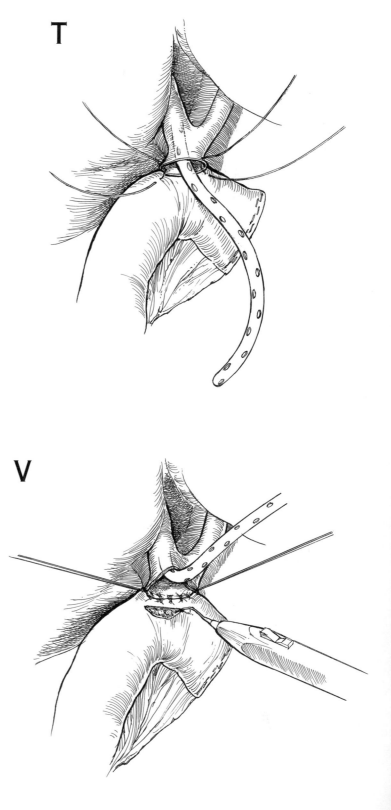

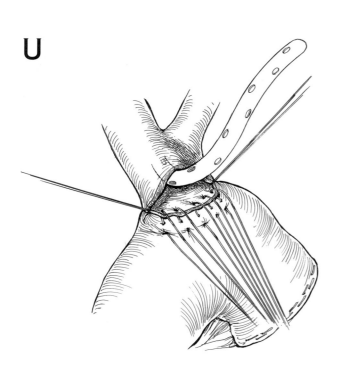

W, X, Y

The Silastic catheter is inserted into the distal limb, and the anterior layer of the anastomosis is completed. Next, the jejunojejunostomy is begun by making an opening for the jaws of the stapler with the fine tip of a cautery.

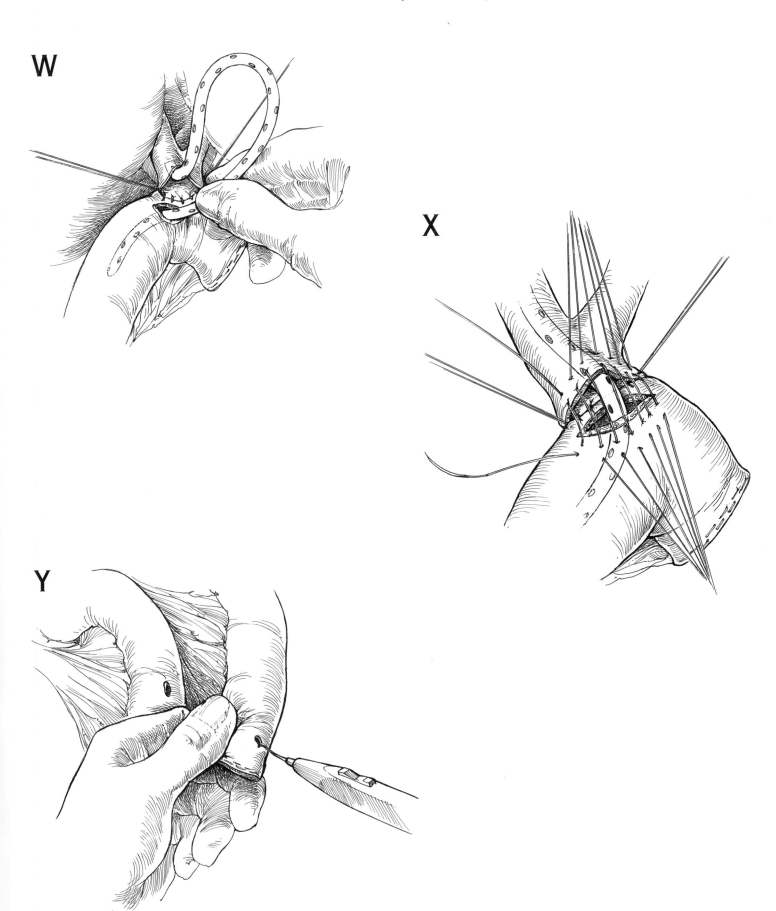

W

X

Y

Z, AA

The separate jaws of the stapler are each introduced into the jejunal loops; the stapler is reassembled and then fired.

Z

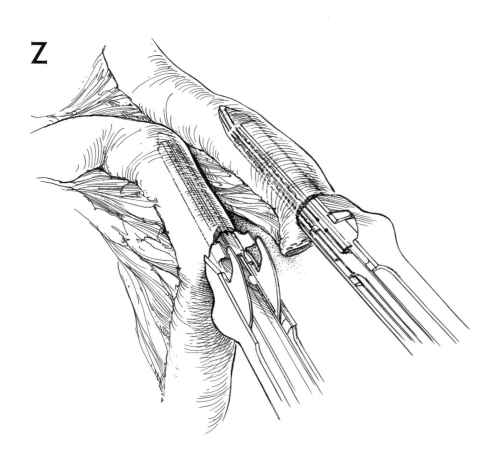

AA

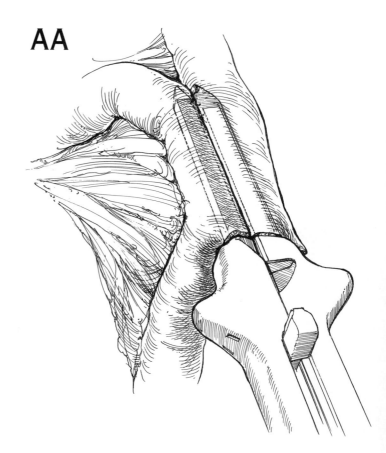

BB, CC, DD

The access holes in the jejunum are closed in two layers, the mucosal layer with a continuous 4-0 Maxon and the seromuscular layer with interrupted simple stitches of 3-0 silk.

BB

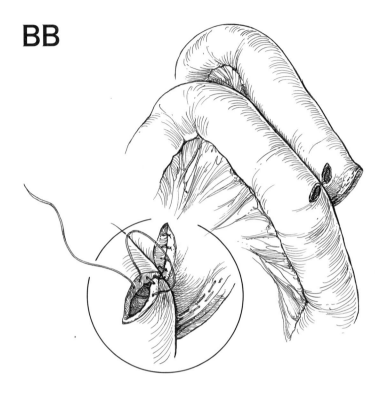

CC

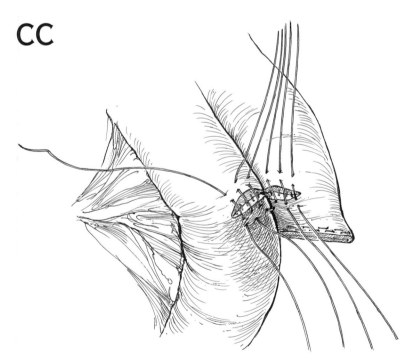

DD

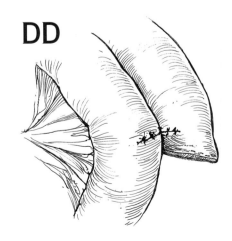

EE

The anastomoses are completed. The mesenteric defect is sutured around the Roux limb. Sometimes the Roux-en-Y limb is anchored to the surrounding tissue with 3-0 silk to lessen the pull on the anastomosis by the weight of the jejunum. A drainage catheter is placed behind the biliary-enteric anastomosis, brought out through a separate incision, and placed on suction. The abdomen is closed in a routine fashion.

EE

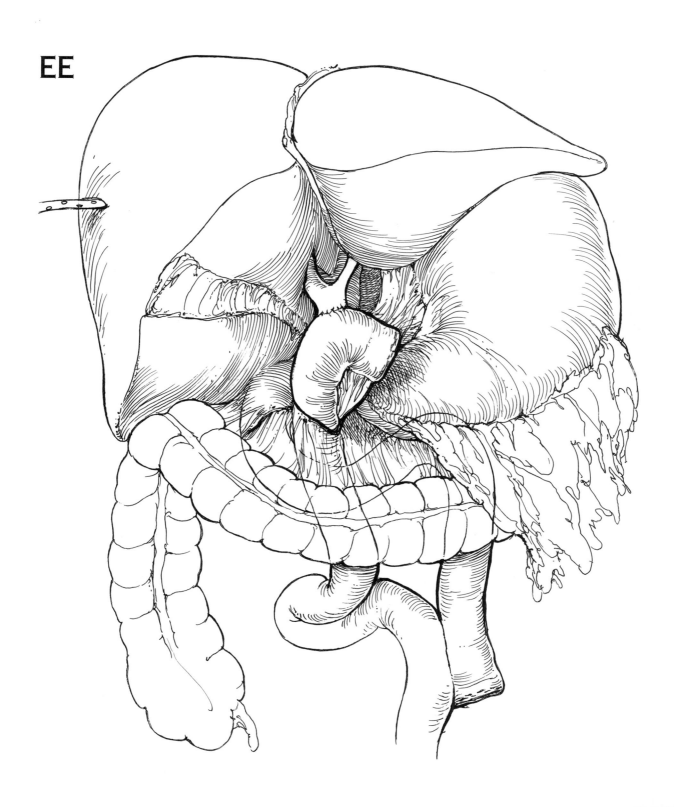

D CHOLEDOCHODUODENOSTOMY—SIDE-TO-SIDE

A

Choledochoduodenostomy is indicated primarily to provide easy passage of retained or new stones into the duodenum of patients who have had multiple large and small stones in the biliary ducts. It is also used to bypass fibrotic stenosis or nonresectable cancer of the terminal duct.

The phantom portion of this illustration (stippled) demonstrates the duodenum that overlies the portion of the duct used during this procedure.

The peritoneum lateral to the duodenum is incised and the duodenum displaced to the patient's left, so that the anastomosis performed in this retroperitoneal area will not be under tension.

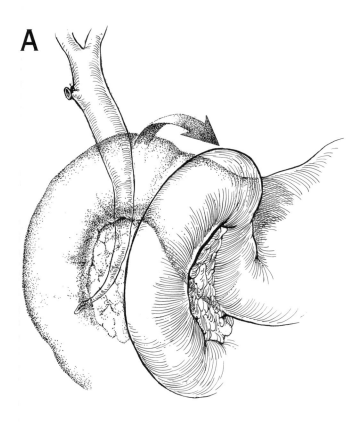

B

With the duodenum reflected, a 1.5-cm longitudinal incision is made over the retroduodenal part of the common duct.

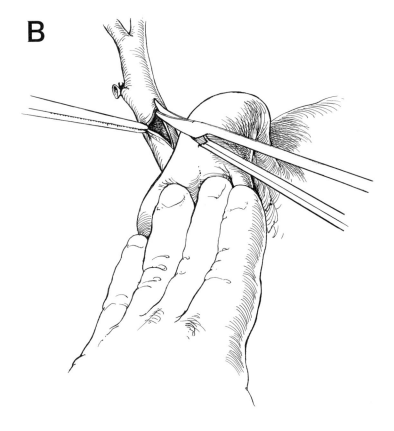

C, D

A duodenotomy of similar dimension or slightly smaller is made opposite the choledochotomy. The anastomosis will be in one layer. Anchoring stitches are placed at the extremes of the anastomotic opening; a stitch using absorbable material is passed between the lower apex of the choledochotomy and the midpoint of the duodenotomy.

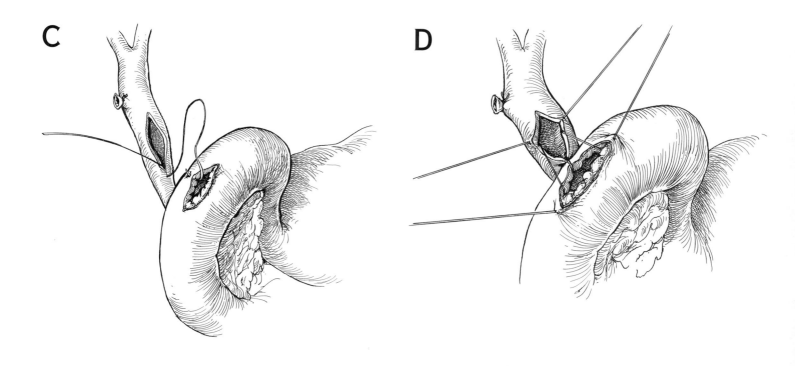

C

D

E, F

The posterior part of the anastomosis using interrupted stitches of 3-0 Maxon is completed with knots tied internally, and the anterior one is begun.

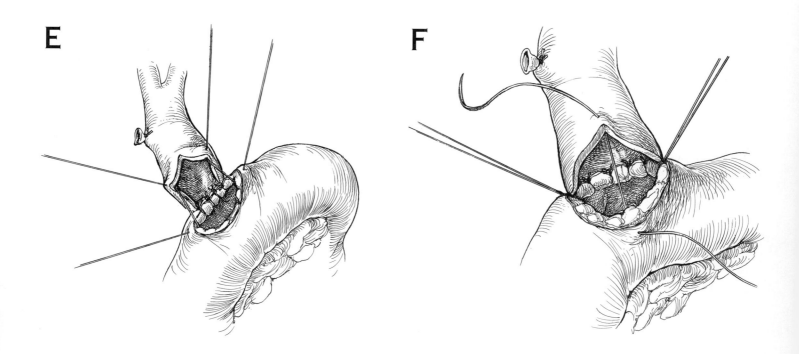

E

F

G, H

The anastomosis is complete. Excessive firm palpation or squeezing to test its patency is not advised; here, pressure by the thumb gives a good idea of patency.

This procedure is relatively contraindicated in patients with normal-sized, thin-walled ducts. Working conditions and results are better if the duct shows signs of chronic obstruction, namely, dilation and thick walls. These characteristics also favor performing anastomosis with a running stitch of fine vascular material.

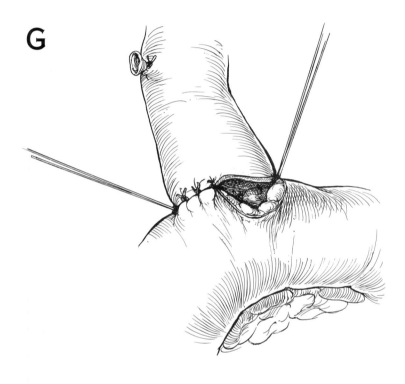

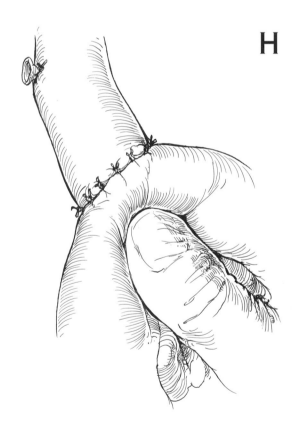

A medium-sized drain is seated adjacent to the anastomosis, exteriorized through a stab wound, and attached to a suction device. The abdomen is closed in the preferred manner.

Chapter

20

PANCREAS

$\bar{\mathrm{A}}$ PANCREATODUODENECTOMY

The pancreas is an endocrine and an exocrine organ, and both of these functions should be kept in mind during pancreatic surgery. Pancreatoduodenectomy for cancer continues to be one of the major operations performed by a general surgeon. Fortunately, the difficulties with the operation and the dismal cure rate of the recent past have improved. Among other changes are new and swiftly improving methods of noninvasive diagnosis and staging. These make it possible to avoid operating on categorically incurable patients so that operations performed are more focused and likely to lead to cure.

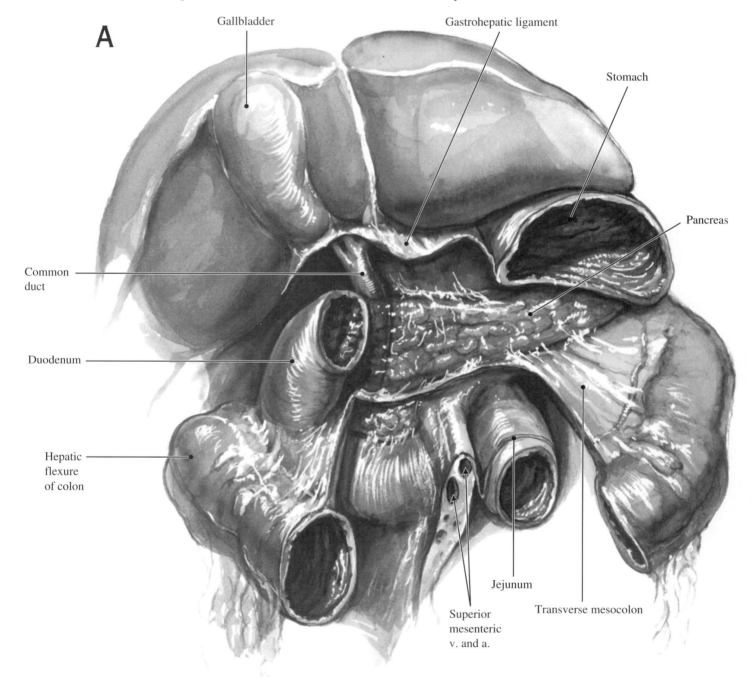

A

The general topographic relationships are shown here. The length of the retroduodenal common duct allows for subsequent sectioning at an adequate distance from an ampullary or duodenal tumor. The hepatic flexure of the colon may overlie some of the second and third portions of the duodenum. The transverse colon and its associated transverse mesocolon have been removed to show some of the underlying anatomy. The transected root of the mesentery of the small bowel makes more obvious the manner in which the duodenum passes under the superior mesenteric artery and vein and over the aorta. The spleen is not shown.

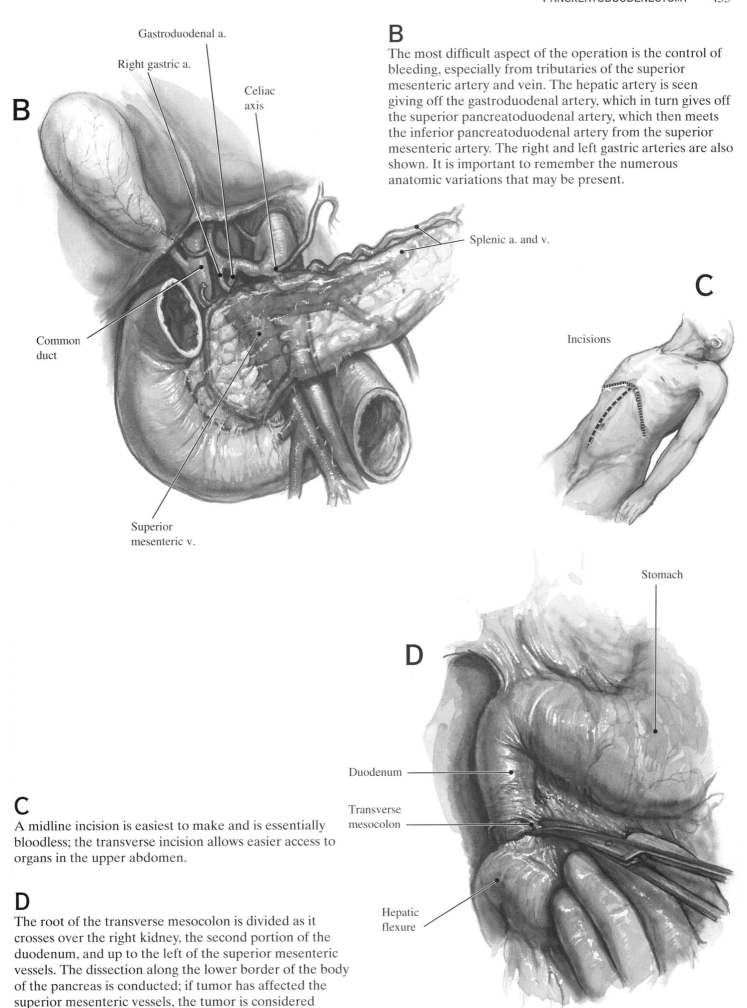

B

Gastroduodenal a.

Right gastric a.

Celiac axis

B

Common duct

Splenic a. and v.

Superior mesenteric v.

C

Incisions

D

Stomach

Duodenum

Transverse mesocolon

Hepatic flexure

B

The most difficult aspect of the operation is the control of bleeding, especially from tributaries of the superior mesenteric artery and vein. The hepatic artery is seen giving off the gastroduodenal artery, which in turn gives off the superior pancreatoduodenal artery, which then meets the inferior pancreatoduodenal artery from the superior mesenteric artery. The right and left gastric arteries are also shown. It is important to remember the numerous anatomic variations that may be present.

C

A midline incision is easiest to make and is essentially bloodless; the transverse incision allows easier access to organs in the upper abdomen.

D

The root of the transverse mesocolon is divided as it crosses over the right kidney, the second portion of the duodenum, and up to the left of the superior mesenteric vessels. The dissection along the lower border of the body of the pancreas is conducted; if tumor has affected the superior mesenteric vessels, the tumor is considered nonresectable and the major procedure is abandoned.

E

The lateral parietal peritoneum is incised, and the duodenum is mobilized by blunt dissection.

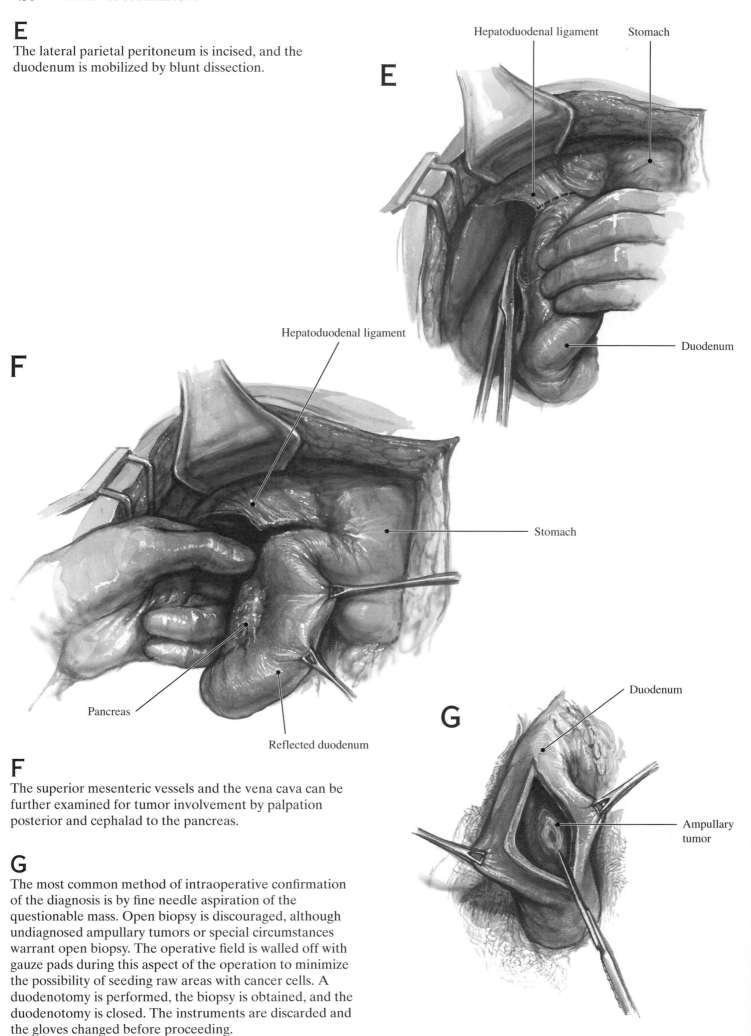

E

Hepatoduodenal ligament   Stomach

Duodenum

F

Hepatoduodenal ligament

Stomach

Pancreas

Reflected duodenum

G

Duodenum

Ampullary tumor

F

The superior mesenteric vessels and the vena cava can be further examined for tumor involvement by palpation posterior and cephalad to the pancreas.

G

The most common method of intraoperative confirmation of the diagnosis is by fine needle aspiration of the questionable mass. Open biopsy is discouraged, although undiagnosed ampullary tumors or special circumstances warrant open biopsy. The operative field is walled off with gauze pads during this aspect of the operation to minimize the possibility of seeding raw areas with cancer cells. A duodenotomy is performed, the biopsy is obtained, and the duodenotomy is closed. The instruments are discarded and the gloves changed before proceeding.

H

The dilated common duct is circumferentially dissected in preparation for its division.

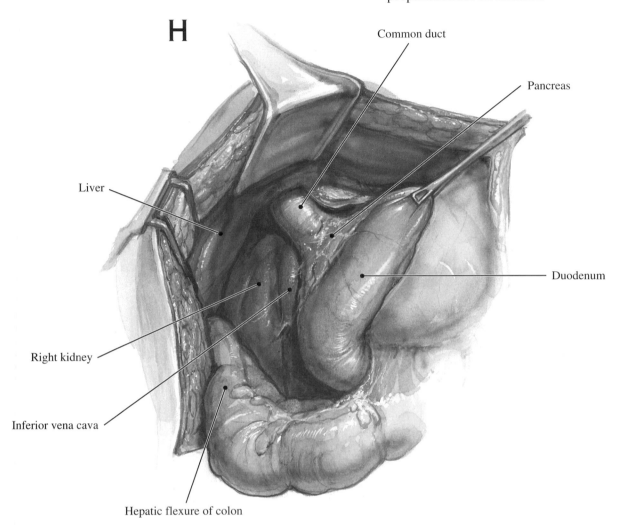

Common duct

Pancreas

Liver

Duodenum

Right kidney

Inferior vena cava

Hepatic flexure of colon

I

The common duct is divided, then encircled with a small rubber drain for retraction and preliminary dissection from the portal vein. The mild inflammatory reaction that is present around a chronically distended common duct means that care is necessary here to prevent injury to the portal vein and consequent serious hemorrhage. The common duct is divided at this time. If it is decided shortly thereafter that the tumor is nonresectable or that the operation must be terminated for other reasons, a choledochoenterostomy can be done.

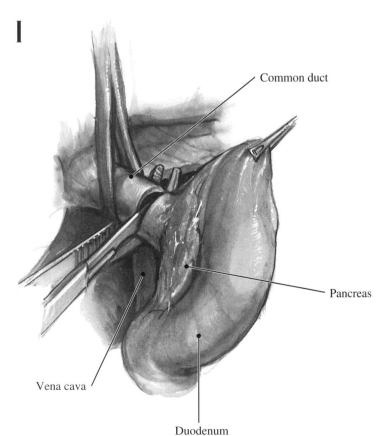

Common duct

Pancreas

Vena cava

Duodenum

J

The head of the pancreas and attached structures are rotated for easier, more accurate ligation of branches from the superior mesenteric vessels, although only the more lateral branches can be adequately exposed at this time. These branches are short and can tear easily from their relatively fixed position in the pancreas; tearing can lead to troublesome bleeding. As shown, vessels are ligated in continuity before being divided.

J

Common duct (proximal)   Portal v.

Common duct (distal)

K

The gastrocolic ligament is divided just outside the gastroepiploic artery through at least the second short gastric branches.

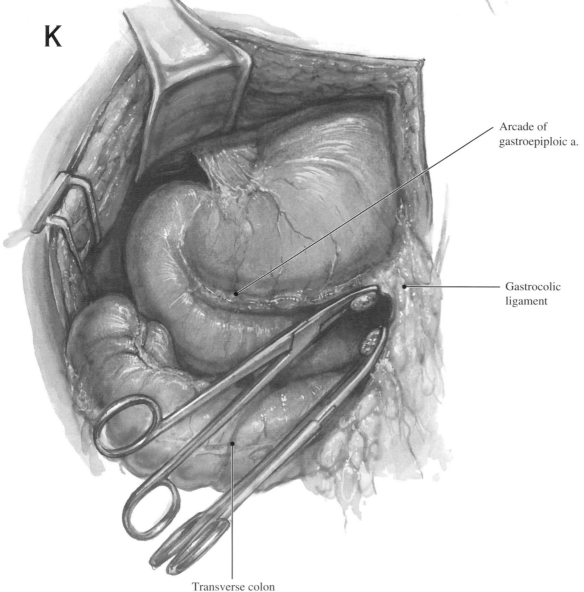

K

Arcade of
gastroepiploic a.

Gastrocolic
ligament

Transverse colon

L

Once the stomach is freed along its greater curvature, it is elevated, fully exposing the pancreas. This exposure makes possible definitive surgery on the pancreas itself and readies the stomach for subsequent transection.

M

The next step involves passing a small soft rubber drain under the body of the pancreas, just to the left of the superior mesenteric artery. This is the safest way to avoid tearing vessels from the superior mesenteric artery and also coincides with the optimum site of division of the pancreas.

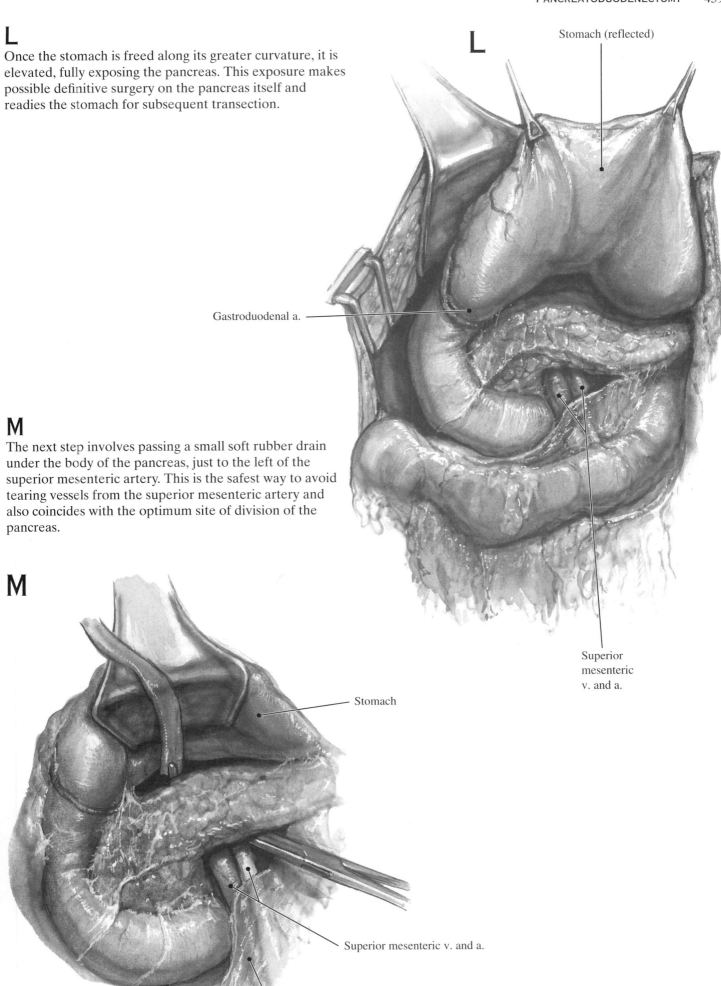

L

Stomach (reflected)

Gastroduodenal a.

Superior mesenteric v. and a.

M

Stomach

Superior mesenteric v. and a.

Middle colic a.

O

The celiac axis and the splenic, hepatic, and gastroduodenal arteries can be seen along the lesser curvature of the stomach. The gastroduodenal artery is occluded with a vascular bulldog clamp on the proximal side and oversewn with 5-0 monofilament suture. The distal end is ligated.

N

The inferior pancreaticoduodenal artery from the superior mesenteric artery should be identified, ligated first, and then divided.

P

The left gastric artery is isolated just above the angula incisura. Because the vessel is adjacent to the stomach, it is necessary to incise the peritoneum of the gastrohepatic omentum to identify it more easily.

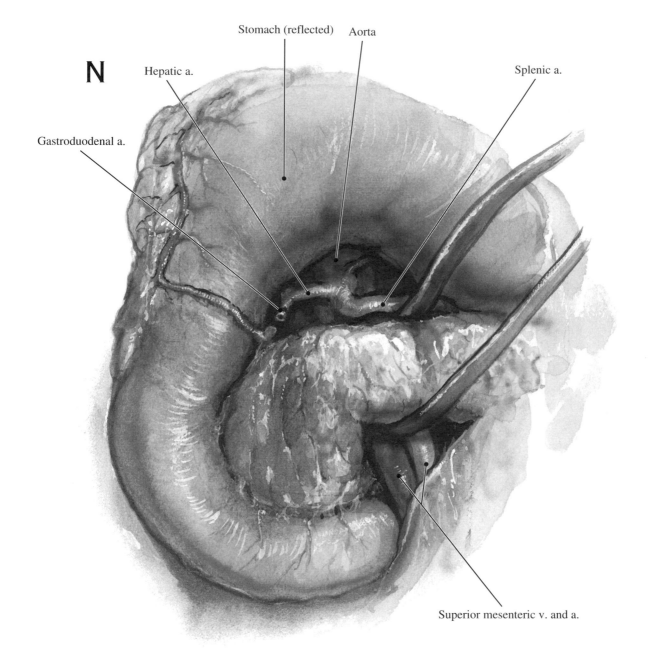

N

Stomach (reflected)   Aorta

Hepatic a.

Splenic a.

Gastroduodenal a.

Superior mesenteric v. and a.

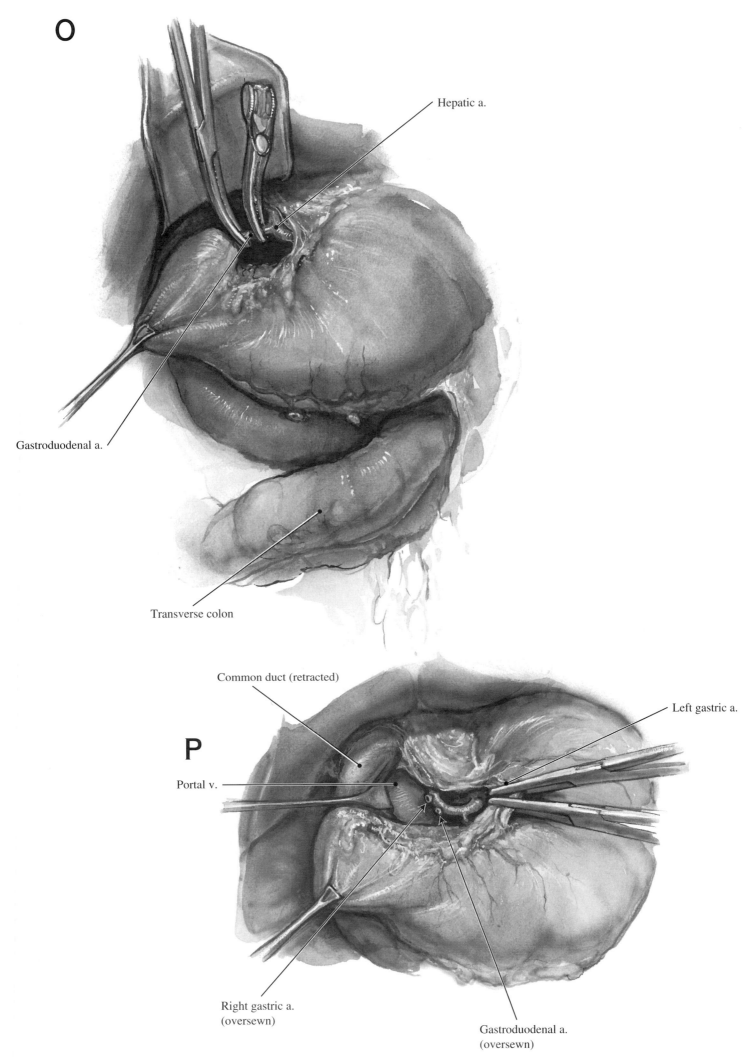

O

Hepatic a.

Gastroduodenal a.

Transverse colon

Common duct (retracted)

P

Left gastric a.

Portal v.

Right gastric a.
(oversewn)

Gastroduodenal a.
(oversewn)

Q

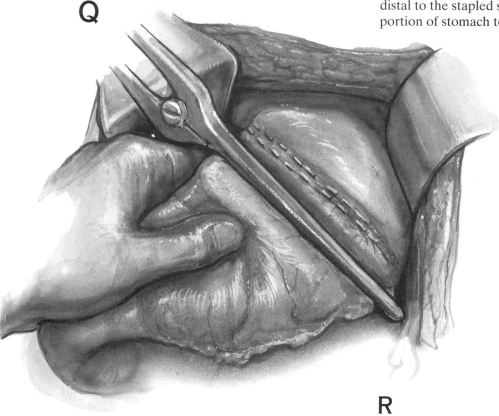

Q

An approximately 50% gastric resection is performed. Just distal to the stapled stomach the Payr clamp holds the portion of stomach to be removed.

R

The antrum is reflected laterally. The stapled stomach along the lesser curvature is inverted with simple interrupted stitches of 2-0 black silk. The staples are trimmed along the greater curvature, leaving an opening of 4 cm for the stoma.

R

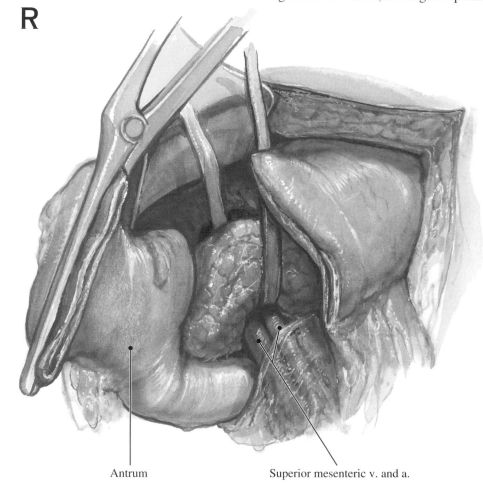

Antrum   Superior mesenteric v. and a.

S

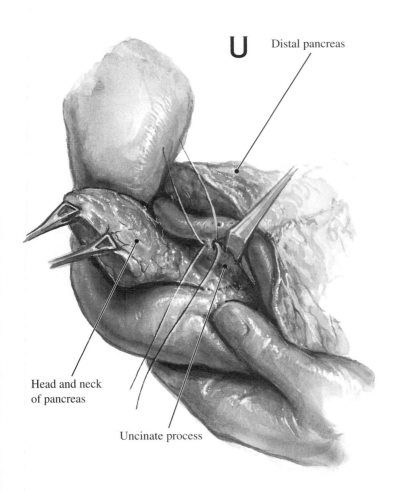

S

The pancreas is now divided. Digital pressure is effective for temporary hemostasis while these vessels are secured with transfixion stitches of 3-0 silk. The pancreatic duct likely will be dilated, and the fluid within it may be under increased pressure.

T

The head of the pancreas is reflected laterally, permitting ligation and division of tributaries from the superior mesenteric vein.

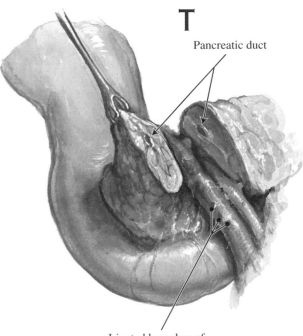

T

Pancreatic duct

Ligated branches of superior mesenteric v.

U Distal pancreas

Head and neck of pancreas

Uncinate process

U

Continued reflection of the head and neck of the divided pancreas to the patient's right and gentle traction on the superior mesenteric vein to the left with a vein retractor facilitate a safe, swift dissection of the uncinate process.

V

The fourth portion of the duodenum and the first portion of the jejunum are mobilized by first dividing the ligament of Treitz. Here this is shown being done from the left of the superior mesenteric vessels. However, gentle traction of the jejunum toward the right from the right side and under the superior mesenteric artery and vein permits a similar dissection.

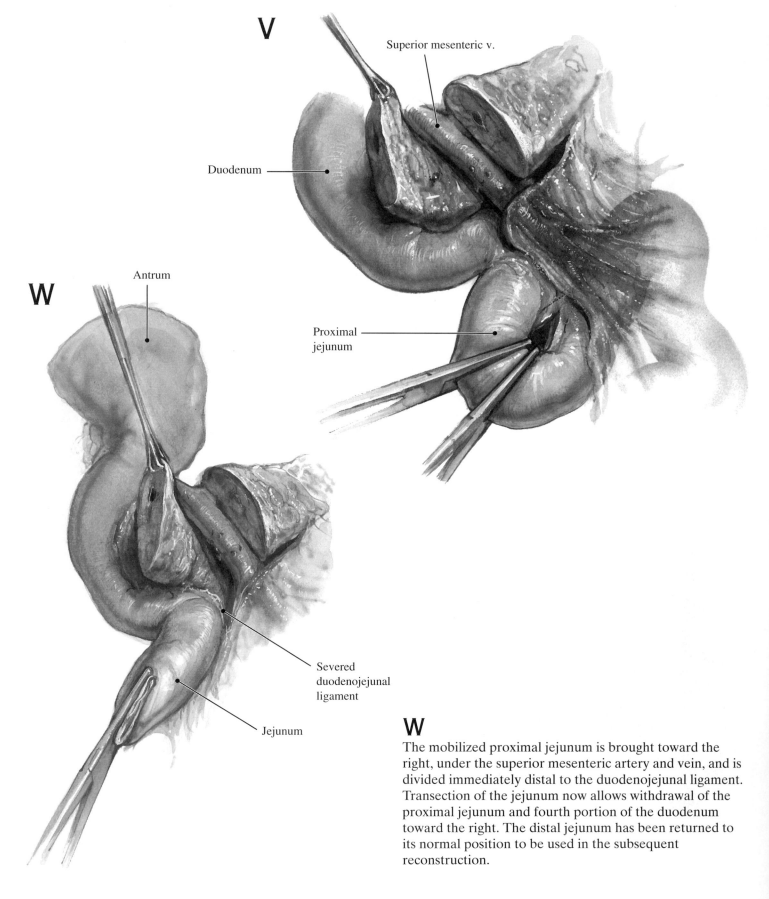

V

Superior mesenteric v.

Duodenum

Proximal jejunum

W

Antrum

Severed duodenojejunal ligament

Jejunum

W

The mobilized proximal jejunum is brought toward the right, under the superior mesenteric artery and vein, and is divided immediately distal to the duodenojejunal ligament. Transection of the jejunum now allows withdrawal of the proximal jejunum and fourth portion of the duodenum toward the right. The distal jejunum has been returned to its normal position to be used in the subsequent reconstruction.

X

The resective part of the operation is complete. In this illustration, the distal stomach, the head and neck of the pancreas, all of the duodenum, some of the proximal jejunum, the gallbladder, the distal common duct, and the accompanying lymph nodes are absent.

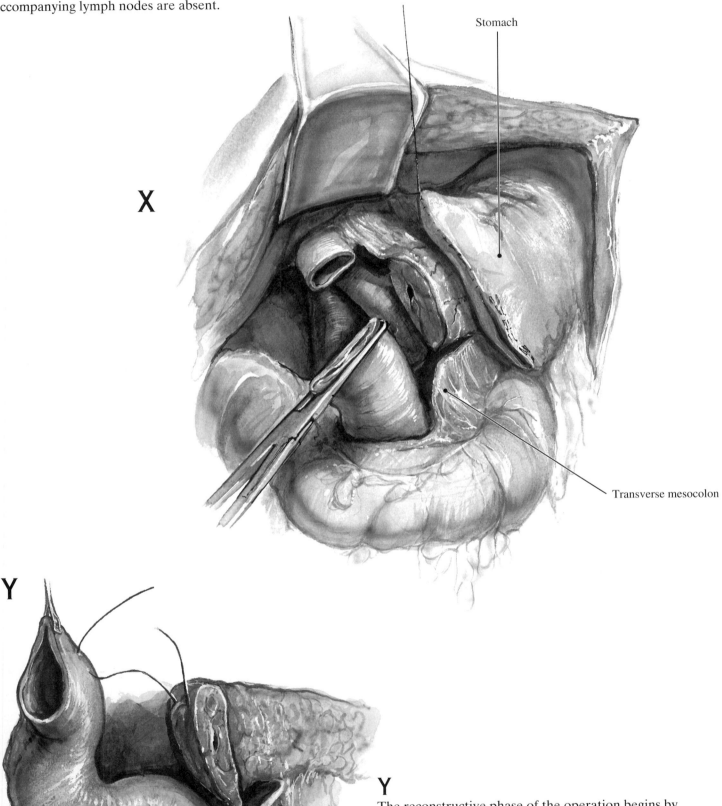

X

Stomach

Transverse mesocolon

Y

Y

The reconstructive phase of the operation begins by passing the proximal jejunum through the mesenteric window. An end-to-end pancreaticojejunostomy is preferred; this anastomosis is performed first. The transected end of the pancreas is inspected and further mobilized as necessary so that the free margin of pancreas measures approximately 2 cm.

Z

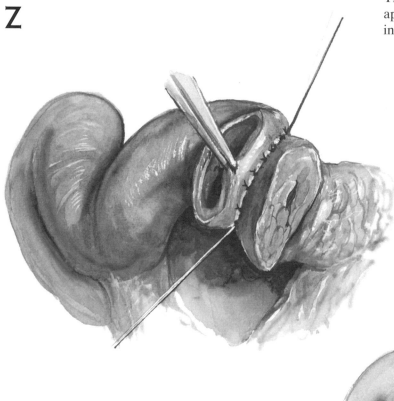

Z, AA

The posterior surfaces of the jejunum and the pancreas are approximated about 1 cm from their respective edges with interrupted stitches of 3-0 black silk.

AA

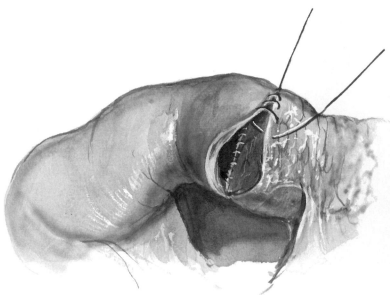

BB

The jejunal mucosa and the capsule of the divided pancreas are approximated with a continuous stitch of atraumatic 3-0 silk.

BB

CC

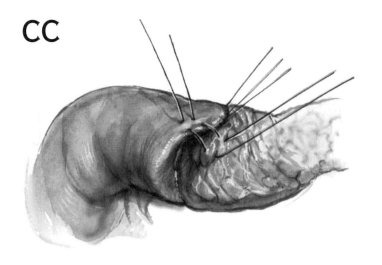

DD

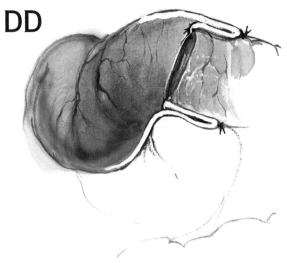

CC, DD

The second anterior row of pancreaticojejunal stitches continues with interrupted atraumatic 3-0 black silk. Stitches also are placed 1 cm back from the respective free edges that engage the seromuscular edge of the jejunum and the capsule of the pancreas. This causes "telescoping" of the free edges so that they lie within the jejunum, creating a broader interface between the pancreas and jejunum.

EE

Pancreaticojejunostomy

FF

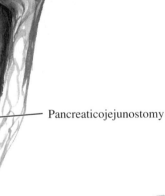

EE, FF

The end-to-side choledochojejunostomy is performed next in two layers. A posterior row of interrupted simple stitches using 4-0 Maxon is followed by a second layer using continuous 4-0 Maxon to appose the mucosa. A continuous suture technique is superior to interrupted stitches because it offers protection against leakage. If the duct is dilated and the walls are thick, the continuous technique can be used in one layer with permanent suture material.

GG

The gastrojejunostomy is performed in two layers—the seromuscular with a continuous stitch using 3-0 silk and the mucosal with a similar stitch of atraumatic 4-0 Maxon. The mesocolic defect is repaired with interrupted stitches of 4-0 Maxon to prevent internal herniation. There should be a sufficient length of jejunum distal to the choledochojejunal anastomosis to prevent the retrograde passage of food up and into the biliary radicles. Ordinarily, a loop of about 25 cm suffices.

GG

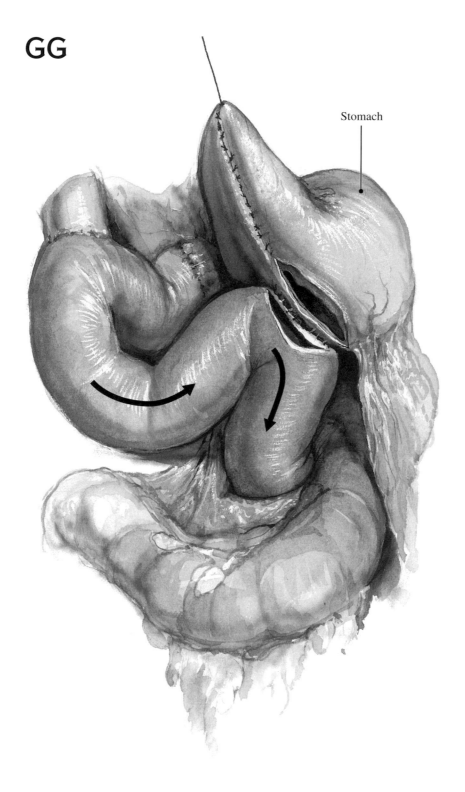

Stomach

HH

The completed operation is shown. Two medium-sized suction tubes are placed adjacent to the pancreaticojejunostomy and include the two other anastomoses in their sweep. They are exteriorized through a counterincision in the right upper quadrant. The incision is closed in a routine manner.

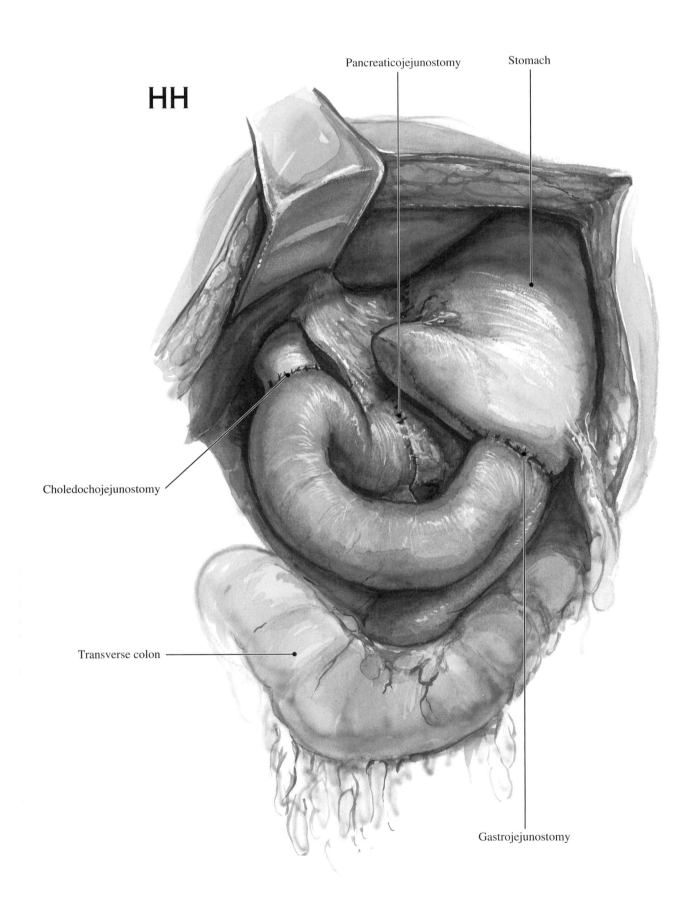

HH

Pancreaticojejunostomy

Stomach

Choledochojejunostomy

Transverse colon

Gastrojejunostomy

B PANCREATICOJEJUNOSTOMY

A

A variety of operations have been devised to relieve pancreatic duct obstruction. This illustration shows the anatomic relationships among the organs that are important in the performance of this operation. The spleen hugs the tail of the pancreas closely, making splenectomy necessary for the several types of pancreaticojejunostomy performed.

The superior mesenteric vein is vulnerable to injury when the pancreas is mobilized. The splenic artery runs along the upper border of the pancreas, giving off branches to the pancreas, with the splenic vein just below the artery. The superior mesenteric artery and vein mark the point to which the pancreas should be mobilized even though the limb of jejunum that will envelop the pancreas will extend farther to the patient's right.

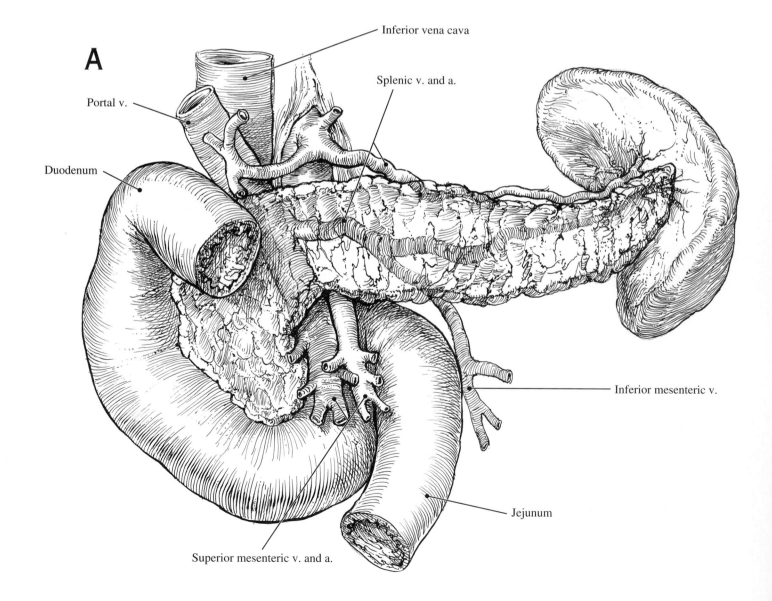

A

Inferior vena cava

Splenic v. and a.

Portal v.

Duodenum

Inferior mesenteric v.

Jejunum

Superior mesenteric v. and a.

B

Many patients with chronic pancreatitis have had previous operations that will influence the abdominal incision to be used. The preferred incision is midline. Portal hypertension, especially in association with adhesions from any previous operation, can make even this incision time consuming. An exploration of the opened abdomen is carried out with particular attention given to the liver and the extrahepatic biliary system.

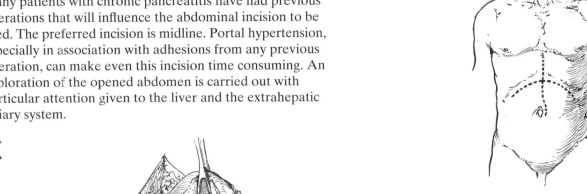

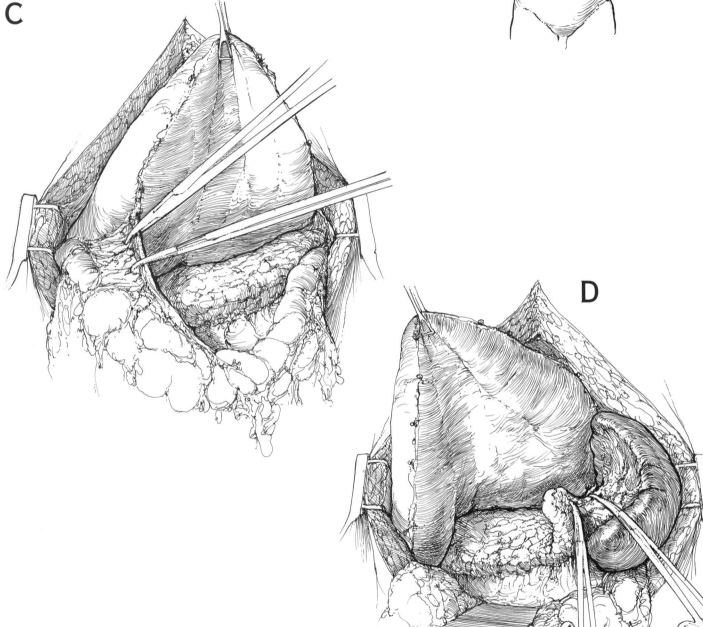

C

The stomach is freed along the greater curvature by separating it from the omentum. This is done by dividing along the relatively avascular area peripheral to the gastroepiploic vessels and extending from the angula incisura of the stomach on the right to the short gastric vessels on the left. Adhesions between the posterior aspect of the stomach and the anterior surface of the pancreas are more numerous than usual but can be lysed without difficulty.

D

The vascular supply to the spleen is interrupted with the spleen in situ or after it has been delivered into the wound, depending on the severity of the perisplenic adhesions. The lesser tributaries are ligated first and then divided. The main vessels can be isolated and divided individually as shown, with tailoring at a later time when the tip of the pancreas is amputated.

E

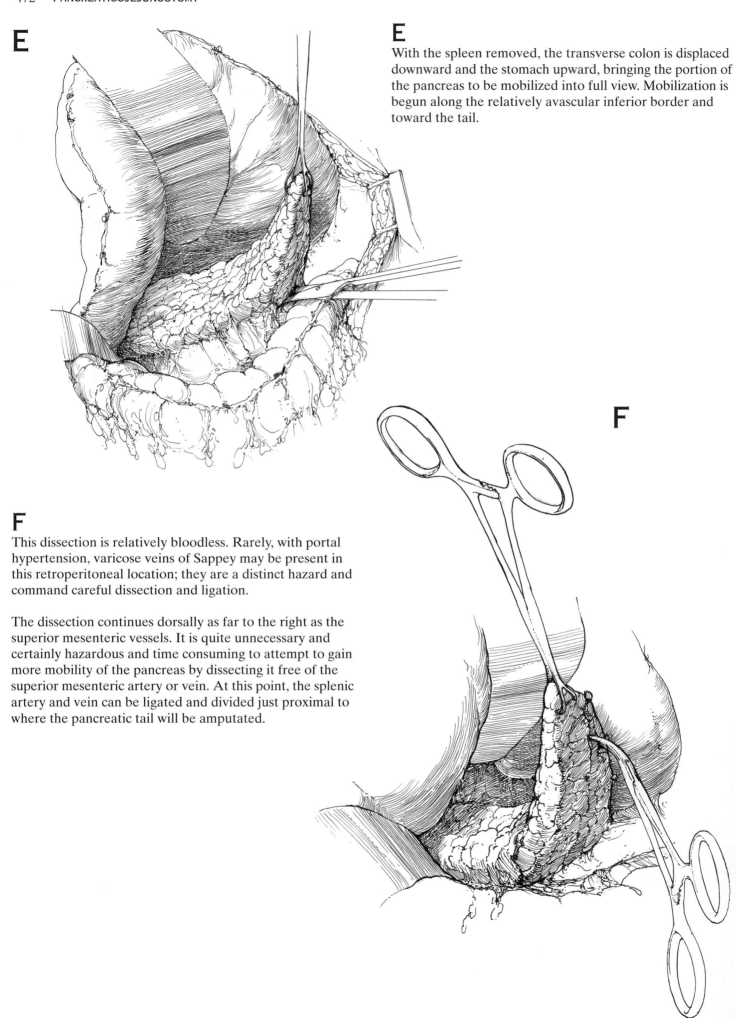

E

With the spleen removed, the transverse colon is displaced downward and the stomach upward, bringing the portion of the pancreas to be mobilized into full view. Mobilization is begun along the relatively avascular inferior border and toward the tail.

F

This dissection is relatively bloodless. Rarely, with portal hypertension, varicose veins of Sappey may be present in this retroperitoneal location; they are a distinct hazard and command careful dissection and ligation.

The dissection continues dorsally as far to the right as the superior mesenteric vessels. It is quite unnecessary and certainly hazardous and time consuming to attempt to gain more mobility of the pancreas by dissecting it free of the superior mesenteric artery or vein. At this point, the splenic artery and vein can be ligated and divided just proximal to where the pancreatic tail will be amputated.

F

G

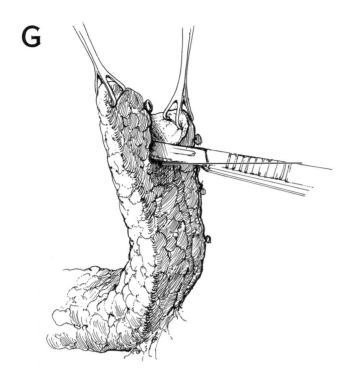

The pancreas is amputated 1 to 2 cm from the tip. Pressure by the fingers of the left hand is the best means of obtaining temporary hemostasis. With periodic release of this pressure, individual bleeding points are detected and secured. The pancreatic duct is usually dilated and can be seen easily, or its presence is indicated by a spurt of pancreatic juice under pressure. Although a dilated duct is almost always found if the surgeon is persistent, further transverse incisions in the tail may be necessary to locate the duct.

H

When the pancreatic duct is found, a blunt-tipped probe is used to determine its direction and degree of patency. There is no point in continuing to probe if an early constriction is met, as the extent of disease will be defined in the subsequent steps.

H

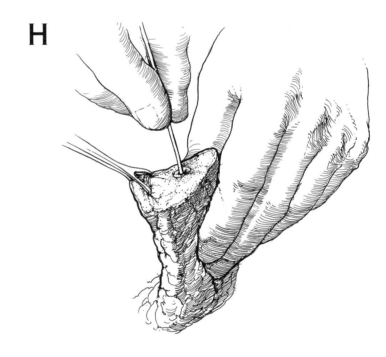

I

With a probe in place, the duct can be opened as illustrated with cautery or with a blunt-tipped scissors. Because the stenotic portions of the duct may be quite narrow, the surgeon must be forceful yet gentle when advancing the scissors. Digital compression remains the most effective way to maintain hemostasis as individual bleeding points along the duct are secured with suture-ligatures of atraumatic 4-0 Maxon. This step continues until the duct is opened to a point at which it appears normal; this usually means going to the right of the superior mesenteric vessels and reaching the ducts of Wirsung and Santorini. If diffuse bleeding occurs along the cut edge of the pancreas, it can be controlled effectively with a continuous suture of atraumatic catgut.

I

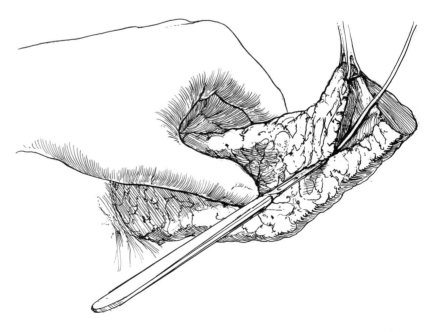

J

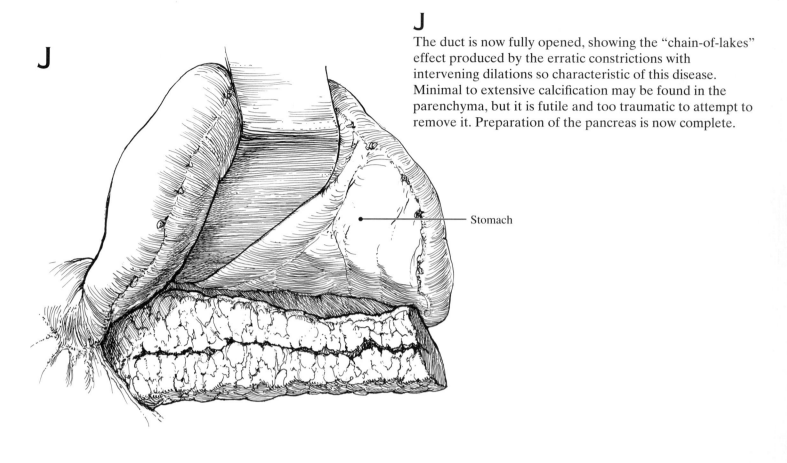

J

The duct is now fully opened, showing the "chain-of-lakes" effect produced by the erratic constrictions with intervening dilations so characteristic of this disease. Minimal to extensive calcification may be found in the parenchyma, but it is futile and too traumatic to attempt to remove it. Preparation of the pancreas is now complete.

Stomach

K

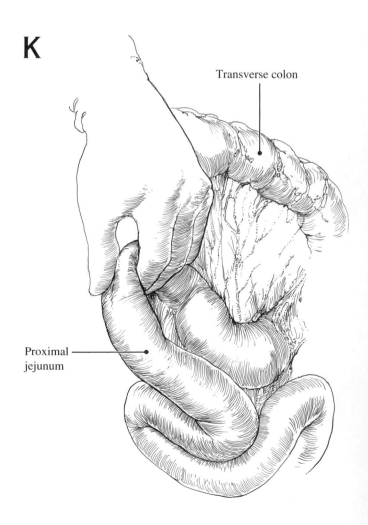

Transverse colon

Proximal jejunum

K

The transverse colon is reflected upward, and the proximal jejunum about 20 cm from the ligament of Treitz is prepared for division. The clamp to be placed on the distal jejunal limb is brought through a window in the avascular portion of the transverse mesocolon, just as it is to be brought back again through this window. This window should not constrict the vasculature of the jejunum passing through it.

L

Some guidance and traction of the transected tail of the pancreas into the jejunum are necessary for the remainder of the procedure. Here, a suture of 3-0 chromic catgut is placed in the pancreas. The needle is held with the point on the convex side of the curved needle holder. It can thus be advanced smoothly inside the jejunum. This distance is predetermined and should exceed by at least several centimeters the length of unroofed pancreatic duct; if this distance is too short, it will thwart the surgeon's attempt to pull the jejunum far enough to the right. The needle holder is now turned so that the point of the needle can be brought through the bowel wall. Both ends of the traction suture may be brought through in the manner shown, or the ends may be brought through separately. In the latter case the ends can be tied and thus will serve as an anchoring suture.

L

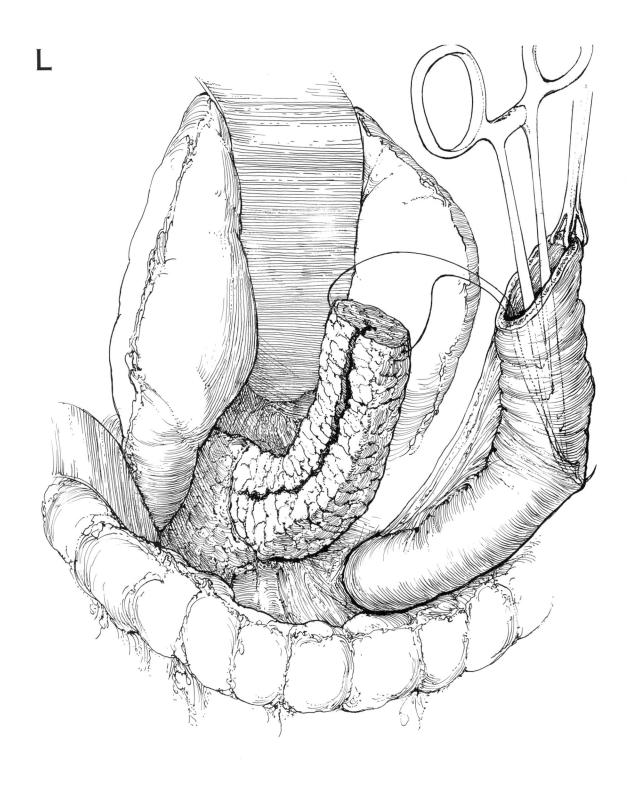

M

The suture attached to the pancreas is held while the accordion-like jejunum, which is beginning to envelop the pancreas, is gently pulled toward the right.

M

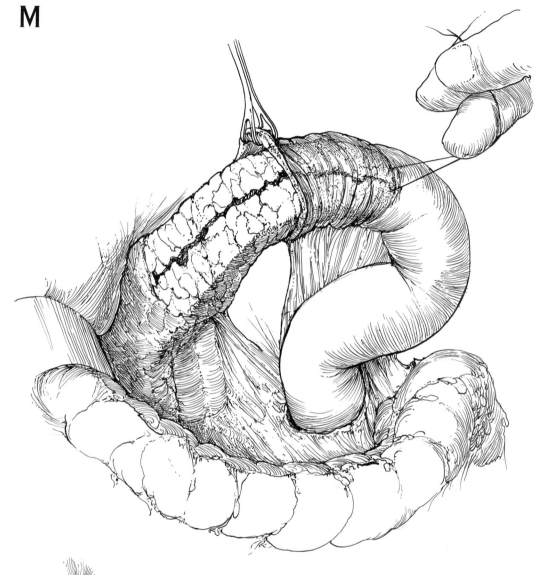

N

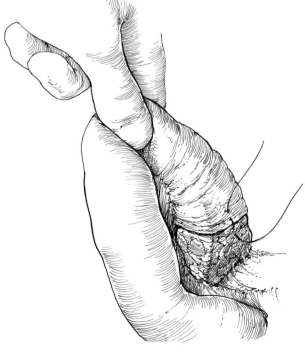

N

The free end of the jejunum is anchored to the pancreas at a point to the right of the unroofed duct with interrupted sutures of atraumatic 3-0 black silk placed about 1 cm apart. The superior mesenteric vessels may sometimes prevent the surgeon from bringing the jejunum far enough to the right, leaving the unroofed cut at the head of the pancreas uncovered. In such a case, the jejunum can be fish-mouthed at the point it comes in contact with the vessels. A slit several centimeters long is usually sufficient for moving the jejunum centrally the several centimeters necessary to cover all the exposed duct. When the placement of sutures on the ventral surface has been completed, the jejunum and pancreas are reflected toward the right and the jejunum sutured to the dorsal surface of the pancreas in a similar fashion.

O

The pancreaticojejunostomy has been completed and the jejunum returned to its normal position. An end-to-side jejunojejunostomy is performed in as proximal a position as possible. A suction drain is placed at the site of the pancreaticojejunostomy and exteriorized through a counterincision. The abdominal incision is closed in the usual fashion.

O

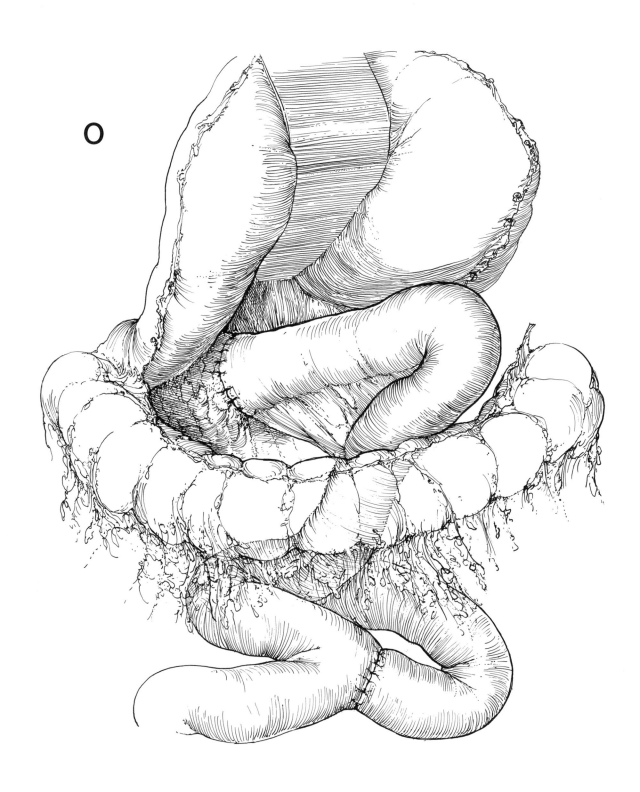

P

The main advantage of side-to-side pancreaticojejunostomy shown here is that the spleen and the tail of the pancreas are not removed. Also, involved pancreatic duct to the right of the superior mesenteric vessels can be uncovered and incorporated in the pancreaticojejunostomy. The suture line is longer and more apt to leak. Nonetheless, this procedure is becoming the clear favorite.

P

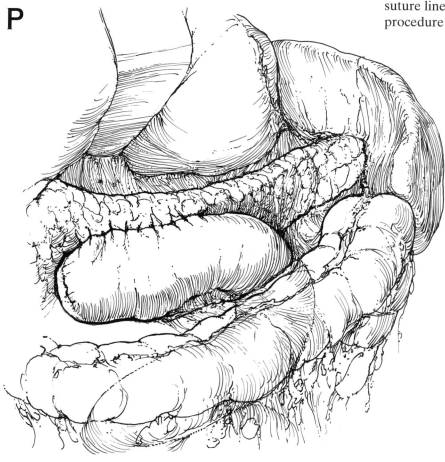

Q

This early operation was used to drain the pancreatic duct in a retrograde direction. It fails to relieve the obstructions created by the chain-of-lakes effect and thus does not relieve the patient's symptoms.

Q

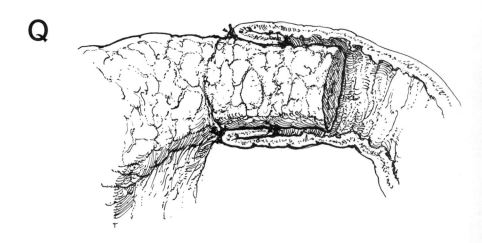

C PANCREATIC CYSTS

A

Pancreatic pseudocyst can occur secondary to infection or trauma anywhere in the pancreas. As can be seen in this panoramic illustration, the pancreas is in intimate proximity to the stomach and duodenum, so most internal drainage procedures are into these organs. Occasionally, a Roux-en-Y limb needs to be brought up; rarely a cystectomy is performed.

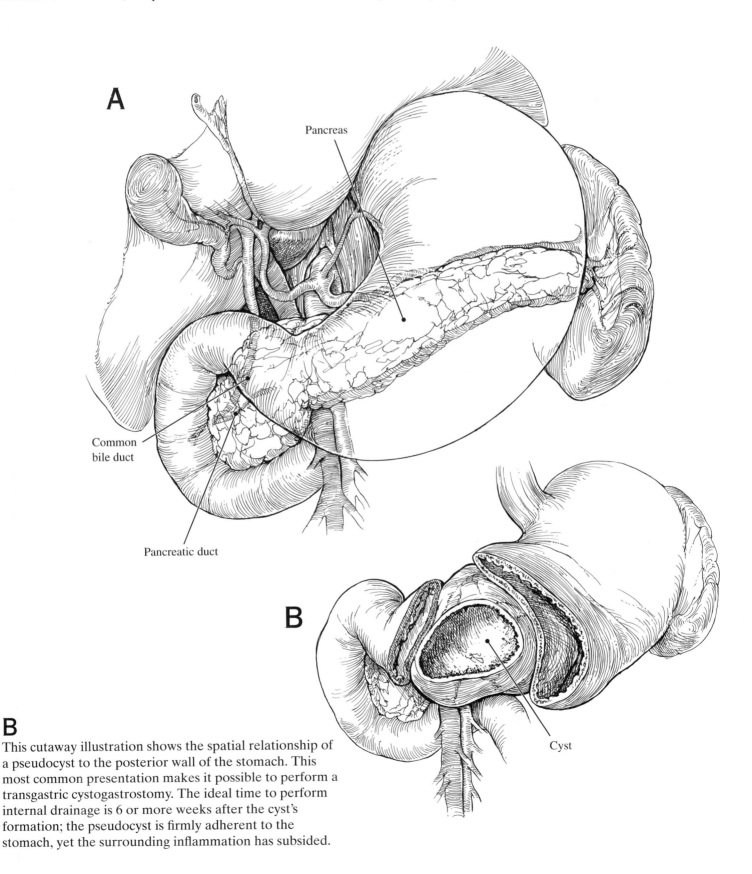

A

Pancreas

Common bile duct

Pancreatic duct

B

Cyst

B

This cutaway illustration shows the spatial relationship of a pseudocyst to the posterior wall of the stomach. This most common presentation makes it possible to perform a transgastric cystogastrostomy. The ideal time to perform internal drainage is 6 or more weeks after the cyst's formation; the pseudocyst is firmly adherent to the stomach, yet the surrounding inflammation has subsided.

CYSTOGASTROSTOMY

C, D

Two Babcock forceps are applied to the anterior wall of the stomach at a point directly over the bulge caused by the pseudocyst. Once the length of the incision is adequate for easy visibility, two additional Babcock forceps are applied and retracted, exposing the posterior wall of the stomach.

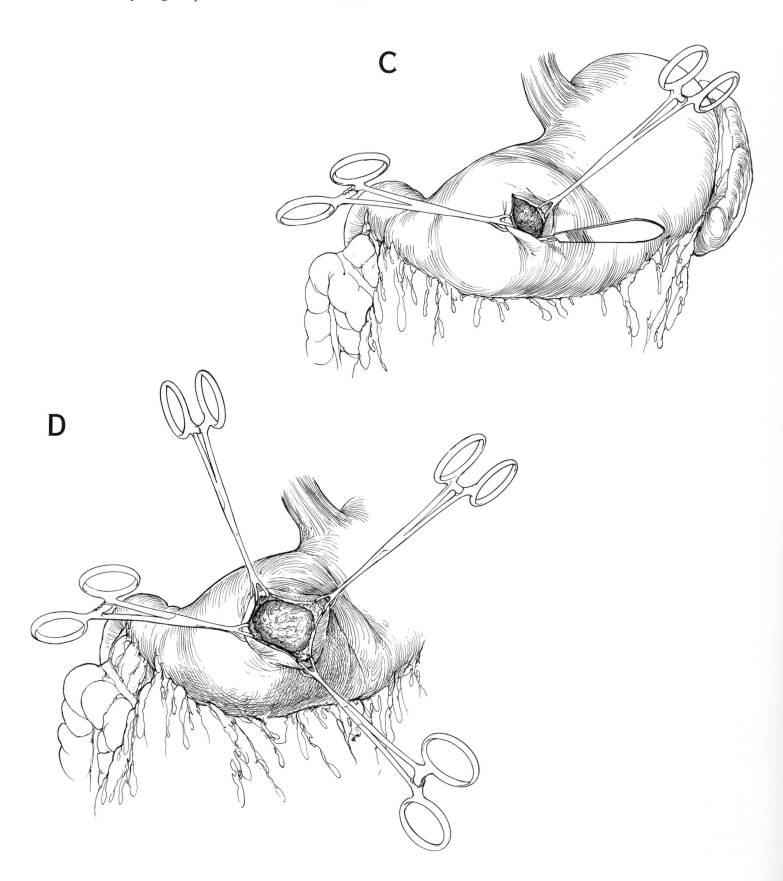

C

D

E

Although preoperative tests and intraoperative palpation provide assurance that a pseudocyst lies deep to the posterior wall of the stomach, aspiration with a needle is used to confirm this.

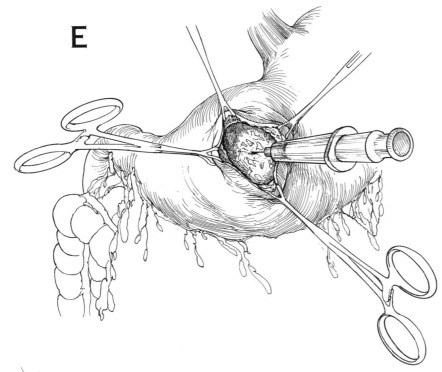

F

Fine-tipped electrocautery is used for formal entry into the pseudocyst, which is emptied of its contents by suction. A disk of tissue containing stomach and pancreas is excised and sent to a pathologist for examination; rarely, it may show cystadenocarcinoma.

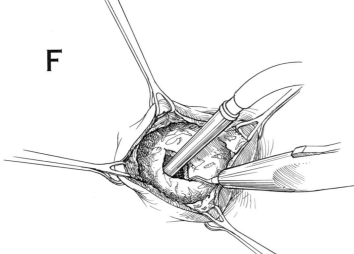

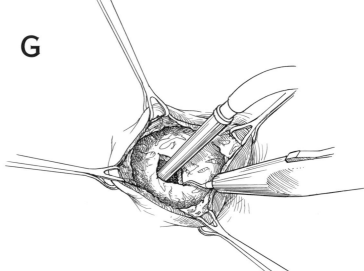

G

The rim of the newly created opening is oversewn with interrupted stitches of 4-0 Maxon. This ensures that the stomach and pseudocyst remain fused to each other. Also, it provides any necessary hemostasis both acutely and even later, should there be progression of the necrotic process.

H

This cutaway illustration demonstrates the completed cystogastrostomy. The opening between the two cavities need not be excessively large. The pseudocyst collapses readily, with minimal risk that it will act as a cesspool for stomach contents that have found their way into it.

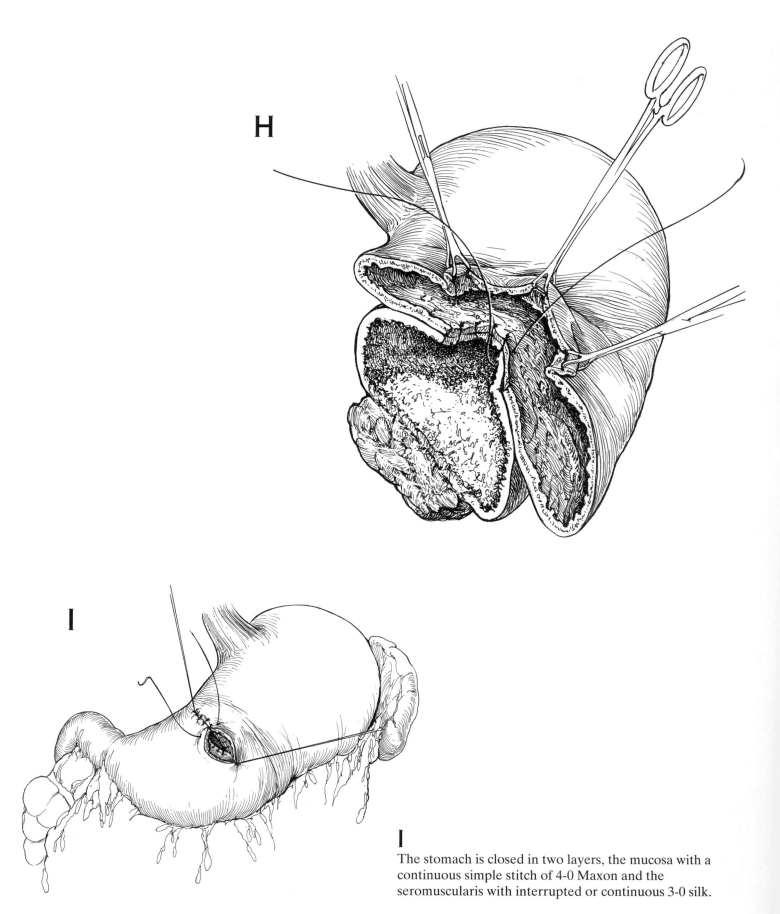

I

The stomach is closed in two layers, the mucosa with a continuous simple stitch of 4-0 Maxon and the seromuscularis with interrupted or continuous 3-0 silk.

CYSTODUODENOSTOMY

A

In this operative setting, draining the pseudocyst into the duodenum is the preferred procedure. The pseudocyst and the duodenum are closely apposed in preparation for a cystoduodenostomy.

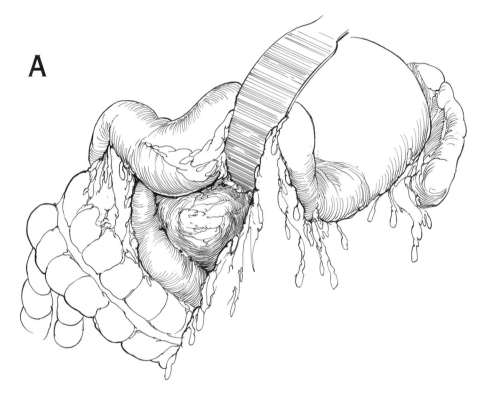

A

B

As in the previous setting, successful aspiration of the pancreatic mass will confirm that it is a pseudocyst.

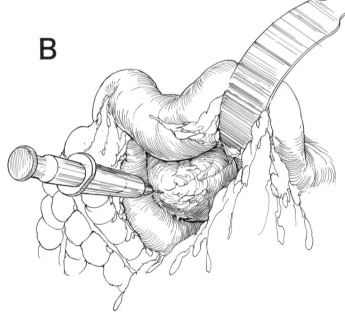

B

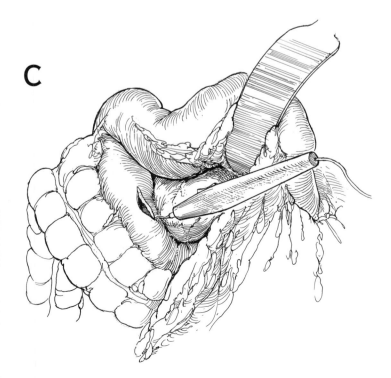

C

C

The duodenum is opened longitudinally and in an area intimately opposite the pseudocyst. This will be the area of anastomosis.

D

In this instance, the determination is made that stenosis of the terminal pancreatic duct is a contributing factor to the problem and that a sphincterotomy should be performed. A small rubber catheter is inserted into the terminal duct and advanced retrogradely.

D

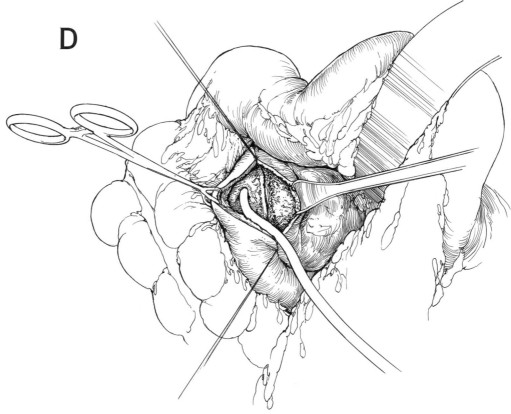

E

The posterior suture line of the cystoduodenostomy is constructed with 3-0 silk and includes all layers.

E

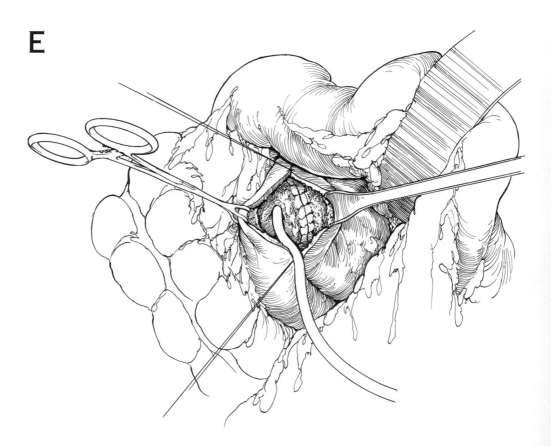

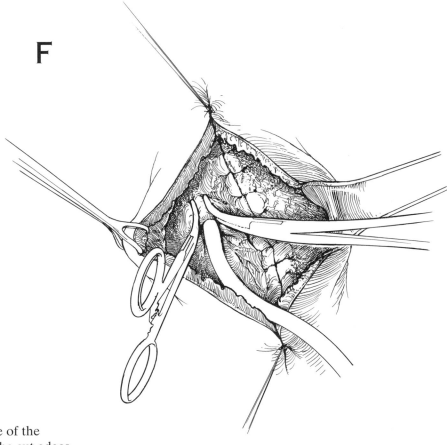

F

F, G

An Adson hemostat is positioned on either side of the
tube, and the tissue between them is divided. The cut edges
of the now patulous sphincter of Oddi are sewn as one
layer with interrupted simple stitches of 4-0 Maxon.

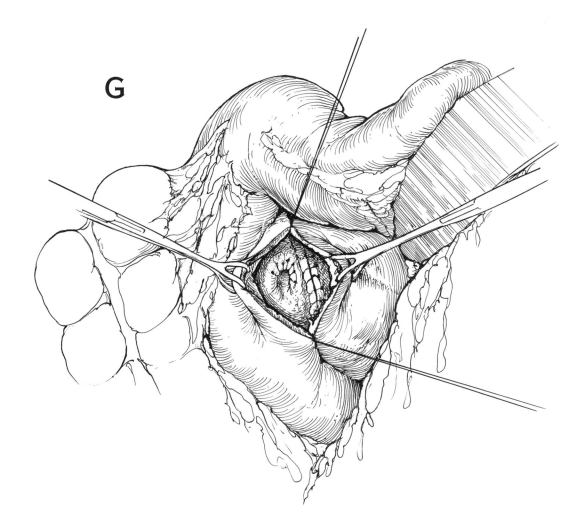

G

H

The anterior anastomosis of simple, interrupted stitches of
3-0 silk completes the anastomosis of the
cystoduodenostomy.

H

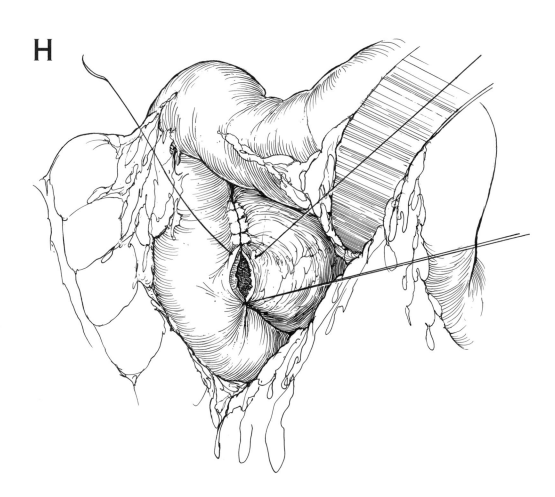

CYSTOJEJUNOSTOMY

A

In the case of a cystojejunostomy, the lack of pliability of the pseudocyst or of adequate tissue to invert for a two-layer anastomosis actually makes it safer to do it in one layer. It is done with interrupted simple stitches of 3-0 silk.

A

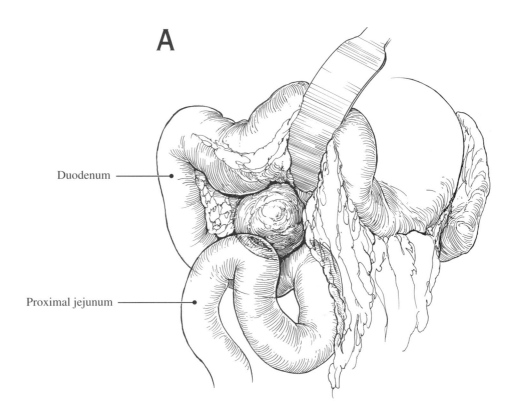

Duodenum

Proximal jejunum

B

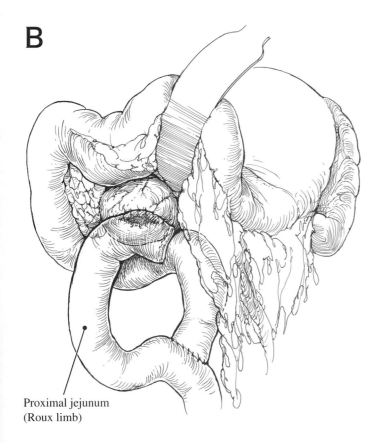

Proximal jejunum
(Roux limb)

B

When performing a Roux-en-Y cystojejunostomy, a segment of jejunum approximately 20 cm from the ligament of Treitz is divided with a linear stapler. The distal limb is brought up to the pseudocyst and anastomosed as one layer with interrupted simple stitches of 3-0 silk. The jejunojejunostomy is done with a continuous mucosal stitch of 3-0 chromic catgut and the serosal one with interrupted simple stitches of 3-0 silk.

CYSTECTOMY

A

Very uncommonly, it is best to excise the cyst. In the example shown in this illustration, the very tail of the pancreas and hilum of the spleen are affected. The splenocolic ligament is divided, some vessels therein requiring ligation with 3-0 silk. The splenic artery and vein are secured with a vascular clamp and oversewn with fine suture material. The method of pancreas division depends on the thickness of the pancreas in this area. For a thin pancreas, stapling and division followed by oversewing of the divided tissue with fine vascular suture material are satisfactory. For a thicker pancreas the division is by scalpel, and individual vessels are suture ligated with fine vascular suture material. A heavy vascular suture material is chosen to oversew the transected pancreas. Sometimes small-vessel oozing can be controlled only by oversewing the full thickness of the pancreas with heavier monofilament suture material.

A

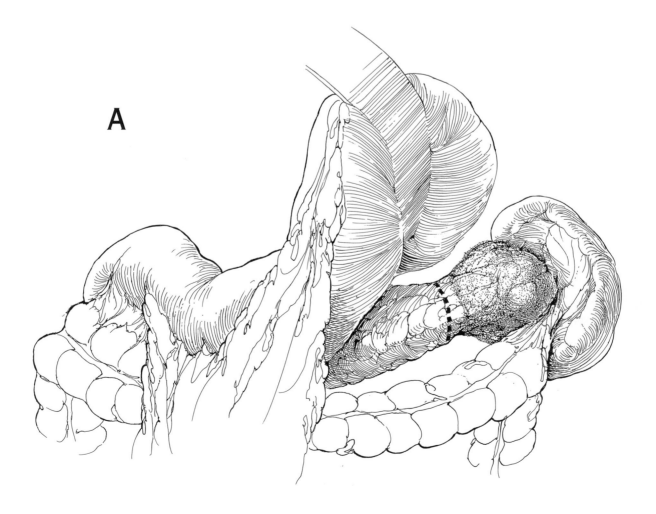

Chapter

21

PORTAL VENOUS SYSTEM

A PORTACAVAL SHUNT

Portal hypertension is a syndrome caused by an increase in portal pressure, leading to esophagogastric varices, splenomegaly, and often ascites. An increase in pressure occurs in the portal system proximal to any obstruction within it. Based on the site of obstruction, portal hypertension is classified as suprahepatic, intrahepatic, or subhepatic.

The surgical treatment of portal hypertension has been directed primarily toward the control of bleeding from esophageal varices and to a much lesser degree toward the control of intractable ascites and severe hypersplenism associated with cirrhosis. The specific procedures used are influenced by the dynamics of portal vein flow and other associated symptoms and findings.

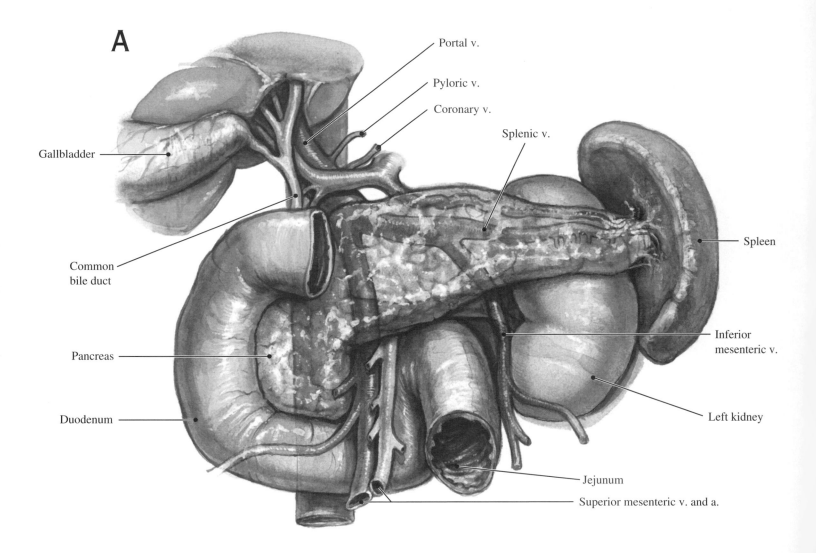

A

Frequently a portacaval shunt must be done on patients already quite ill, so only minimal error in surgical judgment or technique can be tolerated. The surgeon, therefore, must be well versed in the anatomy of this area, the physiologic dynamics of the portal system, and the demanding technical requirements.

The splenic and superior mesenteric veins meet dorsal to the pancreas to form the portal vein, which continues as such for 6 to 7 cm before dividing into left and right branches, each immediately entering the liver. It remains singular in only 10% of patients. The diameter of the portal vein is normally about 1 cm but may be greater in a patient with portal hypertension. Approximately two thirds of the time it is entered into by the coronary and pyloric veins, which form a loop that hugs the lesser curvature of the stomach and receives branches, or is a continuation of the left gastric vein, the esophageal plexus, or the short gastric veins. Whatever tributaries the portal vein has enter on its medial side.

B

The patient is placed in the supine position, and general anesthesia with endotracheal intubation is employed. A subcostal incision is used, sometimes skewed to the right or the left side. The distance from the subcostal margin is dictated by the position of the lower border of the liver.

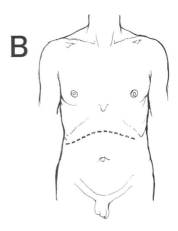

B

C

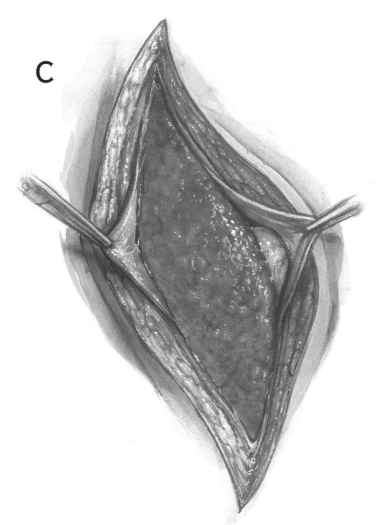

C

Almost invariably, free fluid is found in the peritoneal cavity, even in patients not being operated on for relief of ascites. The usual thorough exploration of the peritoneal cavity is carried out, and the surgeon remains alert to the possibility of a multicentric hepatic malignancy, which can be missed in an already nodular liver. Because ulcers are frequently seen in patients with portal hypertension, the duodenum deserves special attention. If stones are found within the gallbladder, a cholecystectomy should be performed at the conclusion of the operation. This should be done with scrupulous care as there can be troublesome bleeding from the gallbladder fossa. If a liver biopsy is contemplated, it should be obtained earlier rather than later in the course of the operation because the handling of the liver may produce factitious microscopic changes.

D

D

The portal venous pressure is taken at this time through a portal tributary, usually a mesenteric vein. A disposable spinal tap manometer is adequate. The needle is inserted into an exposed vein, and the patency of the saline-filled manometer is determined by fluctuations consonant with respirations. Readings are obtained in at least two vessels.

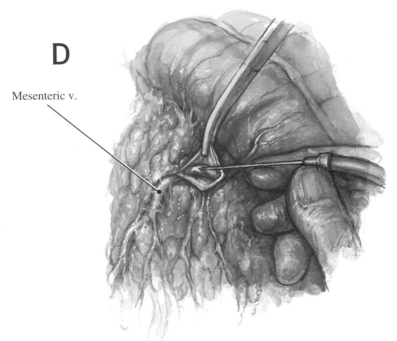

Mesenteric v.

E

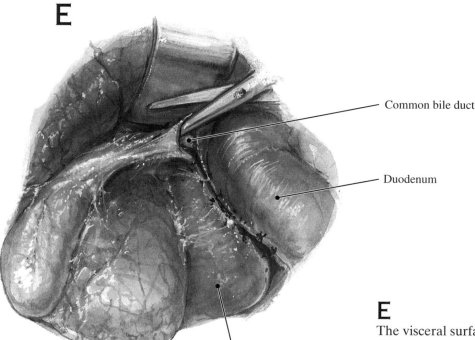

Common bile duct

Duodenum

Posterior parietal peritoneum

E

The visceral surface of the liver is covered with two thicknesses of moist laparotomy pads and retracted cephalad with a wide Deaver retractor. Often a distended gallbladder hampers development of the exposure, but with pressure from the retractors it gradually empties. The hepatic flexure of the colon and the small bowel are retracted caudally. The portal vein can be assessed further and located bidigitally with the index finger within and the thumb over the foramen of Winslow. The turgid vessel can be compressed but refills quickly. The duodenum is mobilized only if necessary. Whereas the posterior parietal peritoneum lateral to the duodenum is ordinarily avascular and can be cut without concern for prolonged bleeding, the collateral veins and venules in such patients create just such a problem. In the drawing, the peritoneum over the portal triad is being cut so that mobilization of the portal vein can begin.

F

The portal vein lies medial and dorsal to the common bile duct and the hepatic artery. These structures run along the right border of the gastrohepatic ligament. The arrow points to the foramen of Winslow. Considerable fibroadipose tissue and some lymph nodes may be found on the intestinal side of the portal vein. This illustration shows how dissection of the portal vein may be carried out by retracting the common bile duct and hepatic artery medially and anteriorly for adequate exposure without performing any dissection on the hepatic artery or common bile duct.

F

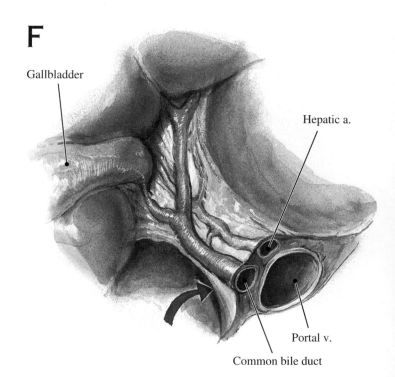

Gallbladder

Hepatic a.

Portal v.

Common bile duct

G

A small soft rubber drain or vessel loop is passed around the portal vein and will be used for gentle retraction to expose the various surfaces of the vein. The parietal peritoneum over the vena cava is incised and dissected free with scissors, and the vena cava is exposed from the level of the renal vein and upward to the liver. Occasionally, collateral vessels coursing through this layer can lead to troublesome bleeding and may require ligation. It is not advisable to expose the posterior and medial surfaces of the vena cava, as to do so may incite unnecessary bleeding.

G

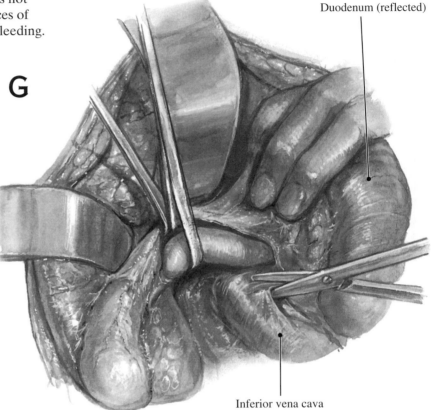

Duodenum (reflected)

Inferior vena cava

H

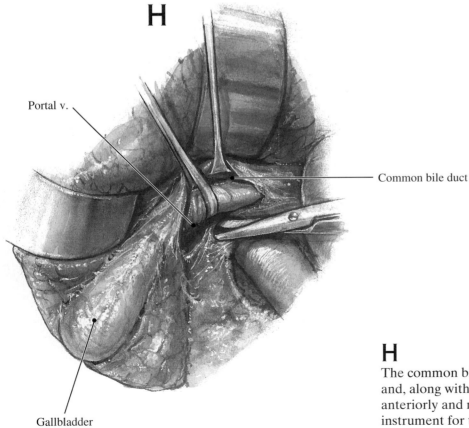

Portal v.

Common bile duct

Gallbladder

H

The common bile duct has been freed from the portal vein and, along with the hepatic artery, is being retracted anteriorly and medially with long vein retractors, the ideal instrument for this.

I

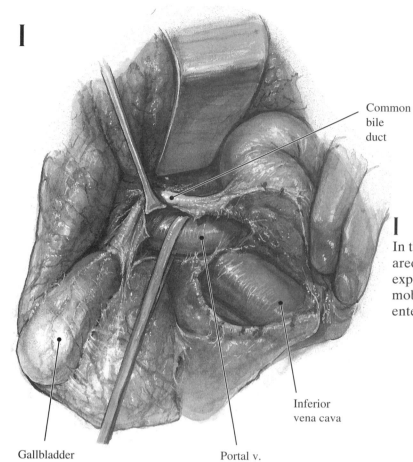

Common bile duct

Inferior vena cava

Gallbladder   Portal v.

I

In the retroduodenal area there may be excessive fatty areolar lymphatic tissue that has to be excised for proper exposure and mobilization. The portal vein is cautiously mobilized circumferentially. The coronary and pyloric veins enter on its medial side.

J

Gallbladder

Inferior vena cava

J

A straight or angled Potts arterial clamp is applied to the intestinal side of the portal vein so that the anastomosis can be performed without tension and with the proper sweep and angle of union with the vena cava. For this reason, the portal vein must be secured as close to the liver as possible. This can be done easily and quickly with a ligature of 2-0 silk; greater safety, probably without additional sacrifice of vein, can be achieved with closure using a continuous stitch of fine monofilament vascular suture.

K, L

Sometimes an enlarged caudate lobe covers the vena cava in such a fashion that it is necessary to bend the portal vein excessively for it to meet the vena cava at a more caudal site. This causes it to kink—a condition that is certain to lead to failure of the procedure and is obviously unacceptable. Before removing a portion of the caudate lobe, it must be freed from the underlying vena cava. A "peanut" dissector can be used to tease apart the liver and vena cava while also looking for and securing one or two pairs of short veins entering this portion of the liver from the vena cava.

K

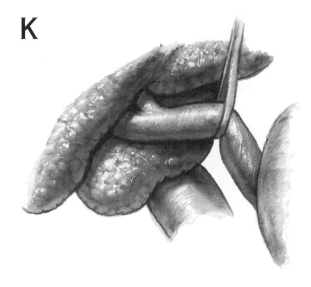

L

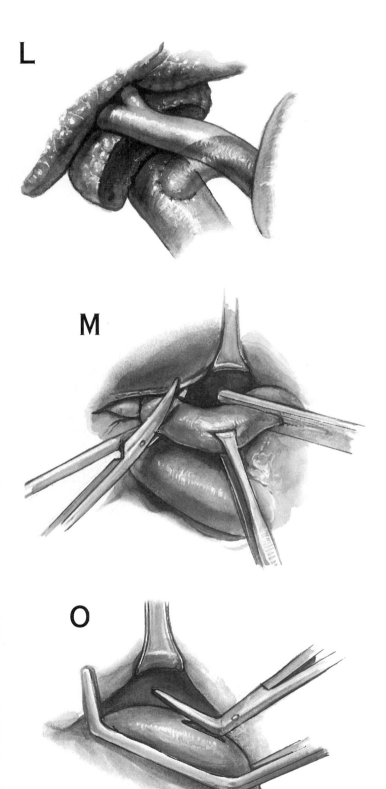

M

The Potts clamp is applied first as close as possible on the intestinal side of the portal vein, and the tie on the liver side is secured. The portal vein is divided cleanly, leaving a 3-mm cuff on the liver side.

N, O, P

A Satinsky clamp is used to isolate that portion of the inferior vena cava that can best meet with the portal vein. Although an oval piece of vena cava can be cut out straight away, the more deliberate method shown is more accurate. *N* and *O* show the opening of the vena cava, which in *P* is being fashioned into an oval that will accommodate the portal vein. The oval is on the long axis of the vena cava. A simple slit in the vena cava has long since been found to be undesirable and is more likely to become occluded. The open vessels are flushed with heparinized saline.

M

N

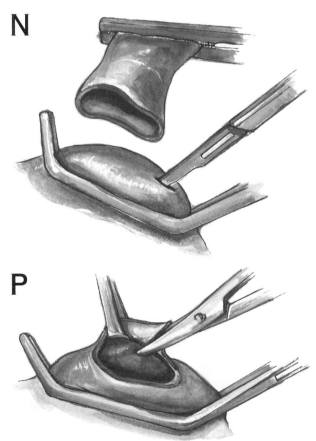

O

P

Q, R, S, T

There are a number of proper and adequate vascular anastomotic techniques; the surgeon will choose the most comfortable one. The stitches are begun on the far or medial sides of the vessels. The two separate strands, or one double-needle strand, of atraumatic 4-0 monofilament suture material are used and so placed that all knots are on the outside. A simple stitch is used. An assistant is charged with holding the Potts and the Satinsky clamps so that there is no tension on the suture line. At one of the corners (*S*), an everting Connell stitch is used so that as the separate strands approach from each end (*T*) they are looping in opposite directions; when they are tied there is no distortion, as is seen when tying strands that have terminated on the same side of a vessel. The guide sutures (*R*) that can be applied before or immediately after beginning the anastomosis (*Q*) are not utilized in the anastomosis. In performing venous anastomoses, it is particularly important that sutures be placed accurately and proper tension be maintained so that a minimum of suture material is "free" inside the lumen to increase the risk of clot formation.

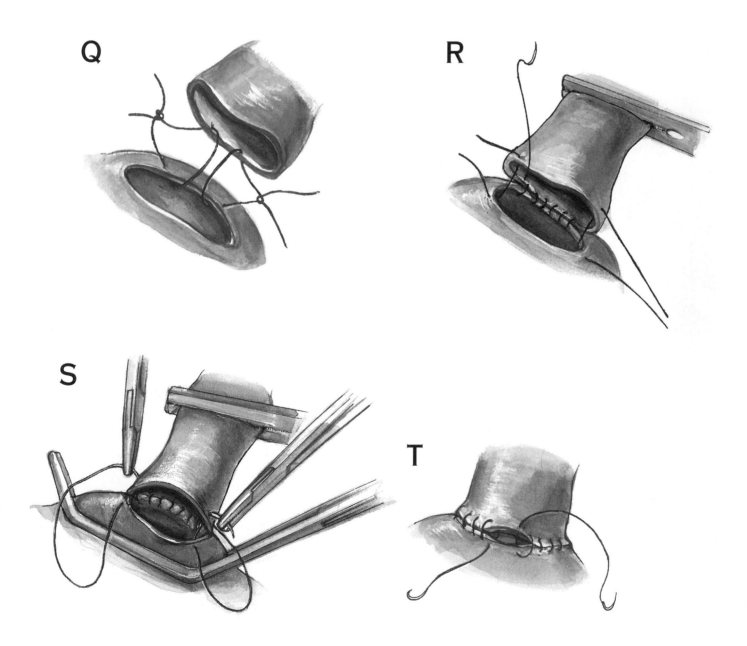

Q

R

S

T

U

On completion of the anastomosis, the caval clamp is removed first, followed promptly by removal of the one on the portal vein. Any oozing from the suture line can be stopped by very gentle pressure for several minutes with a piece of moistened gauze. Any persistent bleeding point can be sealed with individual stitches, but the vessels should not be clamped while this is being done. The wound is not drained routinely. The abdomen is closed in a manner favored by the surgeon.

U

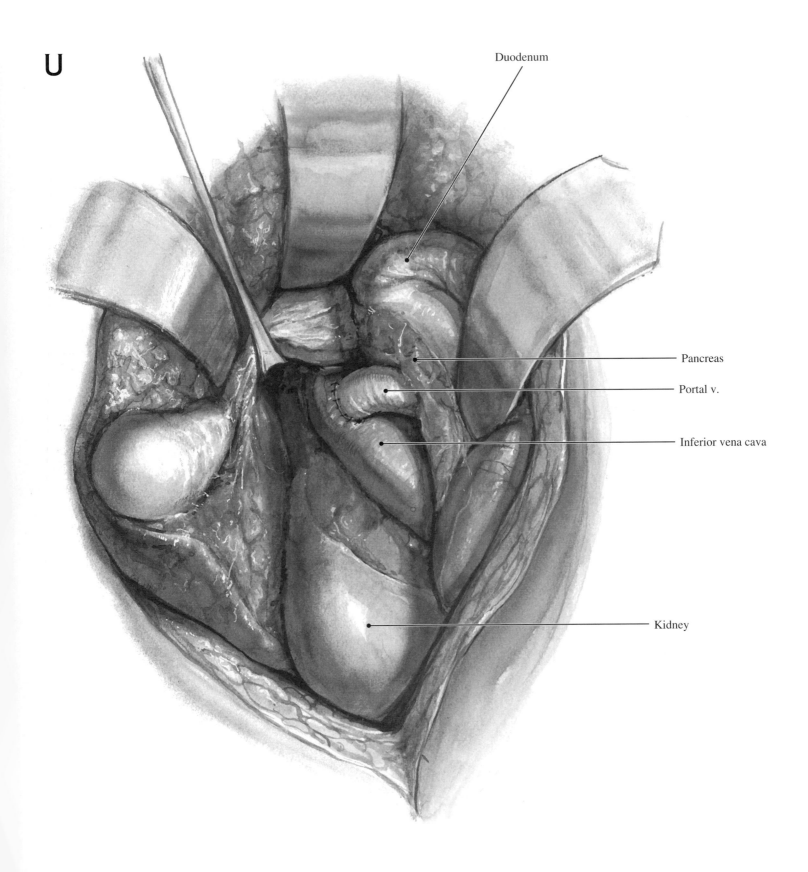

Duodenum

Pancreas

Portal v.

Inferior vena cava

Kidney

V, W, X, Y, Z

A side-to-side anastomosis is performed when complete interruption of portal flow to the liver is not desirable. It is mandatory that the maximal length of vein be mobilized if excessive tension on the suture line is to be avoided. The anastomosis is done as before with special care that the stitches are placed well at the cephalad and caudal aspects of the anastomosis, where the tension is greatest.

V

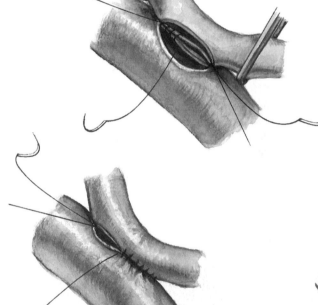

Portal v.

Inferior vena cava

W

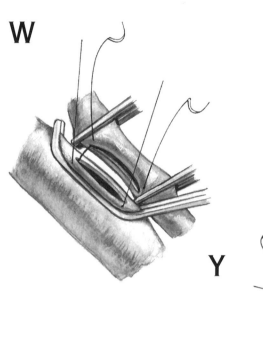

X

Y

Z

AA, BB, CC

A double-barreled portacaval shunt is technically more difficult because the liver and intestinal side of the portal vein must be brought to the vena cava for the anastomosis. It is necessary that the maximal length of vein be mobilized and that neither limb be created at the expense of its partner. The portal vein on the intestinal side is anastomosed first so that its success can be ensured. As with the other types of anastomoses, the course and seating of the vein must be proper so as not to result in twisting or kinking when the clamps are removed.

AA

BB

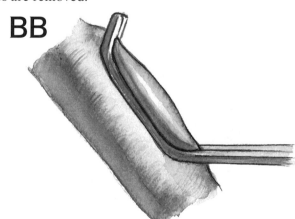

CC

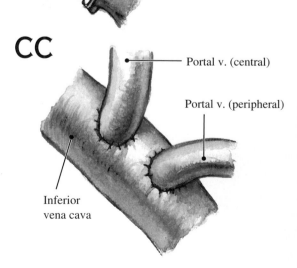

Portal v. (central)

Portal v. (peripheral)

Inferior vena cava

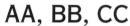

DD, EE

Diagramatic representation of the two most common types
of portacaval shunts.

DD

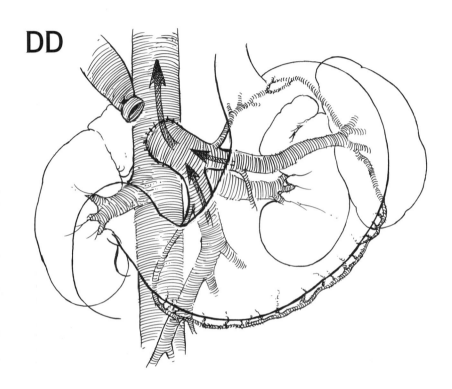

EE

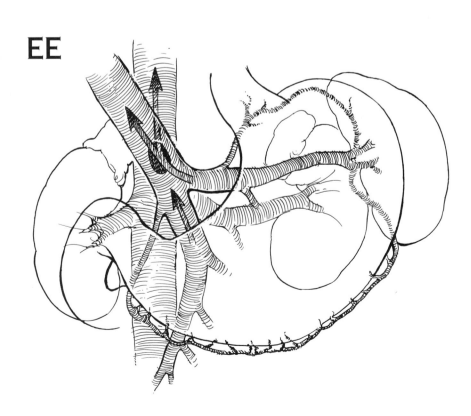

B SPLENORENAL SHUNT

Although a surgeon may prefer a certain type of portal decompression operation, any of several may have to be used depending on the circumstances. Shunt surgery should not be attempted unless the surgeon is able to perform all of them and has a thorough knowledge of the vascular anatomy of the upper abdomen.

A

There may be a variable degree of splenomegaly. The splenic vein issues from the splenic hilus as several tributaries and courses toward the right in a position caudal to the splenic artery, remaining behind the pancreas throughout its course. Emptying into it are the left gastroepiploic vein, the short gastric veins, some pancreatic veins, and the inferior mesenteric vein before it joins with the superior mesenteric vein to form the portal vein. Deep to it lie the left kidney, adrenal gland, and aorta.

A

Portal v.

Hepatic a.

Celiac axis

Superior mesenteric v. and a.

Splenic a. and v.

Left adrenal gland

Inferior mesenteric v.

Vena cava

Spleen

Left gastroepiploic v.

Aorta

Psoas m.

Left spermatic a. and v.

Ureter

Left renal v. and a.

Left kidney

Pancreas (transected)

Adrenal v.

B

The shunt shown in B₁ makes possible retrograde flow between the splenic vein and the renal vein. In this shunt the spleen is removed. The alternative one designed for antegrade flow is shown in B₂.

B1

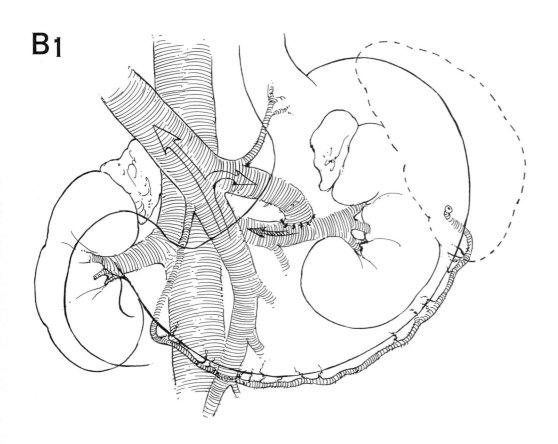

B2

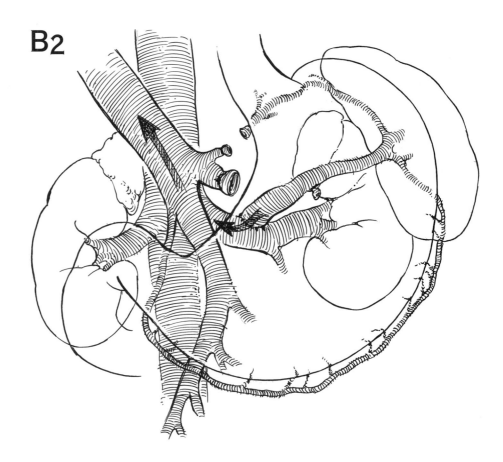

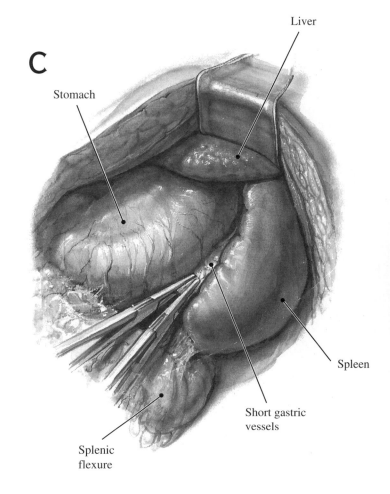

C

The peritoneal cavity is explored. As the status of the splenoportal system must be known, a splenoportogram may be done at this more convenient time under direct vision if there is any doubt on this point. Portal pressures are obtained through a mesenteric vein. Division of the gastrocolic omentum is begun at the midtransverse colon and on the relatively avascular gastric side of the arcades of the gastroepiploic vessels.

The short gastric vessels are divided in their entirety so that the greater curvature of the stomach is entirely free. The splenocolic ligament is clamped and divided. Normally, avascular areas may be traversed extensively by collateral venules, which, owing to portal hypertension, bleed copiously when transected. For this reason, no blunt dissection is carried out in these operations; far more than the usual clamping and ligating of tissue is practiced. Electrocoagulation is used to control small bleeding points.

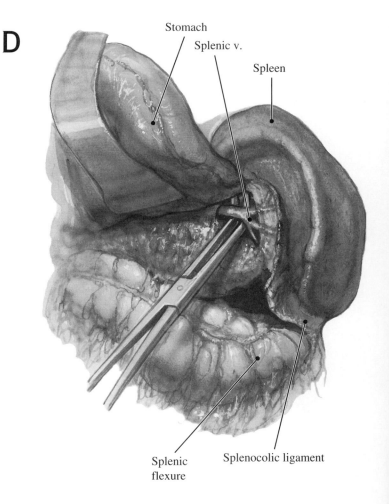

D

The stomach is reflected medially, and the splenic flexure of the colon is displaced downward. The peritoneum over the hilar vessels is incised and dissection of the vessels begun. The artery is isolated first and tied with 2-0 silk or looped with a linen tie and temporarily left open so that it can keep the splenic vein and its tributaries turgid for easier dissection. The splenic vein is isolated next. This is done slightly away from the hilus and over the single vein rather than in a time-consuming dissection of its tributaries off the spleen.

E

The spleen is reflected medially. Although this is normally an avascular area, extensive collateral vessels make it necessary to clamp any tissue here before division and ligation. The problem is aggravated if there are any perisplenic adhesions or if the spleen is quite large. If such conditions are present and blood loss threatens to become excessive, the splenic artery is ligated first.

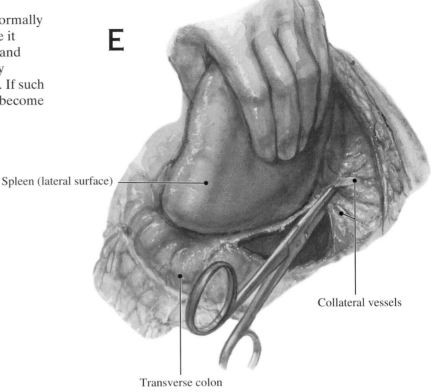

E

Spleen (lateral surface)

Collateral vessels

Transverse colon

F

The spleen is reflected even more to the right and the posterior parietal peritoneum at the tail of the pancreas incised so that this portion of the pancreas can also be reflected. A spring Potts clamp is placed on the splenic vein close to the hilum, and the spleen is amputated. Five milliliters of heparinized saline are injected into the vein immediately proximal to the clamp, and the vein is reclamped just proximal to the needle puncture. All this is done on a portion of the vein that is not to be used subsequently.

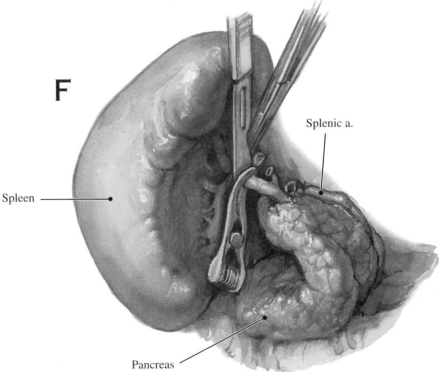

F

Splenic a.

Spleen

Pancreas

G

The splenectomy results in a wide exposure, which is
necessary for proper mobilization of the splenic vein. The
vein is delicately teased away from the pancreas, and the
pancreatic veins are isolated with an Adson hemostat,
ligated first with 5-0 silk, and then divided. The splenic vein
is mobilized medially to the point at which it is joined by
the inferior mesenteric vein.

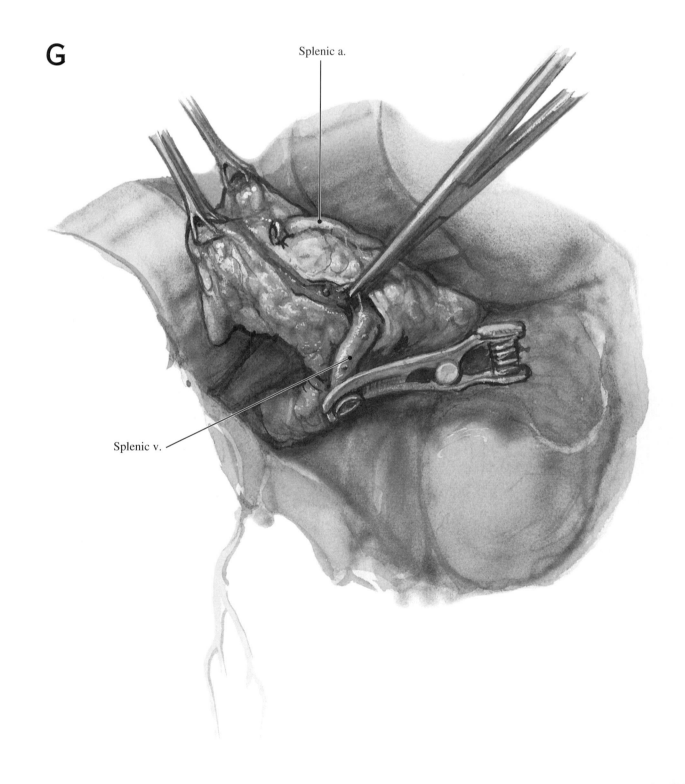

G

Splenic a.

Splenic v.

H

The renal vein is prepared in its middle third for the anastomosis. The tail of the pancreas is temporarily displaced cephalad, and the posterior parietal peritoneum over the renal vein is incised to the vena cava. The entire kidney need not be mobilized. The spermatic and adrenal veins are susceptible to injury and are spared if possible but can be ligated with impunity if they appear to interfere with the contemplated anastomotic site.

H

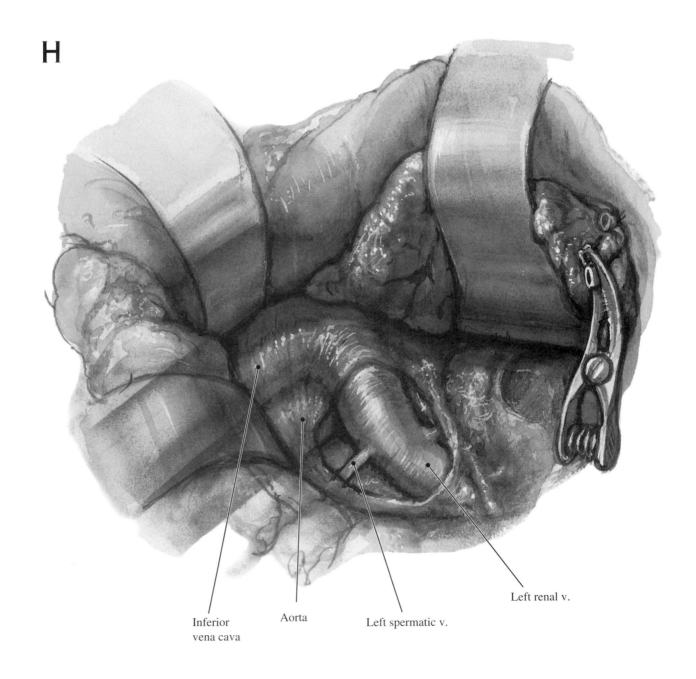

Inferior
vena cava

Aorta

Left spermatic v.

Left renal v.

I

A Satinsky clamp is applied over a portion of the renal vein, and the splenic vein is brought into position. At this time the downward curve of the splenic vein is observed, because the surgeon must feel confident that there will be no kinking or twisting that will encourage thrombosis. If there is any doubt, the vein is mobilized further so that it can make a smooth downward sweep. The tail of the pancreas is held out of the way with a Babcock clamp attached to the peripancreatic fatty areolar tissue.

I

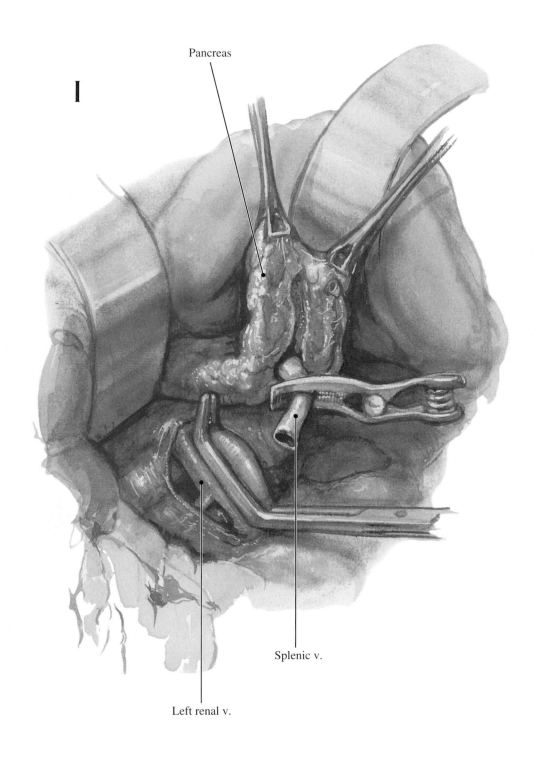

Pancreas

Splenic v.

Left renal v.

J, K, L

An oval window suitable for the splenic vein is cut away from the renal vein with a sharp curved scissors. The vessels are joined by anchoring stitches at the ends of the oval, and the posterior anastomosis is performed first. Atraumatic 6-0 vascular suture is used, with the bites of the needle about 1.5 mm apart and 1.0 mm from the cut edge. Smooth-tipped vein hooks are used to manipulate rather than to grasp the vessel edges during placement of the anterior row of stitches. Often it may not be possible to partially occlude the renal vein during the anastomosis. If total occlusion is necessary, it must be preceded by occlusion of the artery. The short period of renal ischemia during performance of the anastomosis is not harmful if it is limited to 30 minutes or so.

K

Left renal v.

Splenic v.

Vena cava

J

Aorta

L

M

The clamp on the renal vein is removed first, followed promptly by removal of that on the splenic vein. Oozing from the suture line will stop if pressure is applied with a moist sponge for a moment. The pancreas is examined carefully for any trauma. If the tip of the tail has been transected, the defect is sutured with fine atraumatic suture material. Portal pressure is again determined in a mesenteric vessel to assess the immediate effect of the shunt. A drain is placed in the splenic bed and made to pass by the tail of the pancreas on its way to the outside through a counterincision, and suction is applied. The wound is closed in a preferred fashion.

M

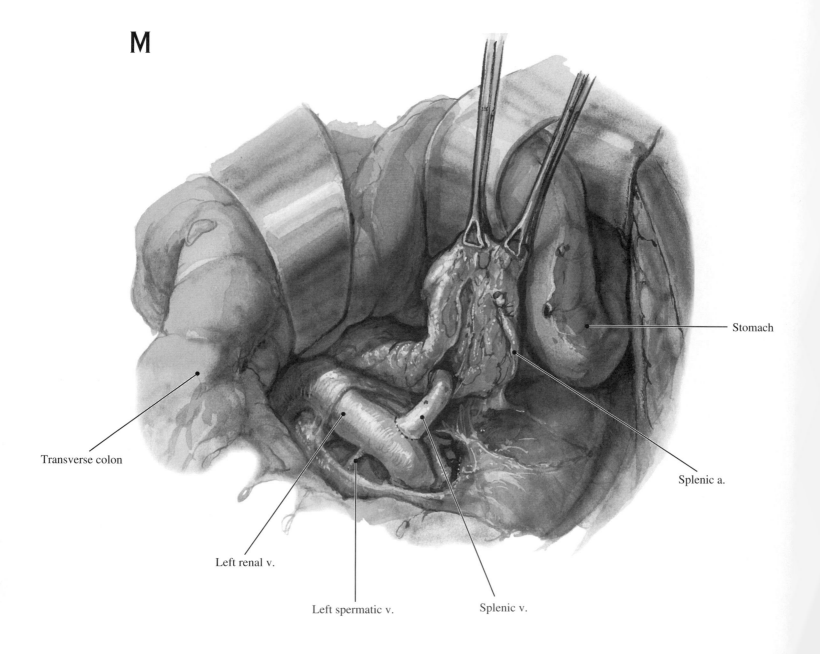

Stomach

Splenic a.

Transverse colon

Left renal v.

Left spermatic v.

Splenic v.

C MESOCAVAL SHUNT

H-GRAFT

In a mesocaval shunt, retrograde flow is expected through the portal mesenteric vessels into the vena cava. This shunt procedure is performed less commonly than is the portacaval or splenorenal; it can be used when the splenic vein is unavailable, as in postsplenectomy patients or in patients whose portal vein is thrombosed or cavernous. In addition, it often is the operation of choice for a cirrhotic patient who is likely to require a liver transplantation at a later date. The reason is that transplantation is markedly more difficult in patients with a portacaval shunt, so this choice should be avoided. A splenorenal shunt is less troublesome in this regard. Also, mesocaval shunting is used more commonly in children in whom other types of shunts are associated with a higher incidence of thrombosis.

The connection between the vena cava and the superior mesenteric vein can be via an interposed graft (*H-graft*), the choice in adults, or by *direct* vessel-to-vessel connection, the choice for children but unacceptable in adults because of the high incidence of leg edema.

A

This illustration highlights the anatomic structures pertinent to the mesocaval shunt operation.

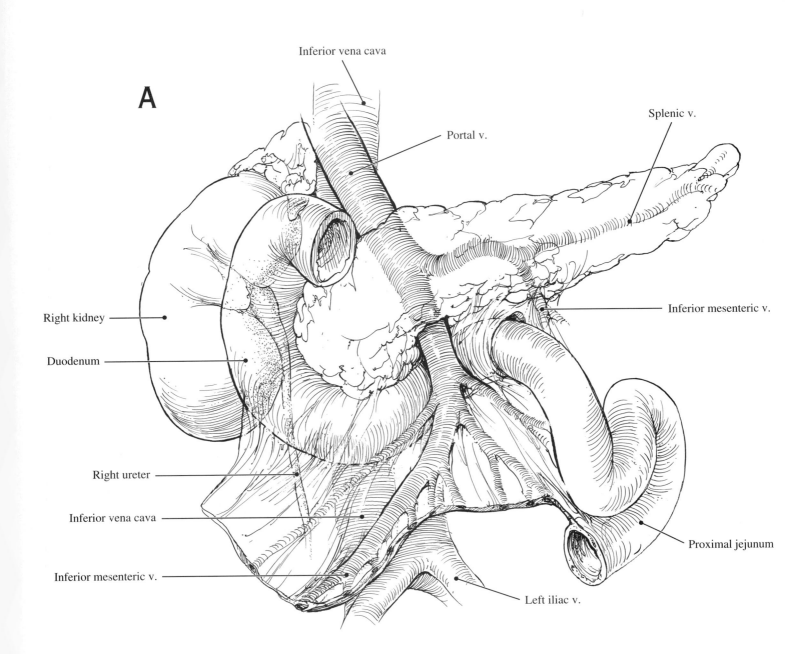

Inferior vena cava

Portal v.

Splenic v.

Right kidney

Duodenum

Inferior mesenteric v.

Right ureter

Inferior vena cava

Proximal jejunum

Inferior mesenteric v.

Left iliac v.

A

B

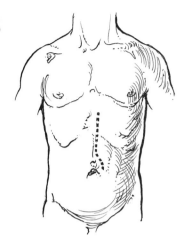

B

A midline incision is preferred.

C

After exploring the opened abdomen, the portal pressure is determined by cannulation of a peripheral mesenteric vein.

C

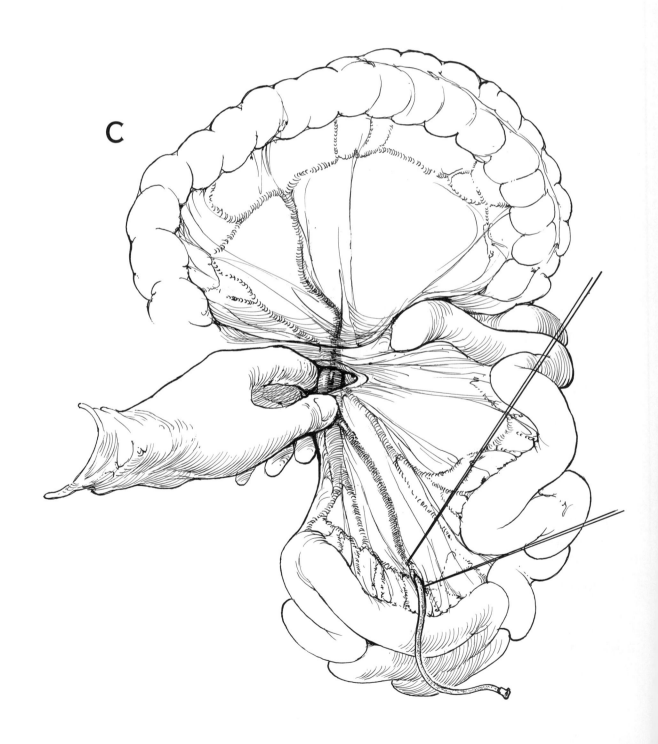

D

With the transverse mesocolon retracted upward, a transverse incision is made over the superior mesenteric vein and vena cava. The superior mesenteric vein is exposed between its first tributary and cephalad to almost the pancreas. The duodenum is mobilized cephalad to adequately expose the vena cava.

D

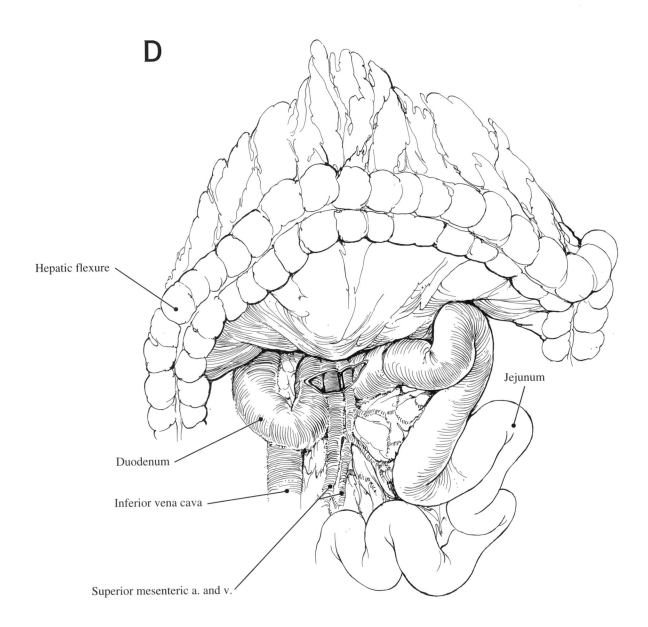

Hepatic flexure

Jejunum

Duodenum

Inferior vena cava

Superior mesenteric a. and v.

E

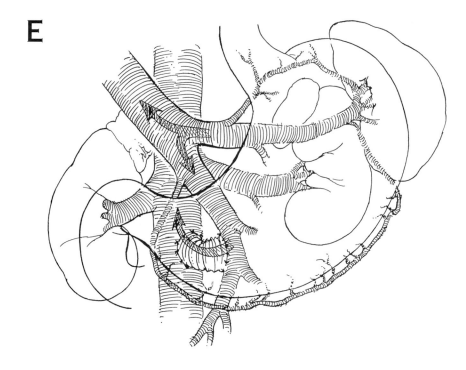

E

This diagnostic rendition illustrates the planned shunt. Splenic vein contribution depends on the presence or absence of the spleen or collateral vessels. Portal vein antegrade flow depends on the degree of outflow blockage. Neither of these considerations applies when this procedure is being performed for potential candidates for later liver transplantation.

F

The vessels are shown exposed and before the bypass site has been selected.

F

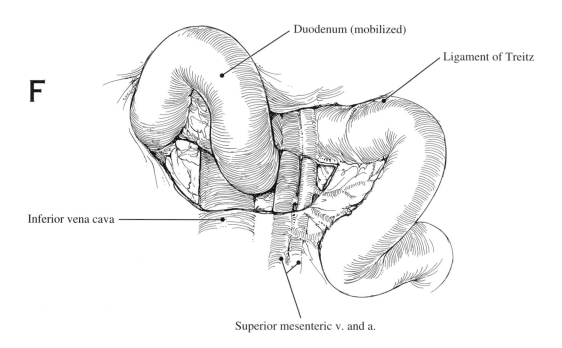

Duodenum (mobilized)

Ligament of Treitz

Inferior vena cava

Superior mesenteric v. and a.

G

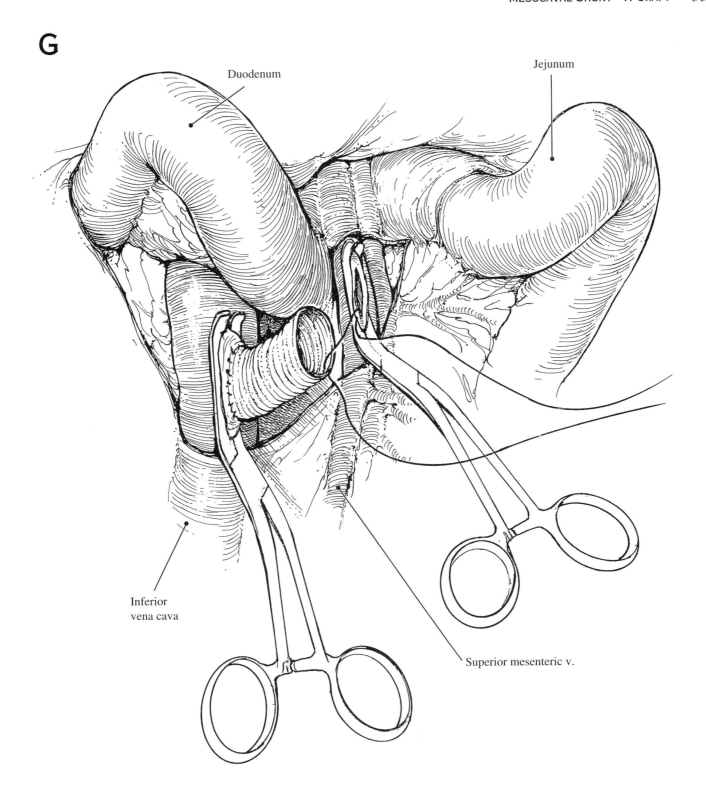

Duodenum

Jejunum

Inferior
vena cava

Superior mesenteric v.

G

When the connecting sites are chosen, a Satinsky clamp is
applied on the anterior surface of the vena cava. The
venotomy is made to accommodate the largest workable
diameter (usually 18mm) of a Dacron graft, and an
anastomosis is made with a continuous stitch of fine
vascular suture material.

H

The graft is clamped at its opposite end, and the caval clamp is released, filling the graft and preclotting it. The caval clamp is reapplied and the blood aspirated from the graft. The graft is trimmed with great care so that it is neither under tension nor too long. A Satinsky clamp is applied over the predetermined area on the superomedial surface of the inferior mesenteric vein, and a venotomy of apppropriate size is made. Th anastomosis again is made with fine vascular suture material employing a continuous stitch. The clamps are removed and the area inspected for adequate hemostasis. No drains are used. Abdominal closure is made in a customary manner.

H

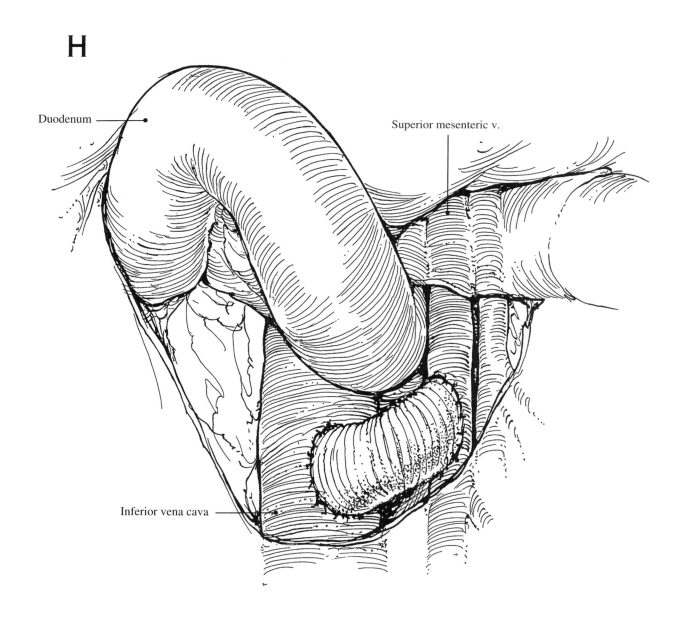

Duodenum

Superior mesenteric v.

Inferior vena cava

DIRECT

A

The intent in creating a *direct* mesocaval shunt is to effect a vessel-to-vessel connection between the inferior vena cava and the superior mesenteric vein. On the caval side, either the left or the right iliac vein can be used or even the vena cava itself. The determining factors are the need for adequate length, proper sweep, and comfortable apposition of the two vessels so that there is no kinking in their course and no tension on the suture line—both factors that predispose to thrombosis.

B

This view is "anatomically clean" for the purpose of identifying organs and structures; it does not reflect the appearance during clinical dissection.

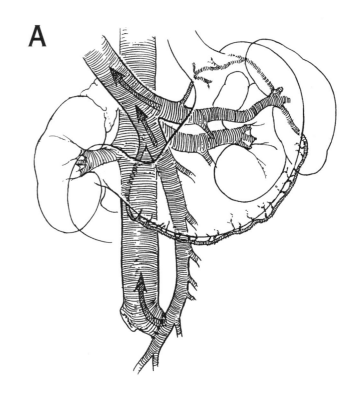

A

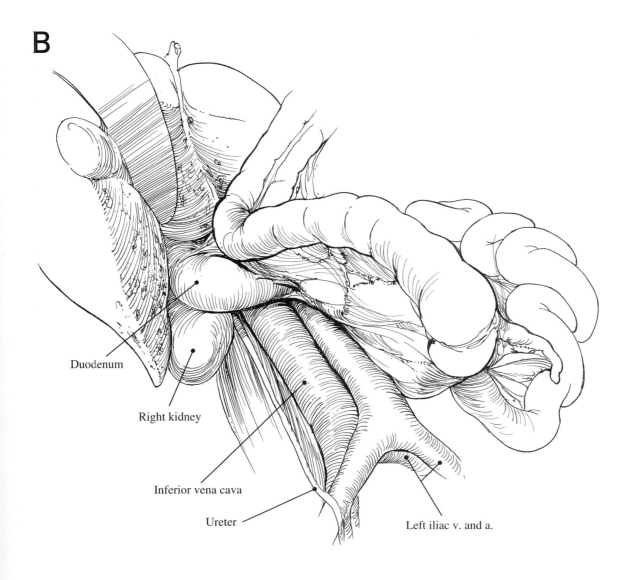

B

Duodenum

Right kidney

Inferior vena cava

Ureter

Left iliac v. and a.

C

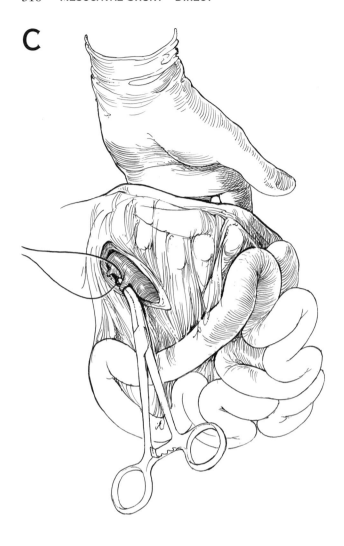

C, D

A portion of the mesenteric vein about 6 cm in length is prepared for the anastomosis. The vessels emanating from the right side are first ligated with 4-0 silk and then divided (*C*). Those on the left side are spared as much as possible, because the anastomosis takes place near them but does not affect most of them. Temporary vessel loop tourniquets can be placed around some of them as needed (*D*).

D

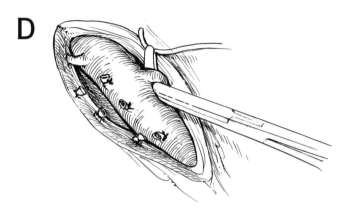

E

Although the inferior vena cava can be approached directly, gaining full exposure of it and of the iliac veins can be awkward. Adequate exposure can be effected by reflecting the right colon to the patient's left as is illustrated here. This approach, however, requires incision of the lateral peritoneal reflection, which is traversed by multiple collateral vessels requiring ligation. The ureter should be identified and protected from harm.

E

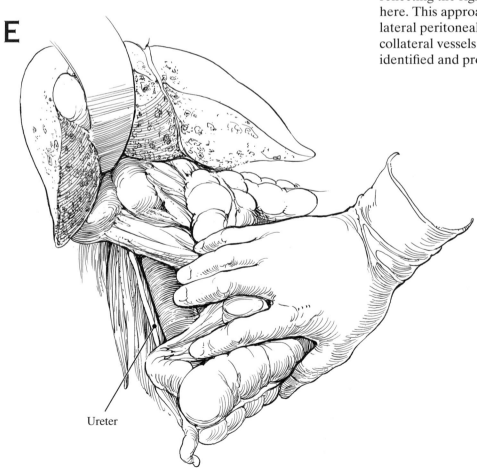

Ureter

F

A window is made in the mesentery of the right colon as a passageway for the iliac vein to the mesenteric vein. The mesentery in such patients is often very edematous, thick, and fibrous, so that even fashioning this passageway may require sharp dissection and careful attention to hemostasis.

F

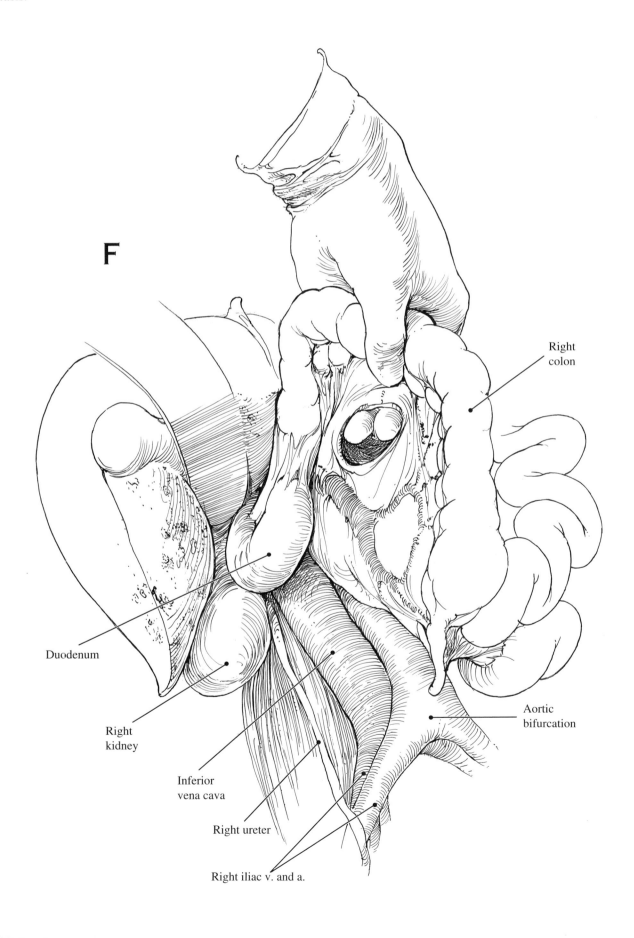

Right colon

Duodenum

Right kidney

Inferior vena cava

Right ureter

Aortic bifurcation

Right iliac v. and a.

G

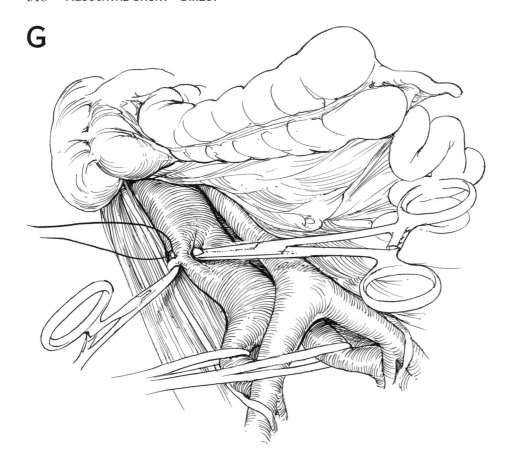

G, H

Vessel loops are placed around the iliac veins. Several lumbar veins are ligated with 2-0 silk and divided; this helps to mobilize the vena cava sufficiently to ease it toward the mesenteric vein if this is needed (*G*). Adjacent lumbar veins are encircled with vessel loops for ready access if necessary (*H*).

H

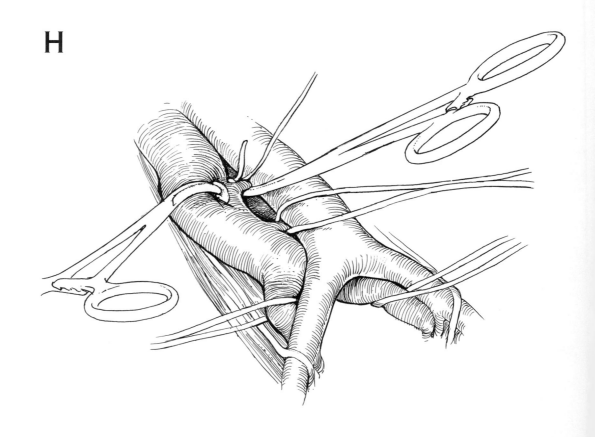

I

Vascular clamps are placed on the left iliac vein as distally as possible, and the vein is divided. The distal limb is oversewn with fine vascular suture. The right common iliac vein is cross-clamped flush with the vena cava at its bifurcation. More proximally, a spring-serrated bulldog vascular clamp is placed across the vena cava.

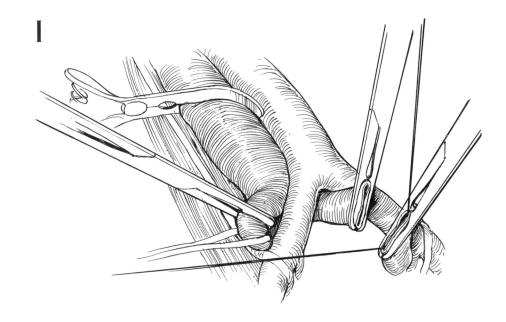

J

The right iliac vein is divided, and both sides of the vessel are oversewn with fine vascular suture. Traction and orientation sutures are placed in each side of the left iliac vein.

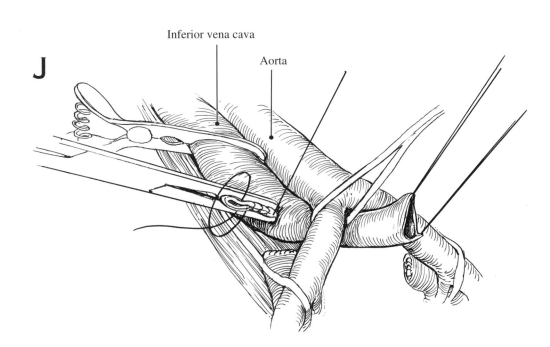

K

The "fashioned" inferior vena cava is brought ventral to
the left common iliac vein.

K

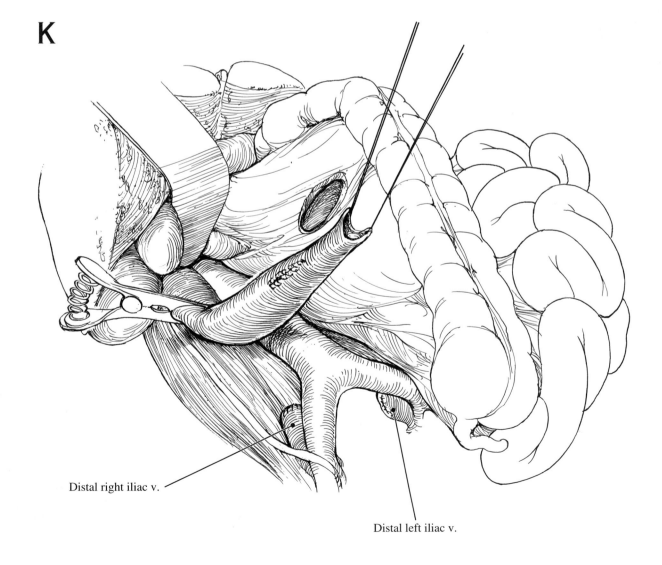

Distal right iliac v.

Distal left iliac v.

L

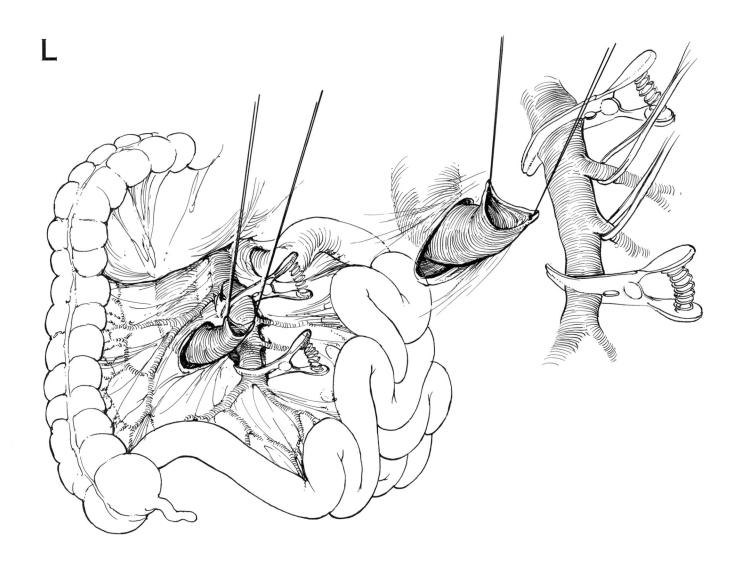

L

The "fashioned" left iliac vein is then brought through the mesenteric window and next to the mesenteric vein, which has been occluded on either side with vascular clamps. Tributaries within the occluded segment of the mesenteric vein are encircled with vessel loops.

M

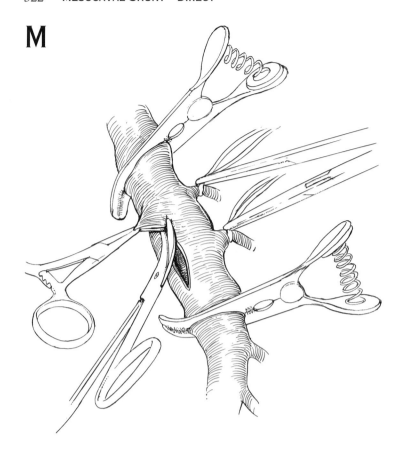

N

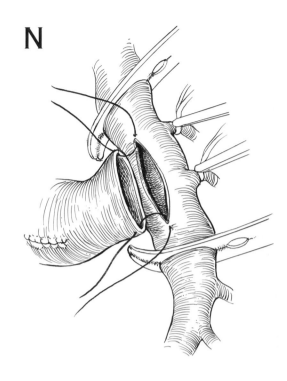

M, N

The vessel loops are tightened, after which an oval window is cut out of the mesenteric vein to match that in the presenting iliac vein.

O, P

Orientation stay sutures of 4-0 Prolene are placed at the proximal and distal ends of the mesenteric vessel opening. The anastomosis is begun posteriorly and completed anteriorly.

O

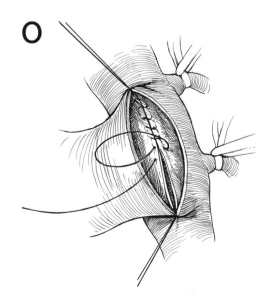

P

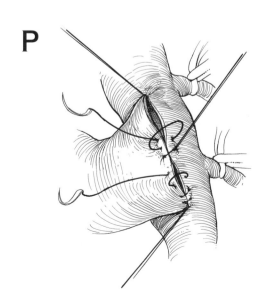

Q

The completed shunt is illustrated. Stray bleeding points are sought and secured. The viscera are repositioned. No drains are used. The abdomen is closed in a customary manner.

Q

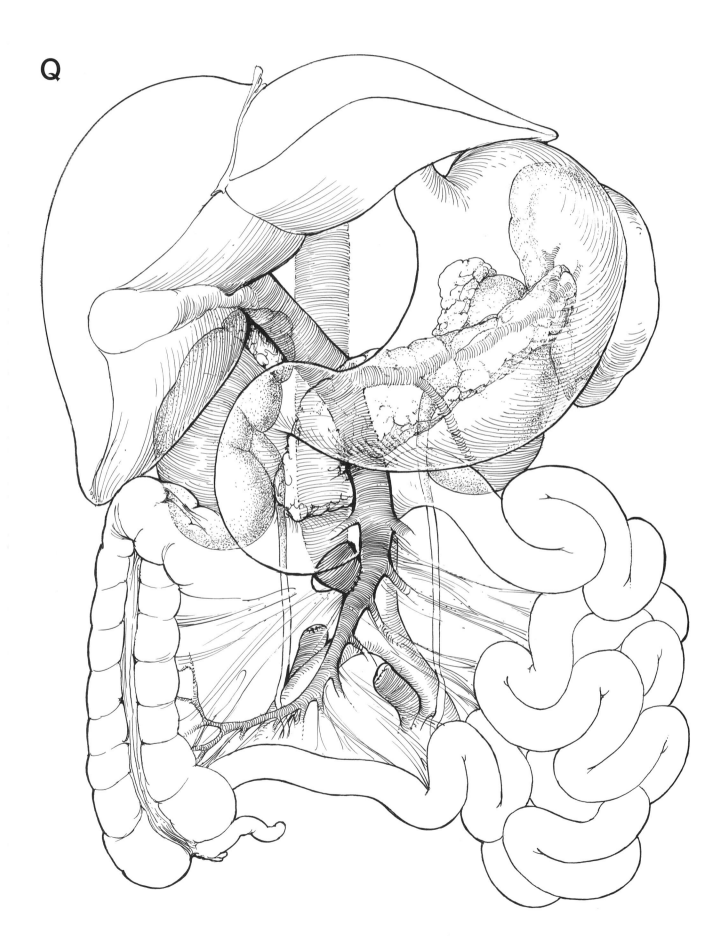

Chapter
22

ADRENAL GLANDS

A ADRENALECTOMY

ANTERIOR APPROACH

Operations on the adrenal gland require certainty of diagnosis, careful preparation, and attention to metabolic needs during the perioperative period. An anterior abdominal approach provides exposure to both the glands and the retroperitoneum but carries greater morbidity. A flank or posterior approach is better tolerated but gives limited exposure. Imaging techniques have become so refined, however, that it is rarely necessary to choose the abdominal approach for the sole purpose of searching for ectopic adrenal tissue.

A

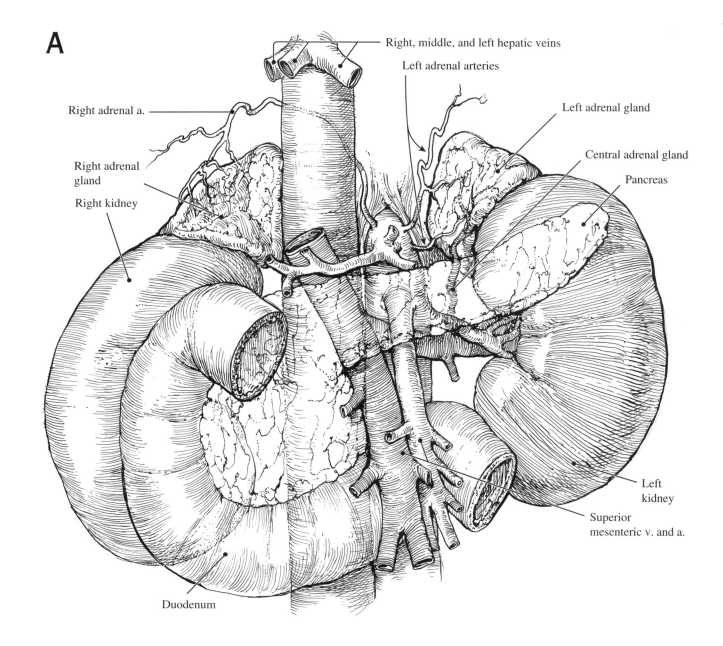

Right, middle, and left hepatic veins

Left adrenal arteries

Right adrenal a.

Right adrenal gland

Right kidney

Left adrenal gland

Central adrenal gland

Pancreas

Left kidney

Superior mesenteric v. and a.

Duodenum

A

The adrenal glands are well ensconced in the body, lying at about the level of the eleventh thoracic vertebra, on lumbar slips of the diaphragm to which they are attached more firmly than to the kidneys. The right adrenal gland is cephalad to the kidney, lateral to the vena cava, and dorsal to the liver. The left adrenal gland is slightly more medial in relation to the top of the kidney and lateral to the aorta. Ventrally, it is covered by the posterior surface of the stomach, the posterior surface of the pancreas, and the splenic vessels. The adrenal glands have a rich blood supply from three arteries that are branches of the aorta, the renal artery, and the inferior phrenic artery.

B

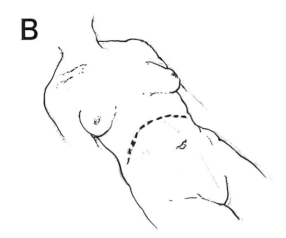

B

Surgical approaches to the adrenal glands are ventral, via the flank, or dorsal, the approach being influenced by the indication for the operation. Generally, the abdominal route is utilized.

ABDOMINAL APPROACH

C

The peritoneal cavity usually is opened through a bilateral subcostal (chevron) incision.

In this instance, the left adrenal gland is being excised first. The gland is exposed by reflecting the spleen, the tail of the pancreas, and the greater curvature of the stomach medially. The surgeon may choose to stand on the patient's right side for a better view of the left suprarenal area; in such instances, the left hand is occupied with retracting the overlying structures. The main disadvantage to reflecting the spleen is that it may be damaged and have to be removed.

An alternative method of exposure is to mobilize the greater curvature of the stomach and to displace it cephalad and the pancreas and splenic vessels caudad for direct access to the adrenal gland: on occasion, with a very low-lying adrenal gland, the body and tail of the pancreas may need to be displaced ventrally to gain the necessary exposure. Although all these efforts may appear to be cumbersome and may fail to provide adequate exposure, they are important considerations when dealing with pheochromocytomas and larger cancers.

C

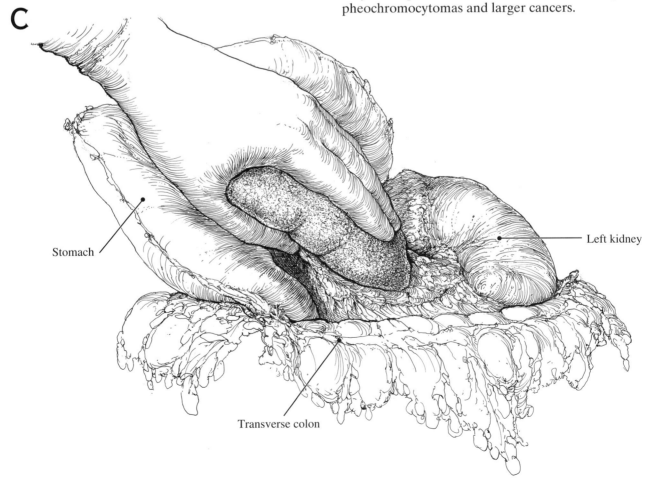

Stomach

Left kidney

Transverse colon

D

This illustration focuses on the vascular supply of the left adrenal gland. If the vessels to and from the adrenal gland (other than the central vein) are divided close to the gland, they can be expected to stop bleeding spontaneously. The central vein most commonly courses caudally to empty into the left renal vein. Familiarity with the venous drainage enables a surgeon to isolate, ligate, and divide the vein early when removing a pheochromocytoma, thus minimizing the wide fluctuations in blood pressure that can be seen during even minimal manipulation of the tumor.

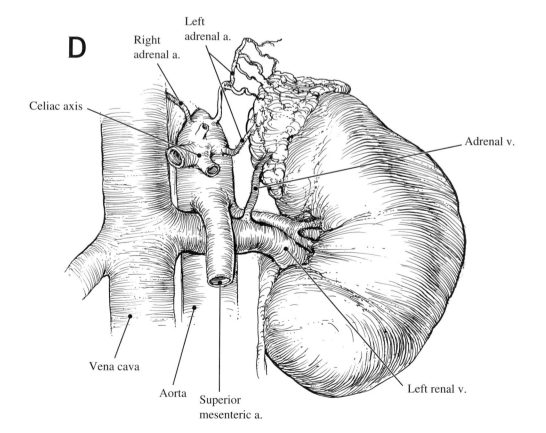

D

Left adrenal a.

Right adrenal a.

Celiac axis

Adrenal v.

Vena cava

Aorta

Superior mesenteric a.

Left renal v.

E

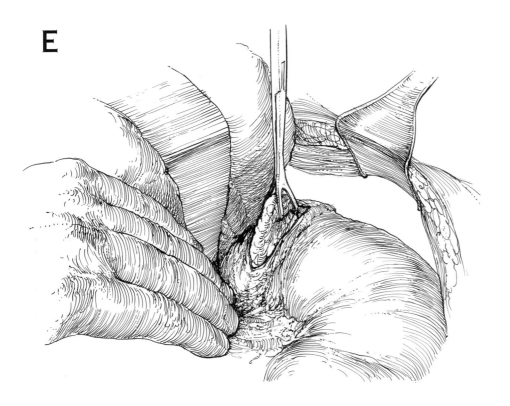

E, F

The exposure of the suprarenal area is excellent with the
abdominal approach. Usually the adrenal gland can be
palpated through the posterior parietal peritoneum. If it
cannot, as may occur especially in obese individuals, the
peritoneum is incised transversely just above the kidney,
the leading edge of the adrenal being delivered easily in
this fashion. Blunt and sharp dissection are used to free the
adrenal, with clips being applied to the arterioles. The
central adrenal vein usually is singular, but considerable
bleeding can occur from lesser accessory veins. The central
vein is tied with 2-0 silk before being divided and the gland
removed.

F

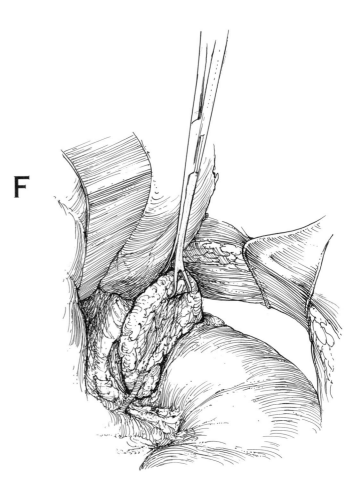

G

Exposure and removal of the right adrenal gland is more difficult than removal of the left gland because of limited accessibility of the central vein.

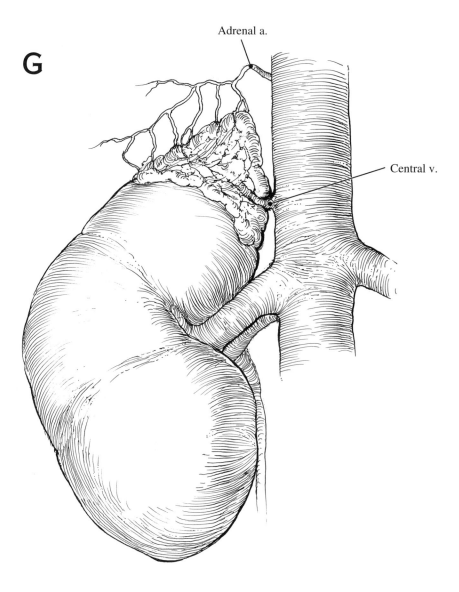

G

Adrenal a.

Central v.

H

A Deaver retractor is used to expose the furthest medial recess of the gland next to the vena cava. The portal triad is retracted medially. The kidney is displaced caudally with the hand, bringing the adrenal gland with it and downward somewhat. The posterior parietal peritoneum over the adrenal is incised, and the gland is dissected as on the opposite side. Again, the arterial supply to the gland is abundant, but the arterioles are not large. They are secured with clips. The central vein, usually singular, is rarely longer than 1 cm and drains directly into the vena cava. As on the left side, it should be tied first with 2-0 silk before being divided. This should be done with care; loss of control of the central vein can result in a major hemorrhage.

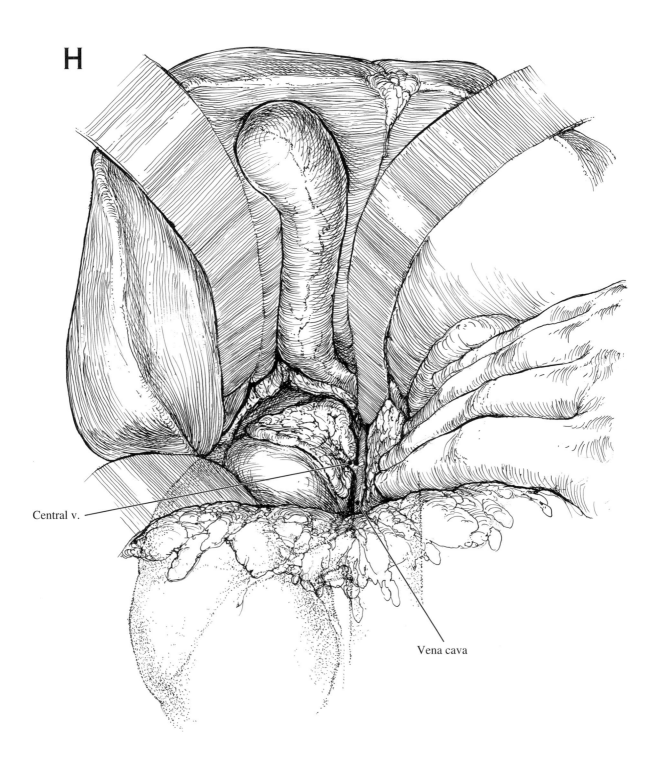

H

Central v.

Vena cava

FLANK APPROACH

A

The flank approach is probably the least traumatic to the patient and should be used if at all possible. In this posterior oblique view of the back, a window has been cut out of the latissimus dorsi muscle, the major muscle. A portion of its lateral edge has to be divided when utilizing this technique. Here the medial portion has been removed to show the underlying muscles. Some fibers of the internal oblique muscle have to be divided anteriorly. The serratus posteroinferior muscles and the intercostal muscles have to be disengaged from the rib while making the incision.

A

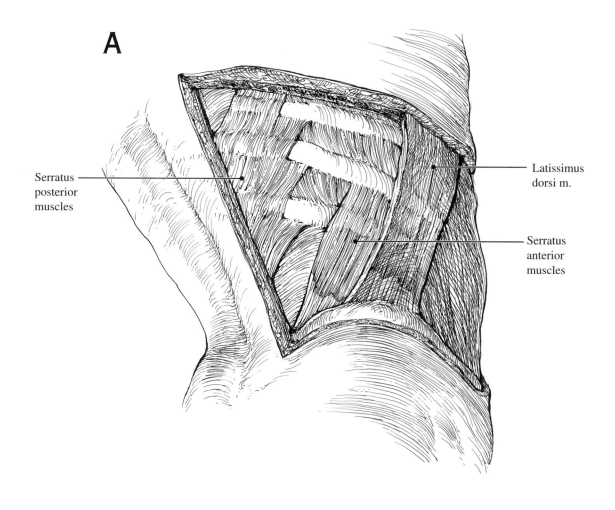

Serratus
posterior
muscles

Latissimus
dorsi m.

Serratus
anterior
muscles

B

In this rendition, a phantom illustrative technique is used to show some of the relationships of the right adrenal gland. The vena cava is on its medial border; inferiorly it lies on the kidney. On its anterior surface the gland is covered by the duodenum, the undersurface of the liver, and sometimes the inferior vena cava. The gland is positioned between the eleventh and twelfth ribs posteriorly, although this relationship varies considerably. The illustration demonstrates how the pleural reflections dip below the body of the twelfth rib laterally and need to be displaced cephalad on the way to the adrenal gland if intrapleural entry is to be avoided. Some fibers of the diaphragm must also be transected, but they are inconsequential.

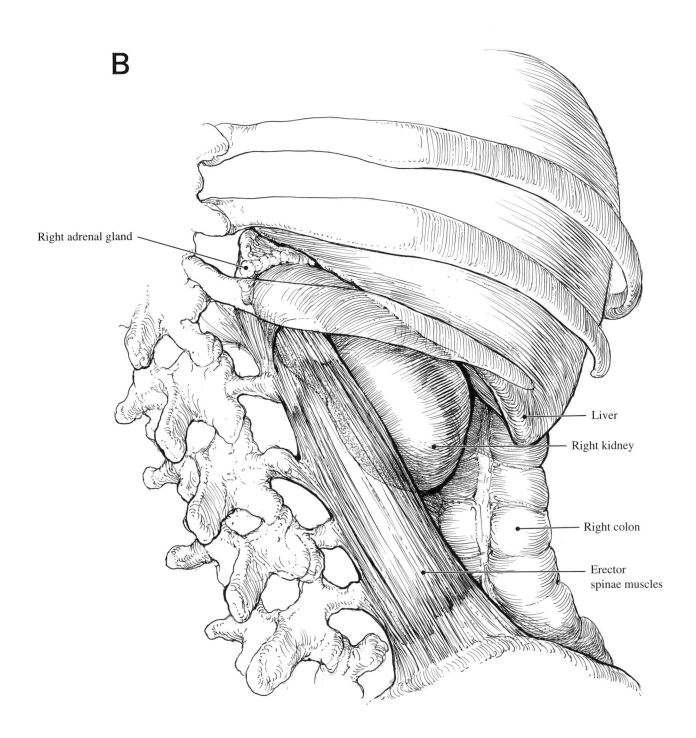

B

Right adrenal gland

Liver

Right kidney

Right colon

Erector
spinae muscles

C

C

Proper positioning of the patient is an important ancillary consideration for optimum exposure of the gland. The patient is placed in the direct lateral position. If the patient is somewhat obese, a slight ventral tilt encourages the abdominal viscera to fall away. The break in the table must be precisely at the level of the twelfth rib; having the table break at a level lower or higher than this is useless or even detrimental in that the kidney rest, when raised, may elevate the chest or pelvis and cause a narrowing rather than a widening of the space between the last rib and the iliac crest. The inferior leg is folded, the superior is kept straight, and a pillow is placed between them. Three-inch tape is placed across the hips and attached to the table to anchor the patient. A similar piece of tape is placed across the shoulder and is used to determine the tilt of the upper torso.

D

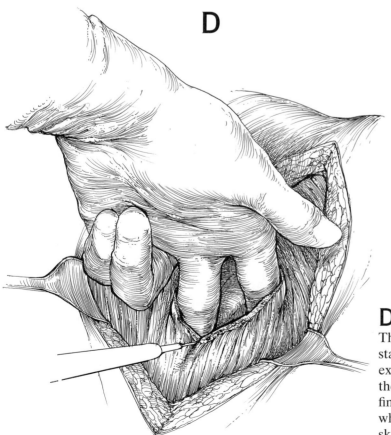

D

The incision is carried along the course of the twelfth rib, starting 3 to 5 cm from the midline in the back and extending to the anterior axillary line. Bleeding points in the skin and subcutaneous fat are electrocoagulated. The fingers are insinuated under the latissimus dorsi muscle, which is divided to the sacrospinalis muscle in line with the skin incision.

E

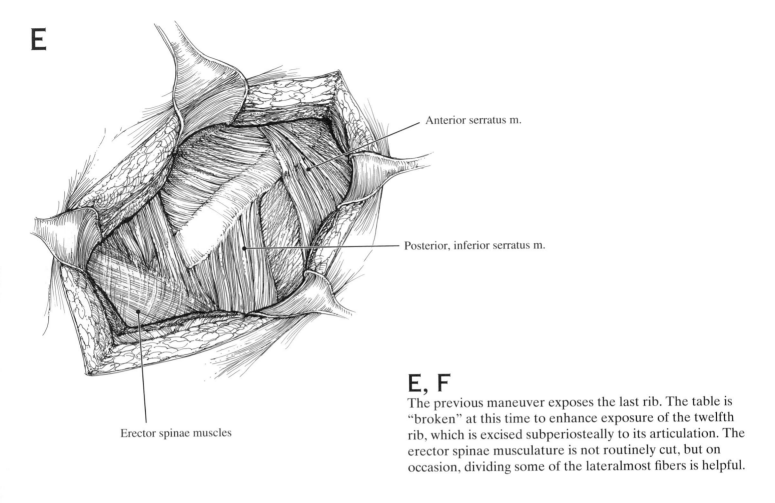

Anterior serratus m.

Posterior, inferior serratus m.

Erector spinae muscles

E, F

The previous maneuver exposes the last rib. The table is "broken" at this time to enhance exposure of the twelfth rib, which is excised subperiosteally to its articulation. The erector spinae musculature is not routinely cut, but on occasion, dividing some of the lateralmost fibers is helpful.

F

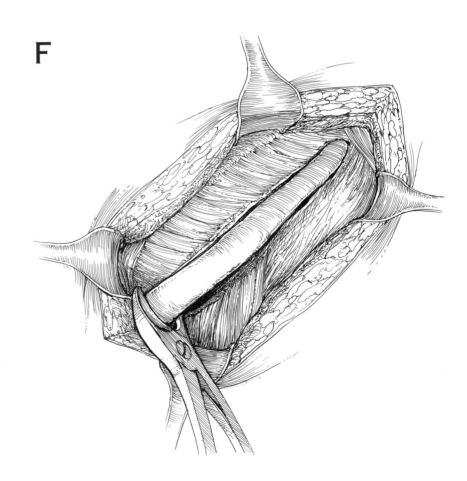

G

As the bed of the twelfth rib is incised, the surgeon should remain alert for the location of the costophrenic sulcus. The two surfaces of the pleura are often difficult to see at this point, and the only signal that the pleural cavity has been entered may be the hissing sound of air being sucked in. It is helpful to have the anesthesiologist inflate the patient's lungs to a maximum so that the extremes of the costophrenic sulcus can be detected as the lungs reach this point. Once the sulcus is identified, it cannot be assumed to follow a course parallel to the rib; it may course more caudally posteriorly.

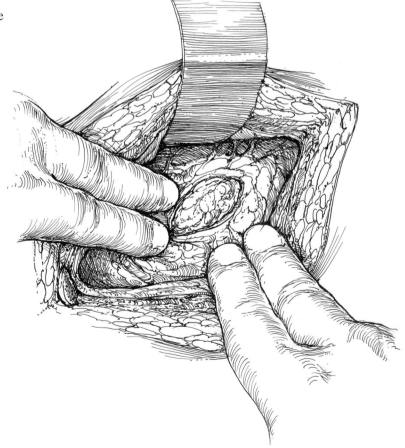

G

H

The kidney rest is now elevated, further helping to push the kidney outward. Gerota's fascia is incised; the perirenal fat is spread with the fingers; and the adrenal gland, which is slightly more orange-yellow in color than the surrounding fat, is sought. In patients with abundant perirenal fat, finding the adrenal gland may not be a simple matter. The adrenal gland is considerably more firm than the surrounding fat. Although this firmness is not so discernible at this stage of the dissection, it can be an important means of identifying the gland in otherwise formless fat. On the left side, an adjacent thin tail of the pancreas may confuse the issue.

H

I

Once an edge of the gland is freed, it is gently grasped with a Babcock clamp, the best means of doing so without tearing; tearing is associated with modest but most annoying bleeding. If the gland is not affected by a pheochromocytoma or cancer, the dissection can best be carried out by staying close to its capsule. The dissection is one of gentle teasing and spreading the periadrenal tissue with scissors, forceps, and even the tip of the suction tube. Most of this dissection is relatively bloodless; arterioles of concern are best secured with clips.

J

On the right side, the central vein can be expected to be about 1 cm long and to course directly medially into the vena cava. On the left side, as shown here, it is longer and courses directly caudally toward the left renal vein. The vein is tied first with 2-0 silk and divided.

J

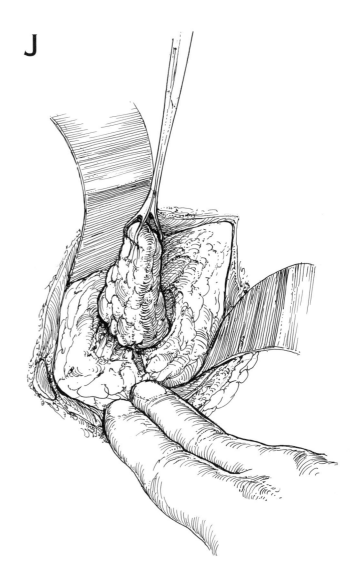

I

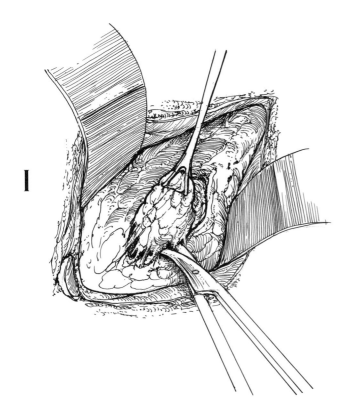

K

Hemostasis must be complete, as there is minimal firmness in the surrounding tissue to restrain bleeding. If the pleura has been opened, a small catheter is inserted into the pleural cavity through the opening and the pleura closed around the catheter with a continuous simple stitch of atraumatic 3-0 chromic catgut. (The catheter is removed after the skin is closed and as the anesthesiologist inflates the lungs maximally.) The table is made flat. Gerota's fascia is closed with continuous 3-0 chromic catgut. If the wound warrants drainage, a simple Penrose drain or closed suction technique is appropriate.

K

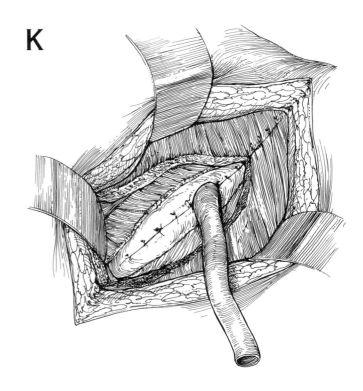

DORSAL APPROACH

A

This semidiagrammatic phantom drawing demonstrates the structures surrounding the adrenal gland that have to be displaced or traversed in removing the adrenal gland through the dorsal approach. The posterior reflection of the pleura is usually at the level of the twelfth rib. If, therefore, the approach is through the bed of the twelfth rib, the pleura often can be reflected upward without intrapleural entry. Notice also that diaphragmatic fibers extend this low, but few have to be cut if entry is made over the twelfth rib. The adrenal gland is more closely subjacent to the eleventh rib; if the dorsal approach at this level is used, then perforce the pleura is entered intentionally and more fibers of the diaphragm must be cut, but exposure is improved.

A

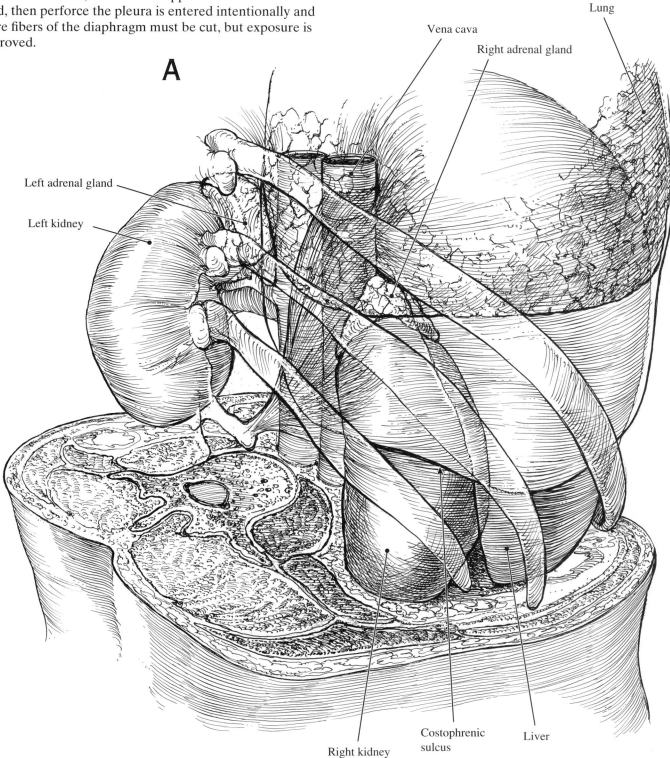

B

Entry usually is through the bed of the twelfth rib. On occasion, it is necessary to approach the gland at a higher level, in which instance the incision is made over the eleventh rib. This choice necessitates entry into the pleural cavity and should be avoided if possible. Because it is a more difficult approach, it will be featured here. The incision is centered over the eleventh rib but is curvilinear and paravertebral from the tenth rib to the iliac crest. It is important to so position the patient that the normal lumbar lordosis is reversed but that ventilation is unimpeded and adequate.

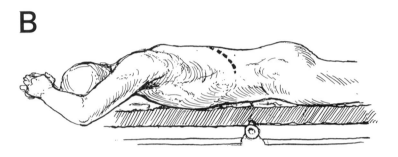

C

The skin and subcutaneous tissue have been incised and bleeding points electrocoagulated. The latissimus dorsi muscle is cut practically transverse to the direction of its fibers. The eleventh rib is excised subperiosteally for its entire length, and the pleural cavity is entered. The lung is displaced cephalad, and the diaphragm is incised along a level with the eleventh interspace where its fibers are sparse. Deep to this, Gerota's fascia is incised to reveal the perirenal fat.

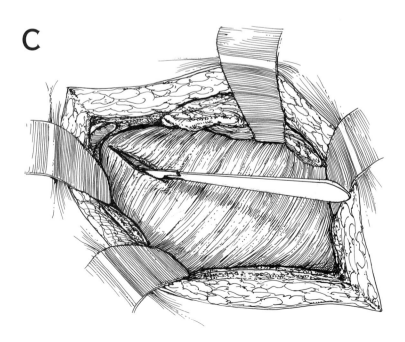

D

The adrenal gland (here the right one) is located and mobilized, with the anticipation that the short central vein will course centrally toward the vena cava. The arterioles to the gland are secured with clips. Less desirably, they can be cut and ignored with assurance that most will stop bleeding spontaneously. The central vein is tied first with 2-0 silk before it is divided. On the left side, the vein courses caudally to enter the left renal vein and is managed in a similar manner.

D

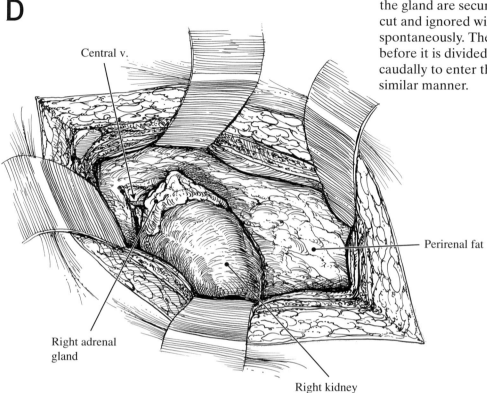

Central v.

Perirenal fat

Right adrenal gland

Right kidney

E

With hemostasis ensured, the wounds are closed in layers. The diaphragmatic incision is reapproximated with interrupted horizontal mattress stitches of 2-0 silk. The periosteal beds are closed with a continuous stitch of 2-0 chromic catgut. Before completion of this closure, medium-sized catheters are exteriorized from each pleural cavity. The divided latissimus dorsi muscles are reapproximated with interrupted 2-0 chromic catgut and the skin with interrupted vertical mattress stitches of 3-0 nylon. The anesthesiologist is then asked to expand the lungs maximally, at which time the catheters are withdrawn.

E

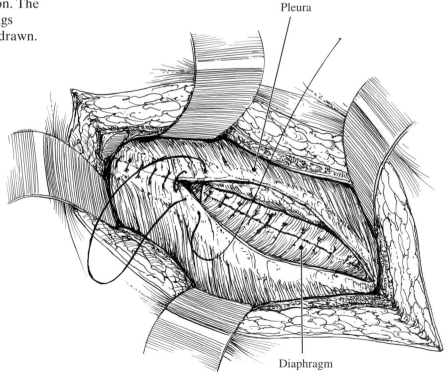

Pleura

Diaphragm

Chapter

23

GENITOURINARY SYSTEM

$\overline{A}$ RADICAL NEPHRECTOMY

Radical nephrectomy is indicated for operable carcinoma of the kidney. The rationale for this extended operation is the tendency of these tumors toward direct perirenal or venous invasion and lymphatic spread. If the tumor is transitional and arises in the collecting system of the kidney, nephroureterectomy and bladder cuff resection should be performed.

A

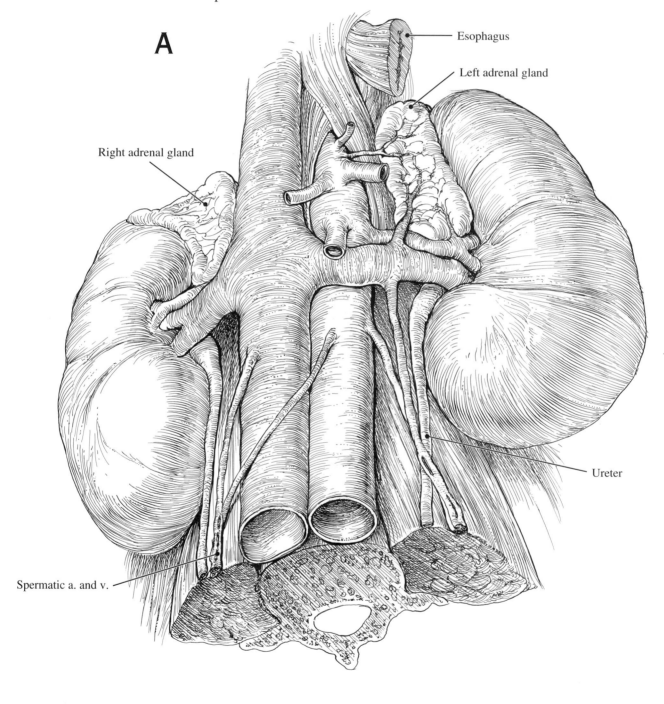

Esophagus

Left adrenal gland

Right adrenal gland

Ureter

Spermatic a. and v.

A

There is a considerable amount of anatomic complexity in both renal areas. A radical nephrectomy involves excision of the perinephric tissue with Gerota's fascia and the adrenal gland and thus mandatory exposure of most of the numerous topographic relationships of these organs. Those that are significant for the surgeon are illustrated here.

B

General endotracheal anesthesia is used. The patient is tilted with the operative side elevated about 25 degrees and supported in this position with several small sandbags. The leg on the operative side is flexed over the opposite leg, which is kept straight, and a pillow is placed between them. The arm is positioned away from the side of the patient and, after it is padded sufficiently, is supported in this position. The incision is made over the course of the eleventh rib.

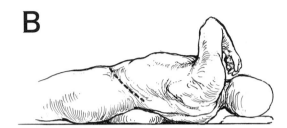

C

Most blood vessels encountered to this point are small and can be electrocoagulated. The incision is carried several centimeters posterior to the latissimus dorsi muscle and parallel to the fibers of the serratus anterior muscle so that very few of the muscle fibers need to be divided. The eleventh rib is excised subperiosteally. The anterior border of the latissimus dorsi muscle is retracted strongly so that as much of the rib as possible can be removed. The lung collapses readily on opening the chest, exposing the diaphragm. The fibers of the diaphragm are divided, usually transverse to their long axis, and the phrenic nerve should be sought and spared.

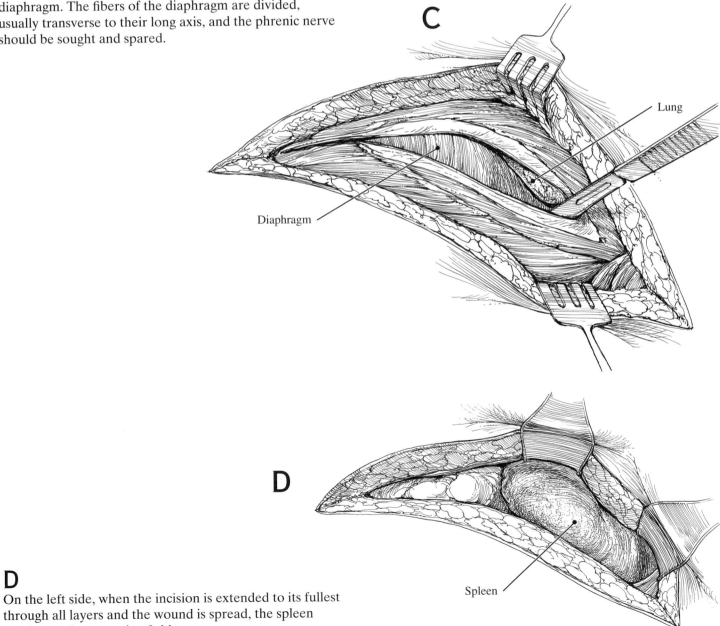

D

On the left side, when the incision is extended to its fullest through all layers and the wound is spread, the spleen dominates the operative field.

E

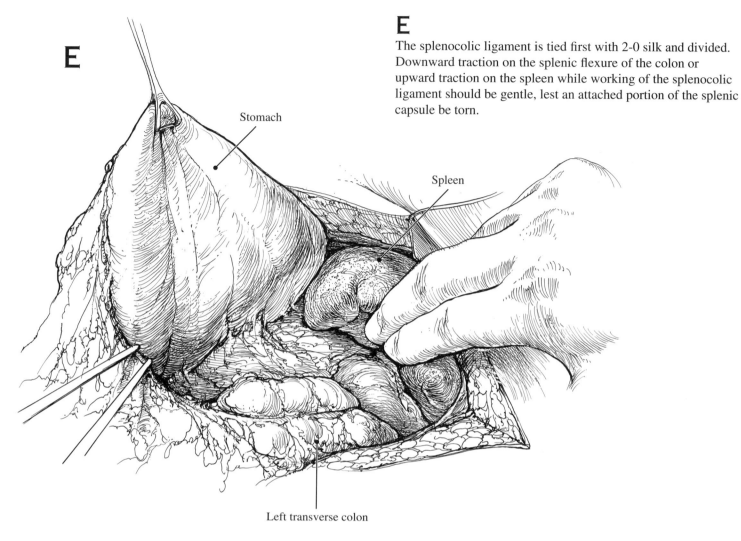

E

The splenocolic ligament is tied first with 2-0 silk and divided. Downward traction on the splenic flexure of the colon or upward traction on the spleen while working of the splenocolic ligament should be gentle, lest an attached portion of the splenic capsule be torn.

F

In the case of very large tumors, the gastrocolic ligament is divided next, the line of dissection located in the relatively avascular area inside the gastroepiploic artery and vein. Following this maneuver, the short gastric vessels are divided and ligated so that the colon and stomach can be displaced downward and medially. The body and tail of the pancreas are also exposed.

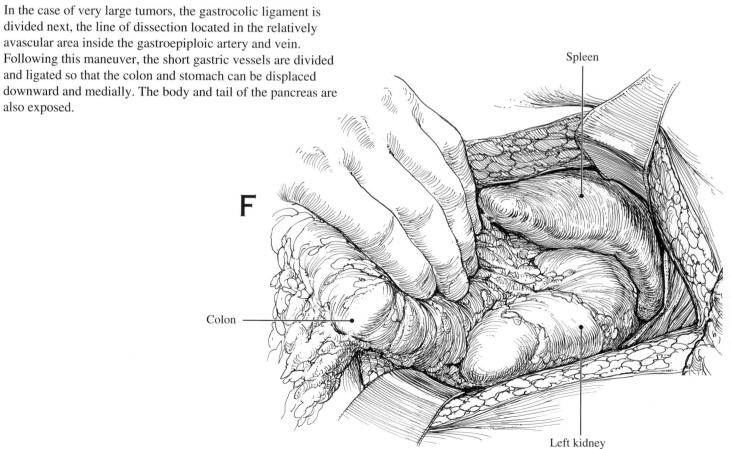

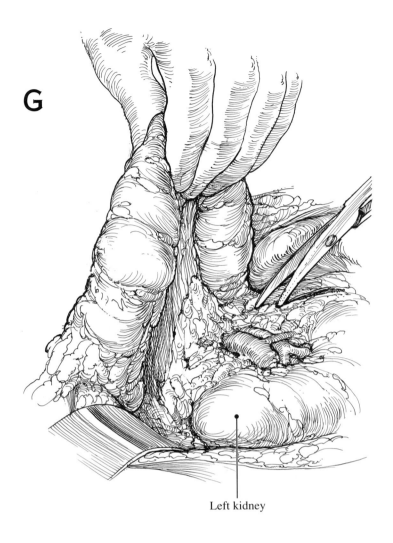

G

Left kidney

G, H, I

Most malignant tumors of the kidney are adenocarcinomas. Generally, extension into the renal vein or inferior vena cava can be determined preoperatively by contrast-labeled computed tomography to allow careful preoperative planning of more extensive exposures. Maneuverability around the kidney is one of the dividends of this generous incision and particular approach.

The immediate next step is to secure the blood supply of the kidney. The posterior parietal peritoneum is incised over the aorta, and any fatty areolar lymph node–bearing tissue is dissected laterally to the edge of the aorta.

The renal artery and vein are doubly ligated, in this order. In *H* and *I* the fatty areolar tissue in the area has been omitted for illustrative purposes. A Mixter clamp is used to encircle these vessels in preparation for the application of vascular clamps on each. A word of caution about a lumbar vein coming off the deep side of the renal vein immediately lateral to the aorta. Avulsing or puncturing it can lead to a major hemorrhage. The renal artery and vein are divided and oversewn with fine monofilament suture material. The internal spermatic vein is ligated and divided. The adrenal gland is excised as part of a proper cancer operation but also because its venous drainage must be sacrificed. During the dissection, the adrenal arteries can be secured with silver clips, but most stop bleeding spontaneously when cut.

H

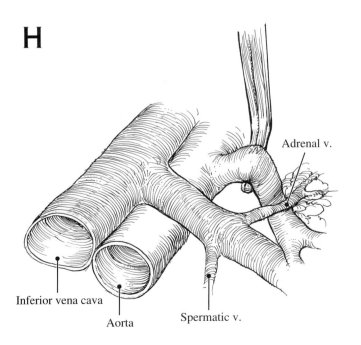

Inferior vena cava

Aorta

Spermatic v.

Adrenal v.

I

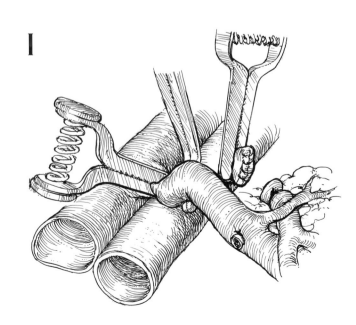

J

Up to this point, the dissection of the kidney has been from a medial to a lateral direction and in keeping with the principle of early sequestration of its blood supply and removal of the lymphatic channels toward their point of origin. Now the kidney is mobilized at its upper pole by incising the peritoneum and perirenal fascia. The adrenal gland lies within the encountered perirenal fat and is excised; at this point, some of the arterioles to the adrenal gland are found. On completion of this portion of the dissection, the base of the operative field will be the posterior insertions of the diaphragm.

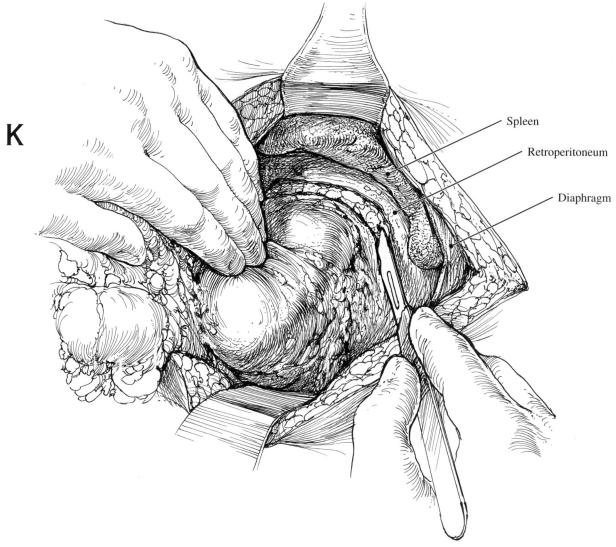

K

Any remaining lateral attachments are severed, and the kidney is lifted so the caudad dissection can continue.

Spleen

Retroperitoneum

Diaphragm

L

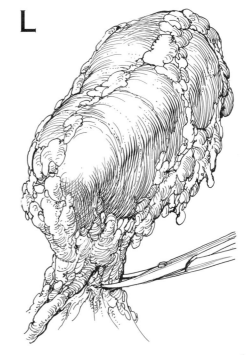

L

The distal point at which the ureter is divided depends largely on the cell type of the cancer being excised. Because in this instance it is an adenocarcinoma, the ureter is divided at its upper one third, and the distal segment is secured with a clip. For tumors of the renal pelvis or ureter, the entire ureter is excised; for ureteral tumors per se, the ureterovesical junction is excised as a button.

M

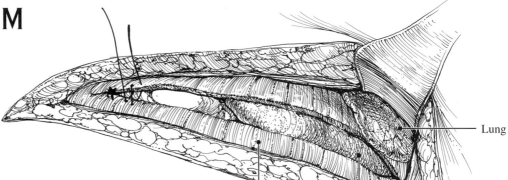

Lung

Diaphragm

Spleen

M

The operative site is checked for residual bleeding. A chest tube is exteriorized at the posterior axillary line at the eleventh interspace and attached to an underwater seal drainage. It is anchored to the skin securely. The lung is examined for areas of atelectasis, and any such areas are aerated. The diaphragmatic incision is reapproximated with interrupted horizontal mattress stitches of 2-0 silk.

N

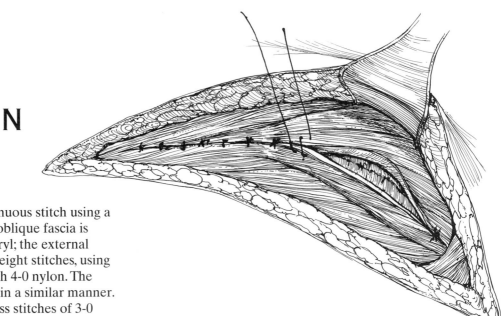

N

The peritoneum is closed with a continuous stitch using a stout absorbable suture. The internal oblique fascia is closed with a running stitch of 1-0 Vicryl; the external oblique fascia is closed with figure-of-eight stitches, using similar material. The skin is closed with 4-0 nylon. The intercostal muscles are approximated in a similar manner. The skin is closed with vertical mattress stitches of 3-0 nylon.

B URINARY CONDUIT

A urinary conduit is frequently needed in the setting of radical surgery to control pelvic neoplasms. Its associated purpose is to provide ready passage of urine to an external receptacle, thus eliminating the sequelae of retrograde infection or of urinary stasis.

A

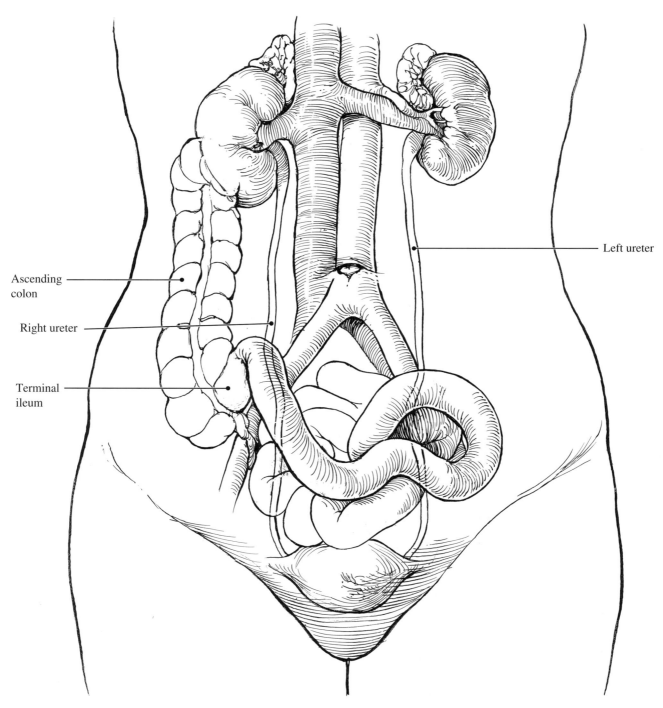

Ascending colon

Right ureter

Terminal ileum

Left ureter

A

Some of the topographic relationships that are helpful in the construction of an ileal conduit are shown. The conduit will lie deep to the reanastomosed ileum, such that its distal end will have to course anteriorly to reach the outside.

B

The ureters have multiple origins of blood supply from the renal, spermatic, hypogastric, and inferior vesical arteries. Even so, they should be dissected for the necessary length only; also, they should not be stripped of their periureteral fat. Both of these factors can lead to ureteral necrosis and urinary leakage postoperatively. The ureters course along the medial borders of the psoas muscles and the bifurcation of the common iliac vessels before entering the pelvis. At the pelvic aperture, the left ureter lies behind the sigmoid colon and its mesentery.

B

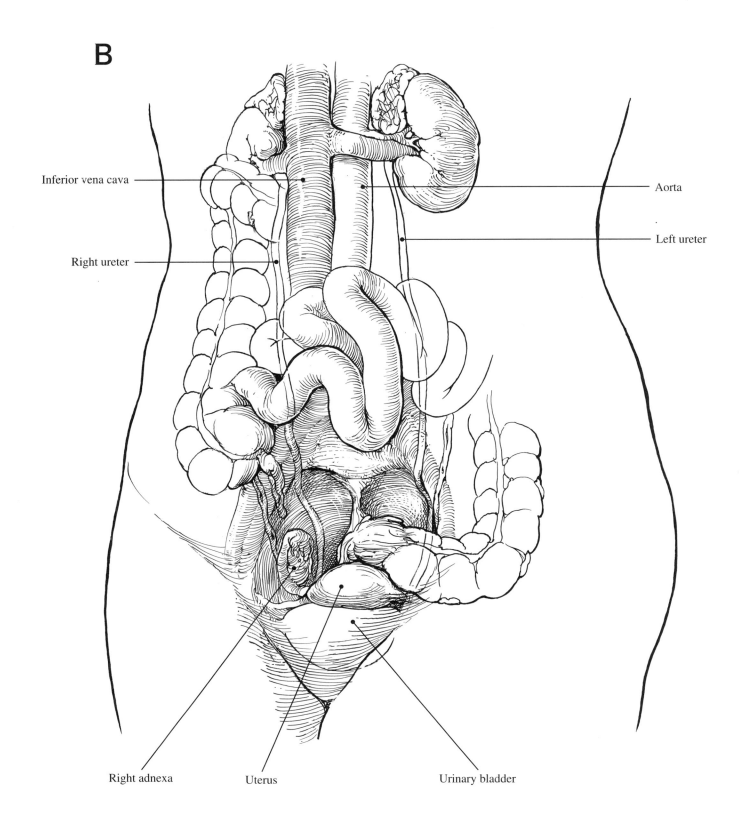

Inferior vena cava

Right ureter

Aorta

Left ureter

Right adnexa   Uterus   Urinary bladder

C

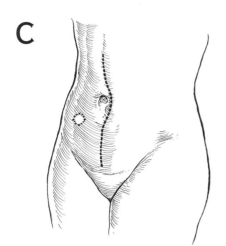

A midline incision is used. It is important to give adequate thought to the site of the ileostomy so that it will be surrounded by flat skin; the functional success of the operation depends on whether the appliance for urine collection is fitted and glued properly postoperatively and does not leak. This means that the stoma should not be too close to the umbilicus or anterior iliac spine and that deep natural skin creases should be avoided. The spot for the stoma should be marked on the patient's abdomen preoperatively and with the patient standing.

D

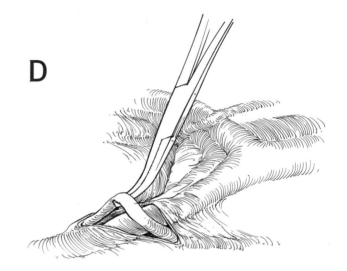

D, E

The posterior peritoneum over the iliac bifurcation is incised to expose and mobilize the ureters, but the dissection must not be so thorough that it removes the periureteral adventitial tissue and the associated nutrient blood vessels or that it invites ureteral ischemia and necrosis. As it would be technically awkward and clinically hazardous to deal with an acute appendicitis in such patients, an appendectomy is performed routinely.

E

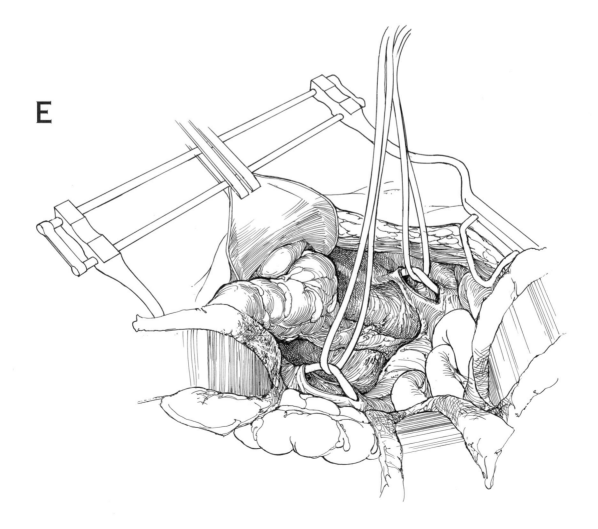

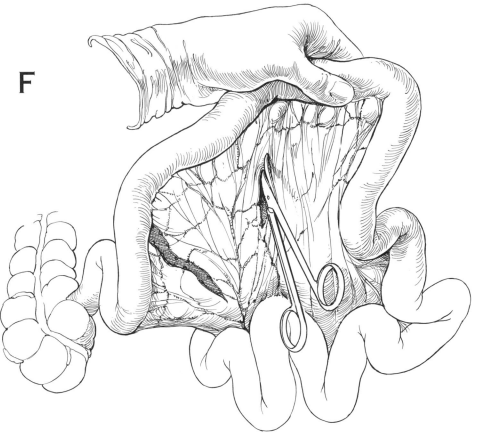

F

A section of terminal ileum about 20 cm in length and 10 cm from the ileocecal valve is selected for the conduit.

G

The mesentery of this ileal segment should be divided toward its root, creating a segment sufficient only to fashion the conduit; excessive dissection may jeopardize its blood supply. The periphery of the mesentery of the proximal end of the conduit is fashioned as shown. The ileum is stapled and divided in three places: the proximal and distal ends and the location indicated by the dashed line. The short, devitalized middle segment is discarded.

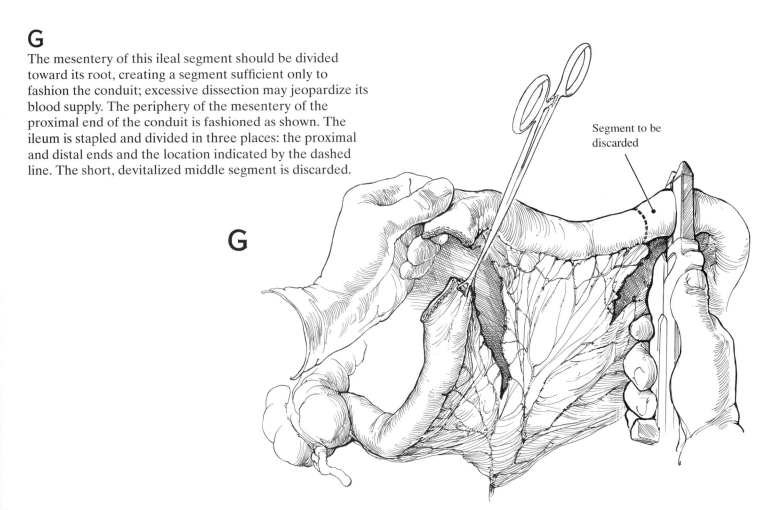

Segment to be discarded

H

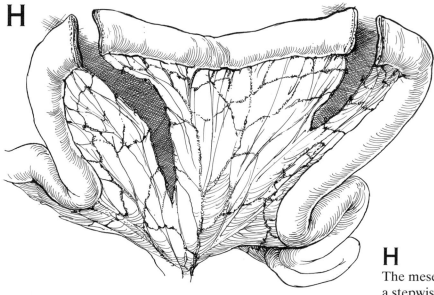

H

The mesentery of the distal portion of the conduit is cut in a stepwise fashion, particularly so in patients with a thick abdominal wall. Such tailoring of the mesentery makes available a few more centimeters of distal ileum with an adequate blood supply so that the ileal stoma can reach the skin surface without undue tension.

I

The isolated segment of ileum is brought dorsal to the segments of ileum whose mainstream will be reestablished. If the conduit were to course ventrally, it would require a longer traverse of the ureter to reach it and also permit small intestine to lie on it. Both invite kinking of the conduit or disruption of the ureteroileal anastomosis.

I

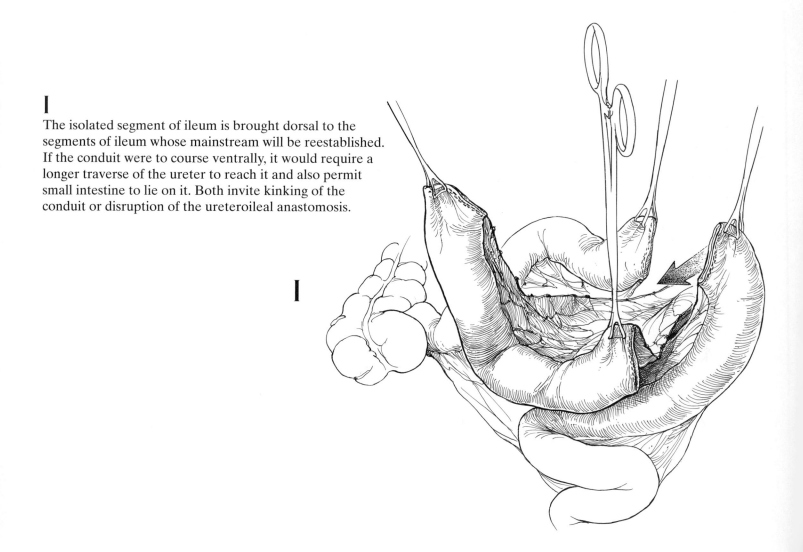

J, K

The ileal stream can be reconstructed in several ways; here it is shown end-to-end and hand sewn. The stapled ileum is trimmed, and a row of interrupted simple stitches of atraumatic 3-0 silk is applied through the seromuscular layer (*J*). The posterior row of stitches through the seromuscularis is completed; the seromuscularis stitches at each end are retained for stabilization. The mucosa is approximated with a continuous stitch or with interrupted simple stitches of 4-0 chromic catgut (*K*).

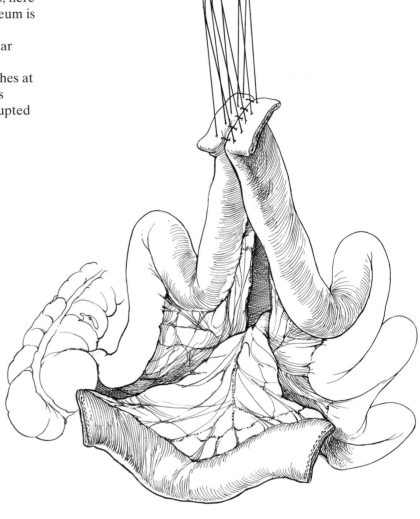

K

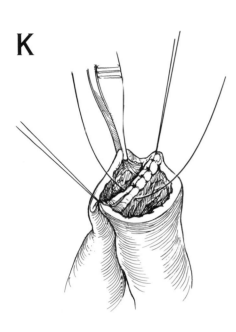

L, M

The anterior row of interrupted seromuscular stitches of 3-0 silk is now applied. Experience and judgment enable the surgeon to do this without invagination of excessive amounts of tissue.

L

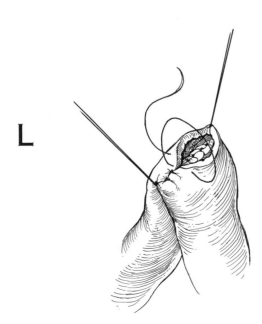

M

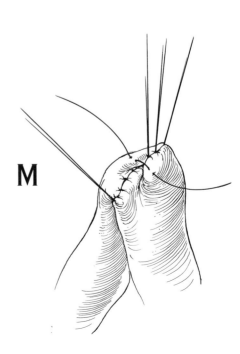

N

The mesenteric defect is closed with a continuous stitch of atraumatic 4-0 Maxon. The mesentery should be caught just inside its cut edge. Sometimes, careless placing of the needle too far from this edge results in occlusion of a marginal vessel, thus posing a threat to the viability of the ileum at the anastomosis. Also, the mesenteric opening should be ample enough that the blood supply to the conduit is not compromised, yet not so generous that intestine can herniate through it.

N

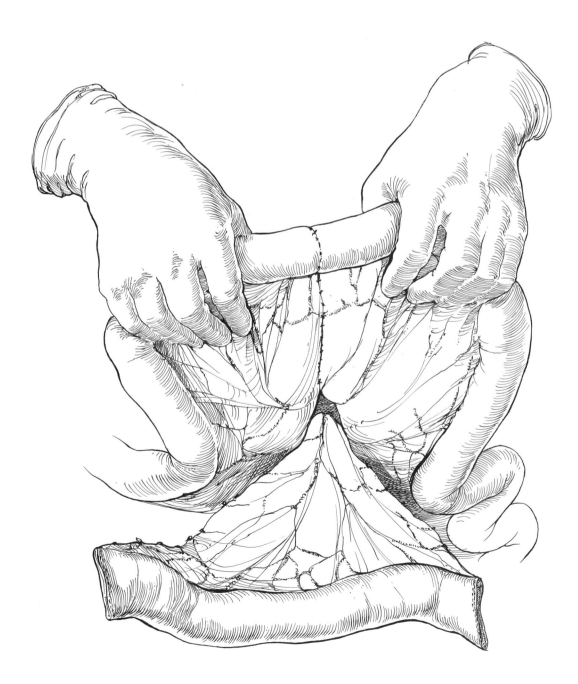

O

The reanastomosed ileum is displaced cephalad with the conduit positioned dorsal to it.

At the beginning of the operation the ureters were identified as they crossed the bifurcation of the iliac vessels. They are now transected 3 to 4 cm beyond this point, and the distal ureters tied with 2-0 Maxon. The proximal ureters are then freed for a distance of 4 or 5 cm. The left ureter is anastomosed first and as it presents itself. An alternative method is to mobilize the left ureter for 8 to 10 cm and to tunnel it retroperitoneally toward the right so that both anastomoses can be made close to the exit of the conduit.

O

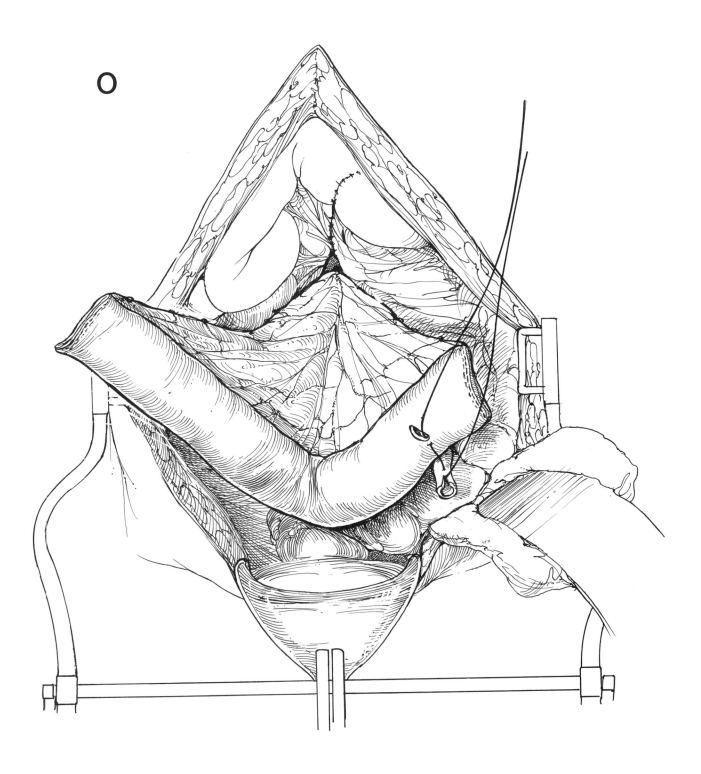

P, Q

A first transverse row of about four stitches of 4-0 vascular suture material is applied between the serosa of the bowel and the adventitia of the ureter (*P*). The stitches should be placed about 1.5 cm from the cut end of the ureter.

The diameter of the terminal ureter is enlarged by making a 1-cm longitudinal slit proximally and on its ventral side. Such spatulation is not necessary, of course, if the ureter already is hydronephrotic. Next, a no. 7 French J-shaped ureteral stenting catheter is advanced up the ureter.

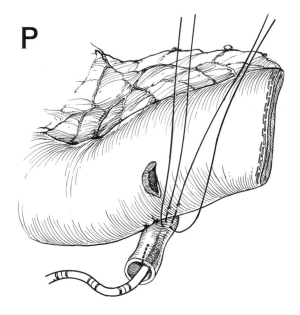

P

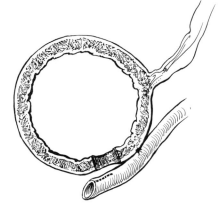

Q

R, S, T

The ileal opening should correspond in size to the diameter of the spatulated ureter. The inner mucosal anastomosis is performed with interrupted 4-0 Maxon. The first stitch is placed between the apex of the spatulating cut in the ureter and the dorsalmost point of the ileal opening. The opposite end of the stenting ureteral catheter is inserted into the conduit and advanced to its distal, open end. This and the remaining stitches—through the entire thickness of the ureter and bowel—are placed 2 mm from each edge (*R*). The anastomosis is completed by placing the anterior row of stitches between the adventitia of the ureter and the seromuscular layer of the ileum (*S, T*). A similar anastomosis is carried out on the right side.

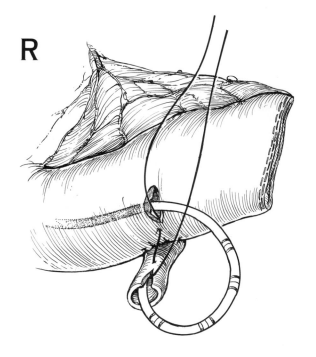

R

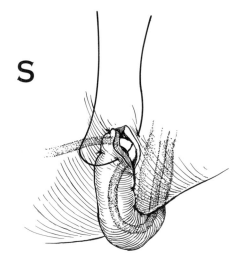

S

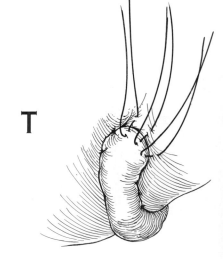

T

U, V, W, X, Y

The site for exteriorization of the conduit will have been chosen before beginning the operation. A button of skin and subcutaneous fat is excised in adequate diameter to allow unrestricted passage of the ileum. Similar pieces of fascia and peritoneum have to be excised, but before this is done, they should be pulled medially so that all the openings are in proper alignment. Otherwise, there may be a shearing effect along the various layers of the abdominal wall, leading to obstruction of the conduit. Alternatively, the opening for the conduit can be fashioned before making the major abdominal incision. The ileum is gently eased through the abdominal wall while the conduit is observed for kinking, twisting, or excess tension.

The stapled ileum is trimmed (*U, V*), and 4-0 chromic catgut is used to anchor it to the abdominal wall in the following manner: the stitch is placed through the seromuscularis; just short of the skin surface, the stitch again is made to engage the seromuscularis; while still at this depth the needle is turned to engage a short distance of the skin, whereupon it is exteriorized. It is tied gently so as not to cut through the conduit. Usually, eight such stitches are necessary to create the proper "nipple" of ileal tissue (*W, X, Y*). The abdomen is closed in a preferred manner.

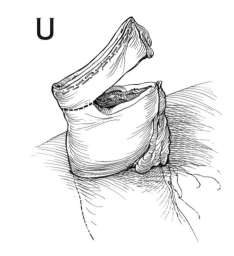

U

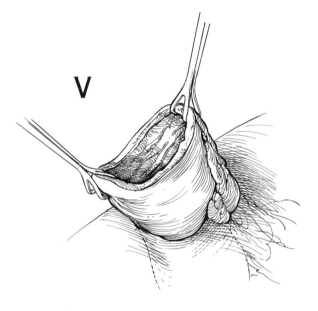

V

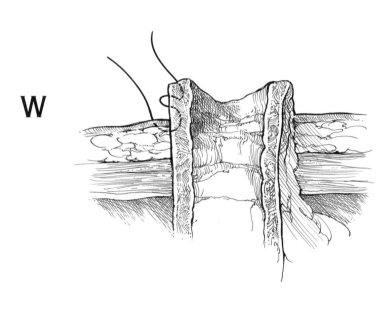

W

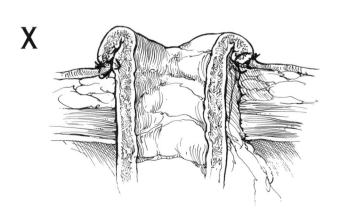

X

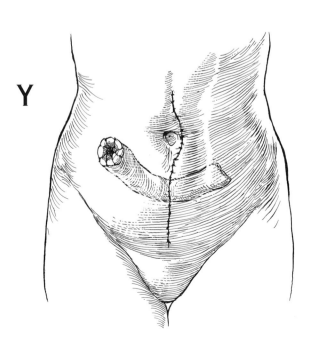

Y

C HYDROCELECTOMY

A

The purpose of this operation is to excise enough of the tunica vaginalis and so reconstruct it that a hydrocele cannot recur. The anatomic structures associated with a hydrocelectomy are straightforward.

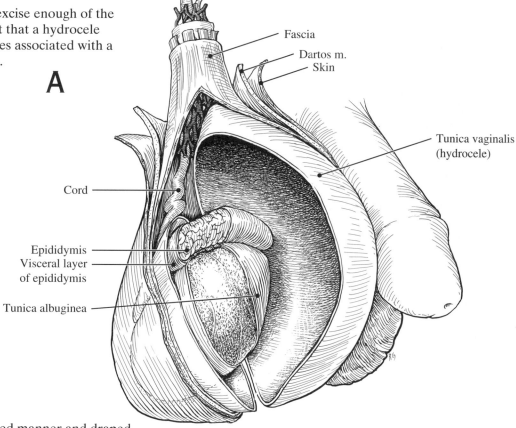

A

Fascia

Dartos m.

Skin

Tunica vaginalis (hydrocele)

Cord

Epididymis

Visceral layer of epididymis

Tunica albuginea

B

The scrotum is prepared in a preferred manner and draped. The scrotum with the contained hydrocele is grasped with one hand and squeezed in a manner that the skin over the hydrocele is stretched. A longitudinal incision about 6 to 10 cm in length is made and carried through the scrotal skin, levator muscle, and cremasteric fascia to the (parietal) tunica vaginalis, which forms the hydrocele.

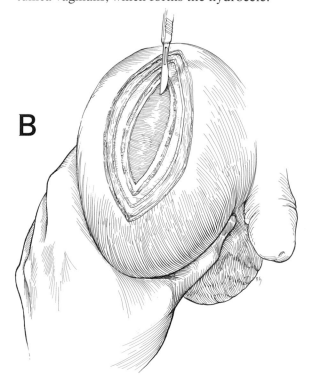

B

C

A medium-sized Metzenbaum scissors is used to dissect along the tunica vaginalis; a fine-tipped cautery is used to coagulate bleeding points, with particular attention to the tissue that is to remain.

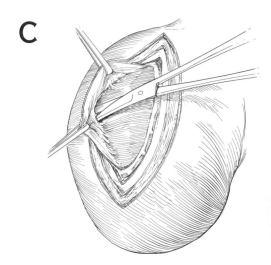

C

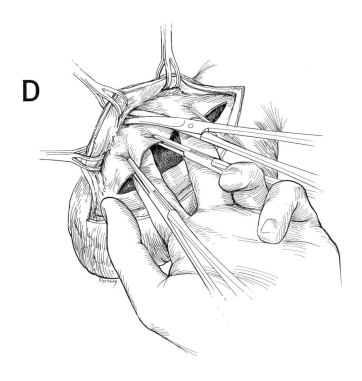

D

D, E

At this point a trocar is used to evacuate the hydrocele, which then is further opened by electrocautery. Hemostats are applied to the cut edge of the tunica vaginalis, and Babcock forceps are used to grasp inclusively the skin, dartos muscle, and cremasteric fascia. With both sets of instruments on traction, the tissue plane is developed further, the dissection of the tunica vaginalis being carried to within 2 cm of the testicle.

E

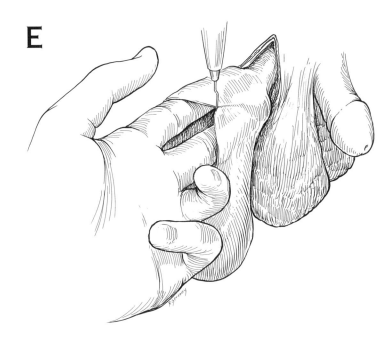

F

The tunica and testicle are grasped as shown and the testicle delivered out of the hydrocele sac in preparation to trimming the sac.

F

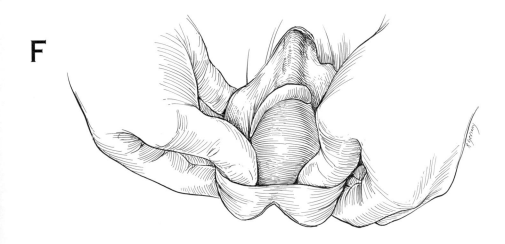

G

The excess tissue of the hydrocele sac is trimmed circumferentially with the electrocautery, maintaining a distance of about 2 cm from the testicle. Concurrent with this trimming of the tunica vaginalis is the oversewing of its free edge with a continuous simple running stitch of 4-0 chromic catgut. Excess tension on the catgut should be avoided so that it does not create a purse-string effect.

H, I

The tunica is inverted on itself to eliminate the risk of reformation of the hydrocele. Flipping the testicle upward provides access to its opposite surface. The edge of the everted tunica vaginalis is approximated to itself with a continuous simple stitch of 4-0 chromic catgut. The upper end of the tunica is left open for escape of serous fluid.

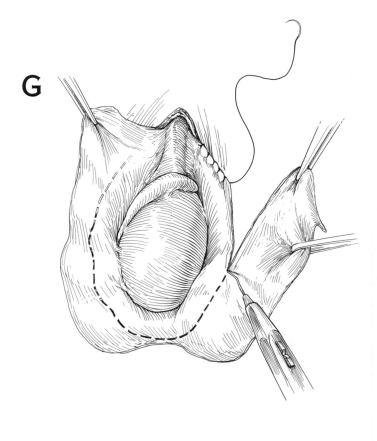

G

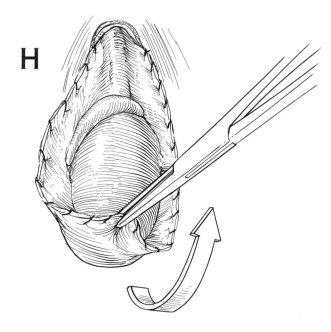

H

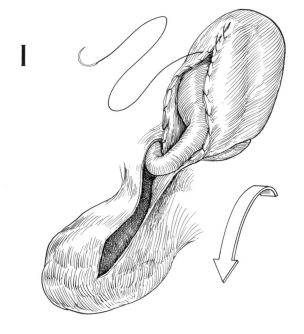

I

J

The entire operative field is carefully examined, and bleeding points are electrocoagulated. Even small bleeding sites in this loose tissue can grow into a large hematoma postoperatively.

The testicle is replaced into the scrotum and carefully positioned so that no torsion is present. A small Penrose drain is exteriorized through the scrotal incision that is closed as one layer using interrupted vertical mattress stitches of 5-0 nylon. An elastic suspensory scrotal support is a simple way to keep a dressing in place and provide some wound pressure and some comfort as well.

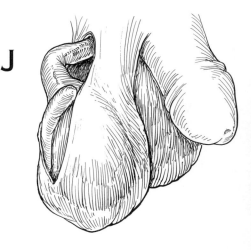

J

A SPLENECTOMY

ELECTIVE

There are a number of indications for splenectomy. In some, the spleen is relatively normal in size, and the patient is in reasonable condition. In others, the surgeon is presented with a seriously ill patient whose spleen is simply enormous. It is essential, therefore, that the surgeon be both fully conversant with the anatomy of this area and the various technical considerations that are applicable and knowledgeable of the disease process making the splenectomy necessary.

A

This illustration shows the complex anatomy of the splenic area.

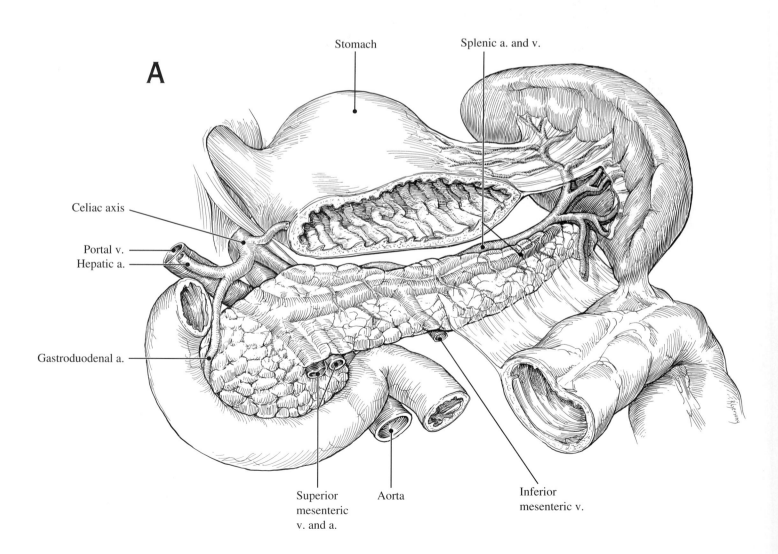

A

Stomach

Splenic a. and v.

Celiac axis

Portal v.

Hepatic a.

Gastroduodenal a.

Superior
mesenteric
v. and a.

Aorta

Inferior
mesenteric v.

B

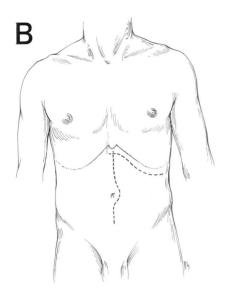

B

For a spleen of average size the incision can be left subcostal, but for gross splenomegaly it should be longitudinal and the full length of the abdomen.

C

The abdomen is opened and first explored for unexpected abnormalities. The splenocolic ligament contains vessels large enough to warrant ligating this tissue in its entirety with 2-0 silk and dividing it.

D, E

Whenever possible, it is advantageous to ligate and divide the short gastric and any accessory vessels before addressing the splenic artery and vein.

Unless it is unavoidable, the spleen is not routinely delivered outside the abdominal cavity to work on its nutrient vessels. Whereas such a step gives quick control of the listed vessels, it is accompanied by the need to lift the pancreas off of its retroperitoneal bed with the attendant leakage of lymph postoperatively. Although the approach described above attempts to avoid this, if utilizing it presents any difficulties the spleen is exteriorized and the vessels handled individually. If for some reason there is brisk bleeding from splenic vessels or the spleen itself, the entire hilus is secured with a vascular clamp, and the spleen amputated. The vessels can then be ligated more specifically and at leisure. Further care should be taken to avoid damage to the tail of the pancreas.

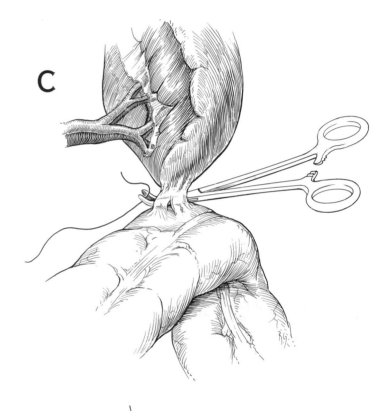

D

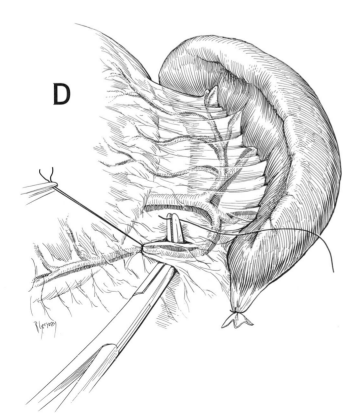

E

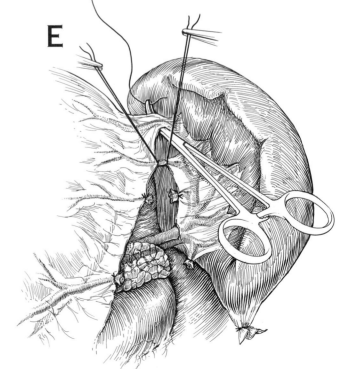

F, G, H

The splenic artery is ligated first and doubly with 2-0 silk (*F, G*). After a few moments to allow for blood within the spleen to reenter the general circulation, the splenic vein is ligated with 2-0 silk and divided (*H*). The short gastric vessels will have been secured; if not, they are attended to now.

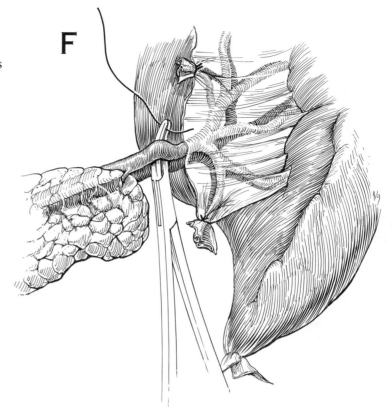

F

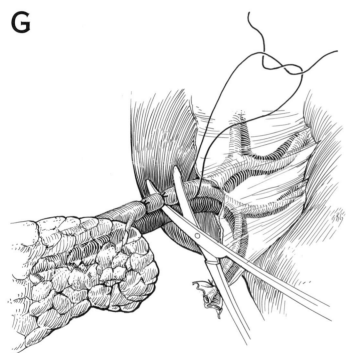

G

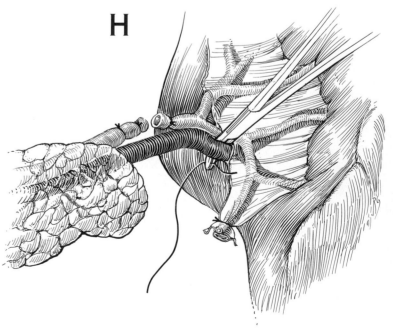

H

I

The devascularized spleen is now removed, and several dry laparotomy pads under mild pressure are placed in the splenic bed. There follows the important step of methodically electrocoagulating any oozing point, however small. Tamponading by other organs in this area is minimal, so even a small amount of oozing can produce a surprisingly sizable hematoma postoperatively.

I

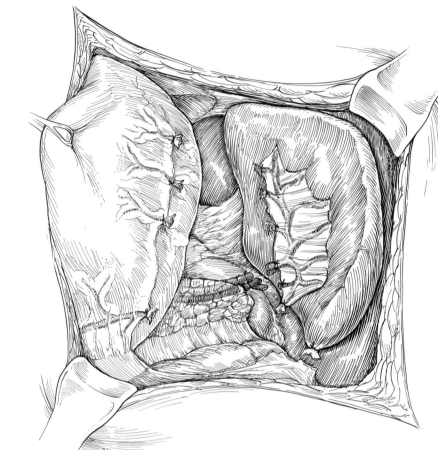

J, K

Occasionally, the spleen and the hilar vessels are so large and sufficiently hazardous to dissect without proximal control that provisional occlusion of the splenic artery along the lesser curvature of the stomach (*J*) permits a more careful and safer dissection of the vessels at the splenic hilum. Such large vessels are best secured with a continuous simple running stitch of fine vascular suture material (*K*).

J

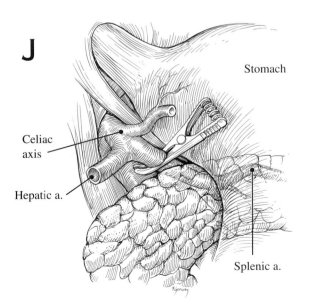

K

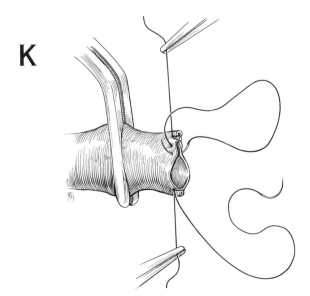

L

If the surgeon's preference is to initiate the resection by mobilizing the spleen to reach the vessels, the spleen is retracted medially while the parietal peritoneum is incised with electrocautery.

L

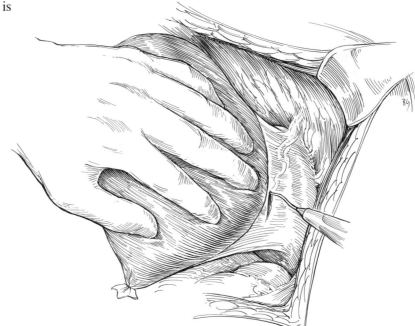

M, N

The splenic vessels are dissected free and the splenic artery ligated first. The spleen is partially lifted, revealing the three or four short gastric vessels, which are ligated with fine silk and divided.

M

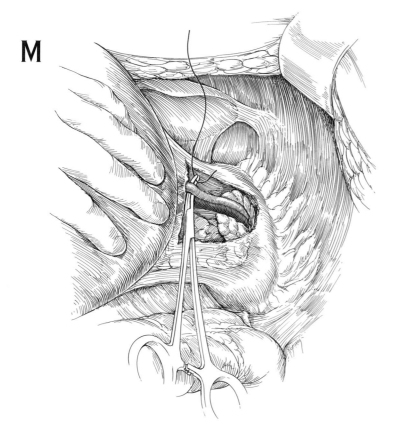

N

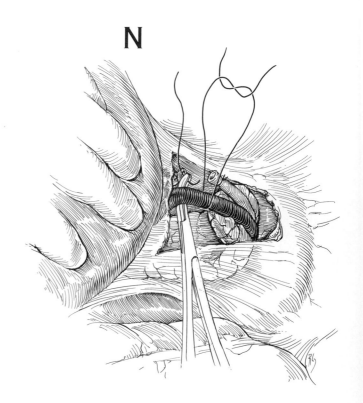

Whichever technique is used, we do not drain the splenic bed but rely on meticulous hemostasis. The incision is closed in a preferred manner.

SALVAGE

Abdominal trauma, especially to the left upper quadrant, is the most common cause of injury to the spleen. This illustration shows one such causative mechanism.

When to perform a splenectomy or to salvage a portion or all of the spleen requires seasoned clinical judgment, experience, and technical skill. Some pertinent anatomic characteristics of the spleen are as follows: The splenic artery divides into three or more branches before entering the spleen, each branch supplying roughly a particular portion of the spleen. The blood vessels generally run in a horizontal plane, which also is the more common plane of fractures in the spleen. The spleen has a secondary blood supply via the short gastric vessels.

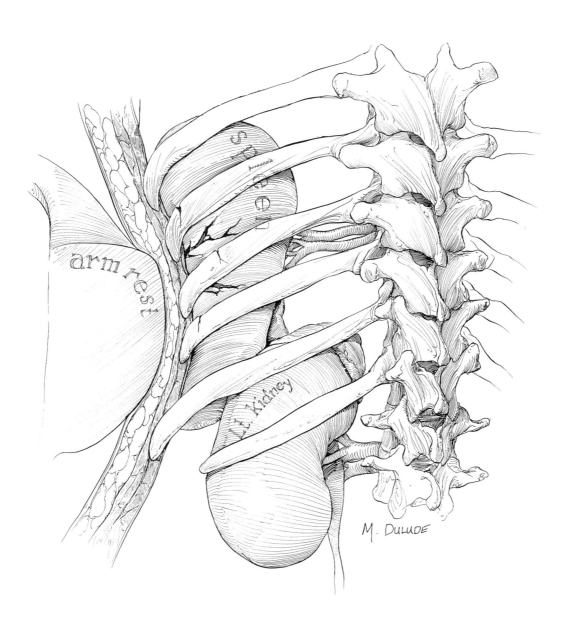

A

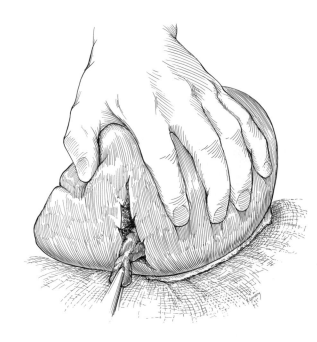

B

C

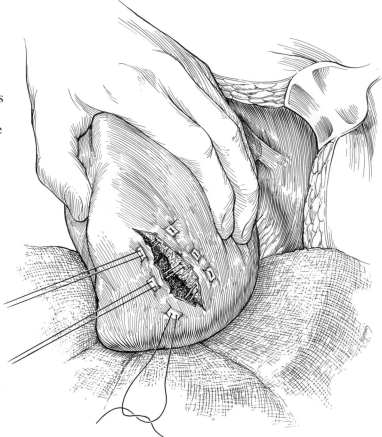

A

Initial operative management of splenic injuries is adequate mobilization of the spleen. Here a spleen that has sustained a horizontal fracture across the lower pole with clot extruding from the fracture but with no bleeding at the moment is mobilized medially by incising the lateral attachments.

B

The spleen is inspected fully, and no other injury is found. Provisional arterial control is established at the hilum. The clot is removed, and obviously devascularized tissue is débrided.

C

Any actively bleeding vessels are secured with suture ligatures of fine vascular suture. Sometimes there is only mild, nonspecific oozing that can be covered with a topical hemostatic agent before closure. Closure is performed with horizontal mattress stitches of vascular material using Teflon bolsters to prevent the sutures from cutting into the spleen.

D

This illustration shows a less common lone vertical tear into which a tongue of omentum has been placed before closure.

E, F

In this example, a portion of the lower pole of the spleen is insufficiently vascularized; it is best to amputate it, incorporating a tongue of omentum over the sutured raw area.

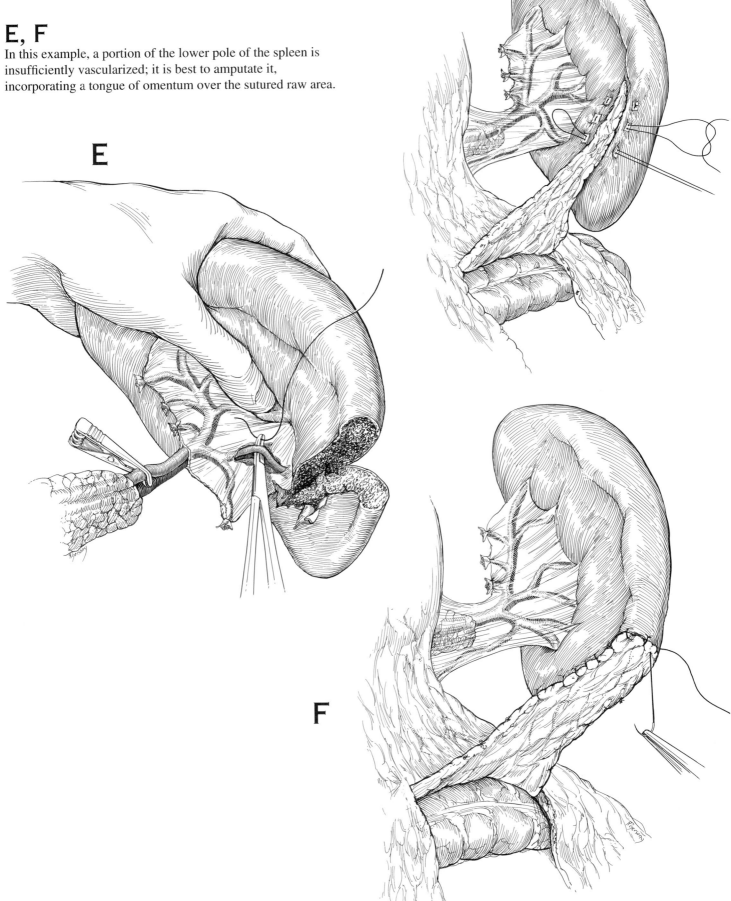

UTERUS AND ADNEXA

A   HYSTERECTOMY AND BILATERAL SALPINGO-OOPHORECTOMY

Hysterectomy with or without bilateral salpingo-oophorectomy is performed for benign disease, most notably for uterine fibroids.

A

The patient is placed in the supine position with provision for some Trendelenburg tilt later. The abdomen is prepared from the midthighs to the groin to include the vagina. The incision is low midline or transverse, depending on body habitus and size of the uterus to be removed.

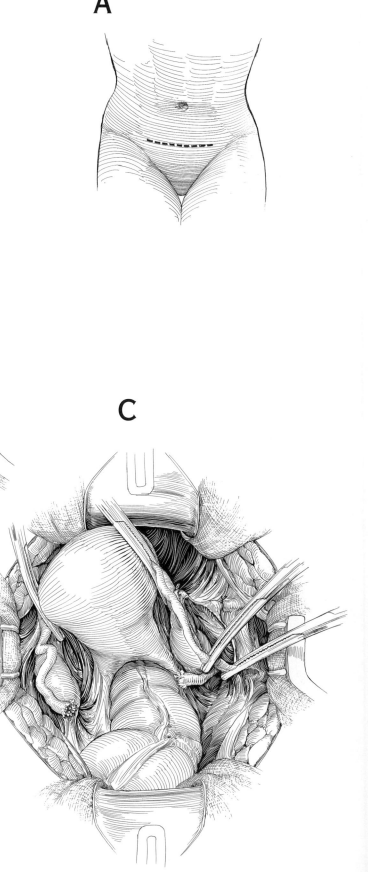

B, C

The location of the ureter should be identified on the medial leaf of the peritoneum before clamping the infundibulopelvic ligament. The infundibulopelvic ligament and the ovarian vessels therein can be clamped before division as shown. Alternatively, a Mixter clamp can be teased through an avascular window and 2-0 silk passed through it for ligation before division.

D–I

The pattern of vessels here makes it valuable to know the several methods of securing them. One method is simple ligation with 2-0 silk, doubly on the proximal side. Another is a transfixion stitch, but because the needle may go through the vessel and provoke a hematoma, a simple ligature is placed more proximal to the transfixion stitch (*D, E, F*). For large vessels, securing them by oversewing them with fine atraumatic vascular suture provides the best security (*G, H, I*).

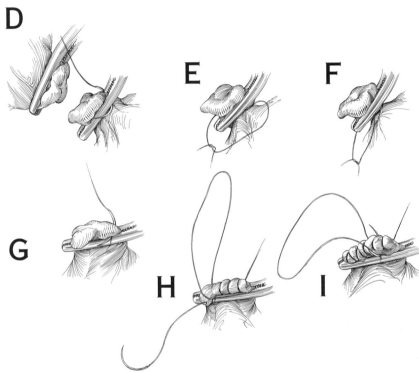

J, K

The peritoneum of the vesicouterine fold is being divided. With continued traction, the peritoneum and the cervicovesical fold are incised and developed with care that the bladder is not entered. A pledget of gauze on a 6-inch forceps (locally referred to as a "peanut") can be used to stay close to the vagina and a safe distance from the urinary bladder (*K*). Alternatively, in patients who have had prior cesarean section and may have scarring of the bladder to the vagina, the bladder may be taken off of the anterior vagina sharply with a Metzenbaum scissors.

L

The uterine artery is identified—preferably entirely visually, but often palpation is necessary—and a clamp is applied. This is done as close as possible to the uterus to lessen the risk to the ureter. Many hemostats for clamping the uterine artery are in vogue. We use one that has stout jaws, is not too long, and has interlocking teeth at its tips. We have developed the safe habit of securing the proximal clamped and divided vessels with a simple over-and-over stitch using vascular suture material. It takes a moment longer but is the most secure. A figure-of-eight stitch is adequate for the uterine side. It is beneficial to remember to attend to each instrument as soon as it serves its function and then to remove it from the field.

L

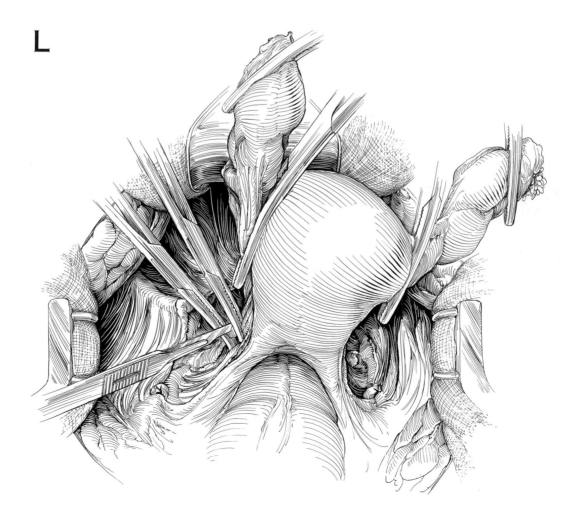

M

The peritoneum is taken down off the uterus posteriorly. One to two more bites with a straight clamp are typically required parallel to the cervix on each side to reach the point where the cervix meets the vagina. The last bite should incorporate the uterosacral ligaments. It is important to place these clamps close to the uterus to avoid damage to the ureter.

M

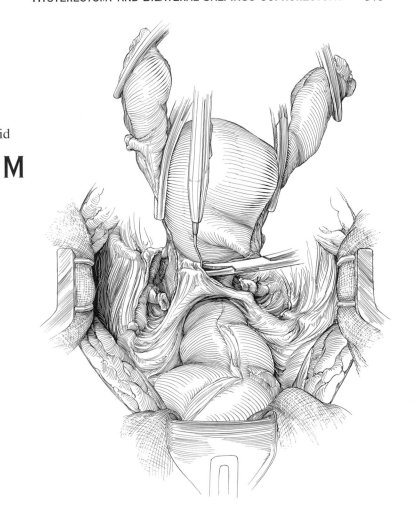

N₁, N₂

The uterus should now be free to just past the cervix. Firm palpation with the thumb and index finger helps delineate this border.

N₁

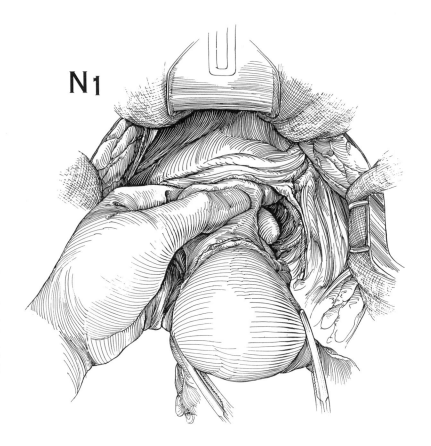

N₂

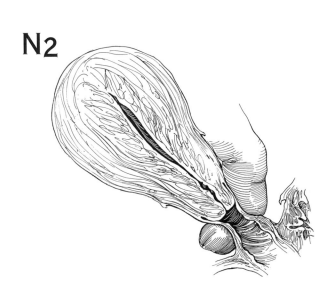

O, P, Q

A forceps is used to hold up the vagina as entry is made into it with the cutting current on the electrocautery unit. Scissors are used to enlarge the opening, leaving about 5 mm of vagina attached to the cervix.

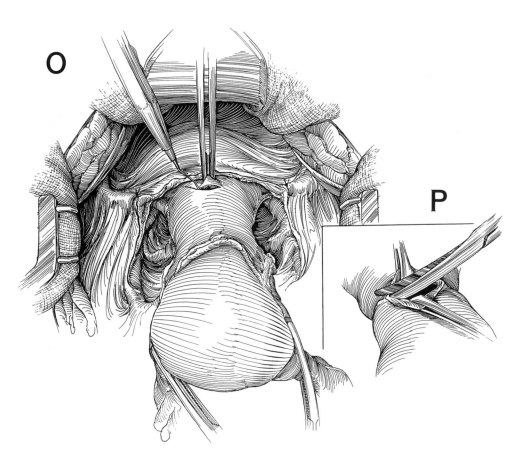

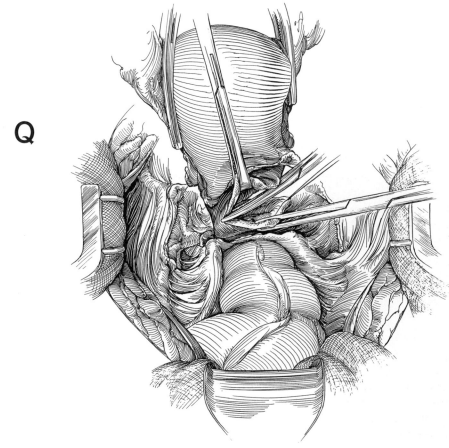

R

Laterally located stabilizing stitches are placed, and a lock stitch of 2-0 chromic catgut is used to obtain hemostasis of the vaginal cuff.

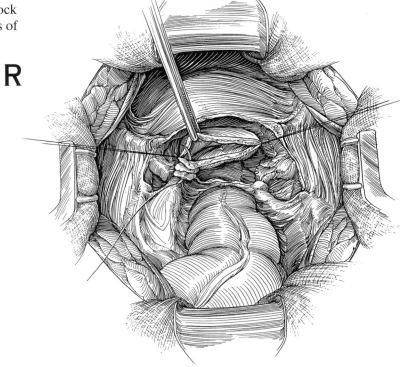

R

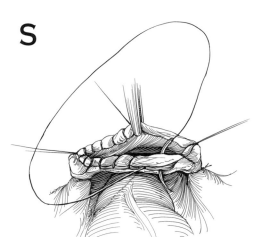

S

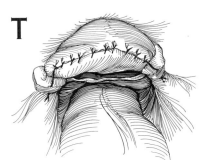

T

S, T

The uterosacral ligament is incorporated into the lateral aspect of the vaginal tissue with separate stitches of 3-0 Maxon (*S*). The vaginal cuff can be closed completely (*T*) with interrupted stitches, but this measure traps fluid that cannot escape into the vagina or out of the pelvic peritoneum, which is about to be sealed. Leaving the cuff open partially helps lessen this problem.

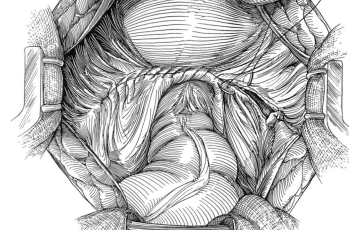

U

U

The pelvic peritoneum is closed with a continuous simple stitch of 3-0 chromic catgut. All raw tissue and stubs should be buried beneath this suture line so that the final surface is smooth and not inviting to the formation of adhesions.

B RADICAL ABDOMINAL HYSTERECTOMY AND PELVIC LYMPHADENECTOMY

A

Radical abdominal hysterectomy with pelvic lymphadenectomy is performed primarily for the treatment of carcinoma of the cervix. Cervical carcinoma spreads by direct extension into the paracervical and paravaginal tissue with concurrent involvement of the intervening lymphatic channels, yet has some tendency to remain confined to the pelvis for a period. For this reason, most surgeons agree that a radical hysterectomy and pelvic node dissection achieve the maximum cure rate provided the cervical cancer is sufficiently confined.

Shown here is the rich anatomy of the female pelvis, about which the surgeon must be thoroughly knowledgeable.

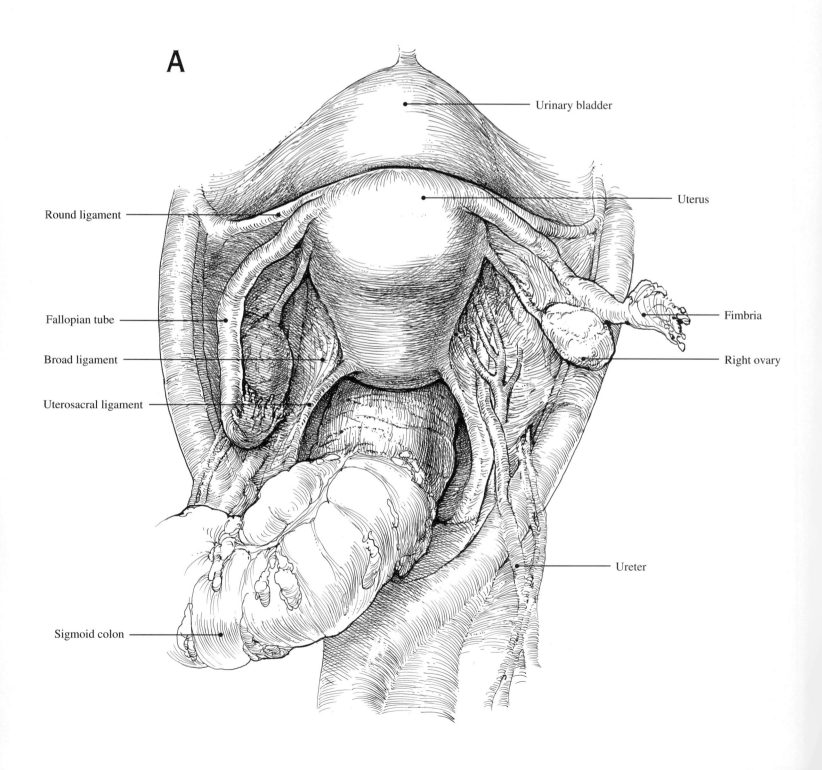

A

Urinary bladder

Uterus

Round ligament

Fallopian tube

Fimbria

Broad ligament

Right ovary

Uterosacral ligament

Ureter

Sigmoid colon

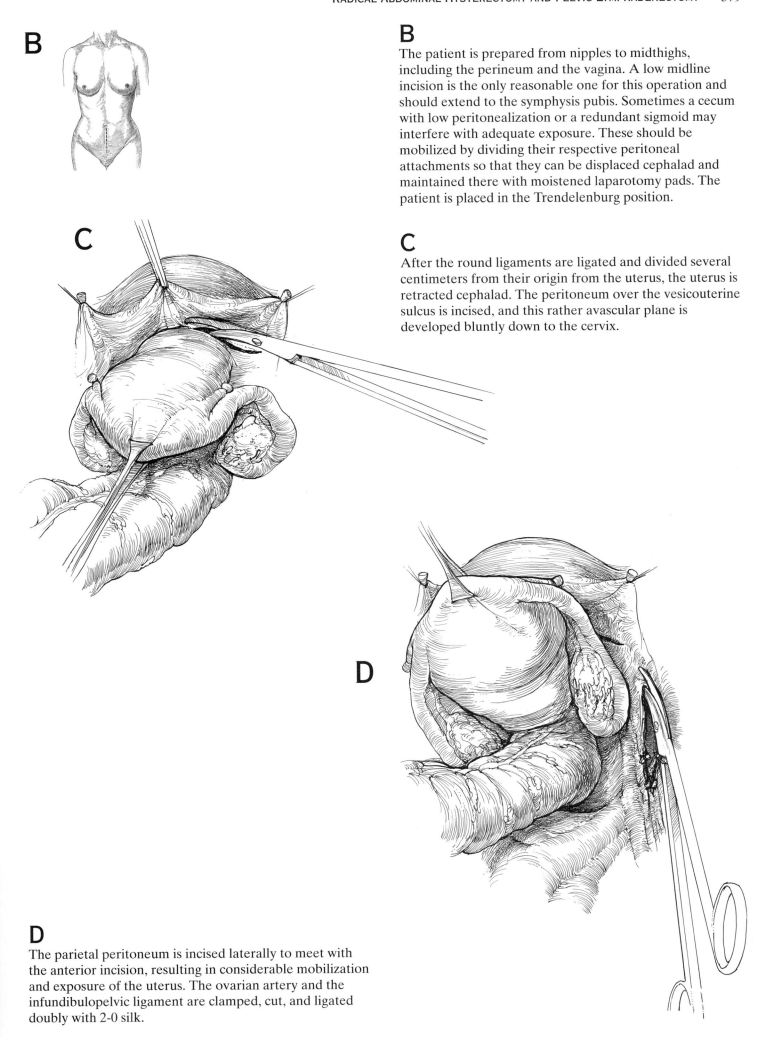

B

B

The patient is prepared from nipples to midthighs, including the perineum and the vagina. A low midline incision is the only reasonable one for this operation and should extend to the symphysis pubis. Sometimes a cecum with low peritonealization or a redundant sigmoid may interfere with adequate exposure. These should be mobilized by dividing their respective peritoneal attachments so that they can be displaced cephalad and maintained there with moistened laparotomy pads. The patient is placed in the Trendelenburg position.

C

C

After the round ligaments are ligated and divided several centimeters from their origin from the uterus, the uterus is retracted cephalad. The peritoneum over the vesicouterine sulcus is incised, and this rather avascular plane is developed bluntly down to the cervix.

D

D

The parietal peritoneum is incised laterally to meet with the anterior incision, resulting in considerable mobilization and exposure of the uterus. The ovarian artery and the infundibulopelvic ligament are clamped, cut, and ligated doubly with 2-0 silk.

E

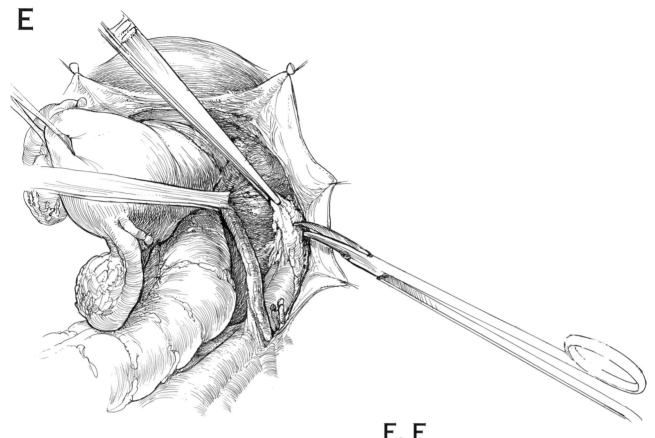

E, F

The ureter is mobilized with constant care not to "strip" it excessively, as this invites avascular necrosis and postoperative fistula formation. The ureter is freed to just past the uterine artery. Dissection beyond this point proceeds later. The web of tissue superior and lateral to the ureter at this point contains the uterine artery, the superior vesical artery, and the obliterated hypogastric artery, all of which arise from the internal iliac artery. The uterine artery is clamped, cut, and ligated at its origin from the hypogastric artery along with the associated web of connective tissue. The superior vesical arteries to the bladder are left intact. A small, soft rubber drain is passed around the ureter and is used to displace it medially while the peritoneum is cut transversely to the lateral border of the iliac artery and then easily freed from the underlying tissue.

F

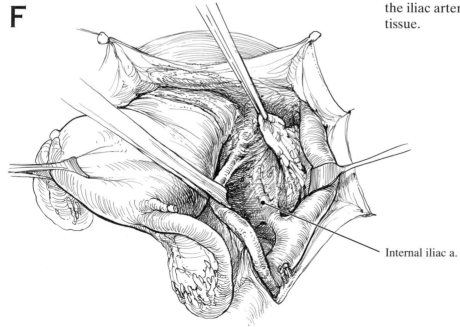

Internal iliac a.

G

The pelvic lymphadenectomy is begun lateral to the iliac artery and toward the medial edge of the psoas muscle. The uterus and ureter are displaced toward the opposite side during the dissection, which is begun at the upper lateral border of the common iliac artery. A plane of dissection is established within the outer adventitia. The fatty areolar lymph node–bearing tissue is then excised easily by a technique that combines spreading and cutting and a sweeping movement with the partially opened scissors. The genitofemoral nerve is frequently encountered during this dissection lateral to the external iliac vessels. If possible, it should be preserved to prevent postoperative groin and medial thigh discomfort.

The dissection of the areolar tissue surrounding the external iliac vessels is carried distally to their termination and then dorsally to the levator muscles. A vein retractor is used to displace the vessels laterally during this dissection. The obturator fascia must next be cleaned of its fatty areolar tissue. The deep portion of the endopelvic fascia that forms the remainder of the vascular sheath is incised to provide access to the obturator veins, which are inconstant in their anatomic location. Careful attention must also be paid to the obturator nerve when removing the node-bearing tissue within the obturator space. This certainly is one area in which it is profitable to spend extra time to perform the dissection with deliberate care.

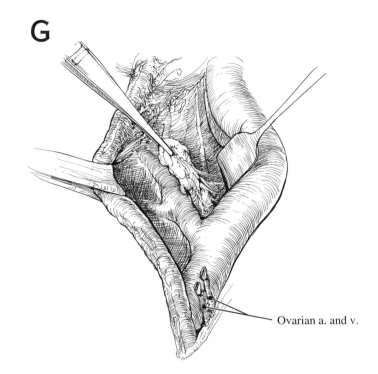

G

Ovarian a. and v.

H

The ureters will have been freed from the pelvic brim to the point at which they are crossed by the uterine artery. This is probably the most awkward area to dissect the ureter adequately and neatly, yet reluctance to do so may jeopardize the adequacy of cancer removal or add to the postoperative morbidity. The medial stump of the uterine artery or the tissue adjacent to it is grasped with forceps and retracted cephalad and medially. This places the cardinal ligament and associated tissue crossing over the ureters under tension, facilitating their deliberate and careful dissection.

I

An Adson hemostat is used to tunnel gently under this tissue, which is the superficial layer of the vesicouterine tissue. If the amount of tissue grasped and ligated each time is excessive, it may distort and possibly obstruct the adjacent ureter. This procedure is continued until the entire ureter is uncovered to the bladder. If the ureteral branch from the uterine artery is encountered at this time, it has to be ligated. Ureteral fistulas occur most commonly in this area, and although many factors contribute to this unfortunate complication, careful attention to detail and gentle handling of tissue are important factors in decreasing their occurrence.

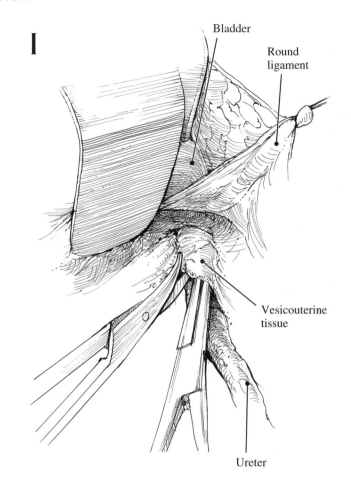

J

All lymph node–bearing tissue has now been dissected off the iliac vessels and their tributaries. The ureter has also been cleared along its entire course until its entry into the bladder. For purposes of anatomic clarity, the fatty areolar lymph node–bearing tissue has been minimized in this illustration.

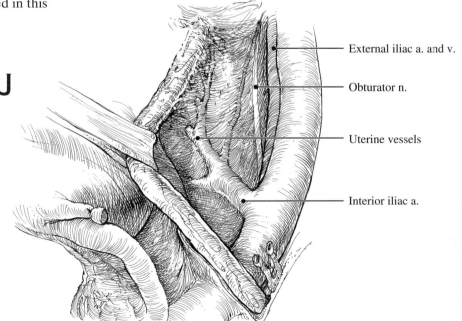

K

With the bilateral lymph node dissection completed, the uterus is retracted cephalad. This brings the vesicouterine sulcus into a more superficial position in preparation for mobilization of the anterior portion of the body of the uterus and the cervix. Sometimes it is advantageous to proceed with the separation of the uterus and bladder after the posterior dissection, which permits the uterus to be pulled farther out of the pelvis, thus appreciably facilitating dissection of the distal ureters. The peritoneum over the vesicouterine junction has already been incised. The dissection is begun with scissors, but in the absence of tenacious fibrosis the tissue can be spread as easily with the fingers. Near the midline, the dissection remains relatively bloodless. The separation is continued to at least 2 cm below the cervix; however, if there is evidence of anterior vaginal involvement, the separation continues to at least 2 cm beyond the cancer.

K

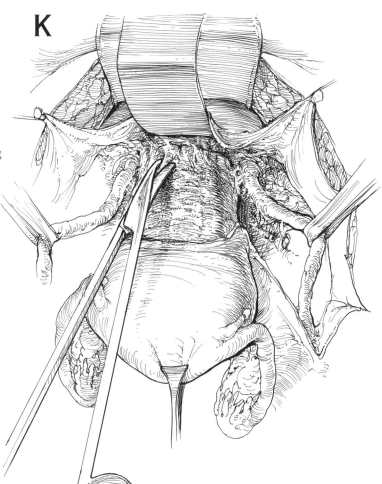

L

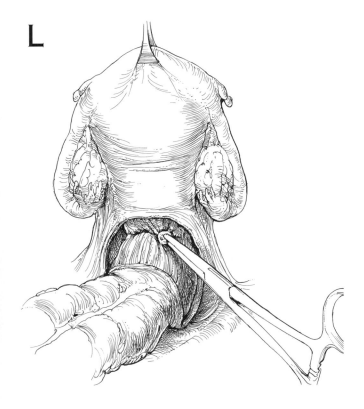

L

The cul-de-sac of Douglas is exposed fully, and the tissues are placed under tension as cephalad traction is applied on the uterus. The peritoneum in the sulcus is incised, and a pledget of gauze on the tip of an 8-inch hemostat is used to separate this tissue. The surgeon will know if the right plane of dissection is not found because of the considerable bleeding and the difficulty in proceeding with the separation of tissue. Care in finding the right plane, therefore, is rewarded by an easy and swift dissection, which is carried to approximately 2 cm beyond the cervix. If difficulty arises in this plane of separation but the operation must continue, the surgeon must be extremely cautious not to enter the rectum. The uterosacral ligaments are clamped as far posteriorly and as close to the ischium as possible and then are divided and ligated with 3-0 Maxon. This completes the major portion of the dissection and leaves the uterus attached only to the vagina.

M

Transection of the vagina is begun. Removal of approximately 2 to 3 cm of vagina is recommended. The paracervical tissue is seen attached to the lateral body of the uterus. One must be mindful not to leave the patient with an unnecessarily short vagina; however, it is entirely improper to compromise the operation on this issue.

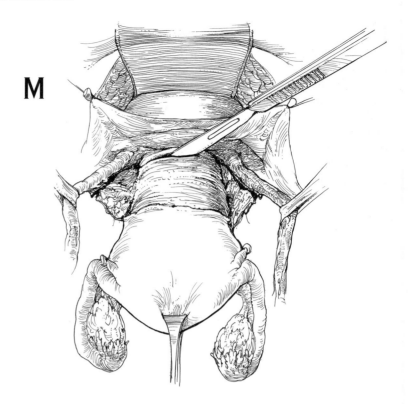

N

As the vagina is incised, its free edges are grasped, if necessary, with Kocher hemostats, which act to keep the rim of the vagina open so that it does not retract. The index finger and thumb encircle the neck of the uterus and pull it somewhat upward, allowing the surgeon to have a direct view of the cervix to make certain that the vagina is being divided an adequate distance from the cancer. After the uterus is removed, small portions of tissue from both edges of the transected vagina are examined histologically for adequacy of excision.

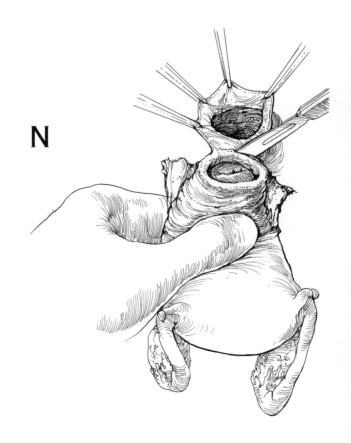

O

A running simple or locking stitch is used, as individual ligation of bleeding vessels in the area is virtually impossible and quite time consuming. Such a hemostatic stitch may cause slight additional necrosis of tissue, but this will be sloughed through the vagina postoperatively. The vagina is closed with 3-0 chromic catgut and without drainage if the operative field is exceptionally dry. Otherwise, the vagina is closed around a catheter, which is placed on suction for 24 hours.

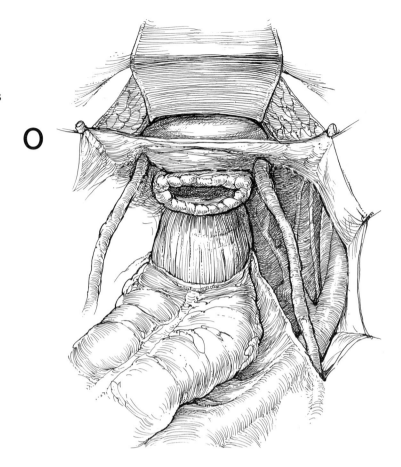

P

A simple stitch of atraumatic 3-0 chromic catgut is used to reperitonealize the pelvis. This is usually accomplished without difficulty, especially if during exposure of the iliac vessels, the peritoneum was not excised widely but rather unfolded with the help of laterally directed cuts. The abdominal wall is closed in a preferred fashion.

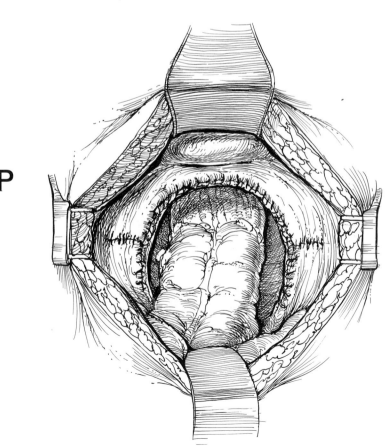

C RECTOVAGINAL FISTULA—REPAIR

Most commonly, rectovaginal fistula is the result of obstetric injury. Although there are more than a dozen methods of repairing it, two types of transvaginal repair are described: these two are more common, and they can be used by a general surgeon who has both a serious interest in such perineal problems and experience in their therapy.

It is important not to have any increase in intrarectal pressure postoperatively, so the patient should have a formal cleansing of the large bowel. The sphincter is gently dilated at the conclusion of the operation so that there will be easier egress of flatus postoperatively.

A

The patient is placed in the lithotomy position. The fistula is identified and sharply circumscribed with a no. 15 blade. The edges of the incised vagina are grasped with Allis clamps and held up as the vaginal mucosa is undercut with a fine Metzenbaum scissors. The process is repeated on the opposite side.

B, C

The fibrous rim of the fistula is excised and the repair of the rectal mucosa begun with interrupted simple stitches of 2-0 Dexon. In an alternative technique, the stitches can be inverted and placed so that the knots are within the rectal lumen, appreciably reducing the bulk of suture material in the healing wound. All sutures are positioned before they are tied snugly. The levator muscles are coapted in the midline to the degree that this can be done without excessive tension.

A

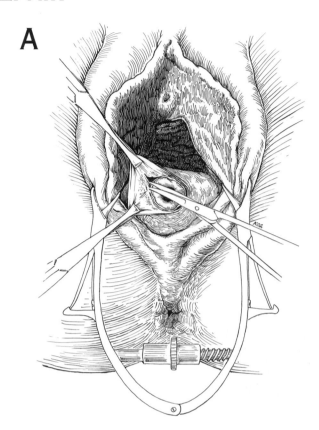

B

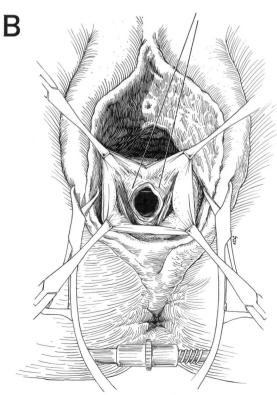

C

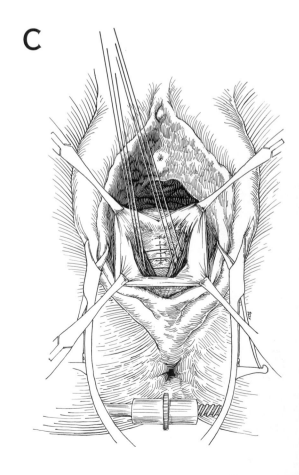

D

Lastly, the vaginal mucosa is coapted with interrupted simple stitches of 2-0 Dexon.

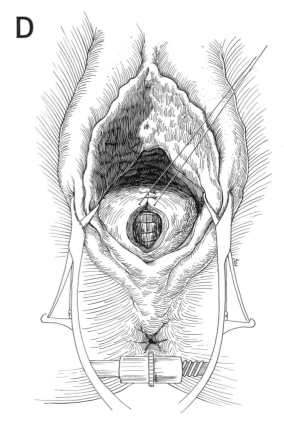

D

E

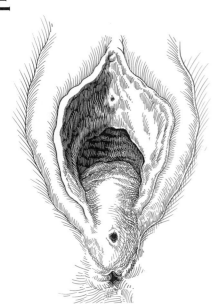

E

When the sphincter has been disrupted and there is significant loss of tissue, the anus will be displaced anteriorly. In addition to the troublesome symptoms caused by the fistula, many women will be incontinent of stool.

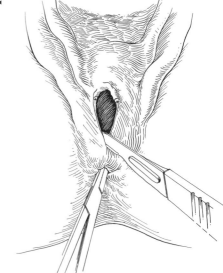

F

F

In such circumstances, it is wisest to convert the fistulous opening to a third-degree tear. This is done sharply between the jaws of a hemostat placed through the anus and out of the fistulous tract in the vagina.

G

The dense fibrous tissue around the fistula is excised so the tissue to be coapted is better vascularized. The vaginal mucosa is undercut, permitting the rectal mucosa to be approximated almost to the anus as a separate layer with interrupted simple stitches of 2-0 Dexon.

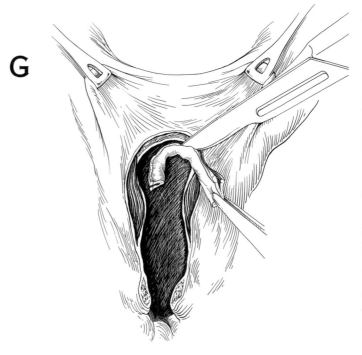

H, I

The divided anal sphincter does not appear as a clean muscle that can be imbricated; usually, fibrous tissue and anal sphincter are intermixed. There must be lateral dissection to free up muscle, as the intent is to imbricate the tissue so that relatively unaffected areas of the sphincter are coapted to each other without too much tension. This is performed with interrupted simple stitches of 2-0 Dexon.

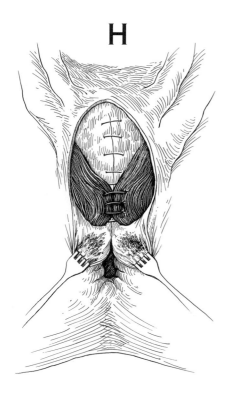

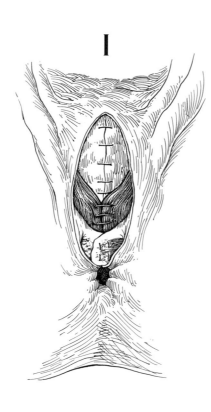

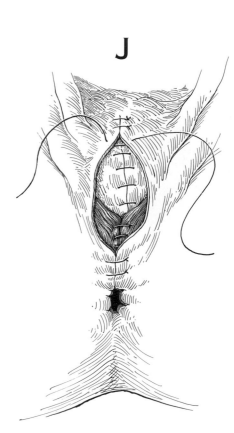

J

The coaptation of the remaining vaginal mucosa is completed with 3-0 chromic catgut. Lastly, the skin is closed with a similar material.

A RADICAL VULVECTOMY

A

Carcinoma of the vulvar skin is by far the most common indication for radical vulvectomy. In addition to removal of the vulva, it has been customary to include in this operation bilateral superficial and deep inguinal lymphadenectomy. Now, however, with numerous aids in staging, from noninvasive techniques to needle aspiration, the radical operation is performed considerably less frequently.

The short transverse suprapubic incision used for the vulvectomy is extended further bilaterally and is utilized for a unilateral or bilateral deep inguinal lymphadenectomy if this is to be done. For the vulvectomy, the patient is placed in the dorsal lithotomy position.

Note: In this chapter, only the vulvectomy is shown. The reader is referred to Chapter 27 on inguinal node dissection for a detailed description of this aspect of the operation if it is to be performed.

A

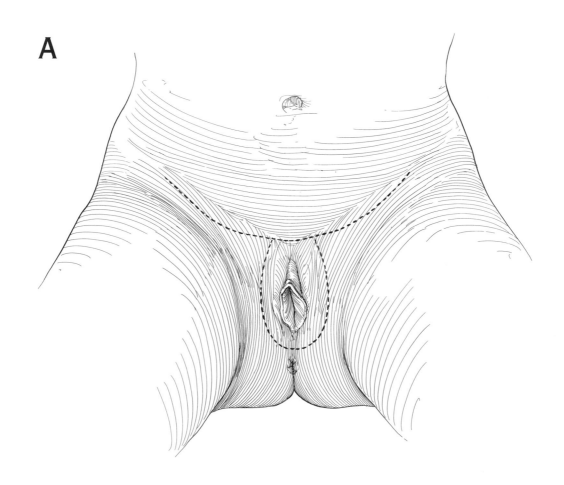

B, C

The vulvar organs are circumscribed as shown with the incision carried down to muscle. At the location of the visible tumor, a 2-cm margin is desirable. The internal pudendal vessels are encountered and are ligated with 3-0 chromic catgut and divided. In addition, multiple small vessels in this very vascular area will require electrocoagulation.

B

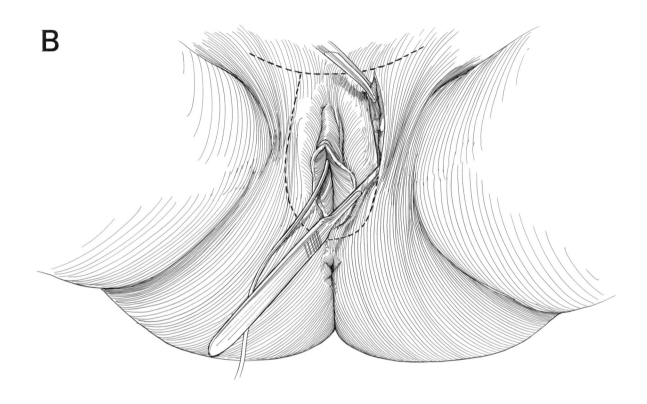

C

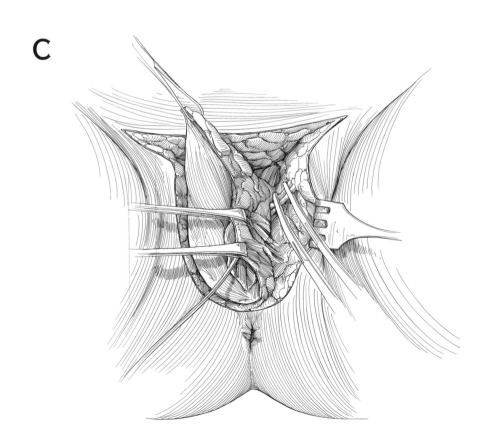

D

The inner vulvar incision is made at the hymenal ring just skirting the urethral orifice. If necessary because of cancerous involvement, the outer one fourth of the urethra may be sacrificed without serious consequences; however, the patient should be counseled preoperatively about the possible development of urinary incontinence.

D

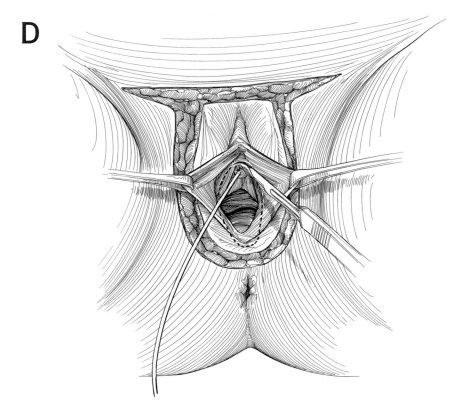

E

The specimen is removed with muscle now occupying the depth of the operative field.

E

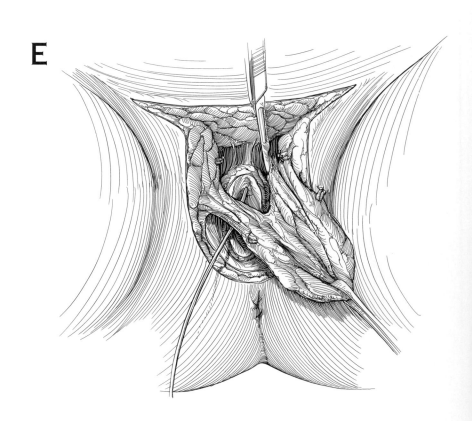

F

For the groin dissection the suprapubic incision is
lengthened some, and skin flaps are mobilized as shown.
With skill and appropriate traction and without insisting on
a "whistle clean" dissection, it can be performed through
this exposure.

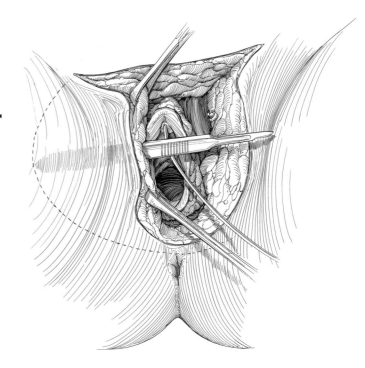

G, H

Throughout the operation, a urinary catheter has been in
place and is kept there now. On the side having the
lymphadenectomy, a drainage catheter is positioned, exited
through a counter skin incision, and connected to a suction
apparatus. It is important to close the incision without
tension as this area is particularly susceptible to wound
dehiscence. The subcutaneous tissue is closed with
interrupted 3-0 chromic catgut and the skin with simple
vertical mattress stitches of 4-0 nylon.

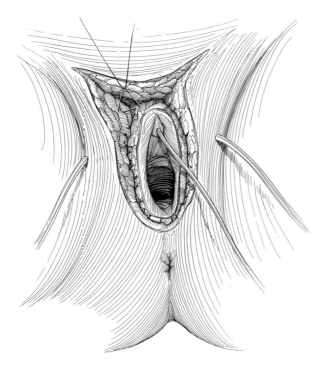

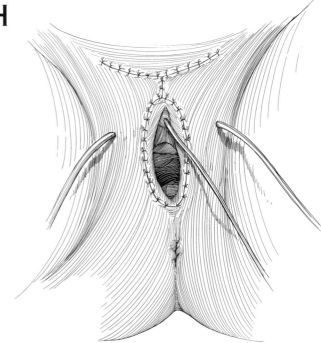

B RECTOCELE

A rectocele is a hernia, and the purpose of the repair is to plicate the perirectal fascia and levator ani muscles over the anterior rectal wall and thus effect a two-layer closure of the hernia.

A

The patient is anesthetized by any of several methods and placed in the dorsal lithotomy position. Although the patient has had the bowel cleansed, a self-adhesive plastic drape applied over the anal opening offers some protection from any anal fecal drainage. The labia are retracted, and a bidigital rectovaginal examination confirms the area requiring repair.

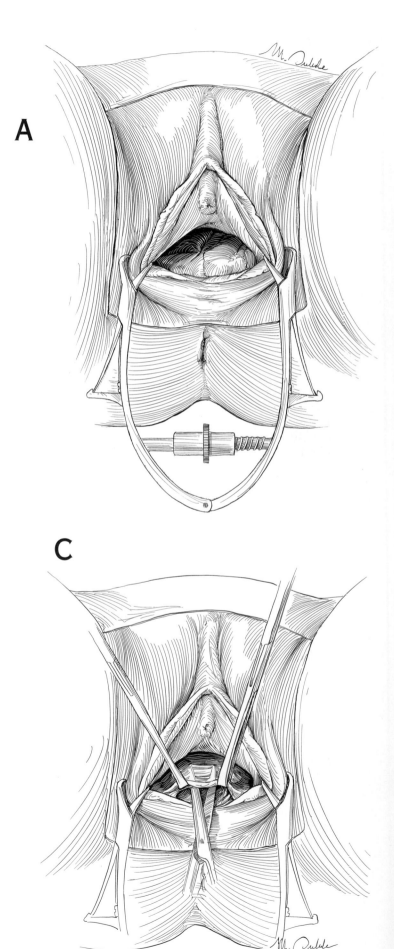

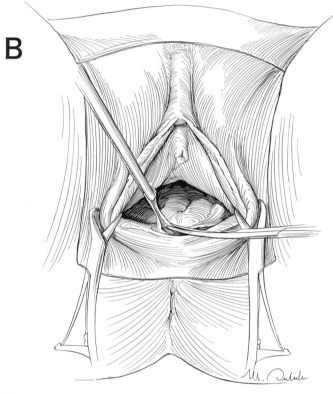

B

The prongs of the self-retaining retractor are at the margins of the original hymenal ring, placing this tissue on a stretch and thus facilitating removal of a strip of the posterior fourchette. Alternatively, Allis clamps may be placed on the hymenal ring at the right and left posterolateral positions and held on traction.

C

The freed vaginal tissue is grasped with Allis forceps and gently undermined to the apex of the herniation, first with a fine Metzenbaum scissors and subsequently with a small, tightly folded pledget of gauze held at the tip of a 6-inch hemostat (a "peanut"). Entering the rectum during this undercutting can have serious consequences because the entire operative field becomes grossly contaminated.

D, E

The vaginal incision is made with a Metzenbaum scissors and carried to the apex of the hernia (*D, E*).

F

The lateral attachments of the rectum to the vagina are freed with a combination using scissors or a "peanut" until the levator ani muscles are identified. Following undermining of the vaginal mucosa, a fine-tipped electrocautery is used to make the field as dry as possible.

D

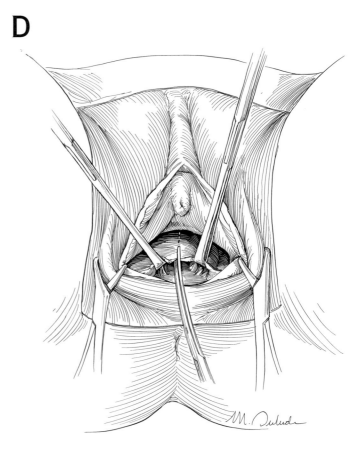

E

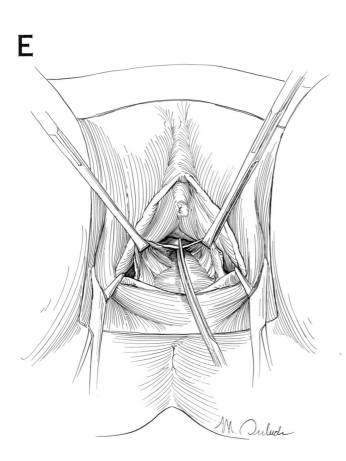

F

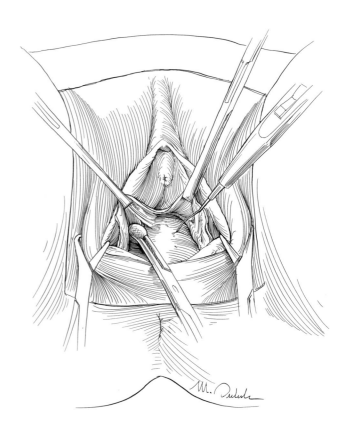

G

A narrow, malleable retractor is used to depress the rectal mucosa and to define the borders of the levator ani muscles, which demonstrate a diastasis. The levator muscles are approximated down to the fourchette with stout absorbable sutures. The surgeon should be careful not to "bunch" the muscles too aggressively, as this may lead to postoperative dyspareunia.

H

The levator ani muscles have been coapted and the field once again inspected for oozing points, which are coagulated.

I

The excess vaginal mucosa is trimmed appropriately with the realization that excessive removal of mucosa can lead to a reduced caliber of the vagina and to sexual dysfunction postoperatively.

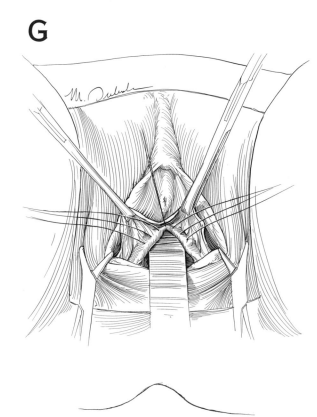

G

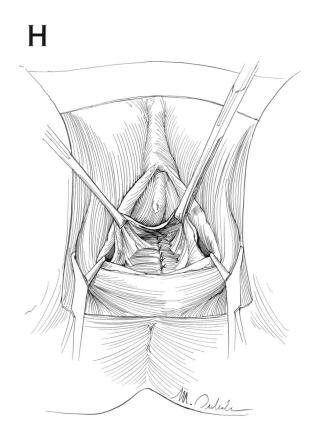

H

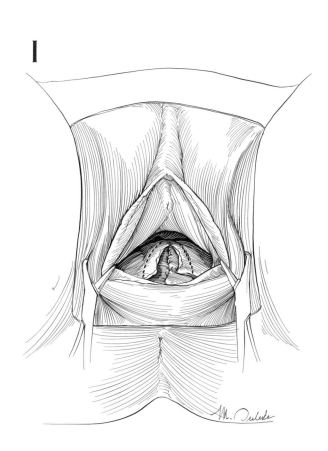

I

J

The mucosa is approximated with continuous simple stitches of 2-0 Dexon interspersed with simple interrupted stitches of similar material.

K, L

The repair is completed with closure of the perineal skin with a subcuticular stitch of fine absorbable suture material.

J

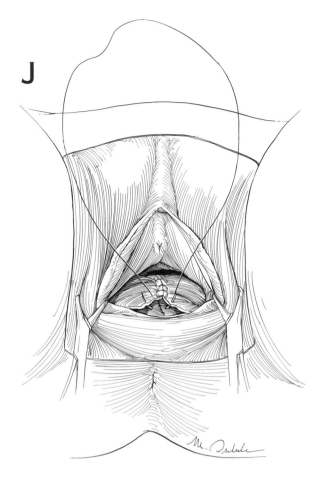

K

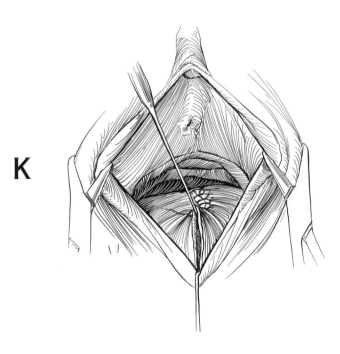

L

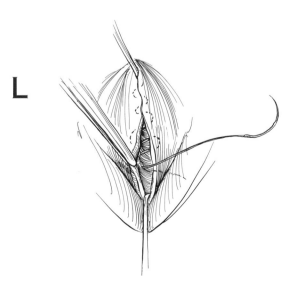

M

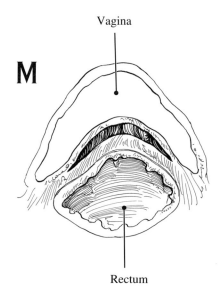

Vagina

Rectum

N

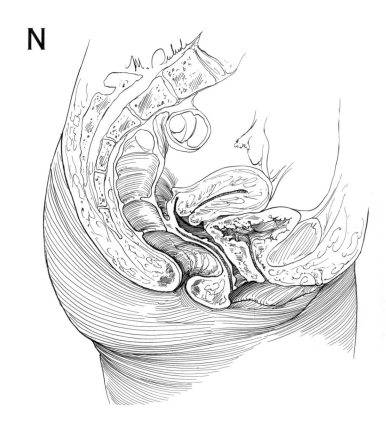

M, N, O, P

This quartet of preoperative (*M, N*) and postoperative (*O, P*) illustrations in sagital and transverse cuts demonstrates the tissue area altered to bring about the repair.

O

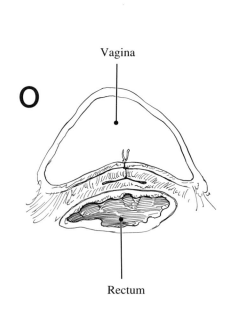

Vagina

Rectum

P

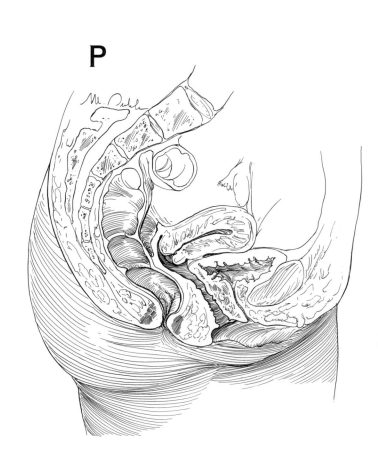

C BARTHOLIN GLAND—EXCISION

Excision of the Bartholin gland is indicated for persistent or recurrent abscess of the gland or cyst.

A

The operation is performed with the patient in the lithotomy position. The labia are grasped with Babcock forceps and spread to expose the gland maximally. The incision is made in an anteroposterior direction centered over the meatus of the gland and as near to the vaginal mucosa (rather than on the labia) as possible.

B

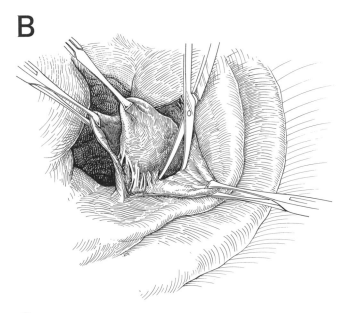

C

The gland has been removed from a bed that generally has myriad oozing points. These need to be coagulated meticulously. The loose tissue does not provide any tamponade, and minimal continued oozing can lead to a large hematoma postoperatively. The best way to coagulate these vessels is to use a fine-tipped electrocautery unit and to persist at the task until hemostasis is complete.

D

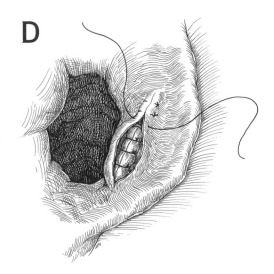

A

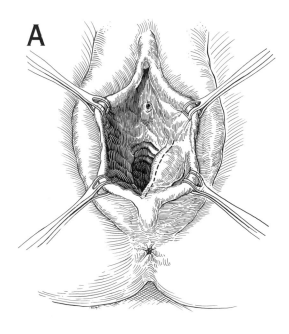

B

The sides of the wound are retracted as the presenting part of the gland is grasped with an Allis forceps and gently pulled downward. A fine Metzenbaum scissors is used to free the gland, all the time staying close to it but not entering it. The rich blood supply from the inferior pudendal artery and the hyperemia caused by the inflammation make this operative field ooze with blood in a very impressive manner. When possible, the small, abundant bleeding points should be coagulated before being divided or should be coagulated promptly after they are severed. This pinpoints their origin more accurately and also reduces blood loss.

C

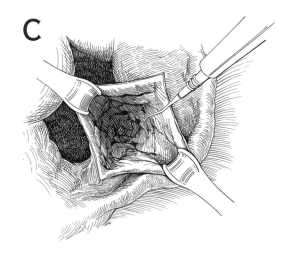

D

The deep aspects of the wound are closed with 4-0 chromic catgut as a continuous or an interrupted stitch in two to three layers. Depending on the wetness of the field and the surgeon's personal preference, a Penrose drain may be used. If it is used, it is anchored with 5-0 nylon and is to be removed in 3 to 4 days.

Chapter 27

ILIOINGUINAL
LYMPH NODES

Ａ DISSECTION

A

The anatomic considerations in the performance of a radical groin dissection are pictured. The tissue to be excised extends from just distal to the bifurcation of the common iliac vessels to the apex of the femoral (Scarpa's) triangle. The femoral triangle is bounded by the inguinal ligament superiorly, the sartorius muscle laterally, and the adductor longus muscle medially. The floor of the femoral triangle is formed by the fascia over the iliopsoas, adductor longus, and pectineus muscles, and the roof is formed by the fascia lata. Actually, most of the lymph node–bearing tissue is to be found in the fatty areolar tissue superficial to the roof of the triangle. The important artery is the common iliac artery. Just before it passes under the inguinal ligament to become the common femoral artery it gives off the deep circumflex iliac artery and the inferior epigastric artery. The common femoral artery bifurcates into the deep femoral and superficial femoral arteries, the latter leaving the operative field just lateral to the apex of the femoral triangle. The femoral vein, as with the artery and nerve, lies deep to the fascia lata.

The femoral nerve appears in the pelvis lateral to the iliopsoas muscle, and as it proceeds distally it is flanked laterally by the iliac muscle. After the femoral nerve exits from under the inguinal ligament, it gives off its multiple branches and proceeds to disappear under the sartorius muscle. The lymph nodes to be excised are the inguinal and the iliac, the former being more numerous.

A

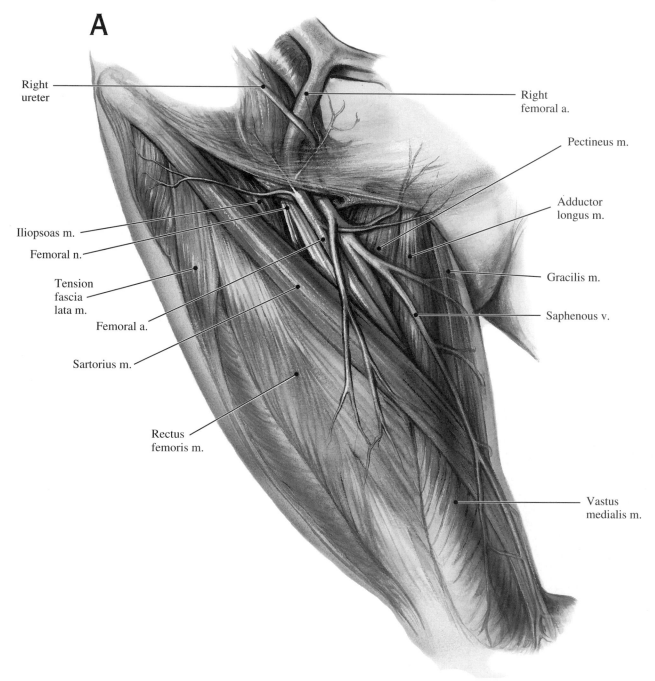

Right ureter

Right femoral a.

Pectineus m.

Adductor longus m.

Iliopsoas m.

Femoral n.

Tension fascia lata m.

Gracilis m.

Femoral a.

Saphenous v.

Sartorius m.

Rectus femoris m.

Vastus medialis m.

B

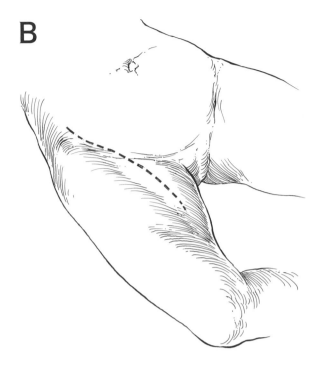

B

The area to be prepared routinely includes the lower abdomen, the perineum and genitalia, and the thigh on the operative side. The patient is placed in the supine position with the leg on the operative side abducted, flexed slightly, and rotated externally. It is supported in this position by a sandbag under the calf. The scrotum and penis are secured to the opposite groin.

The incision is oblique, beginning several centimeters cephalad and medial to the anterosuperior iliac spine, and progresses down to 1 or 2 cm below and then parallel to the inguinal ligament, where, while over the vessels, it curves gently to point to the apex of the femoral triangle.

The depth of the skin incision is about 3 to 4 mm, and the skin flaps are mobilized at this thickness for at least 5 cm from the central portion of the incision. The skin flaps are then tapered so that peripherally they almost blend with the full thickness of the surrounding fat.

C

The subcutaneous fatty areolar tissue over the abdominal area is addressed first, as the dissection is carried down to the aponeurosis of the external oblique muscle.

C

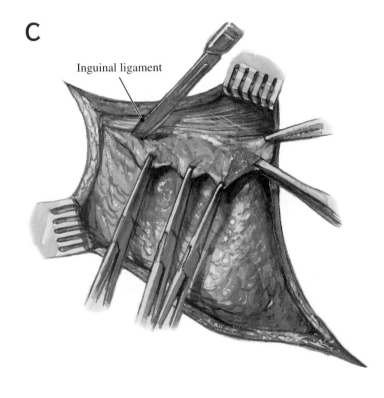

Inguinal ligament

D

Inguinal ligament

Aponeurosis of external oblique m.

Iliopsoas m.

Femoral n.

Sartorius m.

D

The infrainguinal dissection is now begun as the fascia lata is incised along the lateral border of the sartorius muscle. The lateral femoral cutaneous nerve should be sought in the upper aspect of the incision. The tough fascia lata is caught along its free edge and, along with the overlying lymph node–bearing fatty areolar tissue, is retracted medially as it is freed from the underlying sartorius muscle. As the dissecting knife dips slightly at the medial border of the proximal sartorius muscle, care should be taken not to damage the branches of the femoral nerve that are seen disappearing under this muscle.

E

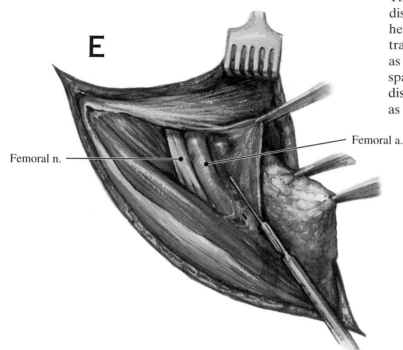

Femoral n.

Femoral a.

E

The superficial surface of the femoral nerve has been dissected free. The femoral sheath will have to be entered here. This sheath is a continuation of the iliac and transversalis fasciae and surrounds both the artery and vein as they pass under the inguinal ligament to the medial space of the femoral arch. Although in this illustration the dissection is being performed with a scalpel, scissors will do as well.

F

As the dissection continues medially, the fascia lata is disengaged from the undersurface of the inguinal ligament. The saphenous vein is divided at the saphenofemoral junction, and the saphenous vein stump is transfixed with 3-0 silk. The femoral vein can then be dissected cleanly along its entire medial aspect, which contains no branches, thus exposing the pectineus muscle.

F

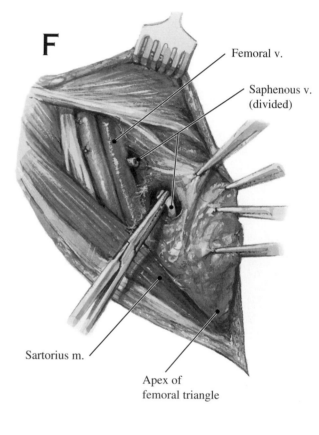

Femoral v.

Saphenous v. (divided)

Sartorius m.

Apex of femoral triangle

G

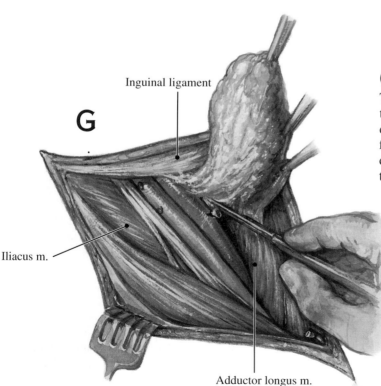

Inguinal ligament

Iliacus m.

Adductor longus m.

G

The previous step will have led to the apex of the femoral triangle, at which point the saphenous vein is ligated and divided a second time. The dissection proceeds toward the femoral canal; all the inguinal tissue to be excised has been dissected free except the part of it that leads directly into the femoral canal.

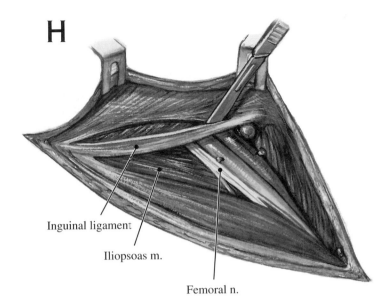

H

Inguinal ligament

Iliopsoas m.

Femoral n.

H

The aponeurosis of the external oblique muscle is divided along its fibers 1 cm above and parallel to the inguinal ligament. The medial extent is the external inguinal ring. The cord is displaced medially and safeguarded.

The aponeurosis of the external oblique muscle is divided, exposing the ilioinguinal and iliohypogastric nerves, which are preserved and subsequently displaced medially as the iliac vessels are exposed.

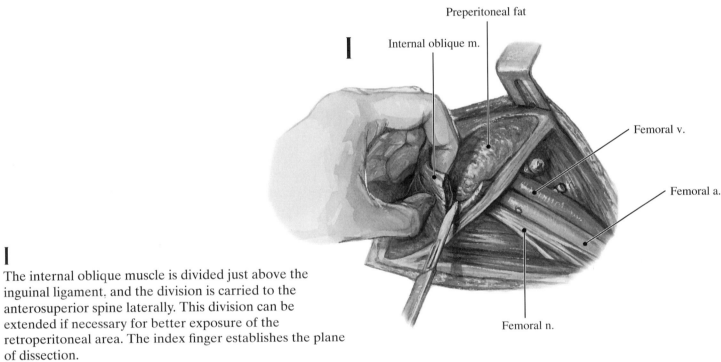

I

Internal oblique m.

Preperitoneal fat

Femoral v.

Femoral a.

Femoral n.

I

The internal oblique muscle is divided just above the inguinal ligament, and the division is carried to the anterosuperior spine laterally. This division can be extended if necessary for better exposure of the retroperitoneal area. The index finger establishes the plane of dissection.

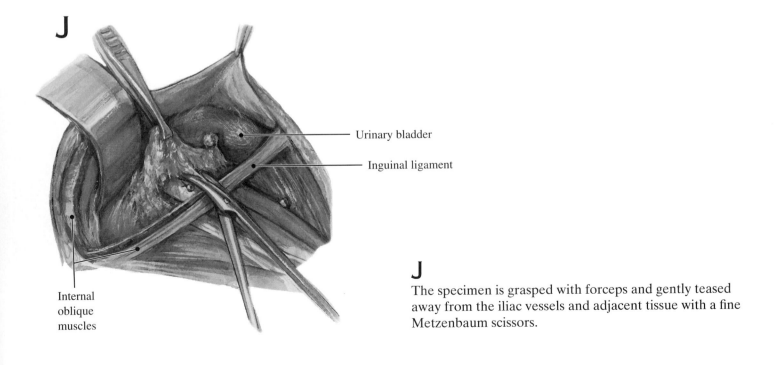

J

Urinary bladder

Inguinal ligament

Internal oblique muscles

J

The specimen is grasped with forceps and gently teased away from the iliac vessels and adjacent tissue with a fine Metzenbaum scissors.

K

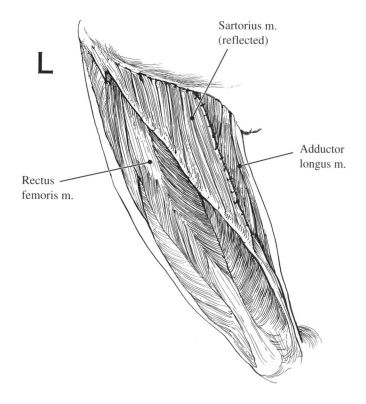

Femoral n.

Deep and superficial
femoral arteries

Femoral v.

K

This is a view of the operative site following the iliac
dissection. The incised suprainguinal tissue is
reapproximated with interrupted stitches of 3-0 silk.

L

Sartorius m.
(reflected)

Adductor
longus m.

Rectus
femoris m.

L

When skin flap necrosis occurs, it is most often at the
middle portion of the wound, which usually is over the
femoral vessels. Exposed vessels are covered with the
sartorius muscle to eliminate the risk of exposure. This
muscle is detached at its origin and folded medially as a
flap but remains hinged on its neurovascular supply, which
is based laterally. It is held in its new rotated position by
suturing the new medial edge to the underlying
musculature with interrupted 3-0 chromic catgut.

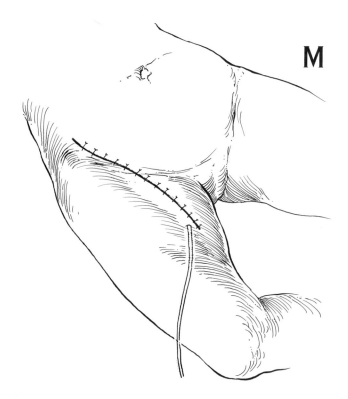

M

M

A catheter is placed next to the vessels and is exteriorized
through a separate incision. It is placed on suction at the
conclusion of the operation. The subcutaneous tissue is
approximated with interrupted simple stitches of 4-0
chromic catgut. The skin is closed with interrupted vertical
mattress stitches of 4-0 nylon.

Chapter

28

AMPUTATIONS

A UPPER EXTREMITY

FOREQUARTER

The intent of a forequarter amputation is to remove the entire upper limb, the shoulder girdle and its numerous muscular attachments, plus the contents of the axilla and the low cervical area. Although it is a logically conceived operation that can be executed with a very low mortality rate, the emergence of limb-sparing operations has displaced amputations in general but especially those that include the shoulder and hip girdle.

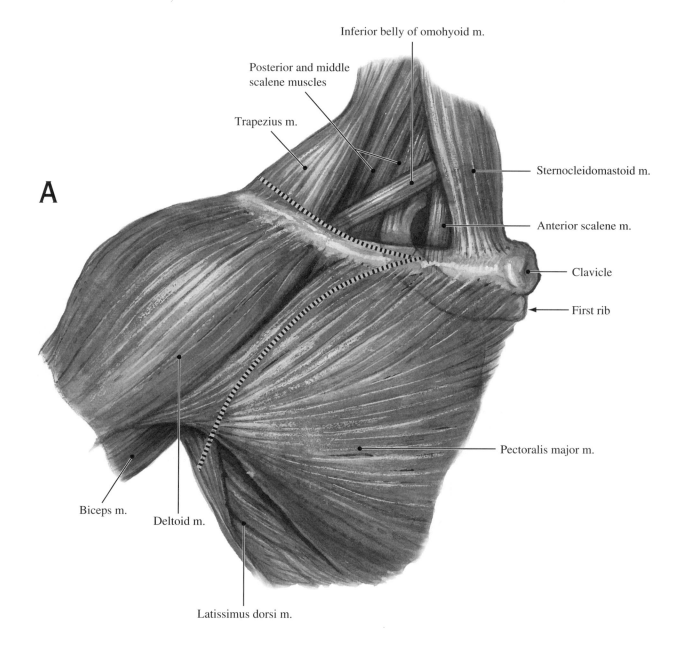

A

A

Shown are the anterior muscle groups that have to be divided in this operation. These include the pectoralis major muscle, which arises from the sternum, and the cartilage of all true ribs and the upper portion of the aponeurosis of the external oblique muscle, which converge to insert into the greater tuberosity of the humerus. Also included is the pectoralis minor muscle, which arises from the third to the fifth ribs and passes upward to insert into the coracoid process. These muscles are divided somewhere along their course, usually closer to their origin than to their insertion. The sternocleidomastoid muscle usually has its lateral clavicular fibers divided; all of them are divided if the clavicle is disarticulated. Posteriorly, the flat triangular trapezius muscle, which arises along a line from the external occipital protuberance to the spinous process of the last thoracic vertebra in the midline, attaches itself to the lateral third of the clavicle, the acromion, and the spine of the scapula. Anteriorly, this muscle is usually divided just cephalad to the clavicle.

B

The abundant vascular cross-traffic, much of it critical and directly relevant to this operation, is shown in this semidiagrammatic illustration. The common carotid artery is shown as it begins at the bifurcation of the innominate artery behind the sternoclavicular joint. On the left, it arises from the highest portion of the arch of the aorta and is intrathoracic at its origin. The vertebral artery and the thyrocervical trunk are given off before the subclavian artery passes under the anterior scalene muscle. The thoracoacromial artery is the pertinent important vessel arising from the axillary artery.

The axillary vein becomes the subclavian vein at the lateral border of the first rib and, as such, receives the anterior and external jugular veins. At the medial end of the clavicle it joins with the internal jugular vein to become the innominate vein.

The composition and complexity of the brachial plexus change swiftly as it proceeds distally. There is not much to be gained by describing this anatomy because, in any case, it will be divided where necessary. The clavicle is usually the only bone worked on; it is sectioned at the junction of its midline and medial third, the point at which the clavicle crosses the vessels leading to the arm. Thus, by disarticulation of the clavicle at the sternum, one can dissect more medially if the occasion calls for it. This is particularly valuable for tumors that impinge on or invade the brachial plexus or for neural tumors that must be resected as far proximally as possible.

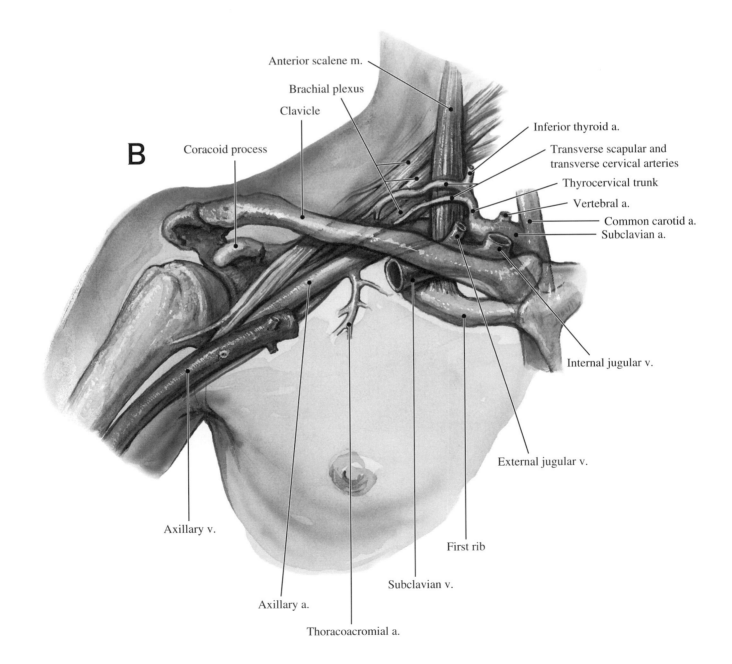

C, D, E

General anesthesia by orotracheal intubation is used. The anesthesiologist must be prepared to cope with deliberate entry into the thorax or even excision of a portion of the chest wall. The patient is placed in the posterolateral position or slightly more toward the supine if a difficult supraclavicular dissection is anticipated. Following preparation of the skin, the patient is draped to leave the thorax exposed beyond the midline on both sides, to the subcostal margin, and to include the lower two thirds of the neck. The arm also is draped in a sterile fashion so that it can be moved during the course of the operation. The racquet-type incision shown is one of several that can be used for a straightforward forequarter amputation, but considerable variations from this may be necessary depending on the clinical findings.

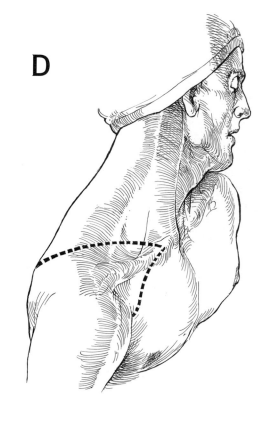

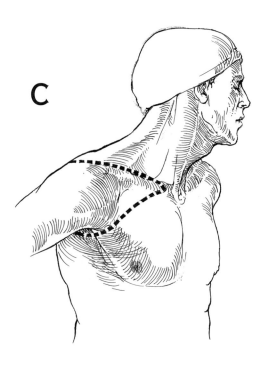

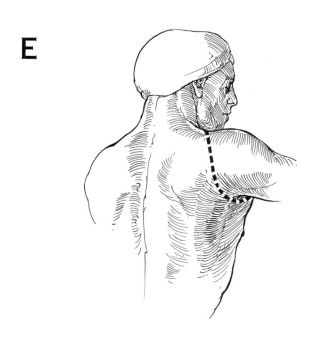

F

The anterior portion of the incision is made first, with the pectoralis major muscle separated from the undersurface of the medial half of the clavicle. The subclavius muscle is divided in line with the anticipated point of division of the clavicle. Division of the tough costocoracoid membrane is also carried out at this time.

The superior aspect of the clavicle is freed next, and the lateral fibers of the clavicular head of the sternocleidomastoid muscle are divided. Deep to the clavicle at this point, the anterior jugular vein is clamped, cut, and ligated.

A passage for the Gigli saw is made. The subclavian vein is closely subjacent, and care should be taken not to tear it during this step because hemorrhage cannot be controlled easily or quickly. The safest way to separate the vein from the overlying clavicle is to proceed subperiosteally. When doing so, however, the periosteum should not be separated from the bone more than is necessary; otherwise denuded bone that is retained is at risk of necrosis. While cutting, the Gigli saw is angled somewhat medially so that the consequent cut edge of the retained clavicle is less sharp. In lesions that affect the shoulder, the entire clavicle is usually removed. In more peripheral lesions, the technique of cutting the clavicle as depicted is satisfactory.

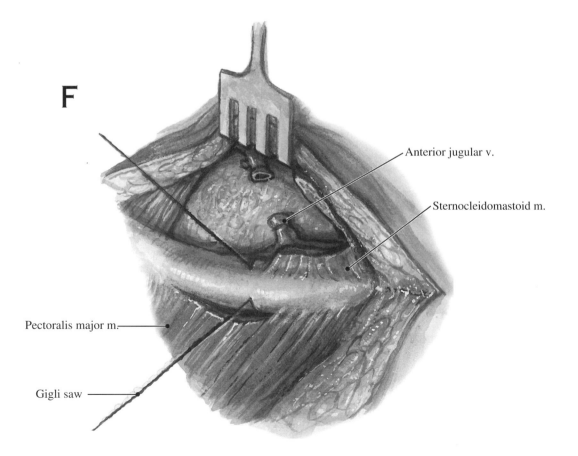

F

Anterior jugular v.

Sternocleidomastoid m.

Pectoralis major m.

Gigli saw

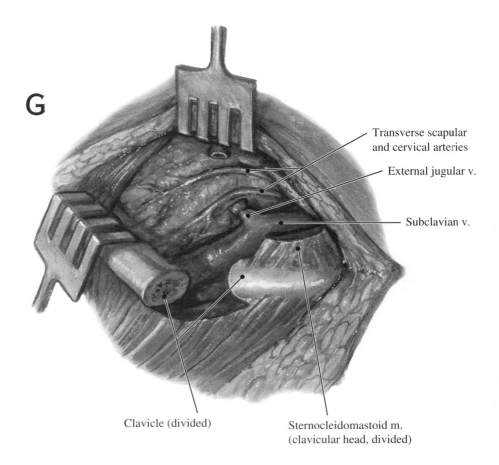

G

Transverse scapular and cervical arteries

External jugular v.

Subclavian v.

Clavicle (divided)

Sternocleidomastoid m. (clavicular head, divided)

G

After the clavicle is divided, the assistant can gently retract the lateral part of it caudally while the surgeon simultaneously frees the underlying tissue that contains the transverse cervical and scapular arteries—usually with the fingers.

H

The subclavian vessels are now addressed. The artery must be ligated before the vein to avoid a congested arm and the consequent waste of the trapped blood. The artery is cephalad to and deeper than the vein. One can expose the artery sufficiently to occlude it with an arterial clamp and then proceed at leisure with the dissection of the overlying veins. The thyrocervical trunk is ligated and divided.

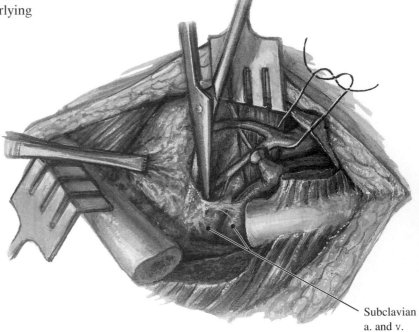

H

Subclavian a. and v.

I

The subclavian artery is doubly stitch-ligated with 2-0 silk. Alternatively, it can be occluded with a vascular clamp and divided and the proximal stump oversewn with fine monofilament vascular suture. Both the artery and the vein should be ligated more medially if the clinical circumstances warrant it.

I

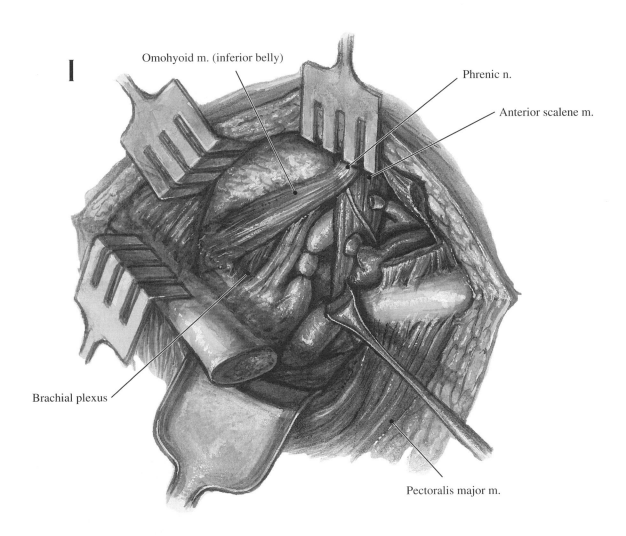

Omohyoid m. (inferior belly)

Phrenic n.

Anterior scalene m.

Brachial plexus

Pectoralis major m.

J

The brachial plexus is simply sectioned without antecedent injection or trying of the nerve trunks. Occasionally, a perineural vessel must be clamped and ligated. The inferior belly of the omohyoid muscle is divided.

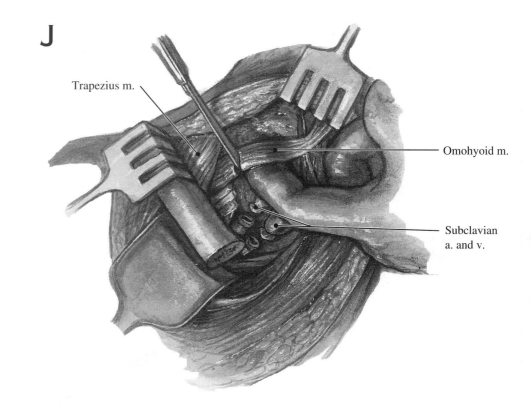

K

Division of the trapezius muscle is begun at its anterior aspect at a point dictated by the extent of the tumor.

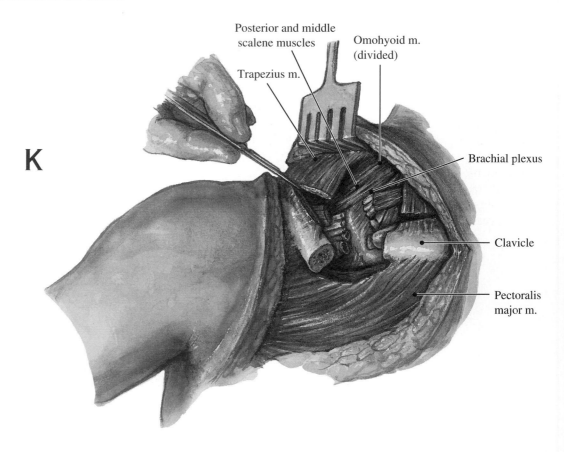

L

The major and minor pectoral muscles are divided next. The muscle incision is slanted so that the cut muscle blends smoothly with the thoracic wall. The pectoralis minor muscle usually is excised in its entirety, but the pectoralis major muscle is not.

The arm is severely abducted by an assistant, and, because the muscular and bony restraints are gone, the entire shoulder girdle can be abducted. The long thoracic nerve will be sacrificed later along with the serratus anterior muscle, which it innervates.

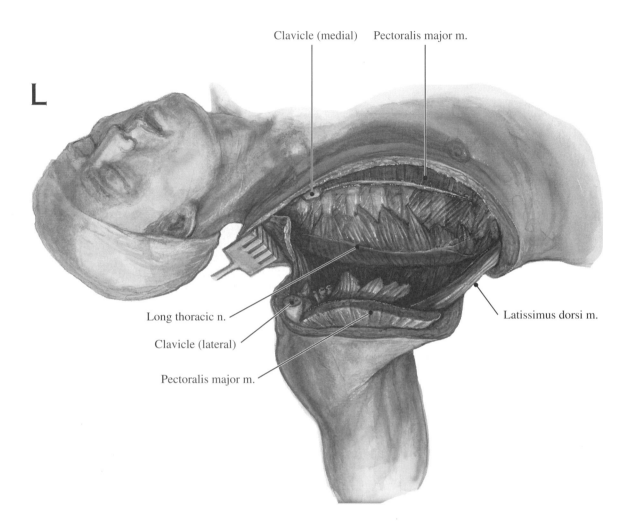

Clavicle (medial)   Pectoralis major m.

Long thoracic n.

Clavicle (lateral)

Pectoralis major m.

Latissimus dorsi m.

M

The field of operation and the view now shift to the dorsal side of the patient. The path of the usual incision is shown. If more skin than that illustrated is to be sacrificed posteriorly, the surgeon should plan initially to compensate by leaving more skin anteriorly. A skin graft can be applied and easily maintained over this rigid convex surface, but one should assiduously avoid placing such a graft over the severed vessels or the brachial plexus.

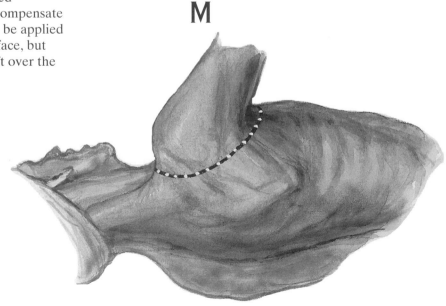

N

The dorsal musculature, some of which is to be divided, is shown. The superficial layer includes the trapezius muscle, which has been described. The latissimus dorsi muscle arises primarily through the lumbodorsal fascia, from the spinous processes of the vertebrae from the midthorax on down, from the posterior iliac crest, and from fleshy digitations of the lower ribs. Its fibers curve around and overlap the inferior border of the scapula as they become a fasciculus inserting into the humerus. The levator scapulae, rhomboideus minor, and rhomboideus major muscles arise at the midline of the back from the transverse processes of the upper cervical vertebrae and proceed in a generally downward direction to insert on the vertebral border of the scapula.

N

Serratus anterior m.

External oblique m.

Trapezius m.

O

The assistant now pulls the arm and shoulder girdle forward so that the muscles attached to the scapulae are under tension. The latissimus dorsi muscle is incised across its greatest thickness. The trapezius muscle is divided along the vertebral border of the scapula so that it meets the incision made during the anterior dissection.

O

Deltoid m.

Rhomboideus minor m.

Levator scapulae m.

Serratus anterior m.

Trapezius m.

Rhomboideus major m.

Trapezius m.

Sternocleidomastoid m.

P

The rhomboideus major, rhomboideus minor, and the levator scapulae muscles now come into view and are divided in a similar fashion. Only the serratus anterior muscle now holds the shoulder girdle in place. The shoulder girdle is lifted, and the serratus anterior muscle is divided.

P

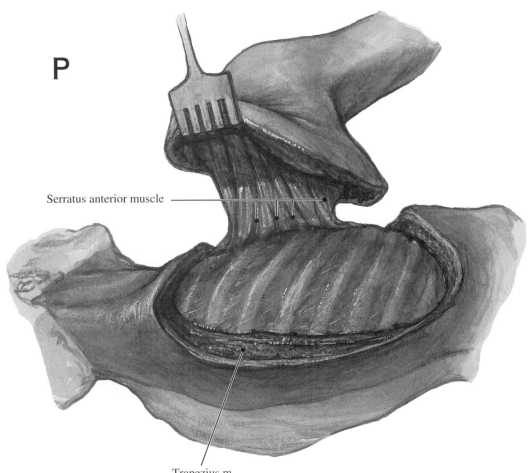

Serratus anterior muscle

Trapezius m.

Q

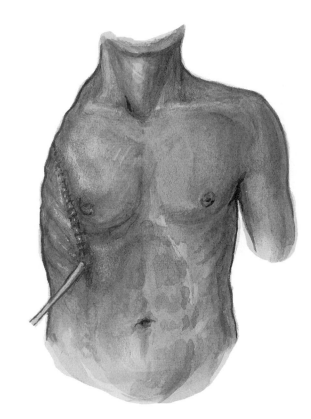

Q

Electrocautery and fine chromic catgut are used to effect complete hemostasis. If the wound closure is snug and the skin flaps are firmly against the chest wall, one drain is exteriorized from the inferior aspect of the wound. If the skin flaps are at all loose, two catheters are positioned, exteriorized through counterincisions, and placed on suction. The skin is closed with interrupted simple and vertical mattress stitches of 3-0 nylon.

B LOWER EXTREMITY

HINDQUARTER

The purpose of this operation is the removal of the lower limb and the ipsilateral half of the bony pelvis, except for the sacrum and the associated muscles. As with the forequarter amputation, the emergence of limb-sparing techniques has lessened its appeal and has made more acceptable a lesser extent of pelvic resection.

A

This illustration demonstrates the excellent exposure that can be obtained for the accurate and deliberate dissection necessary if the operative morbidity of this procedure is to be kept to a minimum. The femoral nerve is shown after it has appeared lateral to the psoas muscle, but it will be divided while still dorsal to this muscle. The obturator artery is seen as the first ventral branch of the internal iliac; the large superior gluteal artery usually appears directly dorsal to it. The ureter and ovarian vessels are displaced medially to gain access to the iliac bifurcation. The psoas muscle is the only major muscle divided across its center.

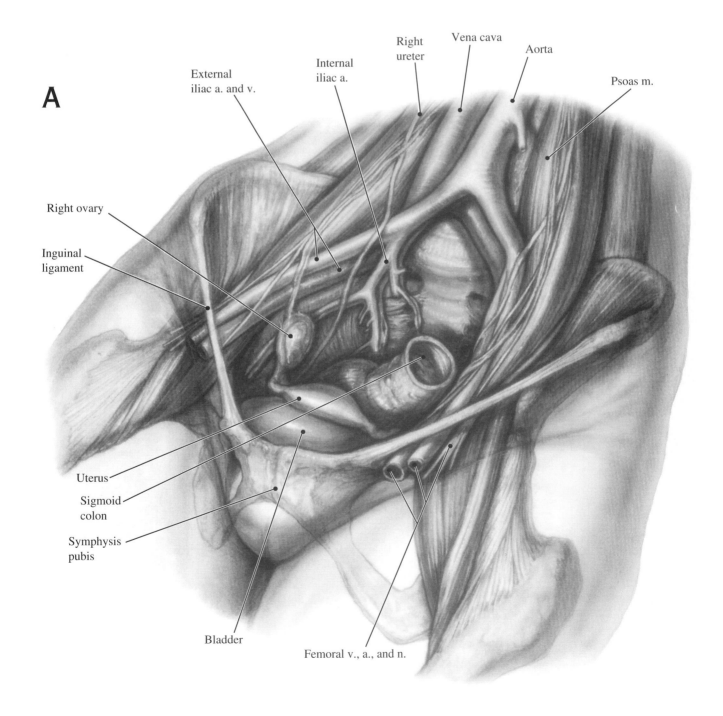

A

B, C, D

General anesthesia is administered endotracheally. A Foley catheter is inserted into the urinary bladder. In the male, it is placed across the opposite leg, keeping the genitalia effectively out of the operative field. The patient is placed in the supine position, with sandbags under the lumbar area and shoulder so that the affected hip is clearly off the table. The skin is prepared in a customary manner. In women, the vagina is prepared as well. The anus is sealed with a purse-string suture of 2-0 silk. The extremity also is prepared in a sterile manner and so draped that it can be moved freely during the operation. Depending on the clinical circumstances, a variety of incisions can be used; the one shown in *B* is most widely applicable and the least likely to result in skin necrosis. Others are shown in *C* and *D*.

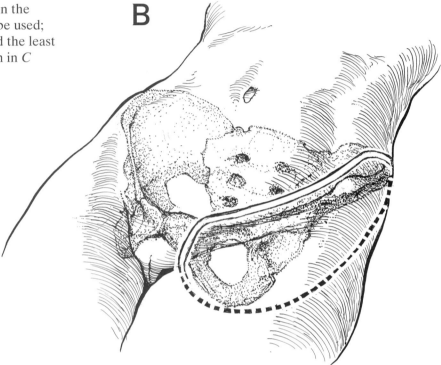

B

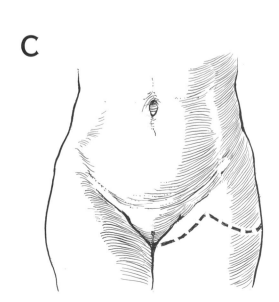

C

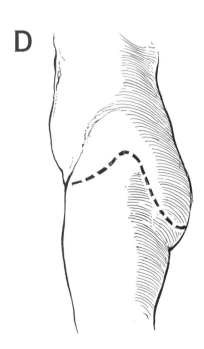

D

E

The incision is started at the iliac crest at the midaxillary line and extended along the inguinal crease. The inguinal ligament and the insertion of the ipsilateral rectus abdominis muscle are detached from the pubic bone. Laterally, the fibers of the external and internal oblique muscles are disengaged from the iliac crest, as are the fibers of the latissimus dorsi muscle at the most posterior extent. The interfoveolar ligament, a thickened extension of the transversalis fascia, is incised to expose the inferior epigastric artery and vein, which are then divided and ligated with 3-0 silk. Throughout this operation the skin flaps are kept full thickness unless there are clinical reasons to do otherwise.

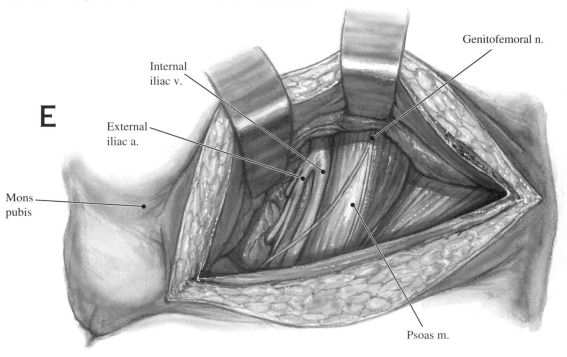

F

Completion of the previous steps permits entry into the retroperitoneal space. This fatty areolar tissue is dissected by blunt technique and displaced medially, thus exposing the iliac area. The surgeon verifies that the ureter remains attached to the peritoneum and is displaced medially.

Much has been made of the necessity of sparing the superior and inferior gluteal vessels if the gluteal flap is to have the best chance of survival. The most important concern, however, is how proximally the vessels need to be divided to encompass the tumor. If the division is to be at the level of the common iliac vessels, a vascular clamp is placed above their bifurcation; they are divided, and the proximal stumps are oversewn with 4-0 arterial suture. The psoas muscle is divided at whatever level is dictated by the operative findings. The femoral nerve is simply divided high and sharply; it will retract under the belly of the psoas muscle.

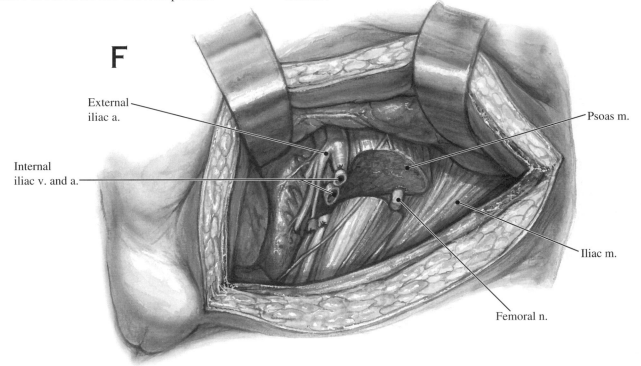

G

The pubic symphysis is visualized and divided with an osteotome. Considerable bleeding may occur from the underlying ischiocavernosus muscle, but it can be controlled with a gauze pack. This largely completes the major aspects of the anterior dissection.

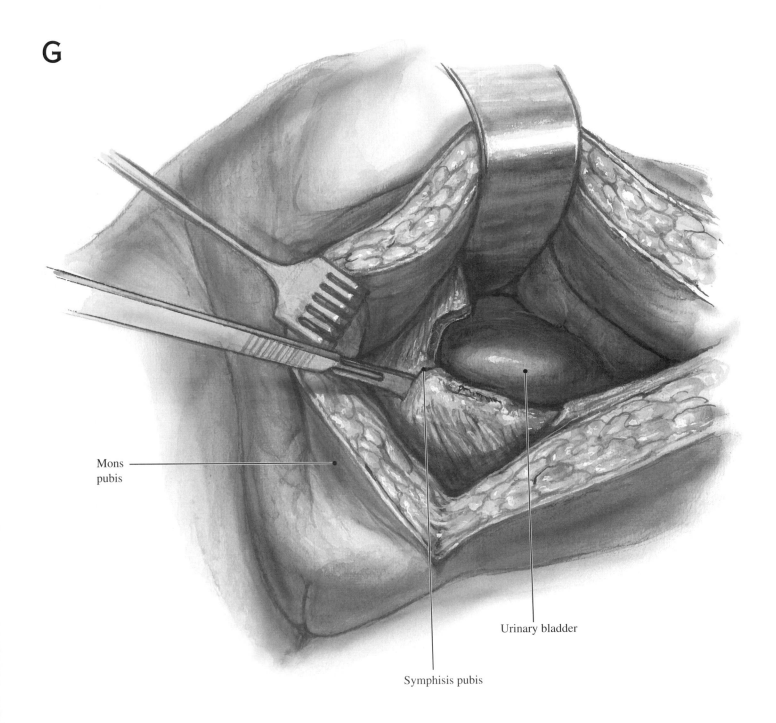

G

Mons pubis

Symphisis pubis

Urinary bladder

H

The posterior portion of the dissection is now performed. The patient has been so positioned and supported initially that the buttock is well off the table on this side. The hip is flexed at least halfway and the leg adducted severely, usually by an assistant simply leaning on it.

This phantom drawing shows some of the structures that are sectioned during the remaining dissection. The areas of origin from which the gluteus maximus muscle has to be separated are the posterior surface of the lower part of the sacrum and the side of the coccyx. The other areas of the origin are within the ilium, as are those of the gluteus medius and gluteus minimus muscles.

The piriformis muscle, which arises mostly from the front of the sacrum, also has to be divided as it passes to the outside through the greater sciatic foramen. The superior and inferior gluteal arteries proceed to their destination from either side of this muscle. The sciatic nerve, which also comes through the greater sciatic foramen, can be seen to pass deep to the piriformis muscle. The portion of the quadratus lumborum muscle that arises from the posterior portion of the iliac crest is divided, as are the lateral fibers of the sacrospinalis muscle that are attached to the posterior iliac crest.

H

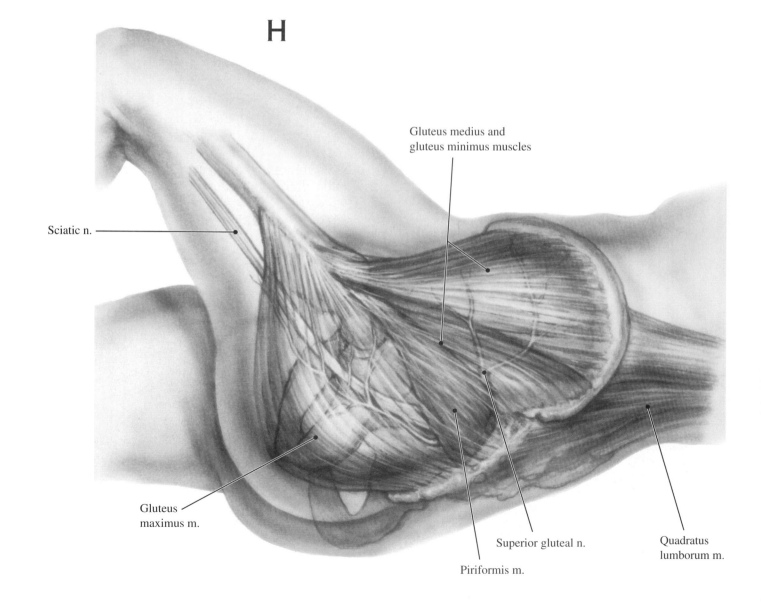

Sciatic n.

Gluteus medius and
gluteus minimus muscles

Gluteus
maximus m.

Superior gluteal n.

Piriformis m.

Quadratus
lumborum m.

I

This drawing shows the sacroiliac joint and the several ligaments that have to be divided in the remaining course of the operation. The sacrotuberous and sacrosciatic ligaments require deliberate sectioning. If cut across near the sacrum, they will be almost as one. The iliolumbar ligament needs to be cut if the Gigli saw is to be seated properly inside the posterior iliac spine to divide the sacroiliac ligaments and synchondrosis.

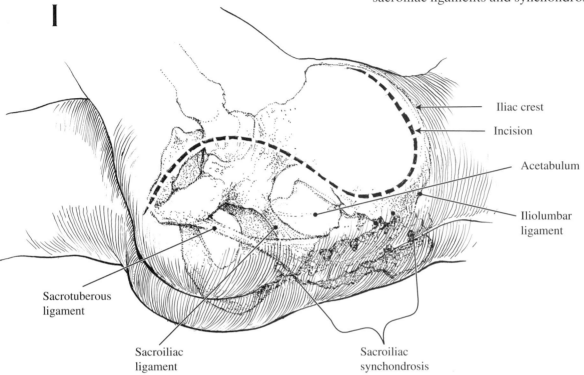

J

The posterior incision is made as planned. Usually it passes over the greater trochanter of the femur. The gluteal flap is kept at full thickness. The fibers of the quadratus lumborum muscle are separated from the iliac crest. More anteriorly along the iliac crest, some of the fibers of the latissimus dorsi muscle and the sacrospinalis muscle will also need to be cut.

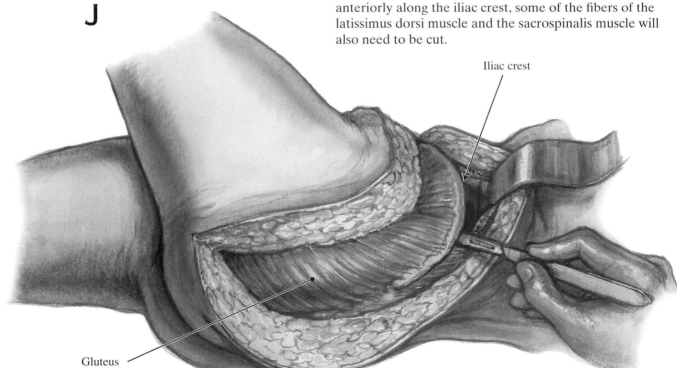

K

The gluteal flap is mobilized to just short of the midline in the back. The fibers of the gluteus maximus muscle are separated from the sacrum, but a few fibers are left on this bone rather than denuding it completely. That part of the gluteus maximus originating from the ilium is not disturbed. The gluteus medius and minimus muscles are not across the path of the scalpel. As the gluteal muscle mass retracts forward, the piriform muscle is exposed. A finger is looped around it to define it before it is cut. The superior and inferior gluteal vessels emerge from the upper and lower aspects, respectively, of the piriform muscle and must be specifically sought and ligated; ligation of the common or internal iliac arteries while they are exposed anteriorly does not eliminate the risk of brisk hemorrhage from the cut gluteal vessels.

K

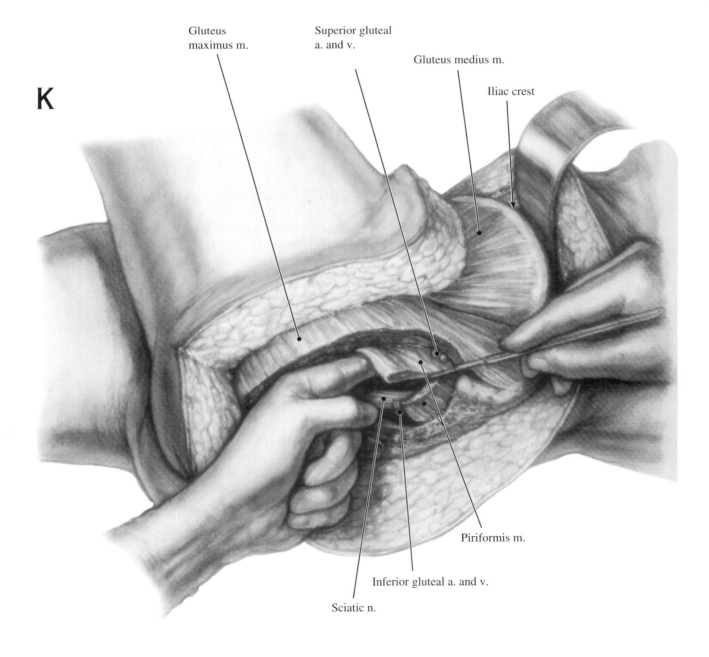

Gluteus maximus m.

Superior gluteal a. and v.

Gluteus medius m.

Iliac crest

Piriformis m.

Inferior gluteal a. and v.

Sciatic n.

L

The piriform muscle has been divided and the gluteal vessels secured. Immediately deep to the divided muscle is the sciatic nerve, which is sharply divided and transected. The tough sacrotuberous and sacrosciatic ligaments are divided close to the sacrum, where they practically fuse.

The sacroiliac division is next. Superiorly, the iliolumbar ligament must be cut so that the Gigli saw may be seated posterior to the posterior iliac spine. Inferiorly, the saw is seated in the sacrosciatic notch; no attempt is made to slant the cut for a smoother surface following closure. Although this cut will almost certainly not pass exactly through the sacroiliac synchondrosis, this is a minor matter.

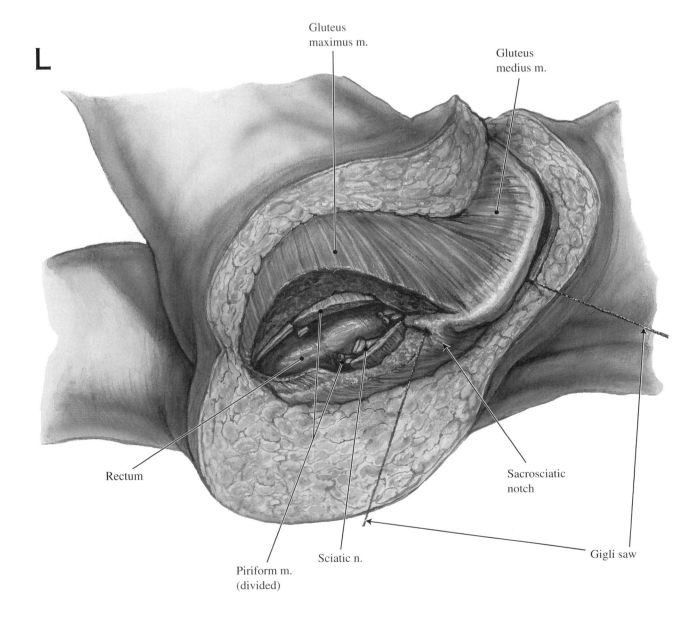

L

Gluteus maximus m.

Gluteus medius m.

Rectum

Sacrosciatic notch

Gigli saw

Sciatic n.

Piriform m. (divided)

M

With the last firm restraints divided, the leg and hemipelvis fall away further, providing an even more generous exposure. Bleeding from the cut bone can be stopped with bone wax. The obturator vessels and nerve also need ligation or division at this time. The levator ani muscles are divided in line with the skin incision, which proceeds toward the perineum. With this, the rectum is brought into view.

M

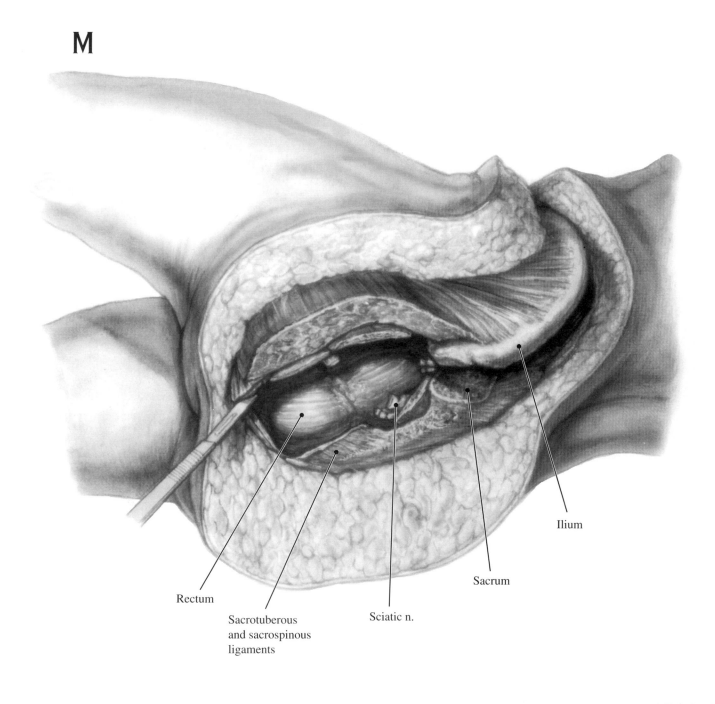

Rectum

Sacrotuberous
and sacrospinous
ligaments

Sciatic n.

Sacrum

Ilium

N

The leg must now be abducted while maintaining some degree of flexion. The skin incision is completed circumferentially, remaining in the crease between the perineum and thigh. The solid line indicates the dorsal incision and the fine broken line the ventral portion of the skin incision. The coarse broken lines indicate points of bone division.

N

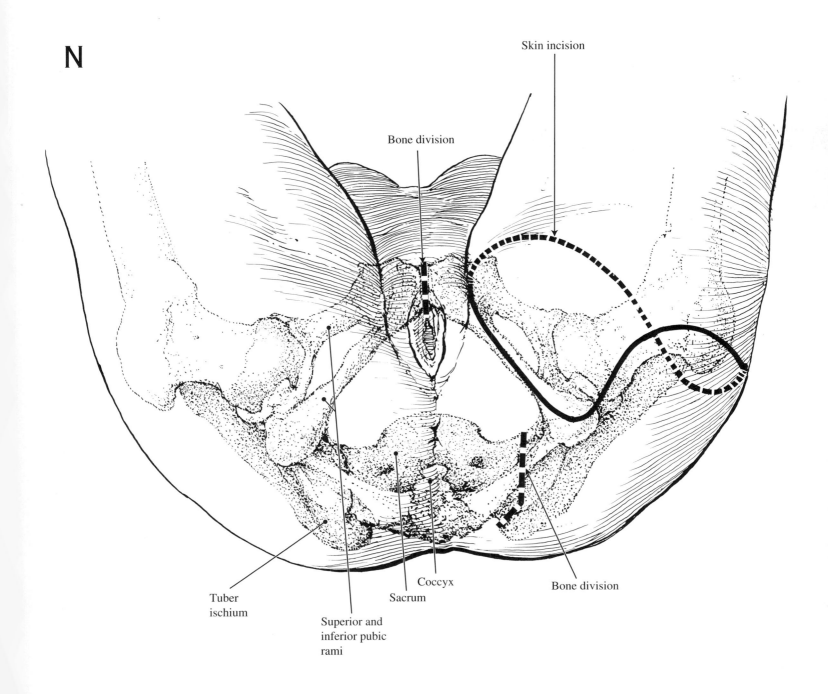

Skin incision

Bone division

Bone division

Tuber ischium

Superior and inferior pubic rami

Sacrum

Coccyx

O, P

The perineal musculature involved in this dissection is shown. Although the skin incision generally runs the course indicated in *N*, the muscles are usually divided more medially. The ischiocavernosus muscle is very vascular and should be ligated before being divided near its medial border. The bulbocavernous muscle is removed in part or entirely if some of the vagina is to be taken. The deep and superficial transverse perineal muscles are taken in their entirety, but a considerable amount of the levator ani muscle is left attached to the rectum. The gluteus maximus muscle is excised in its entirety. The specimen is now free.

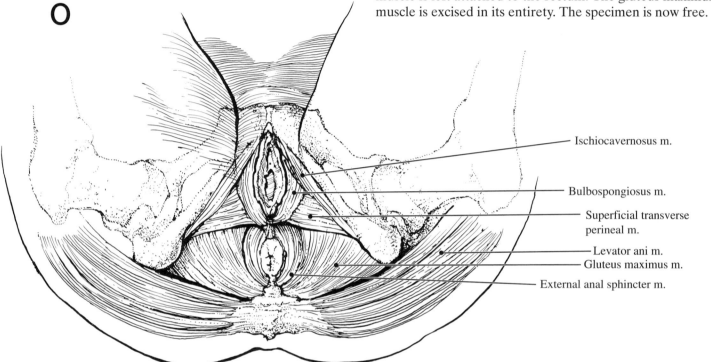

O

Ischiocavernosus m.

Bulbospongiosus m.

Superficial transverse perineal m.

Levator ani m.
Gluteus maximus m.

External anal sphincter m.

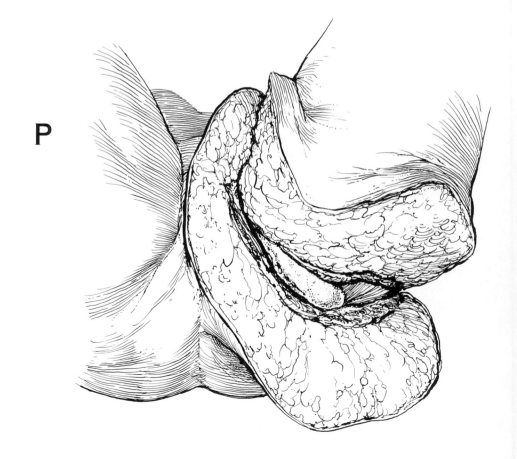

P

Q

The field is wide open for inspection for bleeding points. Bleeding from remnants of the ischiocavernosus muscle can be controlled best with transfixion stitches of 4-0 chromic catgut. If the stump of the sciatic nerve appears too long and threatens to lie within the healing wound, the nerve can be shortened at this time. The closure is begun by approximating the inguinal ligament to the periosteum at the anterior cut edge of the sacrum. This important step utilizes a layer of muscle (the internal and external oblique muscles) to support this weak area, which otherwise would have only peritoneum just under skin.

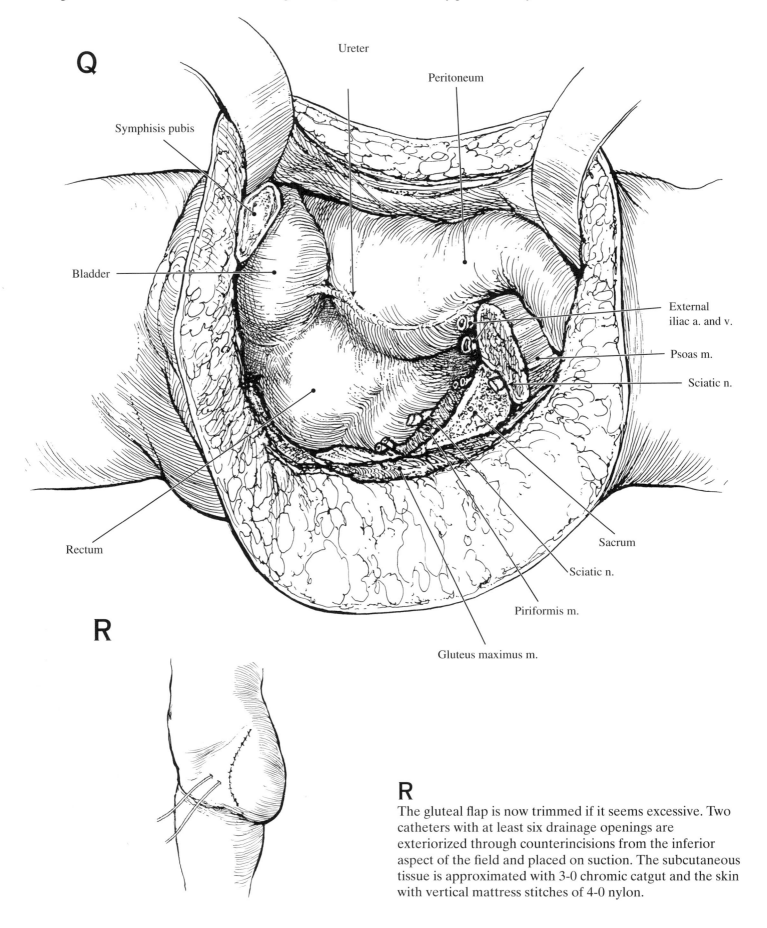

R

The gluteal flap is now trimmed if it seems excessive. Two catheters with at least six drainage openings are exteriorized through counterincisions from the inferior aspect of the field and placed on suction. The subcutaneous tissue is approximated with 3-0 chromic catgut and the skin with vertical mattress stitches of 4-0 nylon.

A

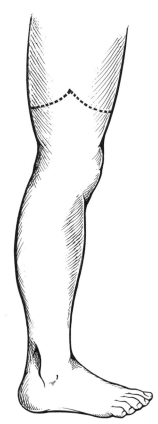

ABOVE KNEE

A, B

The need for a supracondylar amputation is brought about by a number of conditions, including trauma, infection, and lack of vascularity or failure of a lesser amputation. The stump should be as long as is suitable for proper healing, with consideration being given also to the rehabilitative process. The patient is positioned at the edge of the table, permitting full range of motion of the extremity. The leg is prepared with ample exposure for working on the thigh.

The pertinent cross-sectional anatomy is shown.

B

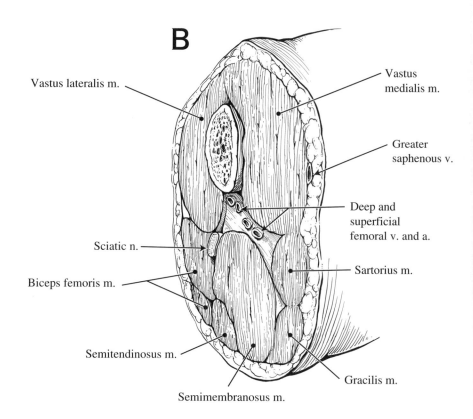

Vastus lateralis m.

Vastus medialis m.

Greater saphenous v.

Deep and superficial femoral v. and a.

Sciatic n.

Sartorius m.

Biceps femoris m.

Semitendinosus m.

Gracilis m.

Semimembranosus m.

C

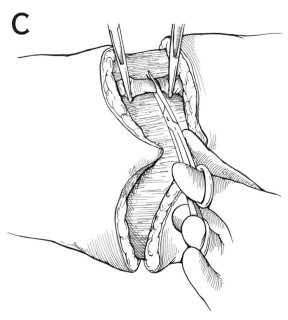

C

The incision is made with some boldness and perpendicular to the skin so that there is no undercutting. The greater saphenous vein is the first major vessel encountered, and it is ligated with 3-0 chromic catgut and divided.

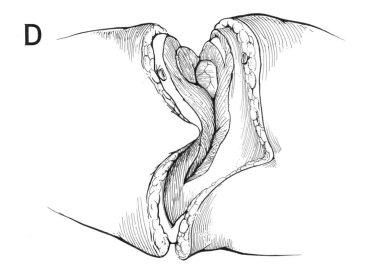

D

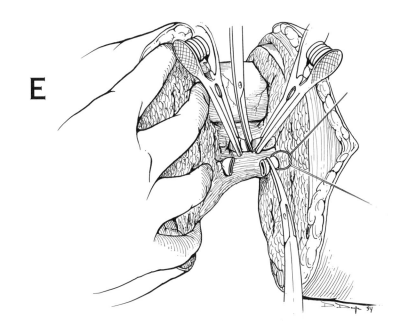

D

The underlying muscles are cut with clean, broad strokes. The muscles will retract somewhat, so the flaps will be devoid of muscle and will consist only of skin and fascia.

E

The femoral artery and vein are identified, dissected free, and ligated with 2-0 silk. If desired, the artery can be oversewn with a simple running stitch using vascular suture material.

E

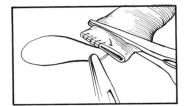

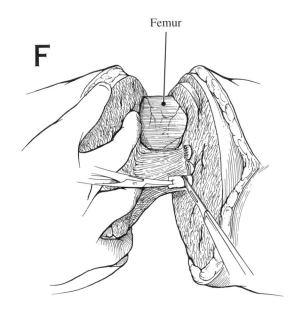

Femur

F

F

The sciatic nerve is identified and prepared for division, a step carried out in many different ways by different surgeons. The method illustrated here is to grasp the nerve, place it on traction, ligate it gently with 3-0 silk to occlude the vessel that overlies it, and then section it just distal to the tie; the nerve will retract deep into the musculature.

G

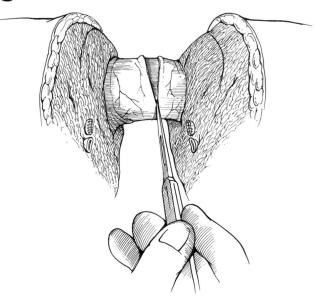

G, H, I

The remaining muscle is cleansed down to the femur; the periosteum is circumferentially incised (*G*). The periosteum is elevated proximally for about 1 cm (*H*). The protective shield is placed about the femur. With the assistant applying proximal retraction, the femur is divided just distal to the most proximal extent of periosteal elevation and the femur is divided (*I*).

H

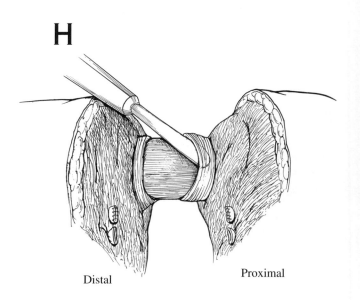

Distal   Proximal

I

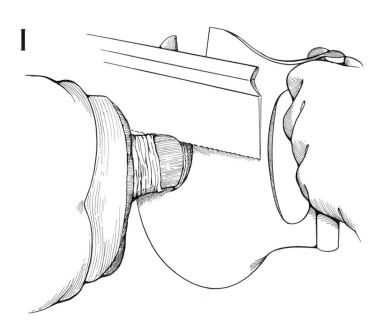

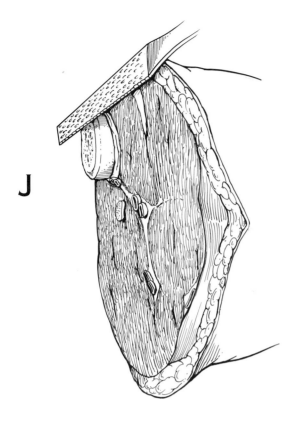

J

Bone wax is used to stop any marrow bleeding. A rasp is used to round off the sharply cut edges of the bone.

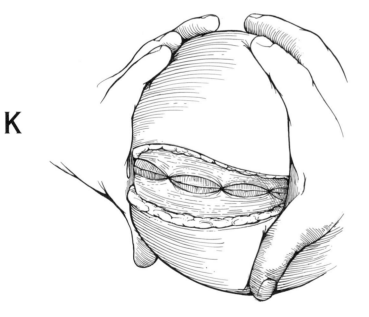

K, L

The assistant's hands bring all the tissue of the thigh together as the fascia is closed with interrupted stitches of 3-0 Maxon and the skin with vertical mattress stitches of 3-0 nylon. The drainage tube, if one is used, is attached to a closed suction apparatus.

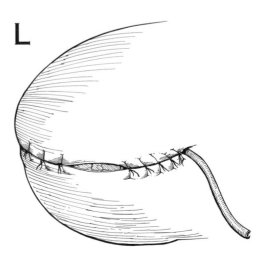

BELOW KNEE

A

Most amputations below the knee are performed for ischemia or for actual gangrene. Several points to keep in mind: If the tibial tubercle and preferably a short length of bone beyond this (10 cm from the knee) can be conserved, then it usually is easier to fit the patient with a functional prosthesis. The posterior of the two flaps is by far the longer and will come to lie over the divided tibia.

The patient's entire leg is prepared and draped so that ready access is provided around the area in which the amputation will be performed.

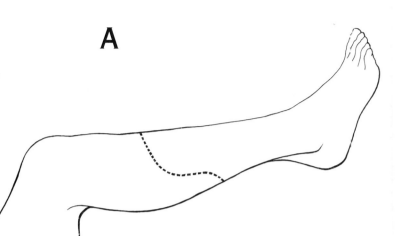

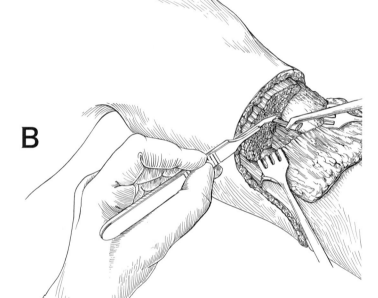

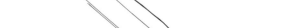

B

The incision is carried directly down to the tibia. The anterior tibial artery and vein are identified, ligated with 2-0 silk, and divided. The nerve is placed under tension and divided, at which point it retracts.

C

The fibula is worked on next, with narrow, deep retractors providing exposure so that it can be divided at least 5 cm proximal to the skin incision. Indeed, often it is desirable, with a short stump, to remove the entire fibula with the aid of double-action cutting rongeurs.

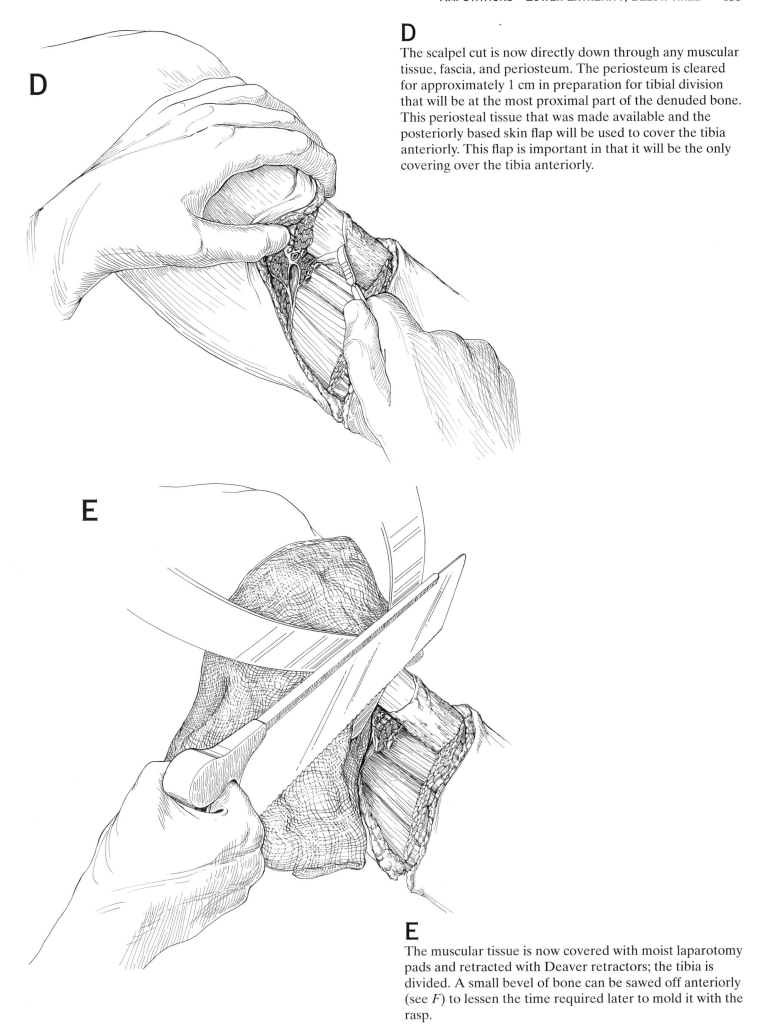

D

The scalpel cut is now directly down through any muscular tissue, fascia, and periosteum. The periosteum is cleared for approximately 1 cm in preparation for tibial division that will be at the most proximal part of the denuded bone. This periosteal tissue that was made available and the posteriorly based skin flap will be used to cover the tibia anteriorly. This flap is important in that it will be the only covering over the tibia anteriorly.

E

The muscular tissue is now covered with moist laparotomy pads and retracted with Deaver retractors; the tibia is divided. A small bevel of bone can be sawed off anteriorly (see *F*) to lessen the time required later to mold it with the rasp.

F

Creation of the posterior flap is important because it is a myocutaneous flap whose proper creation is critical to postoperative function. The assistant now flexes the flail lower leg, creating access to the deep flexor muscles. The tibial artery and vein are ligated with 2-0 silk and divided. The tibial nerve is placed under mild tension, ligated gently with 3-0 catgut, and sectioned sharply just distal to the tie.

The gastrocnemius-soleus muscles are cut at a bevel with smooth, long strokes of the knife. Care is taken not to separate the skin from the musculature.

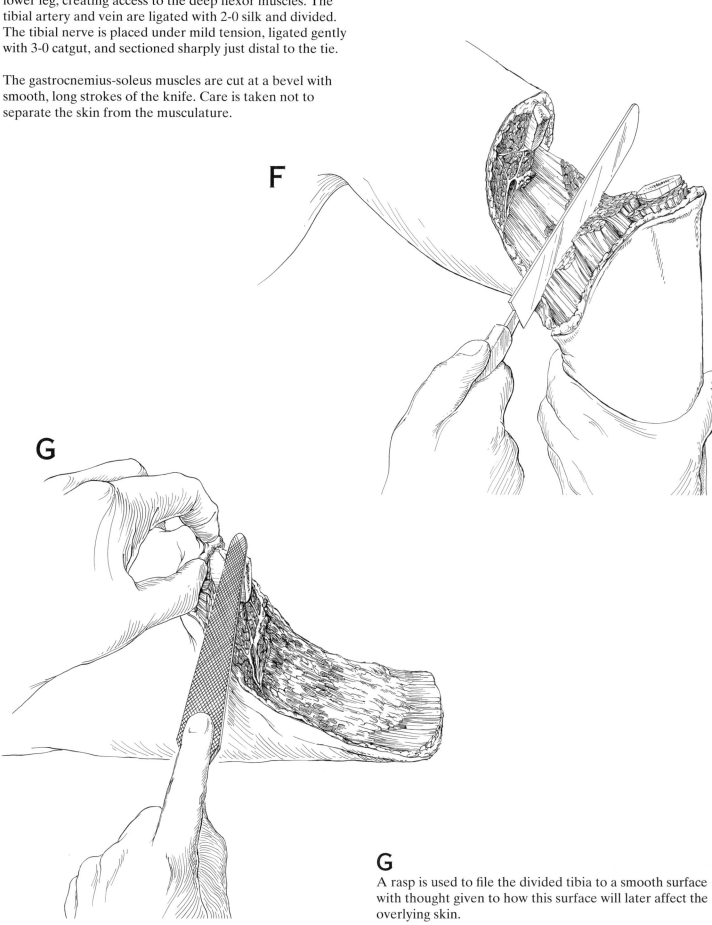

G

A rasp is used to file the divided tibia to a smooth surface with thought given to how this surface will later affect the overlying skin.

H

Fingers instead of forceps are used to handle the flaps as the subcutaneous closure is done with 3-0 chromic catgut.

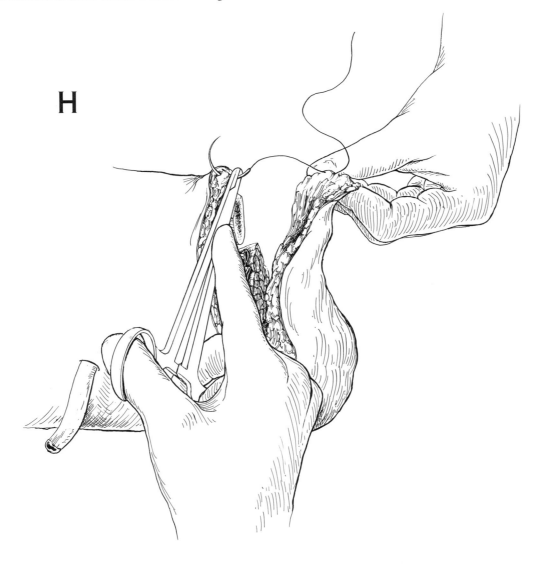

H

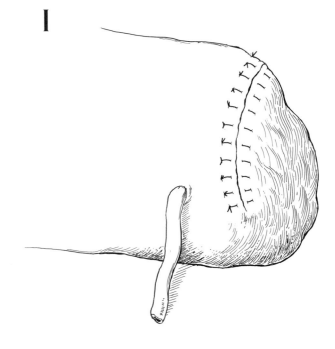

I

I

The skin is closed with vertical mattress stitches of 3-0 nylon. Use of a drain depends on the clinical circumstances. If one is placed, it is exteriorized through a counter incision and connected to a suction apparatus.

A

B

C

TRANSMETATARSAL

Transmetatarsal amputation is most commonly performed for arteriosclerotic gangrene. This operation has the twofold purpose of excising tissue to a level of viability yet leaving the remaining portion of the limb functional. If an amputation higher than one through the metatarsals is necessary, then the realistic level of amputation usually is just below the knee.

A, B

The incision is made at the midmetatarsal level; the plantar flap should be as long and as thick as is practicable.

C

The incision is carried down to the extensor tendons that are divided as proximally as possible. An effort should be made to avoid excessive handling of the tissue that is to remain. The use of fine instruments and precise cuts and not leaving behind devitalized tissue are important in enhancing primary healing.

D

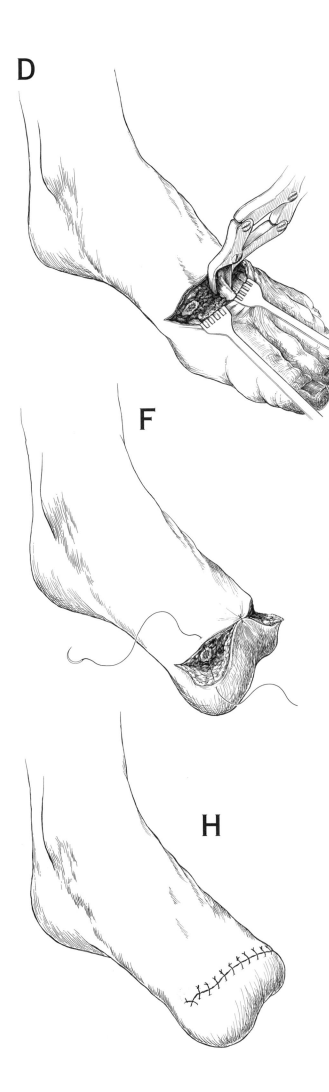

Angled cutting rongeurs are used to divide the metatarsals. The base of the rongeurs is pressed firmly against the ankle side of the metatarsal so that no bone stubs protrude to press against the plantar flap.

E

The tendons are pulled firmly and are serially sectioned sharply, whereupon they retract into the sheath, permitting more vascular tissue to be involved in the healing process of the plantar flap.

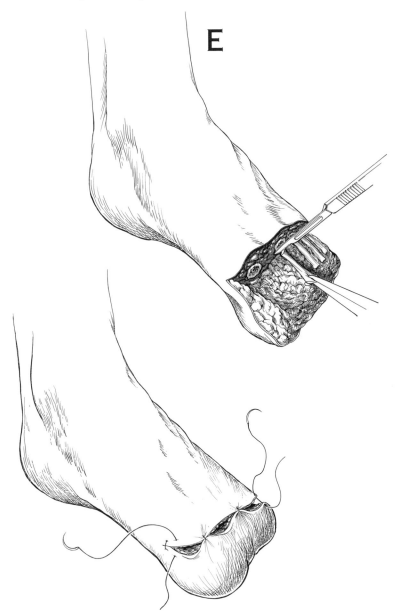

F, G, H

The plantar flap is examined as to appropriate length; small pieces of the avascular fat that are on the flap are carefully trimmed. The use of subcutaneous tissue approximation is a surgeon's preference, influenced somewhat by the ease with which the tissue comes together. The skin closure is carried out with simple interrupted stitches of medium-sized monofilament suture material. A firm but nonconstricting dressing is applied, which helps minimize edema.

AMPUTATION OF THE TOE

Generally, the toe is amputated because its blood supply is sufficiently impaired that it is about to become gangrenous. It is important, therefore, that the surrounding tissue be handled with careful attention so as not to incite a cascade of further necrosis and wider amputation.

A

The racquet incision made can be extended proximally, depending on how much of the metatarsal needs to be removed. Also, it is made on the dorsum of the foot rather than along the instep, where it might be more easily traumatized later with a prosthesis in the shoe.

B

The dissection of the metatarsal is carried just to the point of its amputation. Denuding bone that is to remain should be avoided. The amputation with a double-levered osteotome is on a bias rather than transverse so that following closure the resulting surface is as smooth as possible.

C

No tourniquet is used intraoperatively. Hemostasis is achieved with fine-tipped electrocoagulation or with 4-0 chromic catgut. There is no subcutaneous approximation. The skin is closed with vertical mattress stitches of 4-0 nylon.

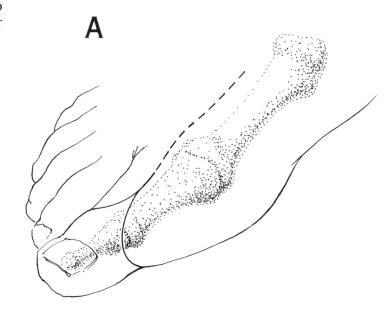

A

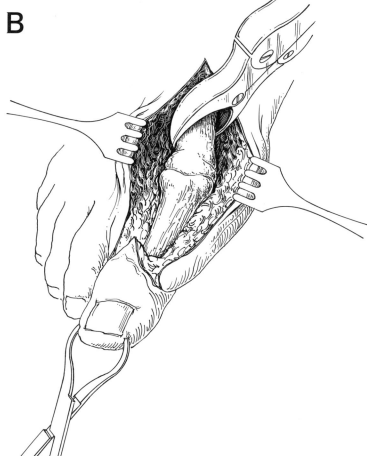

B

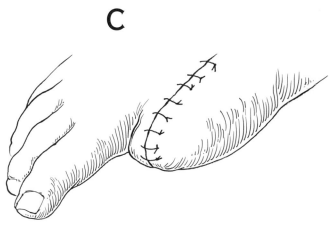

C

VASCULAR PROCEDURES

A CAROTID ENDARTERECTOMY

A

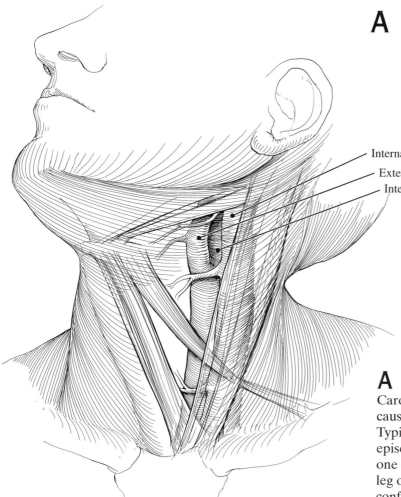

Internal jugular v.

External carotid a.

Internal carotid a.

A

Carotid endarterectomy is performed to prevent stroke caused by atherosclerotic plaque at the carotid bifurcation. Typical symptoms that lead to the diagnosis include episodes of giddiness or dizziness, episodic loss of vision in one eye (amaurosis fugax), loss of function in the hand or leg opposite the side of the lesion, transient aphasia, and confusion with temporary loss of consciousness. The plaque is confirmed by ultrasound and arteriographic studies.

B

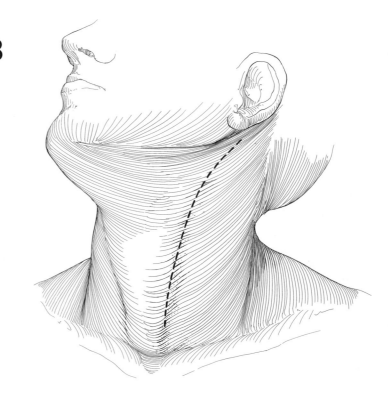

B

The patient is positioned in a "chaise lounge" configuration with the neck extended and the head turned away from the side being incised. The neck should be level.

The incision is made along the anterior border of the sternocleidomastoid muscle. This incision allows maximal exposure of the upper carotid artery high in the neck and beneath the jaw.

The incision is carried down through the platysma muscle to expose the sternocleidomastoid muscle.

C

The anterior border of the sternocleidomastoid muscle is dissected from the deeper structures. The omohyoid muscle is identified first; the medial side of the jugular vein is then separated from the carotid at this site as the dissection proceeds toward the ear. The middle thyroid vein is ligated with 3-0 silk and divided. The common carotid artery is surrounded with a vessel loop. The dissection is most effective if it is carried up behind the internal carotid artery at the bulb area. The external carotid is cleared of its surrounding structures. The superior thyroid artery is temporarily occluded with a clip. The vagus nerve (particularly at the carotid bulb) is identified and protected. The ansa hypoglossus, which leads into the hypoglossal nerve, can be cut with impunity; lifting it helps elevate the hypoglossal nerve out of the way. The dashed lines indicate the site of the intended arteriotomy.

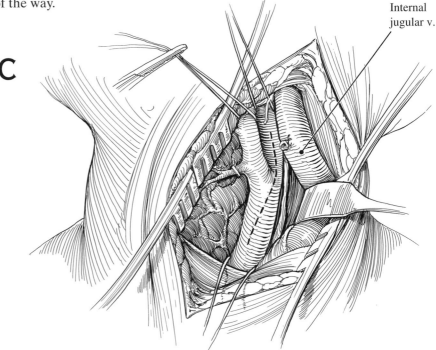

C

Internal jugular v.

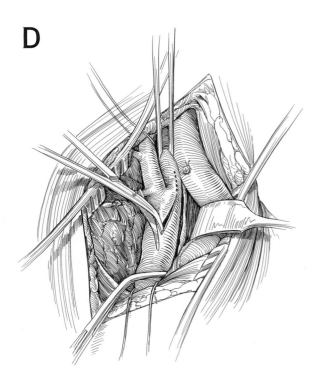

D

D

The common carotid and the external carotid are occluded, and the arteriotomy is made. The initial direction of the arteriotomy is caudal on the common carotid artery and then cephalad into the internal carotid extending beyond the end of the plaque. An important caution is to make certain that the incision in the common carotid artery leading into the internal carotid is laterally positioned to avoid impinging on the carotid body.

E

At this point, a temporary bypass shunt is inserted. It is first inserted into the internal carotid artery to ensure backflow and thereby to clear debris. The narrower end is clamped with Javid clamps to hold the shunt in place after it has been seated. The larger end of the shunt is shown being inserted into the common carotid artery. Again, it is important to have air and debris cleared by the backflow of blood from the internal carotid before gently inserting the shunt into the common carotid artery. A larger shunt clamp holds this in place.

E

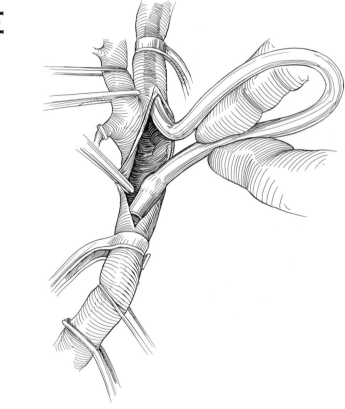

F

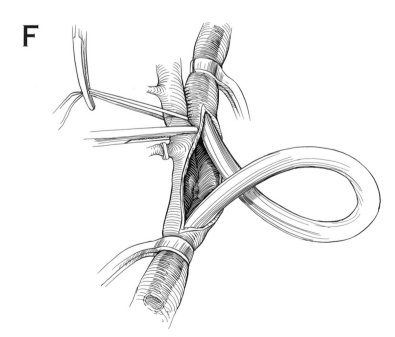

F

The Javid bypass shunt is now in place, providing circulation to the internal carotid artery and to the cerebral circulation. Looping the shunt so it can be uncoiled somewhat allows a clear view of the plaque to be removed and an accurate and unobstructed view of the dissection.

G

The common carotid is shown transected to illustrate the usual depth at which the plaque is separated from the artery wall. The intima and a portion of the media are included in the plaque. A smooth, clean endarterectomized arterial bifurcation is sought.

H

The plaque is removed under clear exposure made possible by the shunt. The surgeon must make certain that the end of the plaque in the internal carotid has a clear tapered aspect with no shelf of intima. After all of the debris and arterial wall strands have been removed, closure of the arteriotomy can be performed. Frequent irrigation of the area with heparinized saline solution removes any blood clots that may form and clears overlooked debris.

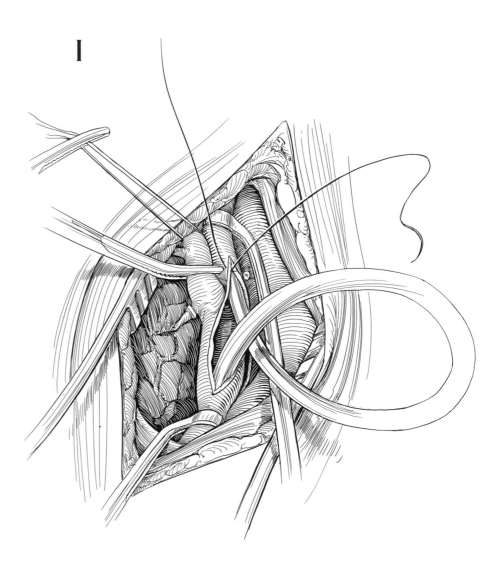

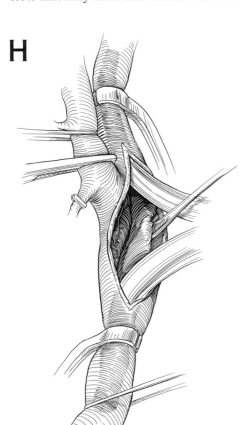

I

The arteriotomy is usually closed with 6-0 vascular suture begun inside the apex of the arteriotomy in the internal carotid and tied. This places the knot outside, and by going out through the apex of the arteriotomy, narrowing at the internal carotid end is minimized.

J

The upper suture line of the internal carotid artery is completed to the level of the external carotid bifurcation. The common carotid is then closed until 1 cm of arteriotomy opening remains around the Javid shunt.

J

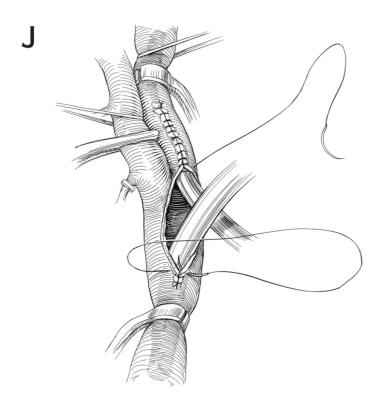

K

The shunt clamp is removed from the internal carotid. The shunt is now extracted and either clamped or pinched off. Bleeding from the internal carotid artery is controlled by simply elevating the vessel loop. As the larger end of the shunt is removed, the common carotid clamp is applied.

K

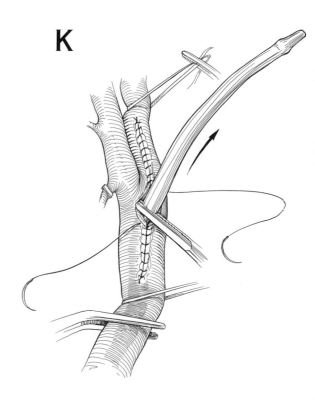

L

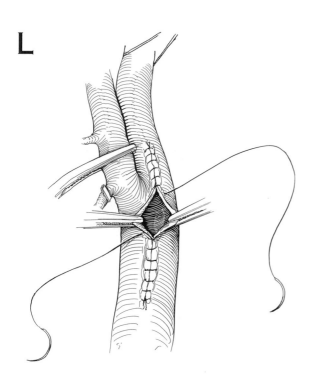

L

The arteriotomy closure is completed by suturing from above and moving down. The vessel loop around the internal carotid artery is intermittently lowered and raised to further remove any clots or debris that might have formed.

M

On completing the closure, the flow is restored to the internal carotid in steps: First, the internal carotid vessel loop is removed; second, a tissue forceps is used to occlude the internal carotid at the bifurcation; third, the external carotid clamp is removed; and fourth, the common carotid clamp is removed.

The initial circulation is directed into the external carotid before removing the internal carotid tissue forceps. This further prevents emboli from entering the cerebral circulation and helps minimize the risk of postoperative stroke. The clip temporarily occluding the superior thyroid artery is removed.

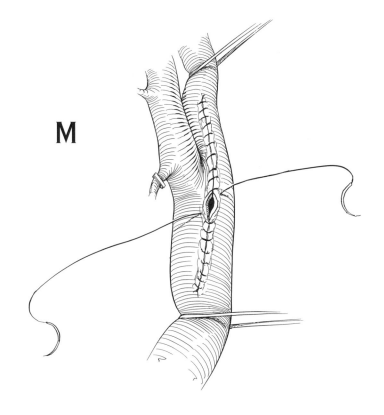

N

When the diameter of the internal carotid is small or when the carotid is friable (or when thrombosis occurs in the recovery room and the patient is returned immediately to the operating room for reoperation), an alternative closure is to use a vein patch. The vein is usually harvested from the greater saphenous vein at the ankle, split longitudinally, and sewn in the direction of flow. With the shunt in place, the medial side of the patch is sewn first, followed by the lateral side. The shunt is removed as previously described, and the final 1-cm defect between the patch and artery is sutured.

Cerebral flow is restored exactly as without a patch.

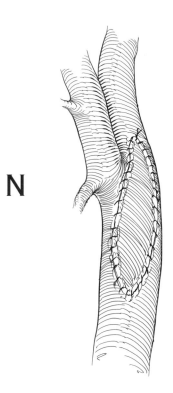

B ABDOMINAL AORTIC ANEURYSMECTOMY

Patients with an abdominal aortic aneurysm generally are operated on electively, and that is the operation featured here. If the aneurysm is ruptured, however, it must have immediate surgical attention if the patient is to be saved. Some steps appropriate to an emergency aneurysmectomy will be commented on during the description of the elective operation.

A

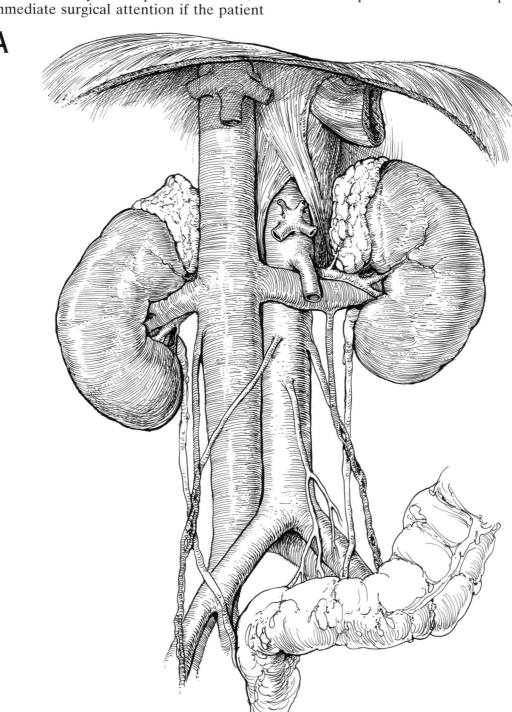

A

The aorta is flanked by the diaphragmatic crura as it makes its appearance in the abdomen at the level of the twelfth thoracic vertebra and continues downward to bifurcate at the level of the iliac crest. It is intimately related to the vena cava at the level of the respective bifurcations and lies somewhat anterior to it. More cephalad, the vena cava separates to enter the thoracic cavity more anteriorly than the aorta. The aorta is crossed obliquely by the base of the mesentery of the small bowel.

The left renal vein, the transverse portion of the duodenum, and the splenic or beginning of the portal vein, come in direct contact with the aorta as they pass anteriorly to it. Much of this topography may be greatly distorted by a ruptured aneurysm.

B

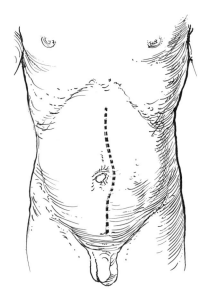

B

In the setting of a ruptured abdominal aortic aneurysm, the chest, abdomen, and groin should be prepared and draped before the induction of general anesthesia. Large bore catheters are inserted peripherally and centrally, with the latter connected to a rapid infusion device capable of delivering large volumes of blood and blood products. With all in readiness, a midline incision is made from the xiphoid to the pubis. The preincision preparations for an elective aneurysmectomy are not as elaborate.

C

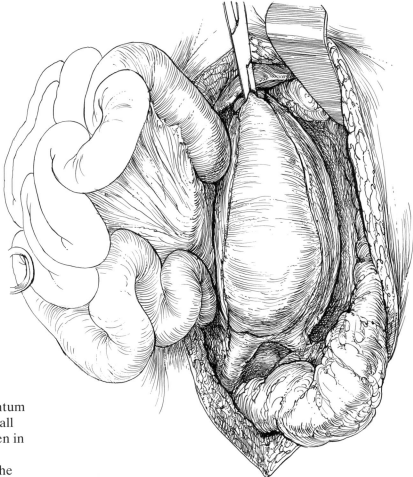

C

A large self-retaining retractor is inserted. The omentum and transverse colon are pulled cephalad and the small bowel and its mesentery retracted out of the abdomen in an upward and right lateral direction. The parietal peritoneum overlying the aneurysm is incised from the duodenal jejunal ligament (Treitz) down to the pelvis. For an elective aneurysmectomy the duodenojejunal ligament is first divided, and the distal duodenum is reflected to the right to expose the aneurysm over its anterior surface. The aorta is encircled with deliberate care before cross-clamping it just below the renal arteries and above the aneurysm. If the aneurysm is ruptured, however, proximal control must be immediate and direct. This is best achieved by retracting the left lobe of the liver cephalad and to the right and entering the lesser omentum near the level of the esophagogastric junction, from which position the aorta is palpated through the fibers of the diaphragm. A large angled aneurysm forceps is maneuvered into position and the aorta occluded. It is unnecessary to dissect and encircle the aorta before clamping.

D

The aorta is dissected between the aneurysm and the renal arteries; only rarely does the aneurysm affect the aorta cephalad to this point. The surgeon should avoid injury to the left renal vein, which may be flattened over the proximal end of the aneurysm. Care should be taken to avoid injury to the iliac vein, which may be closely adherent to the arteriosclerotic arterial wall. This is best avoided by dissecting close to the arterial wall.

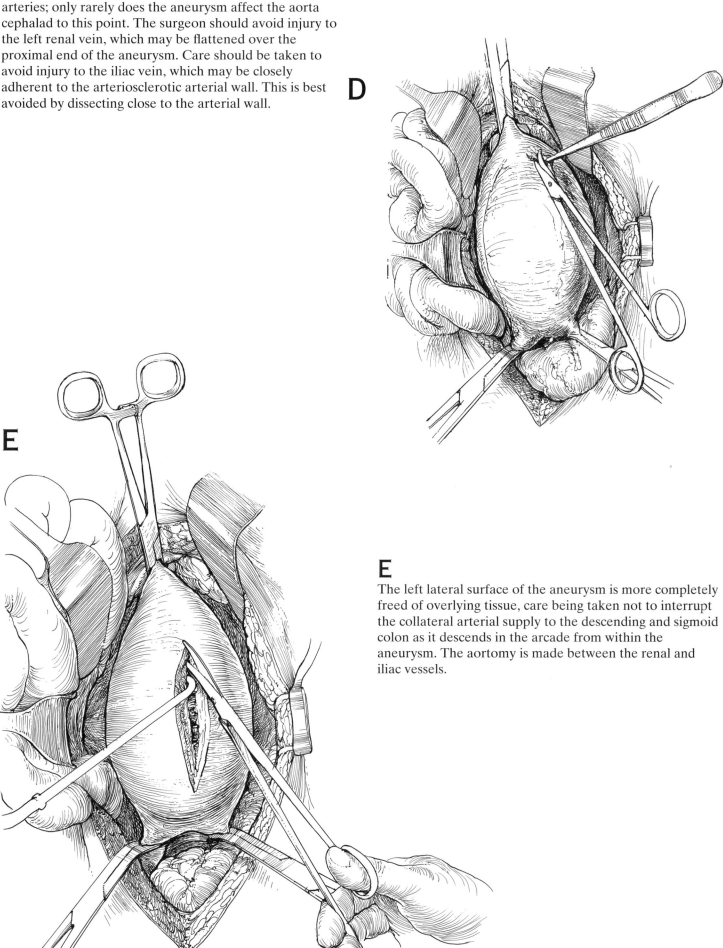

D

E

E

The left lateral surface of the aneurysm is more completely freed of overlying tissue, care being taken not to interrupt the collateral arterial supply to the descending and sigmoid colon as it descends in the arcade from within the aneurysm. The aortomy is made between the renal and iliac vessels.

F

The inner laminated clot and the atherosclerotic material are removed, frequently by a sweep of the finger. Only adventitia and some media remain.

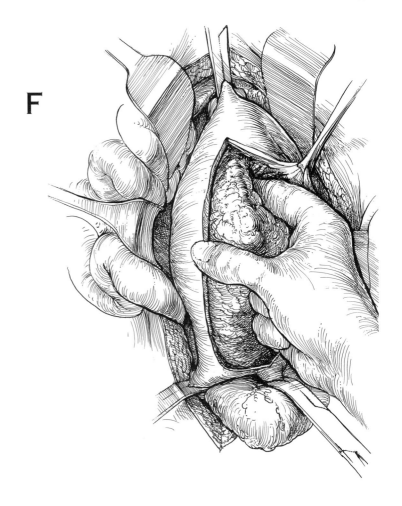

G

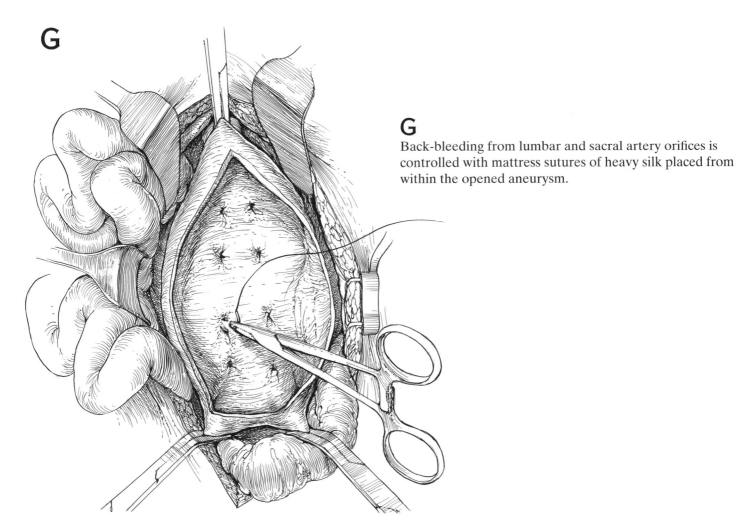

G

Back-bleeding from lumbar and sacral artery orifices is controlled with mattress sutures of heavy silk placed from within the opened aneurysm.

H

The aneurysm is cut transversely just distal to its beginning except for the posterior third of the circumference. There is no objection to complete transection unless the posterior aortic tissues are thin and friable, in which case it is helpful to have the retroaortic prevertebral fascia to aid in holding the posterior suture line.

The aortic portion of the graft is equal—under tension—to the length of the aortic aneurysm. The iliac limbs of the graft are left long and appropriately trimmed just before each is anastomosed.

I

Suturing the graft to the aorta is begun by passing the suture first through the graft and then through the aorta. Again, generously deep bites are taken through the aortic tissue to ensure a strong, blood-tight anastomosis. Several suturing techniques may be used. In this instance, two separate 3-0 monofilament arterial sutures are being started posteriorly with the intention of continuing each laterally and then anteriorly.

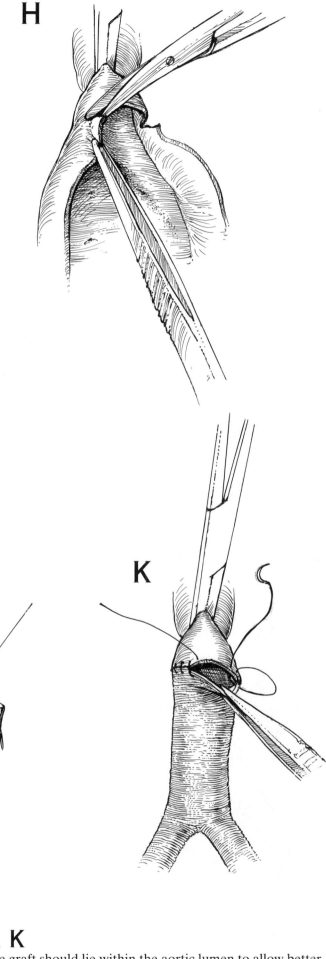

J, K

The graft should lie within the aortic lumen to allow better hemostasis and to prevent dissection beneath an atherosclerotic plaque at the suture line.

L

One can gently test the aortic anastomosis by temporarily loosening the aortic clamp while the graft is digitally occluded. This is the time to be certain that the posterior suture line is secure because it is difficult to expose this area later in the operation.

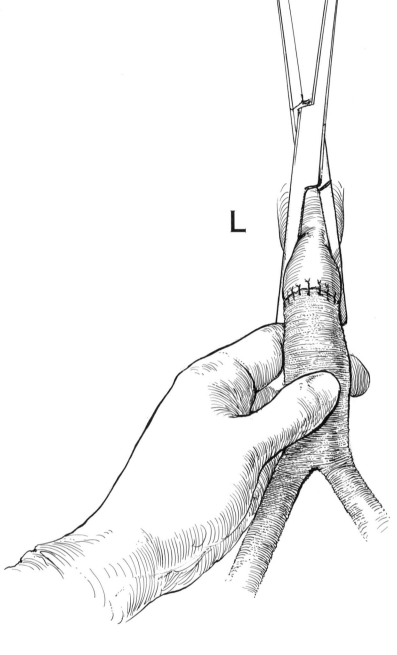

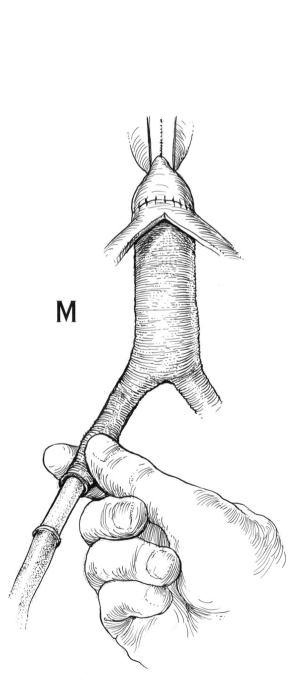

M

Liquid blood, clots, and loose debris are aspirated from within the graft before proceeding with the iliac anastomosis.

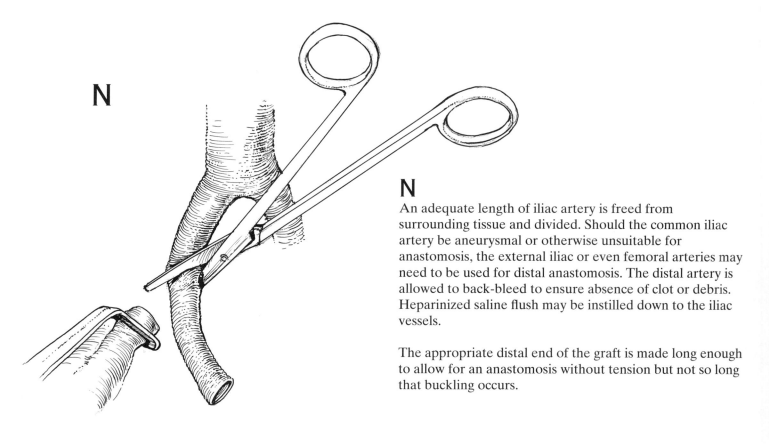

N

An adequate length of iliac artery is freed from surrounding tissue and divided. Should the common iliac artery be aneurysmal or otherwise unsuitable for anastomosis, the external iliac or even femoral arteries may need to be used for distal anastomosis. The distal artery is allowed to back-bleed to ensure absence of clot or debris. Heparinized saline flush may be instilled down to the iliac vessels.

The appropriate distal end of the graft is made long enough to allow for an anastomosis without tension but not so long that buckling occurs.

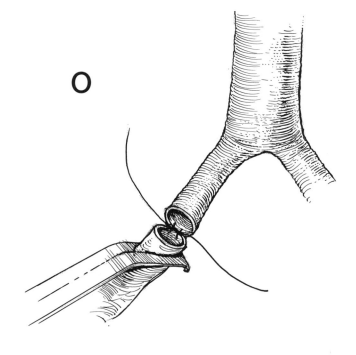

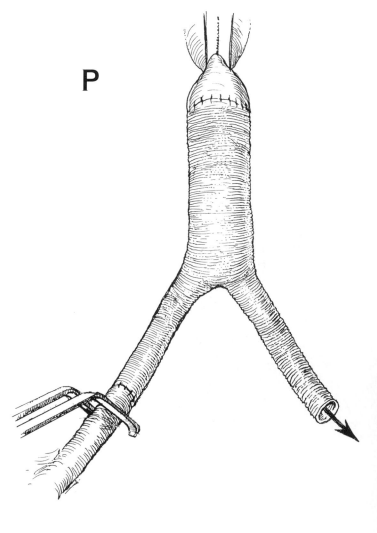

O

The distal anastomoses are performed, again with continuous suturing technique using 5-0 suture material.

P

The order of clamp removal is considered important in the prevention of air or embolic material from passing into the legs. The clamp on the right iliac artery is opened so that there is back-bleeding into the graft and out the unsutured left limb.

Q

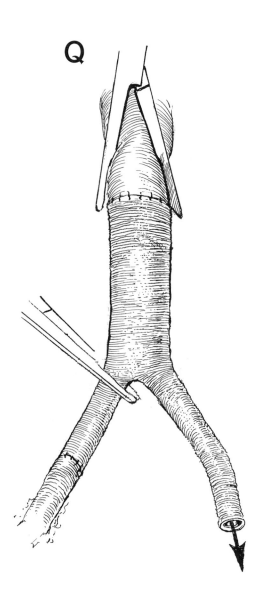

Q, R, S

A rubber-shod vascular clamp is placed on the proximal end of the sutured limb, and the aortic clamp is loosened slightly for a few pulsations, thus flushing the aortic portion of the graft (*Q*). The clamp is now placed across the bifurcation graft practically flush with the aortoiliac junction to avoid any tendency to clot formation in a dead space (*R*). The anastomosis is completed as on the right side (*S*).

S

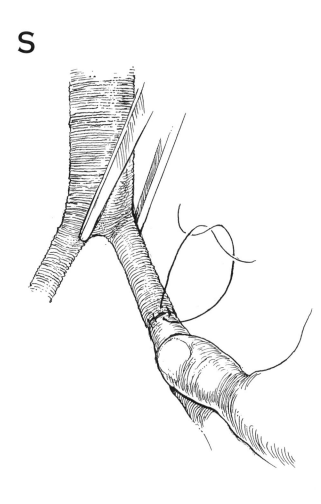

R

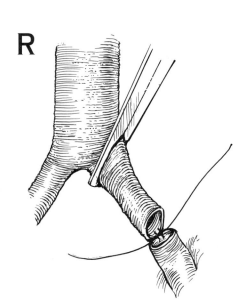

T

U

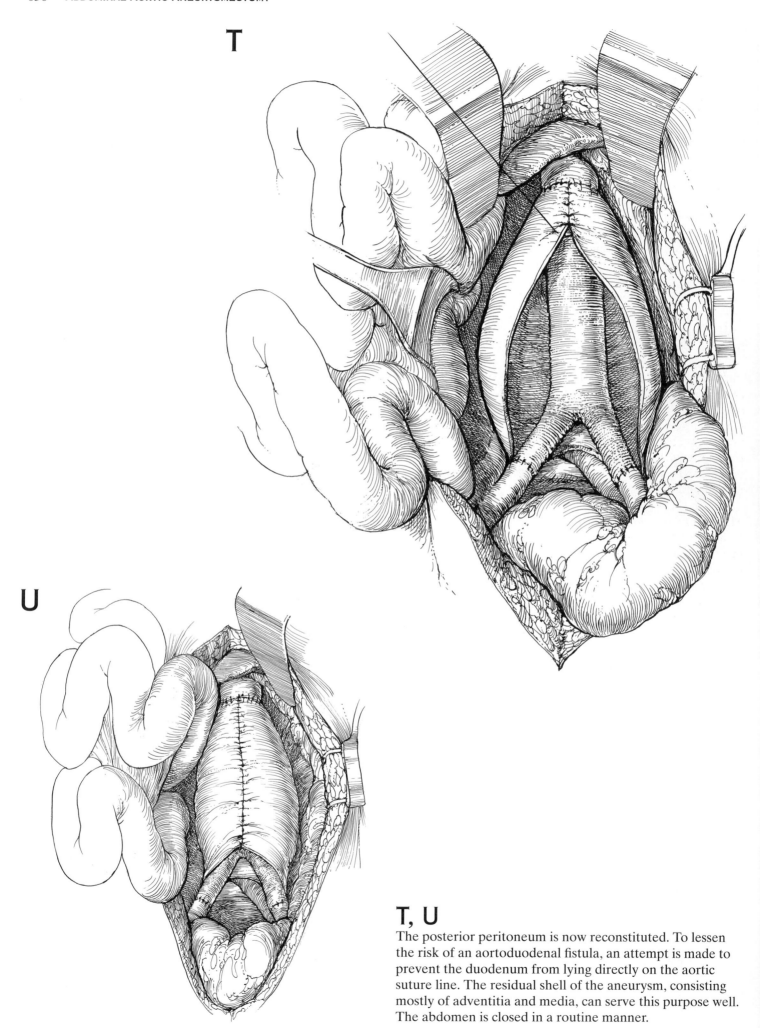

T, U

The posterior peritoneum is now reconstituted. To lessen the risk of an aortoduodenal fistula, an attempt is made to prevent the duodenum from lying directly on the aortic suture line. The residual shell of the aneurysm, consisting mostly of adventitia and media, can serve this purpose well. The abdomen is closed in a routine manner.

C AORTOFEMORAL BYPASS

A₁, A₂

Under general-endotracheal anesthesia, the patient's abdomen, groin, and thighs are prepared and draped in the manner favored by the surgeon. It is important to keep the perineal towel sufficiently narrow and to position it in such a fashion that this portion of the drape does not extend laterally over the groin. Thus, the povidone-iodine (Betadine)®–impregnated self-adherent drape can be positioned over the abdomen and groin area in such a manner as to permit later incisions over the femoral arteries without having the drape become loose on the medial side of the femoral incision; that is, if the towel is too wide, the drape does not have medial wound adherence and the perineum may become confluent with the surgical field, something to be avoided.

Physical examination and arteriography have previously delineated the anatomy and defined the surgical opportunity. If any question exists about whether the femoral arteries with their two-vessel run-off are satisfactory for distal anastomosis, one may choose after the patient is draped to expose a femoral artery and determine its suitability for distal anastomosis before opening the abdomen.

The abdomen is opened through a full-length midline incision, and exploration is begun. The commonest incidental finding is cholelithiasis, but others include hernia, hepatic and pancreatic lesions, Meckel's diverticulum, and lesions of the large bowel. On occasion it is difficult to differentiate between diverticulitis and carcinoma of the colon. If a colon lesion is discovered, the operation may be redirected and the colon lesion given priority. It is never appropriate to perform colon surgery and elective abdominal aortic replacement during the same operation.

A1

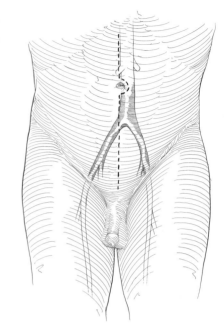

A2

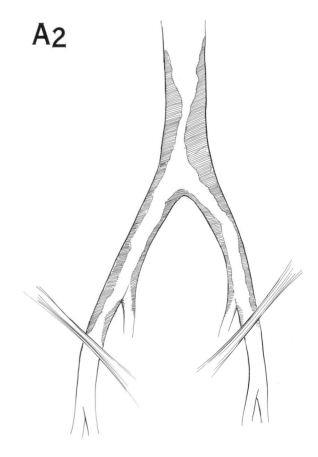

B

After the abdomen has been explored, the colon with the
omentum is pulled downward and then lifted firmly upward
over onto the chest and protected by moist laparotomy
pads (depiction of them in this series is often omitted for
artistic clarity).

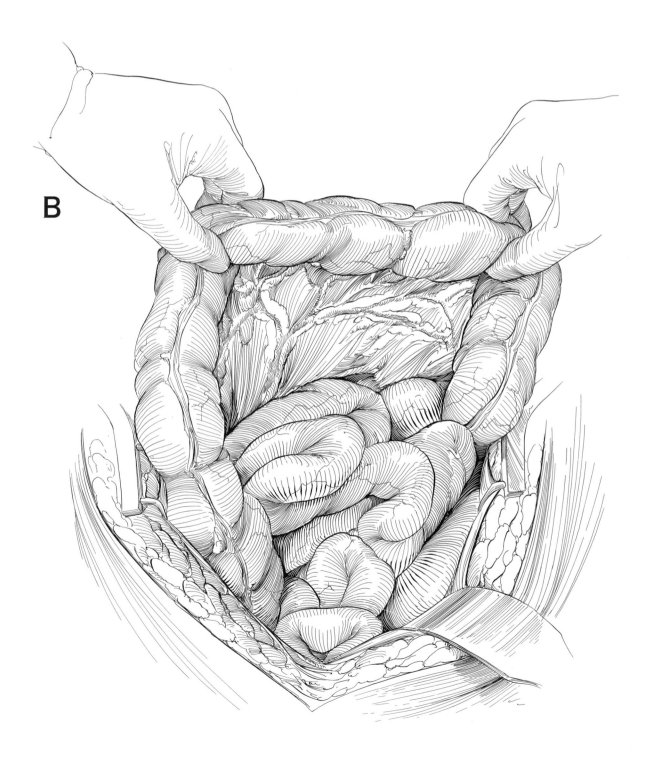

B

C

The retroperitoneal tissues are opened over the upper abdominal aorta with the duodenum and first portion of the jejunum being mobilized toward the patient's right, the intent being to expose the left renal vein. The left renal vein courses anterior to the aorta in the majority of patients, but occasionally it is retroaortic.

C

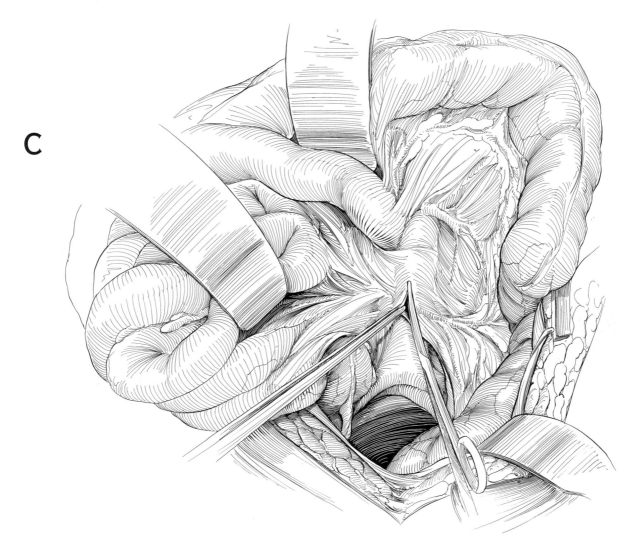

D

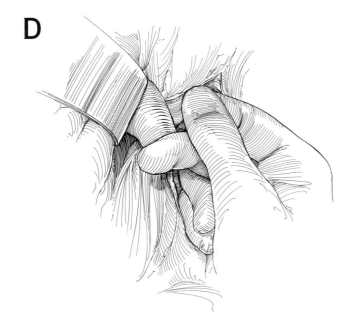

D

The status of the celiac axis and the superior mesenteric and inferior mesenteric arteries has been established previously by aortography, but it is convenient at this point to confirm their patency and adequate flow by palpating these channels through the undissected tissues.

E

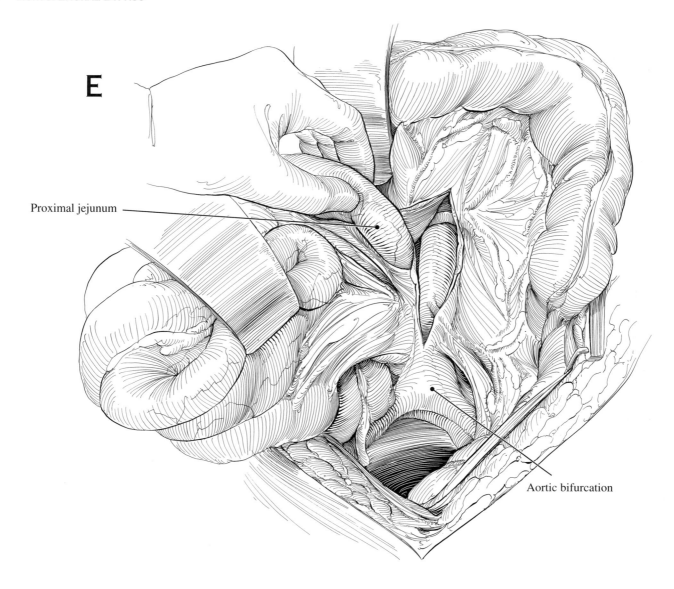

Proximal jejunum

Aortic bifurcation

E, F

Deaver retractors are placed on each side of the upper
portion of the incision to retract the tissues over the aorta
upward and laterally in the process of exposing the aorta
below the left renal vein. A third retractor is placed in the
wound to move the small bowel and its mesentery to the
patient's right.

F

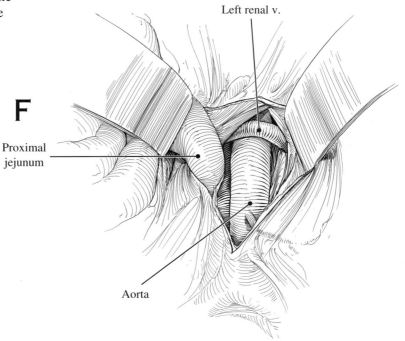

Left renal v.

Proximal
jejunum

Aorta

G

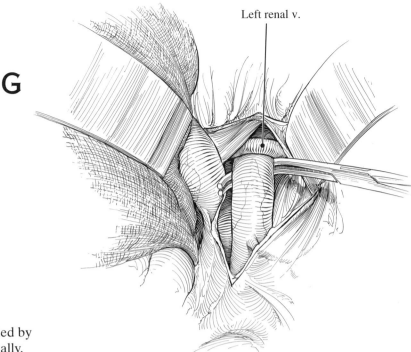

Left renal v.

G, H

The aorta is exposed below the renal vein by scissors dissection and cautery with ligation of small venous channels as they are encountered. The aorta is encircled by using either a finger or a curved instrument. Occasionally, adherence of surrounding tissues may require sharp dissection. The mural quality of the infrarenal aorta is again assessed in preparation for clamping. The disease in the aorta usually extends into the common iliac arteries but may terminate at the common iliac bifurcations. In this instance, both the previously reviewed aortogram and intraoperative palpation of the external iliac arteries may establish that they are suitable for the distal anastomoses.

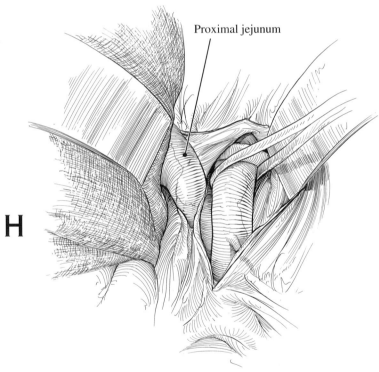

Proximal jejunum

H

I

Common femoral a.

Deep and superficial femoral arteries

I

If these channels are unsuitable, the femoral arteries are then exposed by an incision overlying these channels in each groin. The common femoral artery and its two branches, the superficial and the deep femoral arteries, are then dissected free of surrounding tissue. The superficial femoral channel is single, but the deep femoral artery may be represented by several large posterior femoral branches. It is convenient to encircle these channels with tapes to permit their later control and temporary interruption. The femoral arteries are assessed for their acceptability for distal anastomosis, and the superficial and deep femoral channels are examined to assess their freedom from obstructive orifice disease.

J

Using a finger and, as needed, a ring forceps, channels are then created between the exposed aorta in the abdomen and the femoral arteries in the groin. The diameter of the aorta at the anticipated level of anastomosis is assessed, and then a Dacron bifurcation graft is made available for end-to-end anastomosis to the aorta. Preclotting of the graft may be appropriate in keeping with the manufacturer's instructions.

J

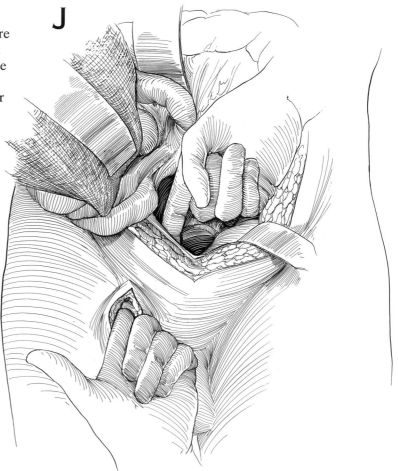

K

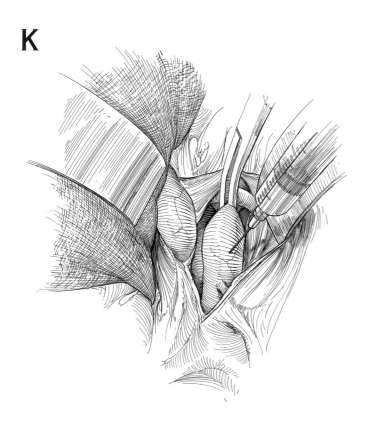

K

The aorta is clamped below the renal arteries so that the calcium plaques in the aortic wall are not fractured. A clamp should be applied to obliterate the distal pulse, but unnecessary forceful ratcheting of the clamp beyond the point of controlling the aortic flow should be avoided. Twenty milliliters of saline containing 2,000 units of heparin are injected into the aorta at the point of intended aortic division. After the heparin has been delivered into the aortic lumen, the aortic clamp is opened for four to five pulsations before the clamp is reapplied.

L, M
The aorta can be handled in one of several ways. Here it is shown being stapled and divided.

L

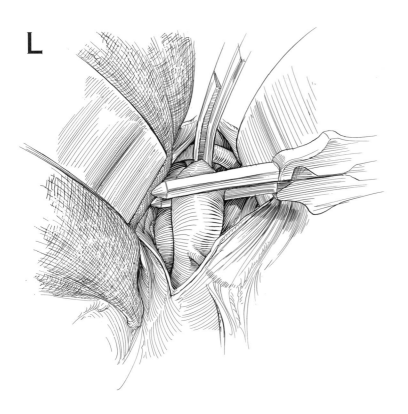

M

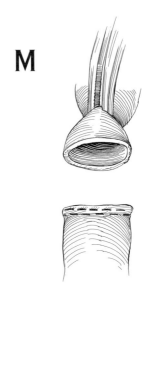

N

N
Alternatively, an angled peripheral vascular clamp can be applied to the aorta proximal to the point of anticipated division (and a second clamp applied more distal to this) and the aorta divided with a scalpel. The distal aorta is oversewn with a heavy suture applied first in mattress fashion and then over and over the cut edge to the point of beginning, where it is tied. The distal aortic clamp is then removed from the field. At this point it may be appropriate to insert a small self-retaining retractor to separate retroperitoneal tissues from around the proximal cut end of the aorta to facilitate exposure and anastomosis.

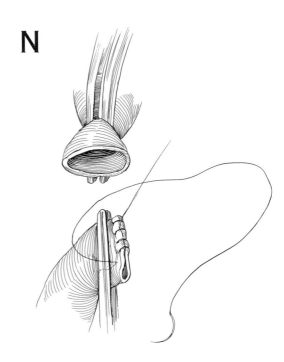

O, P, Q

The common trunk of the aortic bifurcation graft is then trimmed as to length to ensure that after the anastomosis to the aorta has been completed, the iliac limbs at the graft bifurcation will lie in a natural angle on their way through the pelvis to the groin. If the common trunk of the graft is too long, there will be buckling or kinking at the bifurcation that could compromise flow. The graft to aortic anastomosis is then done, usually using a 4-0 monofilament suture. The anastomotic stitching can be done in several ways. If exposure is difficult, as in a large obese patient, it may be best to begin the suture line posteriorly in the midline, as illustrated, and extend it each way laterally to meet in the anterior midline. An alternative is to place a suture at each of the lateral angles, that is, at the 3 o'clock and the 9 o'clock positions. The posterior anastomosis is performed first and the suture tied to its opposite mate, which then is used to complete the anterior anastomosis.

O

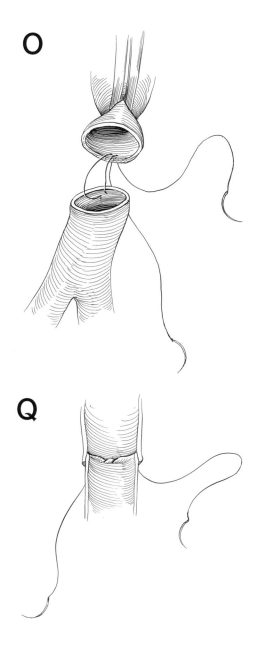

P

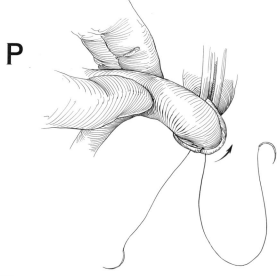

Q

R, S

With each application of a stitch, the graft should be tucked inside of the aortic lumen and each stitch carefully tightened by pulling it at right angles to the aortic wall while supporting the latter by applying counterpressure with the open-jaw needle holder (the suture exits from the aorta between the open jaws of the needle holder). These maneuvers ensure that the anastomosis is secure and that tears do not form in the fragile aortic wall where the suture has been pulled tight.

S

R

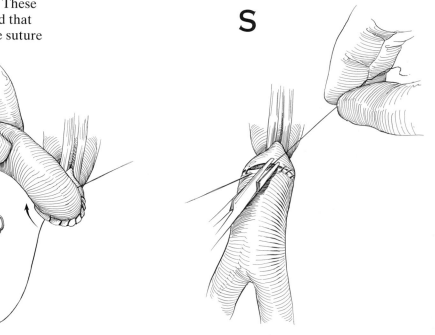

T, U

When the anastomosis is complete, the aortic clamp is released for several beats, allowing for flushing of clots, debris, and air. The limb of the graft to be used is flushed with a heparinized solution.

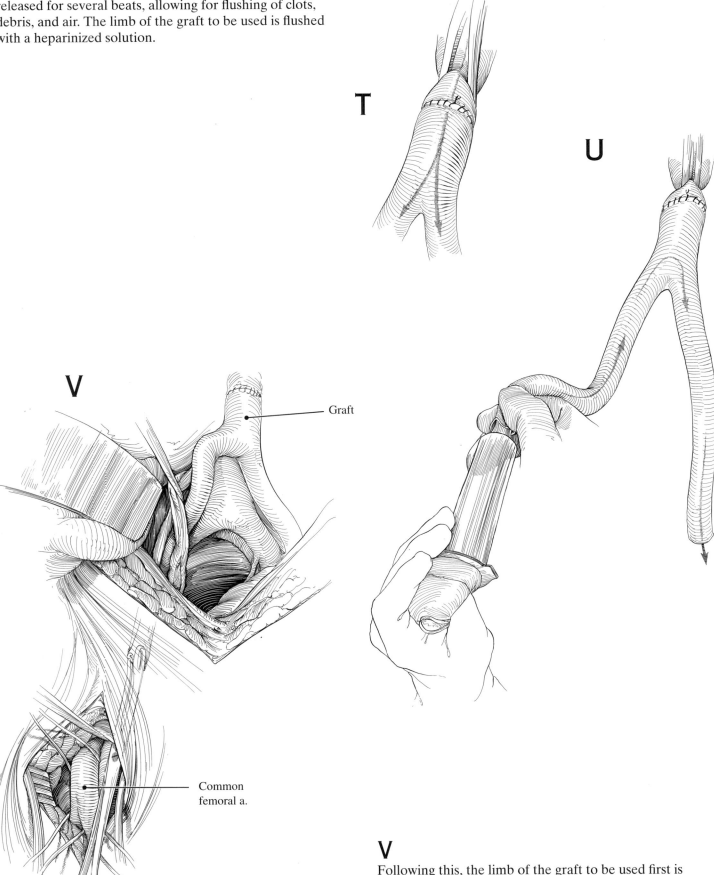

Graft

Common femoral a.

V

Following this, the limb of the graft to be used first is pulled to the groin using a ring forceps placed through the previously constructed retroperitoneal tunnel. The side on which flow was least compromised in the preoperative state usually is the first one selected for restoration of circulation. Care is taken while passing the graft to the groin not to kink or rotate it.

W

The common femoral artery is cross-clamped, usually with a Cooley clamp, and its branches are cross-clamped either with angled peripheral vascular clamps or bulldog clamps.

X

The common femoral artery is then opened in a carefully selected, plaque-free place on its anterior wall, and the lumen is irrigated. The superficial and deep femoral branches are irrigated with heparinized saline solution, which is administered via syringe equipped with a cannula tip that has a bulb that is 3 mm in diameter. This maneuver fills these channels with heparinized saline, establishes that their orifices have adequate continuity with the femoral artery, and gives the operating surgeon information about peripheral resistance.

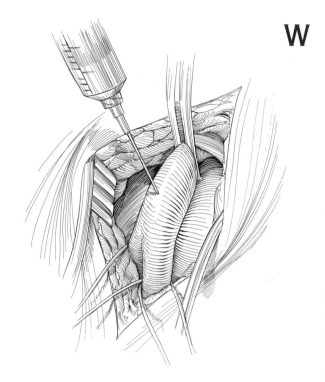

W

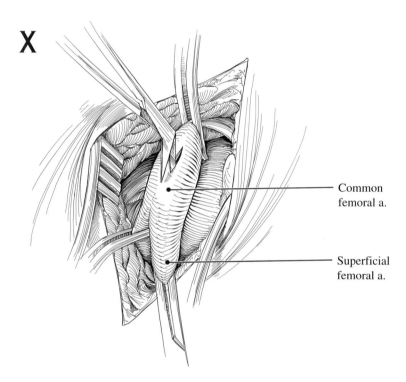

X

Common femoral a.

Superficial femoral a.

Y

The limb of the graft is then tapered at an angle so that the overall length of the graft from aorta to femoral artery is such that it will lie in a natural fashion without redundancy, which could cause stress on the suture lines.

Y

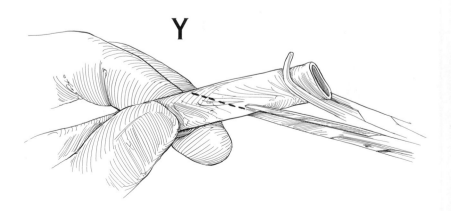

Z

Typically, the anastomosis is 10 to 12 mm long.
Monofilament suture material (4-0 or 5-0) is selected, and
the anastomosis is begun at the heel or most proximal
extreme of the graft femoral artery junction.

Z

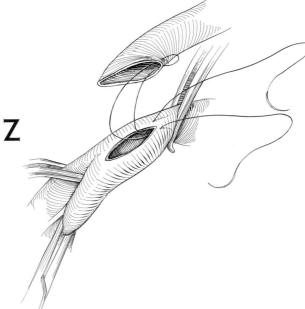

AA

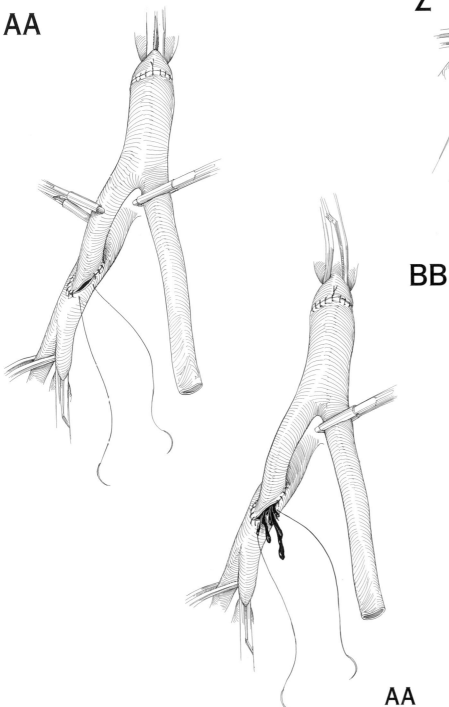

BB

AA

The anastomosis is shown just before completion. The
clamps on the deep and superficial branches of the artery
remain clamped; the one on the common femoral limb of
the graft is loosened.

BB

The clamp on the anastomosed limb is removed, and the
one on the aorta is opened briefly to flush any debris out
through the remaining opening of the anastomosis.

CC

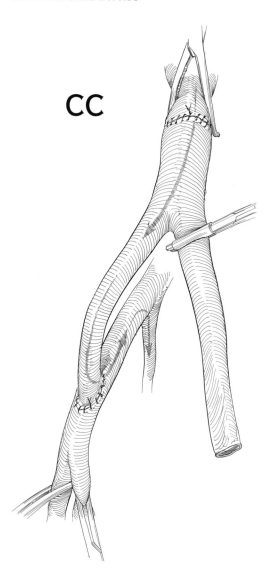

DD

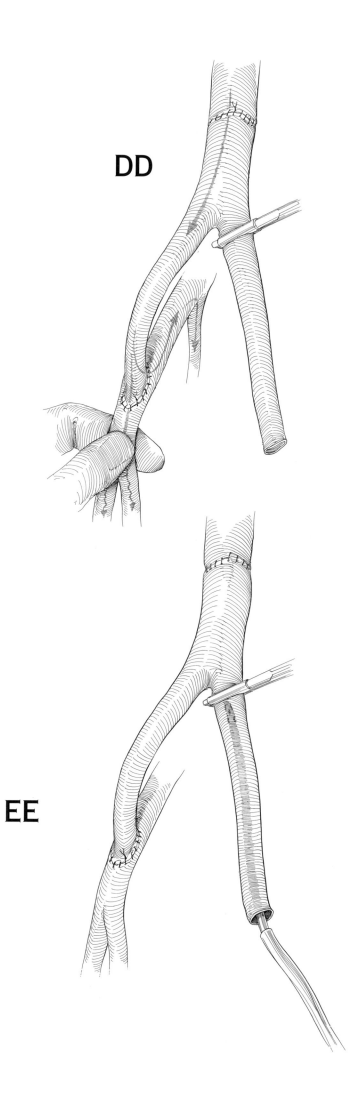

CC, DD

The anastomosis is completed. The clamps on the femoral branches are left in place as the aortic clamp is released. Blood flows through the graft and makes a U turn into the common femoral artery and iliac arteries. This is encouraged by compressing the distal vessel by the thumb and index finger.

EE

A catheter is advanced all the way up the most proximal part of the nonanastomotic limb of the graft and is used to flush it with a saline solution.

FF

The same procedure is carried out on the opposite side.
When the anastomosis is completed, the aortic clamp is
released, but the clamps on the deep and superficial
femoral arteries are left in place. Partial occlusion of the
already anastomosed limb with the fingers encourages flow
down the opposite common iliac and up through the
internal iliacs, carrying with it minor atheromatous debris.

FF

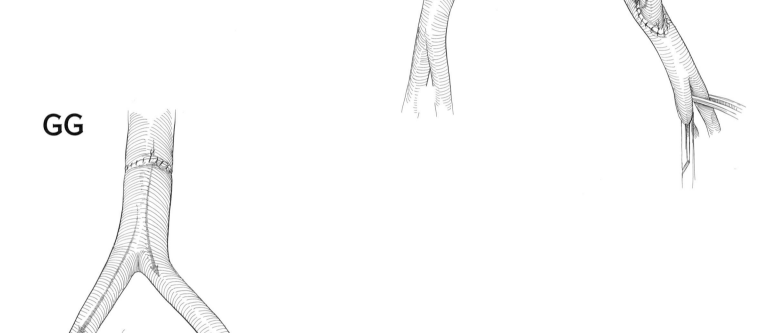

GG

The completed bilateral aortofemoral bypass is shown.

D FEMOROPLITEAL BYPASS

A

The anatomy relevant to a femoropopliteal bypass is illustrated. The ideal graft for use distal to the inguinal ligament is the patient's saphenous vein. If it is not available, a prosthetic graft may be used as in the illustrated procedure.

Following induction of anesthesia in the male patient, the genitalia must be moved away from the surgical site and held in position with paper tape. Although a number of draping techniques can be used, an effective one is to paint the extremity with an antiseptic solution (except for the toes) and to cover it with sterile stockinette. A long window is cut out of the stockinette with the scissors to expose the skin in the surgical area between the knee and the groin. A transparent self-adhering surgical drape is then applied to the skin of the exposed areas; at the same time it secures the margins of the scissor-trimmed edges of the stockinette.

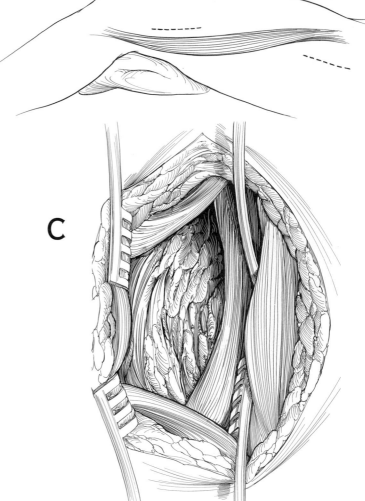

A

Inguinal ligament

Femoral n., a., and v.

Adductor longus m.

Gracilis m.

Greater saphenous v.

Vastus medialis m.

Sartorius m.

B

C

B, C

The location of incisions is illustrated. The distal incision is placed just above the knee in slightly oblique fashion as determined by an imaginary line drawn between the anterior superior iliac spine above and the midlateral point on the knee below. The incision is made about 1.5 cm anterior to this line. There is a tendency to make the incision too far posterior. The inguinal incision is made over the pulsating femoral artery below the inguinal ligament.

The area of the adductor Hunter's canal and the proximal popliteal artery are exposed. The sartorius muscle is located and retracted laterally, and the area of the adductor canal is exposed.

D

Self-retaining retractors are then positioned at both ends of the wound to enhance exposure and retraction of the sartorius muscle. A thyroid retractor placed at the distal end of the wound may enhance exposure of the proximal popliteal artery. The artery is identified at its point of exit from the adductor canal and then mobilized proximally and distally as the local findings may direct. A vessel with an adequate lumen and acceptable mural disease is sought for distal anastomosis. Encircling small veins about the artery are divided as needed to enhance exposure. Small branches of the artery may be interrupted for convenience, and large ones may be preserved to contribute to "run-off."

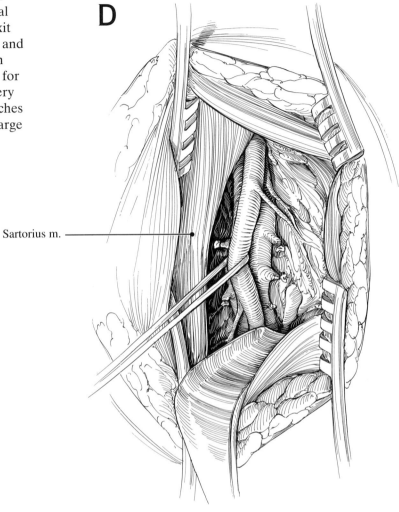

D

Sartorius m.

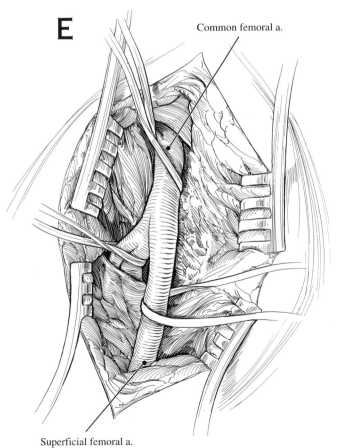

E

Common femoral a.

Superficial femoral a.

E

After an acceptable point for the distal anastomosis has been identified, the surgeon then moves to the inguinal area. A vessel loop is placed around the common femoral artery as well as its superficial and deep branches. The quality of the femoral pulse is assessed, and a satisfactory area of the anterior wall is identified for the proximal anastomosis.

F

A subfascial tunnel is created to connect the two wounds using finger dissection and blunt dissection with a ring forceps.

F

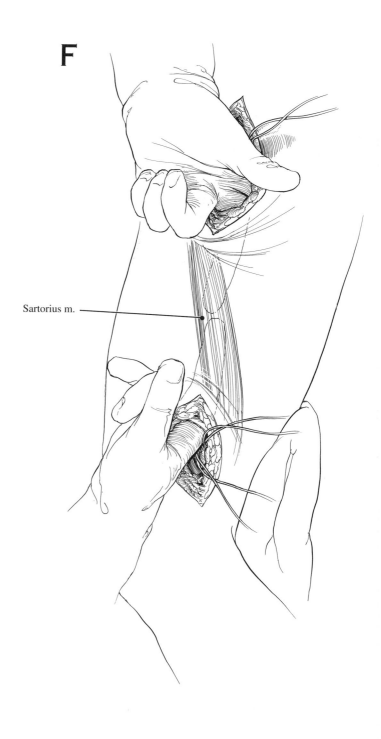

Sartorius m.

G

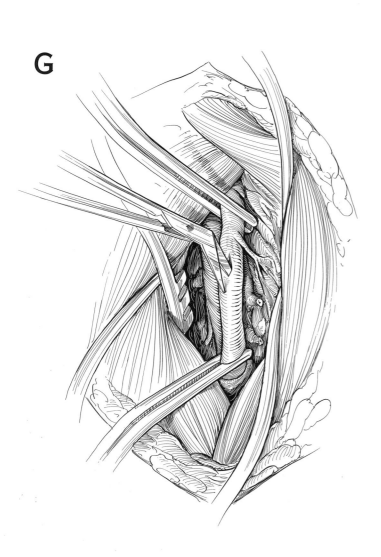

G

The exposed artery in the distal wound is then clamped proximal and distal to the point of intended incision, usually with an angled vascular clamp or a small Cooley clamp. An area has been selected with minimal or no mural disease. The arteriotomy is initiated with a knife and then is enlarged with angled arterial scissors to an average length of 12 to 15 mm. A 20-ml syringe bearing a cannula with a bulb tip that is 3 mm in diameter is then used to flush heparinized saline into the distal artery. The resistance to injection gives the experienced surgeon a measure of the peripheral resistance. A similar amount of solution is then flushed into the proximal artery.

H

The graft is trimmed in oblique fashion to match the size of the arteriotomy.

I

With the arteriotomy rendered dry and the vessel supported for convenience of exposure by the applied vascular clamps, the distal anastomosis is begun. Using monofilament synthetic suture, typically 5-0, the anastomosis is begun at the heel by passing both of the needles from without to within the graft and then out through the proximal corner of the arteriotomy.

J

The suture is then applied over and over from the graft out through the arterial wall. One arm of the suture is continued to the first midpoint halfway the length of the suture line, and then the other arm of the suture is applied from the back corner to the distal corner and on around in its course to meet the first-placed suture.

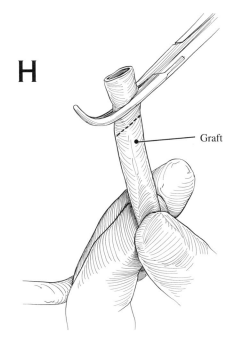

H

Graft

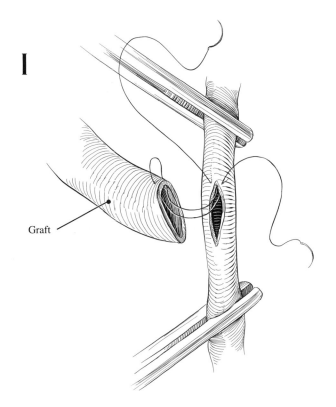

I

Graft

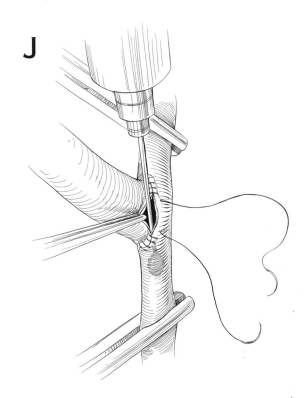

J

K

With several stitches still to be placed, the proximal and distal limbs of the isolated arterial segment are flushed with heparinized saline solution.

L

The suture line is then completed.

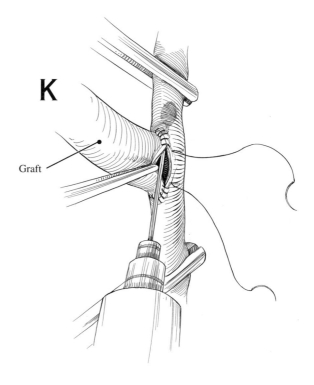

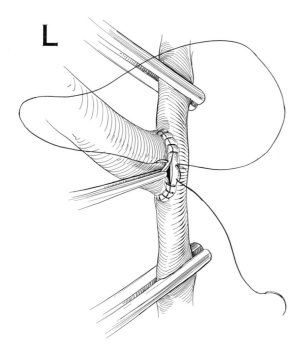

M

The distal clamp is opened, and backflow into the graft can be demonstrated.

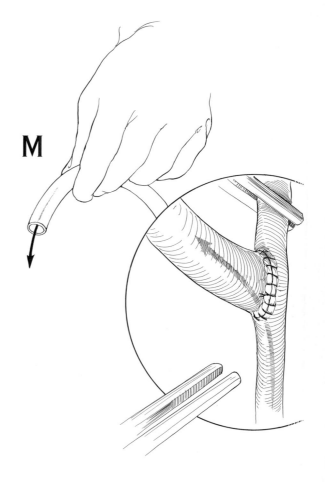

N, O, P

With a vascular clamp applied across the proximal artery, a syringe containing heparinized solution is then used to irrigate the graft from its unattached end and to fill the area of the anastomosis and the popliteal artery below (*N*). The distal clamp is reapplied and the proximal one released very briefly; the graft is open during this maneuver (*O*). The graft is clamped, and both clamps across the artery are released (*P*).

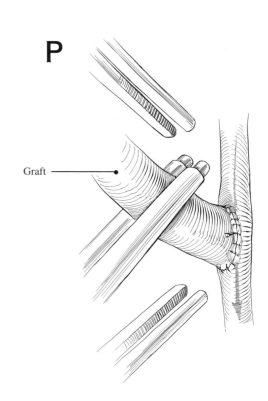

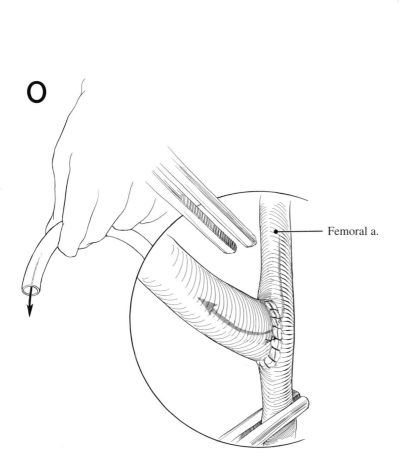

Femoral a.

Graft

Q

Depending on the position of the arteriotomy in relation to the superficial femoral artery occlusion, the surgeon may also wish to irrigate the anastomosis and the proximal artery with its clamp temporarily opened.

Q

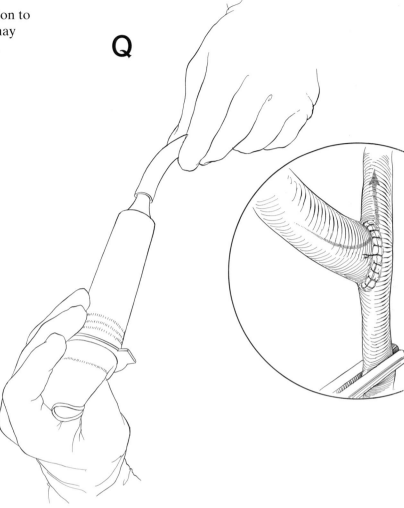

R

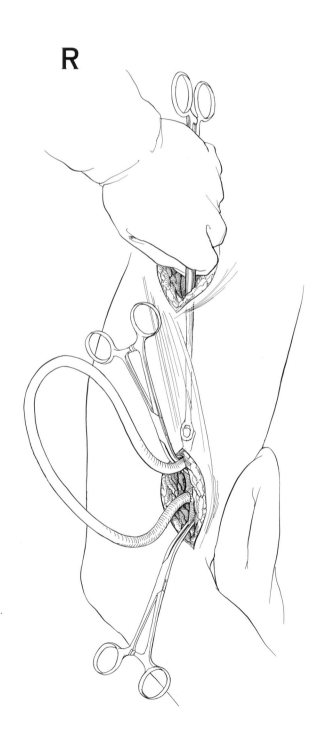

R

The graft is then passed to the groin incision using a ring forceps to move it through the previously created tunnel with care taken to avoid any twisting on its axis.

S

The femoral artery is clamped proximally, usually using a small Cooley clamp, and then 20 ml of heparinized saline is injected into the femoral artery using an 18-gauge needle through the anticipated site of arteriotomy. The site has been selected by palpating the vessel for the area of most favorable mural quality.

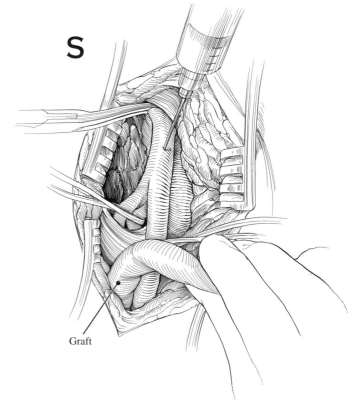

S

Graft

T

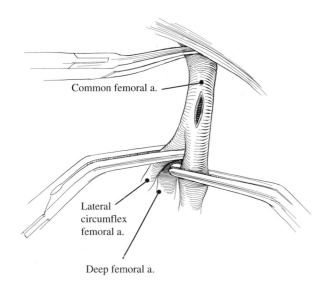

Common femoral a.

Lateral circumflex femoral a.

Deep femoral a.

T

Clamps are then applied to the deep vessels and to the superficial femoral artery if there is proximal patency of the common femoral artery. The femoral arteriotomy is initiated with a knife and then is enlarged with an angled arterial scissors to a length similar to that made for the distal anastomosis.

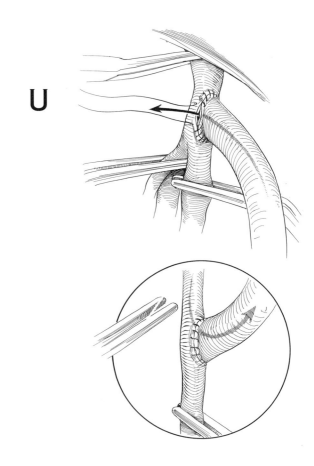

U

U

The graft is cut at an angle so that the circumference of the proximal end of the graft matches that of the arteriotomy and the graft lies in place between groin and knee with neither tension nor redundancy. The proximal anastomosis is performed in a manner similar to that of the distal one, again using fine monofilament, double-armed suture material. The anastomosis is begun at the proximal end of the arteriotomy, with the first suture continued over one fourth of the circumference of the anastomosis and the second suture then applied to the remaining three fourths of the circumference. Before applying the last stitch or two, the arterial clamp placed below the distal anastomosis is released briefly to fill the graft with blood and to evacuate air. In performing both the proximal and distal anastomoses, it is useful to use a small nerve hook to ensure proper lay of the suture and application of the graft to the artery.

V

The clamps are removed to permit flow from the common femoral artery into the deep system. The proximal end of the graft is compressed with the fingers to protect it from flow during this maneuver.

W

The deep channels are then occluded and the clamp proximal to the distal anastomosis removed. Flow is then permitted from the femoral artery through the graft to the distal anastomosis and then retrograde at the adductor canal.

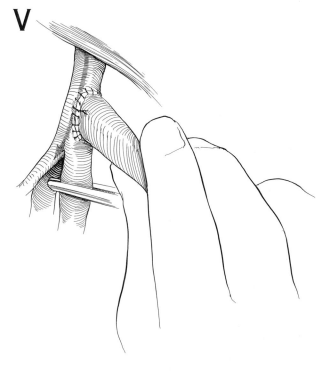

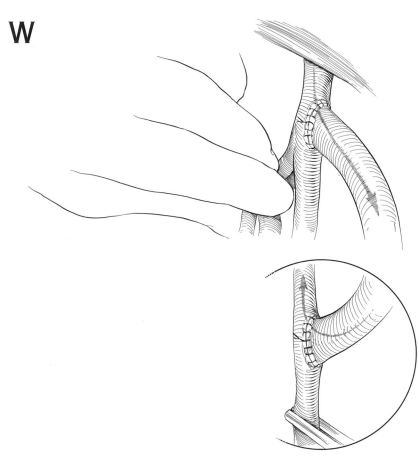

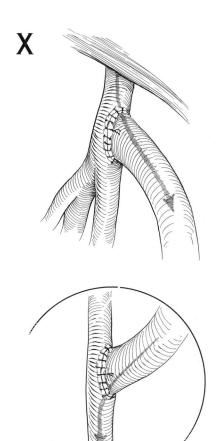

X

The clamps occluding the deep branches are again removed, and, finally, the clamp distal to the distal anastomosis is also removed. At this point, flow through the graft has been achieved, and the pulse in the popliteal artery distal to the reconstruction can be assessed. The presence of a pulse in the foot is assessed by palpation through the stockinette. If a pulse is not immediately present, the stockinette may be opened over the toes and the color of the toes inspected. A completion intraoperative arteriogram may be performed as indicated. After hemostasis has been achieved, the wounds are then closed without drainage, and sterile dressings are applied. Before removing the sterile drapes, the foot is again examined to determine the presence of adequate pulses and color.

INDEX